Great care begins with great CARE PLANNING!

Doenges, Moorhouse & Murr

NURSE'S POCKET GUIDE
Diagnoses, Prioritized Interventions and Rationales

The perfect resource for practitioners and nursing students on the go! Here's everything you need to select the appropriate diagnoses for your patients and develop safe and effective care plans!

Doenges, Moorhouse & Murr

NURSING DIAGNOSIS MANUAL
Planning, Individualizing, and Documenting Client Care

Rely on this complete reference to identify interventions commonly associated with specific nursing diagnoses across the lifespan, and to help plan, individualize, and document care for more than 800 diseases and disorders.

Doenges & Moorhouse

APPLICATION OF NURSING PROCESS AND NURSING DIAGNOSIS
An Interactive Text for Diagnostic Reasoning

Master the nursing process with this interactive, step-by-step, approach to the whys and hows.

Doenges, Moorhouse & Murr

NURSING CARE PLANS
Guidelines for Individualizing Client Care Across the Life Span

Three care plan resources in one—medical surgical, maternity, and psychiatric/mental health—170 customizable plans in all! Take a multimedia approach to care planning with guidelines that make it easier to apply the nursing process and to individualize care.

Schuster

CONCEPT MAPPING
A Critical-Thinking Approach to Care Planning

Master the whys of concept mapping—a clear, visual, and systematic model for gathering and categorizing relevant assessment data, identifying patient problems, and developing patient goals, interventions, and outcomes for each nursing diagnosis.

NURSING CONCEPT CARE MAPS
for Safe Patient Care

Learn to plan individualize

CONDITION
Select the condition or topic you'd like to learn about.

PHYSIOLOGY
Review the physiology summary of your patient's condition. It will serve as the foundation for developing your plan of care.

HANDOFF COMMUNICATION
Follow the SBAR (Situation, Background, Assessment, Recommendation) model to organize your assessment and formulate and implement your plan.

Situation
Summarize what is happening now with the patient/family/population/system in your care.

Background
Complete the pertinent background or past assessment data you need to know in order to develop an effective plan of care.

Assessment
Enter the assessment data which will determine the Nursing Diagnoses that appear on the right hand page.

Recommendation
Each nursing care goal or outcome corresponds with a Nursing Diagnosis on the right-hand page, and describes how you are going to evaluate the care that you have implemented.

CONDITION: Diabetic Ketoacidosis (DKA) and Diabetes Mellitus

PHYSIOLOGY: DKA is a life-threatening emergency caused by a deficiency of insulin. Patients with diabetes type I are prone to DKA. The precipitating factors include illness, infection, inadequate insulin administration, undiagnosed type I diabetes, poor self-management. Symptoms of DKA include dehydration, poor skin turgor, dry mucous membranes, tachycardia, and orthostatic hypotension. As dehydration progresses, the patient becomes weak and eyeballs become sunken. Abdominal pain with nausea and vomiting are common. The patient may have Kussmaul respirations, which are rapid and deep as the body attempts to exhale excessive carbon dioxide and reverse metabolic acidosis. Blood glucose level is greater than 250 mg/dL, arterial blood pH is decreased, bicarbonate levels are decreased, and moderate to large ketones are present in the blood or urine. Complications of diabetes include heart disease, stroke, high blood pressure, blindness, kidney disease, peripheral vascular disease.

HANDOFF COMMUNICATION

S Situation	Assess what is currently happening in a short statement.	Patient presents as _____ VS: LOC:	
B Background	Summarize important past assessment data for your patient here. Place lab results and medications on the concept map.	**Age:** **Gender:** **Allergies:** **Fall Risk:** **Isolation:**	
A Assessment	Use the assessment data to complete your concept map.	**Nursing Diagnosis:** Place the Nursing Diagnoses in prioritized order on the concept map and add any needed for your specific patient. **Plan:** Place any further Nursing Interventions Classifications (NIC) needed on the map.	

Implement Your Plan of Care

		EVALUATE YOUR CARE	
R Recommendation *Evaluate your nursing care and make recommendations related to the achievement of your desired outcomes. Were they met, or do new goals need to be established?*	**Diag**	**Nursing Outcomes Classification (NOC)**	**Outcome met**
	1	Patient demonstrates stable VS, palpable peripheral pulses, good capillary refill, appropriate urine output, and electrolyte levels within normal range.	☐ Yes ☐ No
	2	Patient verbalizes an increase in energy level and displays an improved ability to participate in desired activities.	☐ Yes ☐ No
	3	Patient maintains glucose in satisfactory range and acknowledges factors that lead to unstable glucose and DKA.	☐ Yes ☐ No
	4	Patient identifies interventions to reduce the risk of infection.	☐ Yes ☐ No
	5	Patient reports limited peripheral discomfort or distorted tactile sensation.	☐ Yes ☐ No

Safe and effective nursing care begins with a plan.

Master care planning with concept care maps!

Use this easy-to-construct, visual tool to organize your assessment data, identify patient problems, and see the relationships between the patient's problem, the underlying condition, and your clinical response. You'll also see the relationships between medical and nursing diagnoses, history and physical assessment data, treatments, medications, and laboratory data.

200 easy-to-use templates show you how.

These sample concept care maps cover the diseases and disorders you'll encounter most often in clinical practice.

care for each of your patients.

Nursing Diagnosis 1

Deficient fluid volume related to osmotic diuresis from hyperglycemia evidenced by hypotension, tachycardia, poor skin turgor, increased urinary output.

NIC:
1) Monitor BP lying, sitting, standing, and note orthostatic changes, use of accessory muscles, Kussmaul respirations; **2)** Assess peripheral pulses, capillary refill, skin turgor, mucous membranes; **3)** Monitor I&O, note urine specific gravity; **4)** Weigh patient daily and note changes; **5)** Maintain IV access with large-bore catheter; and **6)** Begin fluid resuscitation with 0.9% NaCl solution until BP stabilizes and urine output is over 30 mL/hr.

Nursing Diagnosis 2

Fatigue related to altered body chemistry, insufficient insulin evidenced by listlessness, overwhelming lack of energy.

NIC:
1) Plan schedule with patient and identify activities that lead to fatigue; **2)** Alternate periods of activity with uninterrupted rest or sleep; **3)** Administer oxygen as prescribed; monitor pulse, respiratory rate, and BP before and after activity; and **4)** Perform active or passive ROM exercises and discuss methods of conserving energy during ADL.

Nursing Diagnosis 3

Unstable blood glucose related to lack of adherence to diabetes action plan, inadequate medication management evidenced by increased ketones.

NIC:
1) Perform fingerstick glucose testing and treat hyperglycemia as needed; **2)** Review patient's dietary program; identify deviations from the therapeutic plan; **3)** Begin continuous regular insulin drip IV as prescribed; **4)** Administer potassium to correct hyperglycemia and sodium bicarbonate for severe acidosis; **5)** Monitor serum glucose and serum potassium levels; and **6)** Provide liquids containing nutrients and electrolytes and progress diet to solid foods when tolerated.

Nursing Diagnosis 4

Risk for infection related to high glucose levels, decreased leukocyte function.

NIC:
1) Observe for fever, inflammation, flushed appearance, wound drainage, cloudy urine, purulent sputum; **2)** Promote good hand-washing techniques by staff, patient, family; **3)** Maintain aseptic technique for IV insertion, site care, and rotate sites as needed; **4)** Reposition patient and encourage coughing and deep breathing; and **5)** Encourage incentive spirometry.

Condition:
Diabetic Ketoacidosis (DKA) and Diabetes Mellitus:

Age:

Link & Explain
• Nursing Interventions Classification (NIC)
• Laboratory and Diagnostic Procedures
• Medications

Nursing Diagnosis 5

Risk for disturbed sensory perception (peripheral neurovascular) related to endogenous chemical alteration: glucose, insulin, electrolyte imbalance.

NIC:
1) Investigate reports of hyperesthesia, pain, sensory loss in feet and legs; **2)** Assess for reddened areas, pressure points, loss of pedal pulses; **3)** Keep hands and feet warm, avoid use of hot water or heating pads; and **4)** Assist with ambulation.

Medications

a. Isotonic (NaCl 0.9%) solution (replaces fluid deficit for the treatment of DKA)

b. Regular insulin (administration by continuous IV infusion to correct hyperglycemia and ketones in the urine or blood; decrease of hyperglycemia should be slow to prevent cerebral edema)

c. Potassium (added to IV as needed to prevent hypokalemia)

d. Bicarbonate (administered IV if pH is less than 7.1 and hypotension is present to correct metabolic acidosis)

Laboratory & Diagnostic Procedures

a. Fasting plasma glucose: used to diagnose elevated blood glucose levels; normal fasting levels are 70–110 mg/dl.

b. Hemoglobin A1c (HgbA1C): determines glycemic control over the past 3–4 months; recommended level is 7%; result greater than 8% indicates changes are needed in treatment.

c. Ketones: measure the amount of acetone in the urine and blood resulting from incomplete fat metabolism; positive results can indicate diabetic acidosis

d. Potassium: in DKA, hyperkalemia results from metabolic acidosis, but potassium is lost in the urine, and the potassium level in the body is depleted; after insulin is replaced and acidosis is corrected, hypokalemia needs to be monitored

NURSING DIAGNOSIS

Each nursing diagnosis on this page corresponds with an outcome box (under the "R" of SBAR) on the left-hand page. You can enter additional diagnoses as needed.

NIC

The NIC section of the box provides a complete list of interventions that go along with the diagnosis, all organized by P-E-S (Problem-Etiology-Signs and Symptoms). You can enter additional interventions as needed.

CONNECTIONS AND LINKS

Think about the relationships between the boxes. The links help you make the connections between what the patient needs, how you are intervening, and what outcomes your interventions are producing.

MEDICATION AND LABORATORY/DIAGNOSTIC

List the important medications and diagnostic tests for your patient...what needs to be completed for the care of your patients.

OUTCOMES

Go back to the 'Recommendation' section on the left-hand page to determine whether the care you provided met each of its goals. The 'Yes' and 'No' checkboxes encourage you to stop and think critically about the outcome of your care, and to revise each step, if necessary, in order to provide the best care for your patient.

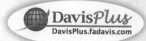
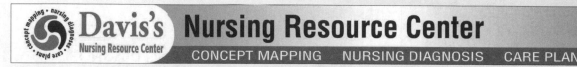

NURSING
Concept Care Maps
for Providing Safe Patient Care

NURSING
Concept Care Maps
for Providing Safe Patient Care

Ruth A. Wittmann-Price PhD, RN, CNS, CNE
Chair, Department of Nursing
Professor of Nursing
Francis Marion University
Florence, South Carolina

Brenda Reap Thompson MSN, RN, CNE
Continuing Nursing Education Coordinator
Assistant Clinical Professor in the College of
    Nursing & Health Professions
Drexel University
Philadelphia, Pennsylvania

Suzanne M. Sutton, MSN, RN
Instructor
Mary Black School of Nursing
University Center Greenville
University of South Carolina–Upstate
Greenville, South Carolina

Sidney Ritts Eskew, BSN, RN
Staff Registered Nurse
Medical/Surgical ICU
Greenville Hospital System University Medical
    Center
Greenville, South Carolina

F.A. Davis Company • Philadelphia

. Davis Company
1915 Arch Street
Philadelphia, PA 19103
www.fadavis.com

Printed in the United States of America

Last digit indicates print number: 10 9 8 7 6 5 4 3 2 1

Publisher, Nursing: Joanne Paztek DaCunha
Director of Content Development: Darlene D. Pedersen
Project Editor: Elizabeth Hart
Design and Illustration: Carolyn O'Brien

As new scientific information becomes available through basic and clinical research, recommended treatments and drug therapies undergo changes. The author(s) and publisher have done everything possible to make this book accurate, up to date, and in accord with accepted standards at the time of publication. The author(s), editors, and publisher are not responsible for errors or omissions or for consequences from application of the book, and make no warranty, expressed or implied, in regard to the contents of the book. Any practice described in this book should be applied by the reader in accordance with professional standards of care used in regard to the unique circumstances that may apply in each situation. The reader is advised always to check product information (package inserts) for changes and new information regarding dose and contraindications before administering any drug. Caution is especially urged when using new or infrequently ordered drugs.

Library of Congress Cataloging-in-Publication Data

Nursing concept care maps for providing safe patient care / Ruth A. Wittmann-Price ... [et al.].
  p. ; cm.
Includes bibliographical references and index.
ISBN 978-0-8036-3052-9
I. Wittmann-Price, Ruth A.
[DNLM: 1. Nursing Care—methods. 2. Models, Nursing. WY 100.1]

610.73—dc23

2012025130

We would like to dedicate this book to Joanne DaCunha for inspiring us with her great idea!

Preface

Dear Students and Faculty,

This book was developed to assist you in organizing the care of your patients. Every day, patient care becomes more complex due to technological and research advances. This book allows you to simplify some of the complex nursing care that you provide in order to deliver care competently and safely.

Each care map begins with a short, focused review of the physiology of the patient's condition (the patient may be an individual, a family, a population, or a system). This physiology review establishes a firm foundation for developing your plan of care. Next, the care map prompts your assessment of the individual patient (or situation) by using the SBAR (Situation, Background, Assessment, Recommendation) format. SBAR is used to organize your assessment and plan because it is a concise method of communicating. In actuality, you are communicating nursing care needs to yourself, other nurses, and interdisciplinary team members. This is the essence of a care plan: communicating the patient's, population's, or system's need to other team members clearly and concisely.

The recommendation section of the SBAR aligns with your nursing care outcomes; these outcomes are how you are going to evaluate the care that you have implemented. The care that you implemented was developed using standard nursing language by choosing priority nursing diagnoses and interventions. Many of those have been done or started for you. These maps can hold up to five nursing diagnoses that can be further developed. We know that the priority for one patient may not be the priority for another, so the diagnoses themselves can be relabeled to reflect that individualization.

The medication and laboratory/diagnostic boxes on the care maps are also a quick reminder of what needs to be completed for the care of your patient. If additional room is needed for any of the areas, forms can be found in the appendix of this book.

The best part comes when you copy your care map. This is when the critical thinking piece comes in and you make the connections and links among what the patient needs, how you are intervening, and what outcomes your interventions are producing. Making the links from a medication to the intervention and then evaluating if your nursing care has accomplished its goal produces a feeling of professional pride and satisfaction.

As you can see, the care maps provide a neat, packaged method of addressing your patient care needs with the ability to individualize them. These care maps will save you time, focus your care and learning, and assist you in your ability to critically think by allowing you to visualize the links.

In addition, we have added forms in the appendices that may be helpful to you in the clinical setting. They include a morning report worksheet, a clinical assessment tool, a patient overview sheet, an extra lab data sheet and medication sheet, and a sheet for nurse's notes. These are provided to help keep you organized during your clinical day.

Included at the end of the introduction is a practice map about you, the nursing student! Use this map as a self-awareness exercise and a concept-map practice tool—it is fun and easy. This will familiarize you with the process of concept mapping.

We hope you enjoy using this book, and we will continue to work on more care maps so nursing students never have to start care plans from scratch again!

Ruth Wittmann-Price
Brenda Reap Thompson

Contributors

Fran Cornelius, PhD, MSN, RN-BC, CNE
Associate Professor
Chair of MSN Advanced Practice Role Department
Coordinator of Informatics Projects
Drexel University
Philadelphia, Pennsylvania

Theresa M. Fay-Hillier, MSN, PMHCNS-BC
Assistant Clinical Professor
Drexel University
Philadelphia, Pennsylvania

Cheryl Mele, MSN, RN
Assistant Clinical Professor
Drexel University
Philadelphia, Pennsylvania

Faye Meloy, PhD, MSN, MBA, RN
Assistant Clinical Professor, Department Chair
Drexel University
Philadelphia, Pennsylvania

Joanne Farley Serembus, EdD, RN, CCRN, CNE
Associate Clinical Professor
Drexel University
Philadelphia, Pennsylvania

Susan Solecki, MSN, FNP-BC, PNP-BC
Clinical Assistant Professor
Drexel University
Philadelphia, Pennsylvania

Brenda Reap Thompson MSN, RN, CNE
Continuing Nursing Education Coordinator
Assistant Clinical Professor in the College of Nursing & Health
    Professions
Drexel University
Philadelphia, Pennsylvania

Ruth A. Wittmann-Price PhD, RN, CNS, CNE
Chair, Department of Nursing
Professor of Nursing
Francis Marion University
Florence, South Carolina

Reviewers

Lois Anderson, MSN, RN
Nursing Professor
South Puget Sound Community College
Olympia, Washington

Pamela D. Andrade, MSN, RN
Nursing Instructor
Delaware Technical and Community College
Dover, Delaware

Debra Backus, PhD, RN, CNE, NEA-BC
Associate Professor of Nursing
State University of New York–Canton
Canton, New York

Kristie Berkstresser, PhD(c), MSN, RN, CNE, BC
Assistant Professor of Nursing
Harrisburg Area Community College
Lancaster, Pennsylvania

Cynthia Gurdak Berry, DNP, RN, CNE
Associate Professor
Ida V. Moffett School of Nursing, Samford University
Birmingham, Alabama

Billie Blake, RN, BSN, MSN, EdD
Professor and Associate Dean
St Johns River State College
Orange Park, Florida

Marylee Bressiem, MSN, RN, CCRN, CCNS, CEN
Instructor Division of Nursing
Spring Hill College
Mobile, Alabama

Amy Brown, PH-CNS, MSN, RN
Assistant Professor of Nursing
Morehead State University
Morehead, Kentucky

Remylin Bruder, MSN, DNP, RN
Associate Professor
Rochester College
Rochester Hills, Michigan

Joy D. Bryant, BSN, MSN, EdD, RN-C (perinatal nursing), IBCLC
Nursing Faculty
Morgan Community College
Fort Morgan, Colorado

Barbara Callahan, RN, NCC, MEd
ADN Faculty
Lenoir Community College
Kinston, North Carolina

Fran Cherkis, MS, RN, CNE
Assistant Professor/Assistant Chairperson
Farmingdale State College
Farmingdale, New York

Deborah J. Cipale, RN, MSN
Online Adjunct Professor
Nursing Resource Lab Coordinator
Des Moines Area Community College
Ankeny, Iowa

Bonnie Colby, RN, BSN, MSN
Nursing Instructor
Central Maine Medical Center College of Nursing & Health Professions
Lewiston, Maine

Sharon L. Davis, MS, RN, CNE
Assistant Professor of Nursing
Roberts Wesleyan College
Rochester, New York

Anne M. DeFelippo, ABD JD MSN RN CNE
Assistant Professor
Salem State University
Salem, Massachusetts

Dinnah Didulo-Masangkay, MS, RN, BC, PHN
Associate Professor
San Diego City College
San Diego, California

Teresa M. Faust, RN, MSN
Nursing Instructor
Neosho County Community College
Ottawa, Kansas

Kathleen S. Fries, PHD, Nursing
Assistant Professor and Program Director UG Nursing
Sacred Heart University
Fairfield, Connecticut

Kelli M. Fuller, DNP ANP-BC
Instructor, Nursing Faculty
Goldfarb School of Nursing at Barnes Jewish College
St. Louis, Missouri

Charlene Beach Gagliardi, RN, BSN, MSN
Assistant Professor
Mount St. Mary's College
Los Angeles, California

Linda Gleason, MSN, FNP, CNE
Professor, Case Manager for Student Success
Saddleback College
Mission Viejo, California

Sue K. Goebel, MS, RN, WHNP, SANE, CLNC
Associate Professor of Nursing
Colorado Mesa University
Grand Junction, Colorado

Judy Hafner, MSN, RN, CNE
ADN Professor of Nursing
Alvin Community College
Alvin, Texas

Donna Herald, BScN, MN
Nursing Instructor
Keyano College/University of Alberta Collaborative Nursing
    Program
Fort McMurray, Alberta, Canada

Minerva Ratliff Holk, RN, MSN
Nursing Faculty
Olympic College
Bremerton, Washington

Ellen S. House, DNSc, RN-BC, CNE
Professor of Nursing and Lead Faculty
Maxine S. Jacobs Nursing Program
Truckee Meadows Community College
Reno, Nevada

Deborah Hunt, PhD, MS, RN
Assistant Professor
College of New Rochelle
New Rochelle, New York

Vicki L. Imerman, MSN, RN
Professor
Des Moines Area Community College
Boone, Iowa

Susan Irvine, MS, RN, CNE
Faculty
Samaritan Hospital School of Nursing
Troy, New York

Alma Jackson, RN PhD, COHN-S
Assistant Professor, BSN Program Director
Colorado Mesa University
Grand Junction, Colorado

Teresa James, MSN, RN, CNE
Assistant Professor of Nursing
Morehead State University
Morehead, Kentucky

Nancy Karnes, RN, MSN, CCRN CDE
Faculty Associate Degree Nursing
Bellevue College
Bellevue, Washington

Kathy Lee, BSBA, MSN, RN
Teaching Assistant Professor
University of Missouri–St. Louis
St. Louis, Missouri

Janice K. Lenehan, RN, MSN
Professor of Nursing
NHTI Concord's Community College
Concord, New Hampshire

Laura Logan, MSN, CNS, RN
Clinical Instructor
Stephen F. Austin State University
Nacogdoches, Texas

Rebecca Luetke, RN, BA, BSN, MSN
Associate Professor Department of Nursing
Colorado Mountain College
Glenwood Springs, Colorado

June McLachlan, RN, Certified Outpost Nurse, MSN, FNP-BC
Instructor
Lake Superior College
Duluth, Minnesota

Kathy J. Mitchell, MSN, RN
Dean, Virginia Appalachian Tricollege Nursing Program
Virginia Highlands Community College
Abingdon, Virginia

Donna Molyneaux, PhD, MSN, BSN, RN
Associate Professor Nursing
Gwynedd Mercy College
Gwynedd Valley, Pennsylvania

Shelly Moore, MSN, RN, CRNP, CNE
Assistant Professor of Nursing
Clarion University of Pennsylvania
Oil City, Pennsylvania

Beth E. Murray, RN, MSN
Assistant Professor, Nursing Science
Lincoln University–Fort Leonard Wood Campus
Fort Leonard Wood, Missouri

Catherine Murray, MSN/ED, RN, CNE
Assistant Professor
Greenville Technical College
Greenville, South Carolina

Sharon S. O'Donnell, MSN, RN
Instructor of Nursing
Radford University
Radford, Virginia

Colleen O'Leary-Kelley, PhD, RN, CNE
Professor and Director of Clinical Simulation
San Jose State University
San Jose, California

Nola Ormrod, RN, MSN
Nursing Director
Associate Professor
Centralia College
Centralia, Washington

Virginia Ousley, RN, MSN
Instructor
Radford University School of Nursing
Radford, Virginia

Donna M. Penn, RN, MSN, CNE
Associate Professor Nursing
Mercer County Community College
Trenton, New Jersey

Norma Perez, MSN, Ed
Ivy Tech Community College–NW
School of Nursing Valparaiso Campus
Valparaiso, Indiana

Susan L. Piva, MSN, RN
Associate Professor of Nursing
Brevard Community College
Coco, Florida

Rebecca Presswood, MSN, RN, PNP-PC
Instructor in Associate Degree of Nursing Program
Blinn College
Bryan, Texas

Colleen M. Quinn, RN, MSN
Assistant Professor of Nursing
Broward College
Pembroke Pines, Florida

Mary K. Rieb, RN, MSN
Nursing Faculty
Central New Mexico Community College
Albuquerque, New Mexico

Carolyn J. Rivard, RN, BScN, Med, EdD
Professor of Nursing Education
Fanshawe College
London, Ontario, Canada

Susan Schwade, MSN
Assistant Professor
Felician College
Lodi, New Jersey

Allison Shields, RN, MS
Instructor of Nursing
Fitchburg State University
Fitchburg, Massachusetts

Lynn M. Simko, PhD, RN, CCRN
Clinical Associate Professor
Duquesne University School of Nursing
Pittsburgh, Pennsylvania

Kathleen M. Sims, PsyD, MN, RN
Professor of Nursing (retired)
George Fox University
Newberg, Oregon

Rebecca Solberg, RN, BSN
Nursing Instructor/Lab Coordinator
St. Johns River State College
Palatka, Florida

Joyce D. Stanley, RN, MSN
Assistant Professor/Adult Health Division Coordinator
University of North Carolina at Pembroke
Department of Nursing
Pembroke, North Carolina

Cheryl Stauffenecker, MS, CNS
Clinical Instructor
University of North Dakota
Grand Forks, North Dakota

Elizabeth Zion Stratton, RN, MS
Assistant Professor of Nursing
Monroe Community College
Rochester, New York

Catherine B. Talley, MSN, RN
Associate Professor
University of South Carolina Upstate
Spartanburg, South Carolina

Marcy Tanner-Garrett, MSN, RN, CNE
Nursing Instructor
Southwestern Oklahoma State University
Weatherford, Oklahoma

Margaret Sorrell Trueman, EdD, MSN, RN, CNE
Assistant Professor
University of North Carolina at Pembroke
Pembroke, North Carolina

Susan Tucker, RN, MSN DNP CNE
Program Director, Nursing Education
Gadsden State Community College
Gadsden, Alabama

Stephanie Turrise, PhD(c), RN, BC, APRN, CNE
Lecturer, School of Nursing
University of North Carolina Wilmington
Wilmington, North Carolina

Kimberly Valich, MSN, RN
Director of Nursing/Department Chair/Nursing Faculty
South Suburban College
South Holland, Illinois

Acknowledgments

A special thanks to Julie Scardiglia for all her organization and assistance in this awesome project.

Contents in Brief

Table of Contents

Introduction

Welcome, Nursing Students and Faculty! We would like to introduce you to our clinical care map book, *Nursing Concept Maps for Safe Patient Care*. This unique book is just what is needed for your clinical learning experience. This book offers *200 concept maps* that perfectly blend current information about frequently encountered health conditions with the flexibility of individualizing the nursing care plan for your specific patient/family, population, or system.

Each concept map is formatted on two pages and provides a holistic snapshot of your patient/family/population/system's needs. The first page contains a brief overview of the assessment data and the goals or outcomes in NOC (Nursing Outcome Classification) format. The second page contains the nursing care plan with the NANDA-I (North American Nursing Diagnosis Association–International) accepted nursing diagnosis and NIC (Nursing Intervention Classification) along with other common nursing interventions. The second page also provides information about commonly used drugs for the condition as well as diagnostic tests. We explain each piece and how to use each care map so that you can critically think about your patient/family/population/system's needs and add and individualize the information to what is already provided in the concept map. When creating your own maps, the two-page format is easy to use in the clinical setting.

The first part of the first page of each concept map starts with a definition and description of the condition or situation straight from *Taber's Cyclopedic Medical Dictionary* (2009) or another reliable source (Figure 1).

The information about the condition that is placed first on every care map provides you with an overview of the condition or situation that your patient/family/population/system is experiencing and brings you up to date on the physiology and specifics. This overview helps you gain confidence in providing nursing care because we know there is so much information to remember and this provides you with a foundational understanding.

Figure 1. Condition and Physiology.

CONDITION: Posttraumatic Stress Disorder (Axis I)

PHYSIOLOGY: Posttraumatic stress disorder (axis I) is intense psychological distress marked by horrifying memories, recurring fears, and feelings of helplessness that develop after a psychologically traumatic event, such as the experience of combat, criminal assault, life-threatening accidents, natural disasters, or rape. The symptoms of PTSD may include re-experiencing the traumatic event (a phenomenon called "flashback"); avoiding stimuli associated with the trauma; memory disturbances; psychological or social withdrawal; or increased aggressiveness, irritability, insomnia, startle responses, and vigilance. Persistent symptoms of increased arousal (not present before the trauma), are indicated by two (or more) of the following: 1) difficulty falling or staying asleep, 2) irritability or outbursts of anger, 3) difficulty concentrating, 4) hypervigilance, 5) exaggerated startle response. Duration of the disturbance is more than 1 month, and the symptoms may last for years after the event but often can be managed with supportive psychotherapy or medications such as antidepressants (*Taber's*, 2009).

Figure 2.   Handoff Communication Tool.

HANDOFF COMMUNICATION

S Situation	Assess what is currently happening in a short statement.	Patient presents with _____	
B Background	Summarize important past assessment data for your patient here. Place lab results and medications on the concept map.	**Age:** **Gender:** **Allergies:** **Social Alerts:** **Mental Status:** **Safety Risk:**	
A Assessment	Use the assessment data to complete your concept map.	**Nursing Diagnosis:** Place the Nursing Diagnoses in prioritized order on the concept map and add any needed for your specific patient. **Plan:** Place any further Nursing Interventions Classifications (NIC) needed on the map.	

Implement Your Plan of Care

	Evaluate your nursing care and make recommendations related to the achievement of your desired outcomes. Were they met, or do new goals need to be established?	**EVALUATE YOUR CARE**	
R Recommendation		**Diag**	**Nursing Outcomes Classification (NOC)**	**Outcome met**

Diag	Nursing Outcomes Classification (NOC)	Outcome met
1	The patient will identify ineffective coping behaviors and consequences. Verbalize awareness of own coping and problem-solving abilities. Meet psychological needs evidenced by appropriate expression of feelings, identification of options, and use of resources. Make decisions and express satisfaction with choices.	☐ Yes ☐ No
2	Patient will appear relaxed and report anxiety is reduced to a manageable level. Verbalize awareness of feelings of anxiety. Identify healthy ways to deal with and express anxiety. Demonstrate problem-solving skills. Use resources/support systems effectively.	☐ Yes ☐ No
3	Report improvement in sleep or rest pattern. Verbalize increased sense of well-being and feeling rested.	☐ Yes ☐ No
4	Patient discusses trauma without experiencing panic. Patient has fewer flashbacks/nightmares. Patient can sleep without medication. Patient demonstrates use of adaptive coping strategies.	☐ Yes ☐ No
5		☐ Yes ☐ No

The second portion of the first page of each concept map is the Handoff Communication tool (Figure 2). This section is arranged in the SBAR (Situation, Background, Assessment, Recommendation) format to organize the important aspects of your care.

The *S* in this section is the situation or what is happening now with the patient/family/population/system you are caring for. An example is provided in Figure 3.

Next is the *B* box of the Handoff Communication, which is the pertinent background or past assessment data that is important to know in order to develop an effective plan of care. It may be data gained from the history, physical assessment, or observation. It can be both objective and subjective data that relates to the current condition (Figure 4).

Now that the situation and background are done, a complete plan of care is needed that includes nursing diagnosis and intervention (Figure 5).

Figure 3.   S: Situation.

HANDOFF COMMUNICATION

S Situation — Assess what is currently happening in a short statement.

Patient presents with _____

Figure 4.   B: Background.

HANDOFF COMMUNICATION

B Background — Summarize important past assessment data for your patient here. Place lab results and medications on the concept map.

Age: **Gender:**
Allergies:
Social Alerts:
Mental Status:
Safety Risk:

Figure 5.   A: Assessment and Concept Map.

HANDOFF COMMUNICATION

A Assessment — Use the assessment data to complete your concept map.

Nursing Diagnosis: Place the Nursing Diagnoses in prioritized order on the concept map and add any needed for your specific patient.
Plan: Place any further Nursing Interventions Classifications (NIC) needed on the map.

Figure 6.   Nursing Diagnoses, Medications, Laboratory and Diagnostic Procedures, and Identifying Information.

Nursing Diagnosis 1

Ineffective coping related to incapacitating stress evidenced by lack of ability to carry out activities of daily living (ADL).

NIC:
1) Assess level of anxiety experienced by the patient; **2)** Assess patient's perceptions and expectations; **3)** Observe early signs of distress; **4)** Evaluate patient's current coping and problem-solving patterns; **5)** Assess for abuse of drugs or alcohol; **6)** Assess and promote presence of positive coping skills and inner strengths, such as use of relation techniques, willingness to express feelings, and use of support systems; and **7)** Establish a therapeutic nurse-patient relationship.

Nursing Diagnosis 2

Anxiety related to constant stress evidenced by verbalizations, and lack of attention.

NIC:
1) Assess degree and reality of threat to patient and level of anxiety; **2)** Stay with the patient and remain calm; **3)** Use simple explanations; **4)** Maintain low-stimuli environment; **5)** Review coping mechanisms used in the past, such as problem-solving skills and asking for help; **6)** Encourage verbalization of current situation; **7)** Maintain frequent contact and therapeutic communication; and **8)** Administer sedatives and tranquilizers as indicated.

Nursing Diagnosis 3

Disturbed sleep pattern related to stress evidenced by insomnia.

NIC:
1) Ascertain usual sleep patterns and changes that are occurring; **2)** Provide comfortable bedding and some of own possessions such as a pillow or an afghan; **3)** Establish new sleep routine incorporating old pattern and new environment; **4)** Encourage light physical activity during the day; and **5)** Promote bedtime comfort regimens and avoid caffeine.

Nursing Diagnosis 4

Stress overload related to diagnosis evidenced by flashback symptoms.

NIC:
1) Accept patient; establish trust; **2)** Stay with patient during flashbacks; **3)** Encourage verbalization about the trauma when patient is ready; **4)** Discuss coping strategies; and **5)** Assist patient to try to comprehend the trauma and how it will be assimilated into his or her persona.

Condition:
Posttraumatic Stress Disorder (Axis I)

Age:

Link & Explain
- Nursing Interventions Classification (NIC)
- Laboratory and Diagnostic Procedures
- Medications

Nursing Diagnosis 5

NIC:

Medications

a. Anxiolytics (e.g., benzodiazepam, BuSpar)

b. Antidepressant medications (e.g., SSRIs, MAOIs)

c. Antihypertensive agents (e.g., beta blockers, alpha2-receptor agonists, clonidine).

d.

Laboratory & Diagnostic Procedures

a. Blood alcohol level, ABGs, electrolytes

b. Renal function tests

c.

d.

This is where the second page of the map comes in (Figure 6). No longer will you need pages and pages of care planning! You can accomplish a complete plan of care that is individualized to your patient/family/population/system by looking through the premade diagnoses and interventions and altering them to fit the situation.

First, each nursing diagnosis box is numbered so you can prioritize your diagnosis (Figure 7).

In the NIC box of the diagnosis is a complete list of interventions that go along with the diagnosis, all organized by P-E-S (Problem-Etiology-Signs and Symptoms). If any of the nursing interventions are not applicable to your patient, you can cross them off and add as many as you need. Of course, if it is a risk diagnosis, there will not be any symptoms.

Figure 7.   Sample Completed Nursing Diagnosis box.

Nursing Diagnosis 1

Ineffective coping related to incapacitating stress evidenced by lack of ability to carry out activities of daily living (ADL).

NIC:
1) Assess level of anxiety experienced by the patient; **2)** Assess patient's perceptions and expectations; **3)** Observe early signs of distress; **4)** Evaluate patient's current coping and problem-solving patterns; **5)** Assess for abuse of drugs or alcohol; **6)** Assess and promote presence of positive coping skills and inner strengths, such as use of relation techniques, willingness to express feelings, and use of support systems; and **7)** Establish a therapeutic nurse-patient relationship.

There are five boxes on your concept map for nursing diagnosis, and we have typically filled in between three and five of them depending on the condition, which may leave you with one or more diagnosis boxes that can be used, if needed, for a specific nursing need you have identified for your patient/family/population/system. If there is a diagnosis that is not listed, you can fill in your own (Figure 8).

Figure 8.   Sample Blank Nursing Diagnosis box.

Nursing Diagnosis 5

NIC:

Each nursing diagnosis on page 2 corresponds with an outcome box (under the *R* of SBAR) on the first page (Figure 9).

During or at the end of the clinical day, you can determine if that outcome has been met or if it needs revision. This is the evaluation of your nursing care. The outcomes are written in NOC language or outcome-specific terminology. The numbered area on each outcome box can be used to match the nursing diagnosis. The student also has the option of checking *yes* or *no* in the Implement Your Plan of Care section. This feature gives you a self-reflective mechanism for each part of your plan. The yes-or-no mechanism encourages you to stop and critically think about the outcome of your care, leading you to accept it or revise it to best care for your patient/family/population/system.

Figure 9.   R: Recommendation.

Implement Your Plan of Care

			EVALUATE YOUR CARE		
R Recommendation	Evaluate your nursing care and make recommendations related to the achievement of your desired outcomes. Were they met, or do new goals need to be established?	**Diag**	**Nursing Outcomes Classification (NOC)**		**Outcome met**
		1	The patient will identify ineffective coping behaviors and consequences. Verbalize awareness of own coping and problem-solving abilities. Meet psychological needs evidenced by appropriate expression of feelings, identification of options, and use of resources. Make decisions and express satisfaction with choices.		☐ **Yes** ☐ **No**
		2	Patient will appear relaxed and report anxiety is reduced to a manageable level. Verbalize awareness of feelings of anxiety. Identify healthy ways to deal with and express anxiety. Demonstrate problem-solving skills. Use resources/support systems effectively.		☐ **Yes** ☐ **No**
		3	Report improvement in sleep or rest pattern. Verbalize increased sense of well-being and feeling rested.		☐ **Yes** ☐ **No**
		4	Patient discusses trauma without experiencing panic. Patient has fewer flashbacks/nightmares. Patient can sleep without medication. Patient demonstrates use of adaptive coping strategies.		☐ **Yes** ☐ **No**
		5			☐ **Yes** ☐ **No**

Page 2 of each care map has some added information for clarifying your plan of care. The center box (Figure 10) has an identifying data area that can be used according to your school policy.

Figure 10.   Identifying Information.

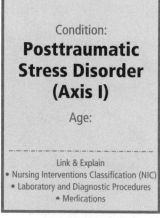

Condition:
Posttraumatic Stress Disorder (Axis I)

Age:

Link & Explain
• Nursing Interventions Classification (NIC)
• Laboratory and Diagnostic Procedures
• Medications

Medications and Laboratory & Diagnostic Procedures boxes (Figure 11) are included at the bottom of page 2 so that you can list your important medications and diagnostic tests for your patient/family/population/system.

We understand that in today's health-care world, multiple medications and tests are completed. Use the supplemental forms located in the appendices to include them.

Figure 11. Medications and Laboratory and Diagnostic Procedures.

Medications

a. Anxiolytics (e.g., benzodiazepam, BuSpar)

b. Antidepressant medications (e.g., SSRIs, MAOIs)

c. Antihypertensive agents (e.g., beta blockers, alpha2-receptor agonists, clonidine).

d.

Laboratory & Diagnostic Procedures

a. Blood alcohol level, ABGs, electrolytes

b. Renal function tests

c.

d.

For many of the patients/families/populations/systems that you care for, you can organize your care on your care map and critically think about it. Once you have your care map filled in, you can explain the links or draw the links. Links are lines that you draw from one item on the map to another to show there is a relationship. Some of the common links include:

• Interventions to assist with one or more nursing diagnosis
• Medications to diagnosis
• Medications to diagnostic tests
• Nursing interventions to other interventions
• Diagnostic test to nursing diagnosis

The possibilities are endless! Each link provides insight into the organization of the nursing care priorities and outcomes for the patient/family/population/system. Additional forms are included in the appendices in case they are needed:

A: Morning Report Worksheet
B: Clinical Assessment Tool
C: Patient Overview
D: Lab Values and Diagnostic Tests
E: Medications
F: Nurse's Notes

The good news is that these care maps will make your clinical nursing experience easier by organizing and prioritizing your care. You will enjoy having some of the information to start with while being able to individualize it to your patient/family/population/system care needs. These care maps also reduce the paper burden for the student, faculty, and the earth! What was previously accomplished on multiple pages can be reduced to two pages.

Included at the end of this introduction is a practice map about you, the nursing student! Use this map as a self-awareness exercise and a concept map practice tool—it is fun and easy. It will familiarize you with the process of concept mapping.

This publication is an ongoing process. Although we have developed 200 expertly reviewed concept maps, we realize there are other conditions that need to be addressed on the health–illness continuum. We invite you to submit any new ideas for concept maps, e-mail your suggestions to ConceptCareMaps@FADavis.com. These care maps are made to assist us all to provide the very best nursing care! Let's get started.

CONDITION: Nursing Student Self-care Concept Map

PHYSIOLOGY: Self-care is a conceptual model of nursing developed by Dorethea Orem. The person (in this case YOU the nursing student) is a self-care agent who has therapeutic self-care demands made up of universal, developmental, and health care demands. The goal of nursing is to help people to meet their therapeutic self-care demands (Taber's, 2009). For this practice concept map you are the nurse and the patient (or the student in a nursing education program)!

HANDOFF COMMUNICATION

S	Situation	Assess what is currently happening in a short statement.	The student nurse presents as _____.
B	Background	Summarize important past assessment data for your patient here. Place lab results and medications on the concept map.	**Age:** **Gender:** **Allergies:** **Fall Risk:** **Isolation:** **Social Alerts:**
A	Assessment	Use the assessment data to complete your concept map.	**Nursing Diagnosis:** Place the Nursing Diagnoses in prioritized order on the concept map and add any needed for your specific patient. **Plan:** Place any further Nursing Interventions Classifications (NIC) needed on the map.

Implement Your Plan of Care

		EVALUATE YOUR CARE		
R	Recommendation	Evaluate your nursing care and make recommendations related to the achievement of your desired outcomes. Were they met, or do new goals need to be established?	**Diag**	**Nursing Outcomes Classification (NOC)**	**Outcome met**
			1	Identify positive and negative factors affecting management of current and future stressors. Have an established plan in place to deal with various contingencies. Report a measurable increase in ability to deal with potential events.	☐ Yes ☐ No
			2	Express feelings freely. Demonstrate individual problem-solving process directed at appropriate solutions to the situation. Encourage family members to handle situation in their own way.	☐ Yes ☐ No
			3	Identify necessary health-maintenance activities. Verbalize factors contributing to current situation. Develop plan to meet specific needs.	☐ Yes ☐ No
			4	Identify resources within yourself to deal with the situation. Participate positively in patient care within limits of ability. Engage in problem-solving with other direct-care providers to meet patient's needs.	☐ Yes ☐ No
			5		☐ Yes ☐ No

Nursing Diagnosis 1

Coping: Readiness for enhanced coping related to nursing education demands evidenced by active planning for predictive stressors.

NIC:
1) Review your previous plans to cope with nursing education; **2)** Assess current stressors; **3)** List your strengths and weaknesses related to upcoming stressors; **4)** Reassess plans for needed alterations; **5)** Prioritize interventions; and **6)** Develop a calendar for time management purposes.

Nursing Diagnosis 2

Risk for interrupted family processes related to nursing education demands.

NIC:
1) Note family members who are affected by you going for a nursing education; **2)** Assess role expectations of family while you are going to school; **3)** Deal with family members in a warm, caring manner while explaining your current situation and priorities; and **4)** Set aside quality time for family when possible.

Nursing Diagnosis 3

Risk for ineffective health maintenance related to long study and clinical hours.

NIC:
1) Explore how your health was maintained prior to starting school; **2)** Set up normal health exams on your time line; **3)** Establish an exercise schedule for nonclinical days and place on your time management calendar; **4)** Monitor nutritional intake by packing healthy lunches and snacks; **5)** Limit caffeine intake; and **6)** Schedule at least 7 hours of sleep per night.

Nursing Diagnosis 4

Risk for caregiver role strain related to clinical experiences that deal with intense human needs.

NIC:
1) Assess your anxiety level through reflection (journaling); **2)** Establish a professional rapport with your peers in your clinical group; **3)** Own the problem by being fully prepared for clinical by role playing therapeutic communication and practicing in the skills lab; **4)** Facilitate collection of data by clarifying any information with nurses on the unit or faculty; and **5)** Understand the professional growth experience as outlined by Patricia Benner's novice to expert theory.

Patient Initials:

Condition:

Nursing Student Self-care Concept Map

Age:

- - - - - - - - - - - - - - - -

Link & Explain: -
- Nursing Interventions Classification (NIC)
- Laboratory & Diagnostic Procedures
- Medications

Nursing Diagnosis 5

(Use the nursing diagnosis list for any others that are specific to YOU!)

P _____

E _____

S _____ (If not a risk diagnosis)

NIC:

Medications:

a. N/A

b.

c.

d.

Laboratory & Diagnostic Procedures:

a. N/A

b.

c.

d.

Concept Maps for Infants

This chapter provides care maps that describe common health conditions experienced by both preterm and term infants. For some of these conditions, the patient may be treated in the neonatal intensive care unit (NICU). The nursing plan of care for the infant in the NICU, as well as in low-risk or intermediate newborn nurseries, always includes the parents or caregivers. The nurse is responsible for the family's understanding of the condition and care required in order to promote a safe discharge situation for the infant. Therefore, the nursing diagnoses for our youngest patients should always include the caregivers or parents in the plan.

The conditions included in this chapter are:

1. Apnea of Prematurity (AOP)
2. Circumcision
3. Cytomegalovirus (CMV) Inclusion Disease
4. Fetal Alcohol Syndrome (FAS)
5. Hyperbilirubinemia of the Newborn
6. Low-Risk Newborn (Neonate)
7. Neonatal Abstinence Syndrome (NAS)
8. Patent Ductus Arteriosus (PDA)
9. Preterm or Premature Infant
10. Respiratory Distress Syndrome (Neonatal)
11. TORCH

CONDITION: Apnea of Prematurity (AOP)

PHYSIOLOGY: AOP is a condition of the preterm infant marked by repeated episodes of apnea lasting longer than 20 seconds. The diagnosis of AOP is one of exclusion, made when no treatable cause can be found. Increased frequency of apneic episodes directly relate to the degree of prematurity. AOP is an independent risk factor for sudden infant death syndrome (SIDS). Apneic episodes may result in bradycardia, hypoxia, and respiratory acidosis (*Taber's*, 2009).

HANDOFF COMMUNICATION

S Situation	Assess what is currently happening in a short statement.	Infant presents as _____
B Background	Summarize important past assessment data for your patient here. Place lab results and medications on the concept map.	**Age:** **Gender:** **Allergies:**
A Assessment	Use the assessment data to complete your concept map.	**Nursing Diagnosis:** Place the Nursing Diagnoses in prioritized order on the concept map and add any needed for your specific patient. **Plan:** Place any further Nursing Interventions Classifications (NIC) needed on the map.

Implement Your Plan of Care

		Diag	**EVALUATE YOUR CARE**	
R Recommendation	Evaluate your nursing care and make recommendations related to the achievement of your desired outcomes. Were they met, or do new goals need to be established?		**Nursing Outcomes Classification (NOC)**	**Outcome met**
		1	Maintain movement of air in and out of lungs and exchange of carbon dioxide and oxygen at the alveolar level.	☐ **Yes** ☐ **No**
		2	Monitor infant development.	☐ **Yes** ☐ **No**
		3	Enhance preterm infant organization.	☐ **Yes** ☐ **No**
		4	Regain or maintain appropriate body temperature for age and size.	☐ **Yes** ☐ **No**
		5		☐ **Yes** ☐ **No**

Nursing Diagnosis 1

Impaired gas exchange related to effects of cardiopulmonary insufficiency evidenced by apnea and decreasing pulse oximetry reading.

NIC:
1) Monitor rate, rhythm, depth, and effort of respirations; 2) Note chest movement and use of accessory muscles; 3) Auscultate breath sounds; 4) Monitor ventilator or oxygen readings; 5) Institute respiratory therapy treatments as prescribed; 6) Monitor chest x-rays; 7) Place infant in supine position; and 8) Institute resuscitation efforts as needed: tactile stimulation or bag and mask if unresponsive to tactile stimulation.

Nursing Diagnosis 2

Delayed growth and development related to decreased oxygen consumption, prematurity, environmental and stimulation deficiencies evidenced by cognitive, somatic, and/or psychosocial delays.

NIC:
1) Monitor weight and growth; 2) Encourage parents to verbalize understanding of growth patterns; 3) Monitor intake and output and nutritional status each day; 4) Provide appropriate age-adjusted stimulation and prevent overstimulation; 5) Protect sleep cycles; and 6) Teach caregivers to understand cues of preterm infant.

Nursing Diagnosis 3

Disorganized infant behavior related to prematurity evidenced by disrupted metabolic processes and sleep disruption.

NIC:
1) Observe infant for cues that suggest stress or discomfort and avoid if possible; 2) Encourage caregivers to provide kangaroo care (KC); 3) Model gentle behavior for caregivers; 4) Support and encourage caregivers; 5) Provide consistent caregivers; 6) Provide infant with opportunity to suck; and 7) Position infant in nested positions.

Nursing Diagnosis 4

Risk for ineffective thermoregulation related to immature CNS (central nervous system) development (temperature regulating center), decreased ratio of body mass to surface area, decreased subcutaneous fat, limited brown fat stores, inability to shiver or sweat, poor metabolic reserves, muted response to hypothermia, or frequent interventions.

NIC:
1) Note conditions of infection or environment that would decrease body temperature; 2) Measure temperature; and 3) Adjust linen into a nest to conserve energy.

Condition:
Apnea of Prematurity (AOP)

Age:

Link & Explain
• Nursing Interventions Classification (NIC)
• Laboratory and Diagnostic Procedures
• Medications

Nursing Diagnosis 5

NIC:

Medications

a. Methylxanthines: caffeine, theophylline, and aminophylline

b.

c.

d.

Laboratory & Diagnostic Procedures

a. Arterial blood gases

b. Continuous cardiopulmonary monitoring

c. Continuous pulse oximetry

d. Chest x-rays

CONDITION: Circumcision

PHYSIOLOGY: Circumcision is the surgical removal of the end of the foreskin of the penis. Circumcision is usually performed at the request of the parents, in some cases for religious reasons. Considerable controversy exists over whether the procedure has medical benefits; some authorities suggest that circumcision is associated with reduced risk of HIV, urinary tract infections, penile carcinoma, and sexually transmitted infections. Other authorities dispute these findings, suggesting that the procedure may have adverse effects on sexual, emotional, or psychological health. If the procedure is preformed, anesthesia should be used (*Taber's*, 2009).

HANDOFF COMMUNICATION

S — Situation — Assess what is currently happening in a short statement.

Infant presents as _____

B — Background — Summarize important past assessment data for your patient here. Place lab results and medications on the concept map.

Age: **Gender:** Male
Allergies:

A — Assessment — Use the assessment data to complete your concept map.

Nursing Diagnosis: Place the Nursing Diagnoses in prioritized order on the concept map and add any needed for your specific patient.
Plan: Place any further Nursing Interventions Classifications (NIC) needed on the map.

Implement Your Plan of Care

R — Recommendation — Evaluate your nursing care and make recommendations related to the achievement of your desired outcomes. Were they met, or do new goals need to be established?

EVALUATE YOUR CARE

Diag	Nursing Outcomes Classification (NOC)	Outcome met
1	Pain control is assessed and recorded.	☐ Yes ☐ No
2	No extra bleeding is noted from surgical site.	☐ Yes ☐ No
3	Surgical site is clean and dry.	☐ Yes ☐ No
4	Parents (caregivers) verbalize appropriate care of the surgical site and understand when to call infant's primary care provider for complications.	☐ Yes ☐ No
5		☐ Yes ☐ No

Nursing Diagnosis 1

Acute pain related to surgical procedure evidenced by crying.

NIC:
1) Use EMLA cream to anesthetize the area before the surgical procedure; **2)** Medicate immediately before the procedure with sucrose concentrate 24% and provide nonnutritive sucking (NNS); **3)** Do not restrain infant longer than necessary; **4)** Make sure restraints do not pinch or tug on infant's skin; and **5)** Expose only necessary areas of body.

Nursing Diagnosis 2

Risk for bleeding related to surgical trauma.

NIC:
1) Monitor in the nursery per postsurgical procedure policy; **2)** Teach parents to monitor thereafter; **3)** Maintain lubricated gauze dressing unless a bell circumcision was done; and **4)** Lubricate diaper area to prevent gauze from sticking and pulling off.

Nursing Diagnosis 3

Risk for infection related to surgical wound.

NIC:
1) Monitor infant's temperature postprocedure; **2)** Assess surgical site for appropriate healing; and **3)** Maintain clean diapers and diaper area.

Nursing Diagnosis 4

Ineffective health maintenance related to knowledge deficit (parental or caregiver) regarding care of surgical area evidenced by questions.

NIC:
1) Explain surgical procedure fully to parents or caregivers, noting all the advantages and disadvantages; **2)** Differentiate between types of circumcisions as needed (surgical or bell); **3)** Describe healing process and changes expected to occur over the next week; and **4)** Teach parents to care for site and demonstrate diaper change.

Condition:
Circumcision
Age:

Link & Explain
• Nursing Interventions Classification (NIC)
• Laboratory and Diagnostic Procedures
• Medications

Nursing Diagnosis 5

NIC:

Medications

a. Lidocaine/prilocaine (EMLA) cream

b. Sucrose concentrate 24%

c.

d.

Laboratory & Diagnostic Procedures

a.

b.

c.

d.

CONDITION: Cytomegalovirus (CMV) Inclusion Disease

PHYSIOLOGY: CMV inclusion disease is a persistent, latent infection of white blood cells caused by CMV, a beta-group herpesvirus, human cytomegalovirus (HCMV) or human herpesvirus 5 (HHV-5). Approximately 60% of people of 35 years of age have been infected with CMV, but the primary infection is usually mild in people with healthy immune function. CMV can be reactivated and cause overt disease in pregnant women and can be isolated in saliva, urine, breast milk, feces, blood, and vaginal secretions, and the infected secretions can retain the virus for months to years. During pregnancy, the woman can transmit the virus transplacentally (usually during a primary infection) to the fetus with devastating results. Ten percent of infected infants develop CMV inclusion disease marked by anemia, purpura, hepatosplenomegaly, microcephaly, and abnormal mental and motor development; 50% of these infants die (*Taber's*, 2009).

HANDOFF COMMUNICATION

S	Situation	Assess what is currently happening in a short statement.	Infant presents as _____
B	Background	Summarize important past assessment data for your patient here. Place lab results and medications on the concept map.	**Age:** **Gender:** **Allergies:**
A	Assessment	Use the assessment data to complete your concept map.	**Nursing Diagnosis:** Place the Nursing Diagnoses in prioritized order on the concept map and add any needed for your specific patient. **Plan:** Place any further Nursing Interventions Classifications (NIC) needed on the map.

Implement Your Plan of Care

		EVALUATE YOUR CARE		
R	Recommendation — Evaluate your nursing care and make recommendations related to the achievement of your desired outcomes. Were they met, or do new goals need to be established?	**Diag**	**Nursing Outcomes Classification (NOC)**	**Outcome met**
		1	Maintain current visual field and acuity.	☐ Yes ☐ No
		2	Identify behaviors to prevent and reduce infection.	☐ Yes ☐ No
		3	Communicate thoughts and feelings utilizing available support systems, such as family, spiritual leaders, and other resources. Demonstrate coping behaviors that reduce anxiety.	☐ Yes ☐ No
		4	Parents (caregivers) verbalize understanding of disease, diagnosis, treatment options, and prognosis.	☐ Yes ☐ No
		5		☐ Yes ☐ No

Nursing Diagnosis 1

Risk for disturbed visual sensory perception related to inflammation of the retina.

NIC:
1) Assess type and degree of visual loss; **2)** Recommend environmental changes to assist patient to manage visual impairment; and **3)** Instill eye medications as prescribed.

Nursing Diagnosis 2

Risk for infections related to exposure to, or contact with, blood or body fluids.

NIC:
1) Maintain aseptic techniques such as good hand washing; **2)** Monitor maternal temperature; and **3)** Obtain body fluid specimen for culture and sensitivity.

Nursing Diagnosis 3

Parental anxiety related to infant condition evidenced by increased tension, apprehension, feelings of helplessness, inadequacy, and worry.

NIC:
1) Ascertain what information the parents have about the diagnosis and expected course of the condition; **2)** Provide an atmosphere of concern and anticipatory guidance; **3)** Encourage questions and provide information; and **4)** Explore spiritual support.

Nursing Diagnosis 4

Deficient knowledge related to lack of information regarding disease process, diagnostic testing, and treatment evidenced by questions and information gathering.

NIC:
1) Assess understanding of disease process and treatment; **2)** Identify and communicate community resources, Web sites, and additional sources of information and support; **3)** Discuss diagnostic evaluation procedures as indicated; **4)** Explain treatment regimen and treatment options and provide related information; **5)** Include family/support systems in informational sessions; **6)** Explain the importance of adherence to follow-up visits and screening; and **7)** Provide education regarding health maintenance practices.

Condition:
Cytomegalovirus (CMV) Inclusion Disease

Age:

Link & Explain
• Nursing Interventions Classification (NIC)
• Laboratory and Diagnostic Procedures
• Medications

Nursing Diagnosis 5

NIC:

Medications

a. Antiviral drugs, such as ganciclovir and acyclovir, are used to decrease viral load.

b.

c.

d.

Laboratory & Diagnostic Procedures

a. IVIG (intravenous immunoglobulin), CytoGam titers

b.

c.

d.

CONDITION: Fetal Alcohol Syndrome (FAS)

PHYSIOLOGY: FAS presents with birth defects to infants born to mothers who consumed alcoholic beverages during gestation. Characteristic findings include a small head with multiple facial abnormalities: small eyes with short slits, a wide flat nasal bridge, a midface that lacks a groove between the lip and the nose, and a small jaw related to maxillary hypoplasia. Affected children often exhibit persistent growth retardation, hyperactivity, and learning deficits and may have signs and symptoms of alcohol withdrawal a few days after birth (*Taber's*, 2009).

HANDOFF COMMUNICATION

S Situation	Assess what is currently happening in a short statement.	Infant presents as _____
B Background	Summarize important past assessment data for your patient here. Place lab results and medications on the concept map.	**Age:** **Gender:** **Allergies:**
A Assessment	Use the assessment data to complete your concept map.	**Nursing Diagnosis:** Place the Nursing Diagnoses in prioritized order on the concept map and add any needed for your specific patient. **Plan:** Place any further Nursing Interventions Classifications (NIC) needed on the map.

Implement Your Plan of Care

R Recommendation	Evaluate your nursing care and make recommendations related to the achievement of your desired outcomes. Were they met, or do new goals need to be established?	**EVALUATE YOUR CARE**		
		Diag	Nursing Outcomes Classification (NOC)	Outcome met
		1	Demonstrates absence of untoward effects of withdrawal and experiences no physical injury.	☐ Yes ☐ No
		2	Demonstrates increased organization in infant's behavior.	☐ Yes ☐ No
		3	Demonstrates appropriate attachment behaviors.	☐ Yes ☐ No
		4	Attains steady gains in growth patterns as supported by established norms.	☐ Yes ☐ No
		5		☐ Yes ☐ No

Nursing Diagnosis 1

Risk for injury (CNS damage) related to external chemical factors (alcohol intake by mother).

NIC:
1) Assess and identify if infant is actively withdrawing; **2)** Monitor for seizure activity; **3)** Protect from excoriating skin; **4)** Closely monitor vital signs; **5)** Administer O_2 as needed; and **6)** Medicate as prescribed.

Nursing Diagnosis 2

Disorganized infant behavior related to alcohol effects evidenced by twitching, irritability, inconsolability, and sleeplessness.

NIC:
1) Assess family interactions and mother's ability to care for infant; **2)** Provide parental teaching on comforting interventions; **3)** Protect infant's skin with cream or transparent overlays; **4)** Provide opportunity for positive parent-infant interaction; **5)** Decrease environmental stimuli; **6)** Decrease handling; **7)** Nest and bundle; **8)** Correlate stress and disorganized behavior to internal factors such as pain, hunger, discomfort; and **9)** Medicate as indicated using appropriate abstinence scale.

Nursing Diagnosis 3

Risk for impaired parenting related to maternal mental or physical illness.

NIC:
1) Evaluate family's current emotional status; **2)** Encourage parents to express feelings; **3)** Remain nonjudgmental; **4)** Encourage mother to understand and capitalize on infant's ability to interact; **5)** Appraise mental resources and availability of support systems; **6)** Model age-appropriate care; and **7)** Refer to case manager.

Nursing Diagnosis 4

Risk for delayed growth and development related to effects of maternal alcohol use.

NIC:
1) Consider the use of early screening tools to indicate delay of growth or development; **2)** Regularly compare length, weight, and physical features with established age-appropriate norms; **3)** Promote appropriate sleep and nutrition; and **4)** Refer to physical and occupational therapy when indicated.

Condition:
Fetal Alcohol Syndrome (FAS)

Age:

Link & Explain
• Nursing Interventions Classification (NIC)
• Laboratory and Diagnostic Procedures
• Medications

Nursing Diagnosis 5

NIC:

Medications

a. Sucrose 24%

b. Camphorated tincture of opium (paregoric)

c. Phenobarbital (phenobarbitone)

d.

Laboratory & Diagnostic Procedures

a.

b.

c.

d.

CONDITION: Hyperbilirubinemia of the Newborn

PHYSIOLOGY: Hyperbilirubinemia of the newborn is an excessive amount of bilirubin in the blood; the condition is seen in any illness causing jaundice, including diseases in which the biliary tree is obstructed and those in which blood formation is ineffective. Jaundice is seen in 60% of term infants and 80% of preterm infants. Unconjugated bilirubin accumulates in the blood stream, and the condition is related to the short life span of red blood cells in infants and the decreased activity of the enzyme transference. Jaundice is usually first present in the face and then progresses to the abdomen and legs and feet. It gives the newborn a yellow or orange color, and the infant may appear lethargic and have feeding difficulties (*Taber's*, 2009).

HANDOFF COMMUNICATION

S	Situation	Assess what is currently happening in a short statement.	Infant presents as _____
B	Background	Summarize important past assessment data for your patient here. Place lab results and medications on the concept map.	Age: Gender: Allergies:
A	Assessment	Use the assessment data to complete your concept map.	**Nursing Diagnosis:** Place the Nursing Diagnoses in prioritized order on the concept map and add any needed for your specific patient. **Plan:** Place any further Nursing Interventions Classifications (NIC) needed on the map.

Implement Your Plan of Care

		EVALUATE YOUR CARE		
R	Recommendation — Evaluate your nursing care and make recommendations related to the achievement of your desired outcomes. Were they met, or do new goals need to be established?	**Diag**	**Nursing Outcomes Classification (NOC)**	**Outcome met**
		1	Maintain weight and increase excretion of bilirubin.	☐ Yes ☐ No
		2	Modify environment and correct hazards to ensure safety.	☐ Yes ☐ No
		3	Parents verbalize understanding of condition and participate in treatment regimen.	☐ Yes ☐ No
		4	Maintain a urine output of 2–5 mL/kg/hr. Maintain skin turgor and moist mucous membranes.	☐ Yes ☐ No
		5		☐ Yes ☐ No

Nursing Diagnosis 1

Nutrition: Less than body requirements related to neonatal transition to extrauterine life and exposure from being under the bili lights evidenced by less than 2–5 mL/Kg/hr of urine.

NIC:
1) Increase frequency of feeding; **2)** Maintain I&O; **3)** Provide rest between feeds; **4)** Keep diaper count; and **5)** Check urine specific gravity.

Nursing Diagnosis 2

Risk for injury related to phototherapy, invasive procedures, and chemical imbalances.

NIC:
1) Maintain eye shields and cover genitals; **2)** Record light output q4h; and **3)** Provide limited time out of lights for feeding and bonding.

Nursing Diagnosis 3

Knowledge deficit related to condition and prognosis; information misinterpretation evidenced by questions, statements of concern, or inaccurate follow-through of instructions.

NIC:
1) Review the condition; **2)** Teach side effects and treatment protocol; and **3)** Discuss alternative feeding pattern.

Nursing Diagnosis 4

Risk for fluid volume deficit related to bili lights and insensible water loss.

NIC:
1) Monitor I&O; **2)** Provide frequent feeds (q3h); and **3)** Maintain body temperature.

Condition:
Hyperbilirubinemia of the Newborn

Age:

Link & Explain
• Nursing Interventions Classification (NIC)
• Laboratory and Diagnostic Procedures
• Medications

Nursing Diagnosis 5

NIC:

Medications

a.

b.

c.

d.

Laboratory & Diagnostic Procedures

a. Direct and indirect bilirubin levels.

b. Urine specific gravity of <1.005

c.

d.

CONDITION: Low-Risk Newborn (Neonate)

PHYSIOLOGY: Low-risk newborn (neonate) usually refers to a term infant less than 28 days old. This is a period of transition from intrauterine to extrauterine life. Human newborns are dependent on care provided to them to maintain their normal physiological functioning that promotes appropriate growth and development (*Taber's*, 2009).

HANDOFF COMMUNICATION

S	Situation	Assess what is currently happening in a short statement.	Infant presents as _____
B	Background	Summarize important past assessment data for your patient here. Place lab results and medications on the concept map.	**Age:** **Gender:** **Allergies:**
A	Assessment	Use the assessment data to complete your concept map.	**Nursing Diagnosis:** Place the Nursing Diagnoses in prioritized order on the concept map and add any needed for your specific patient. **Plan:** Place any further Nursing Interventions Classifications (NIC) needed on the map.

Implement Your Plan of Care

			EVALUATE YOUR CARE	
R	Recommendation Evaluate your nursing care and make recommendations related to the achievement of your desired outcomes. Were they met, or do new goals need to be established?	**Diag**	**Nursing Outcomes Classification (NOC)**	**Outcome met**
		1	Demonstrates improved ventilation and adequate oxygenation of tissue, evidenced by appropriate skin color, arterial blood gases (ABGs), or pulse oximetry within normal limits (WNL), and is free of symptoms of respiratory distress.	☐ **Yes** ☐ **No**
		2	Regains or maintains appropriate body temperature for age and size.	☐ **Yes** ☐ **No**
		3	Demonstrates expected weight loss in the immediate period postbirth and then appropriate weight gain.	☐ **Yes** ☐ **No**
		4	Demonstrates signs of positive attachment by responding appropriately to infant's cues.	☐ **Yes** ☐ **No**
		5		☐ **Yes** ☐ **No**

Nursing Diagnosis 1

Risk for impaired gas exchange related to prenatal or intrapartal stressors, excess production of mucus, or cold stress.

NIC:
1) Assess respiratory rate and depth; **2)** Maintain supine position; **3)** Assess oximetry reading and vital signs (VS) as well as ABGs if ordered; **4)** Auscultate breath sounds; and **5)** Administer O_2 as prescribed.

Nursing Diagnosis 2

Risk for hypothermia related to large body surface in relation to mass, limited amounts of insulating subcutaneous fat, nonrenewable source of brown fat and few white fat stores, thin epidermis with close proximity of blood vessels to the skin, inability to shiver, and the change from a warm to a cooler environment.

NIC:
1) Note conditions of infection or environment that would decrease body temperature; **2)** Measure temperature; and **3)** Adjust linen and dress appropriately.

Nursing Diagnosis 3

Risk for imbalanced nutrition (less than body requirements) related to rapid metabolic rate, high caloric requirement, increased insensible water loss through pulmonary and cutaneous routes, fatigue, and a potential for inadequate or depleted glucose stores.

NIC:
1) Assess nutritional status continuously by recording I&O; **2)** Weigh daily; **3)** Weigh diapers; and **4)** Encourage mother to feed when infant gives cues.

Nursing Diagnosis 4

Risk for impaired attachment related to developmental transition (gaining a family member), anxiety associated with the parent role, or lack of privacy.

NIC:
1) Provide role model for parents; **2)** Educate parents on normal infant behavior, growth, and development; and **3)** Involve appropriate support services.

Condition:
Low-Risk Newborn (Neonate)

Age:

Link & Explain
• Nursing Interventions Classification (NIC)
• Laboratory and Diagnostic Procedures
• Medications

Nursing Diagnosis 5

NIC:

Medications

a. Vitamin K prophylactically due to a deficiency at birth.

b. Erythromycin ointment in eyes prophylactically to prevent ophthalmia neonatorum.

c. Hepatitis B vaccine before discharge as the first of three immunizations in the series.

d.

Laboratory & Diagnostic Procedures

a. Glucose monitoring by heel stick at 1 hour old

b. Bilirubin test for direct and indirect bilirubin levels after 24 hours old

c. Metabolic and supplemental screening for inborn errors of metabolism and congenital disorders after 24 hours old

d. Newborn hearing screening before discharge

CONDITION: Neonatal Abstinence Syndrome (NAS)

PHYSIOLOGY: NAS is a cluster of adverse consequences in the newborn due to exposure to addictive or dangerous intoxicants during fetal development. The consequences include, but are not limited to, preterm delivery; intrauterine growth retardation; asphyxia; low birth weight; and behavioral, psychiatric, and learning disabilities later in life (*Taber's*, 2009).

HANDOFF COMMUNICATION

S	Situation	Assess what is currently happening in a short statement.	Infant presents as _____
B	Background	Summarize important past assessment data for your patient here. Place lab results and medications on the concept map.	**Age:** **Gender:** **Allergies:**
A	Assessment	Use the assessment data to complete your concept map.	**Nursing Diagnosis:** Place the Nursing Diagnoses in prioritized order on the concept map and add any needed for your specific patient. **Plan:** Place any further Nursing Interventions Classifications (NIC) needed on the map.

Implement Your Plan of Care

			EVALUATE YOUR CARE		
R	Recommendation	Evaluate your nursing care and make recommendations related to the achievement of your desired outcomes. Were they met, or do new goals need to be established?	**Diag**	**Nursing Outcomes Classification (NOC)**	**Outcome met**
			1	Identify hazards contributing to risk for injury and institute corrective measures.	☐ Yes ☐ No
			2	Decrease pain and maintain pain control.	☐ Yes ☐ No
			3	Conserve energy and increase well-being.	☐ Yes ☐ No
			4	Fluid balance and appropriate weight gain.	☐ Yes ☐ No
			5		☐ Yes ☐ No

Nursing Diagnosis 1

Risk for injury related to CNS agitation evidenced by irritability and muscle spasticity.

NIC:
1) Maintain appropriate supervision at all times; **2)** Keep side rails up and cardiorespiratory monitor on as prescribed; **3)** Take sudden infant death syndrome (SIDS) precautions; and **4)** Teach family safety measures.

Nursing Diagnosis 2

Acute pain related to biochemical changes associated with cessation of drug use evidenced by grimacing, crying, or irritability.

NIC:
1) Monitor for pain every 1–3 hours using age-appropriate pain scale; **2)** Teach parents pain relief techniques; **3)** Facilitate the appropriate use of analgesics; and **4)** Decrease environmental stimuli.

Nursing Diagnosis 3

Fatigue related to altered body chemistry, sleep deprivation, malnutrition, poor physical condition evidenced by irritability.

NIC:
1) Monitor physiological responses to care; **2)** Plan care around rest periods; and **3)** Provide relaxation techniques such as infant massage if tolerated.

Nursing Diagnosis 4

Fluid volume deficit related to increased perspiration and uncoordinated food intake evidenced by lack of weight gain.

NIC:
1) Monitor I&O; **2)** Provide frequent feeds (q3h); **3)** Medicate before feeds; and **4)** Position in nested vestibular position to conserve energy.

Condition:
Neonatal Abstinence Syndrome (NAS)

Age:

Link & Explain
• Nursing Interventions Classification (NIC)
• Laboratory and Diagnostic Procedures
• Medications

Nursing Diagnosis 5

NIC:

Medications

a. Sucrose 12%

b. Camphorated tincture of opium (paregoric)

c. Phenobarbital (phenobarbitone)

d. Dolophine (methadone)

Laboratory & Diagnostic Procedures

a.

b.

c.

d.

CONDITION: Patent Ductus Arteriosus (PDA)

PHYSIOLOGY: PDA is a communication between the main pulmonary artery and the aorta that persists after birth. This condition in preterm infants has been treated successfully with drugs such as indomethacin (Indocin) that inhibit prostaglandin synthesis (*Taber's*, 2009)

HANDOFF COMMUNICATION

S	Situation	Assess what is currently happening in a short statement.	Infant presents as _____
B	Background	Summarize important past assessment data for your patient here. Place lab results and medications on the concept map.	**Age:** **Gender:** **Allergies:**
A	Assessment	Use the assessment data to complete your concept map.	**Nursing Diagnosis:** Place the Nursing Diagnoses in prioritized order on the concept map and add any needed for your specific patient. **Plan:** Place any further Nursing Interventions Classifications (NIC) needed on the map.

Implement Your Plan of Care

R	Recommendation	Evaluate your nursing care and make recommendations related to the achievement of your desired outcomes. Were they met, or do new goals need to be established?	**EVALUATE YOUR CARE**	
			Diag **Nursing Outcomes Classification (NOC)**	**Outcome met**
			1 Displays hemodynamic stability such as stable blood pressure and cardiac output.	☐ **Yes** ☐ **No**
			2 Maintains an effective breathing pattern free of cyanosis and other signs and symptoms of hypoxia, with breath sounds equal bilaterally and lung fields clearing.	☐ **Yes** ☐ **No**
			3 Infant maintains optimal growth and developmental milestones.	☐ **Yes** ☐ **No**
			4 Caregiver verbalizes understanding of treatment/therapy regimen, identifies individual risk factors, and demonstrates behaviors and techniques to prevent skin breakdown.	☐ **Yes** ☐ **No**
			5	☐ **Yes** ☐ **No**

Nursing Diagnosis 1

Risk for decreased cardiac output related to PDA.

NIC:
1) Monitor and document trends in heart rate (HR) and blood pressure (BP); 2) Observe for changes in behavior; 3) Monitor pulse oximeter readings; 4) Measure and document I&O; 5) Promote uninterrupted rest periods; and 6) Inspect for edema.

Nursing Diagnosis 2

Risk for ineffective breathing pattern related to diminished O_2-carrying capacity of blood.

NIC:
1) Evaluate respiration rate, rhythm, and depth; 2) Monitor for signs of distress: nasal flaring, retractions, and grunting; 3) Inspect skin for cyanosis and blanching; 4) Refer to respiratory therapy; 5) Monitor pulse oximeter readings; 6) Increase rest periods and do not stress at feeding time; and 7) Inspect for edema.

Nursing Diagnosis 3

Delays in growth and development due to hospitalization and chronic illness evidenced by cognitive, somatic, and/or psychosocial delays.

NIC:
1) Perform baseline developmental assessment such as Denver Developmental Assessment; 2) Monitor developmental milestones and provide appropriate developmental tasks; 3) Involve play therapist with selection of activities; 4) Plan for play periods with rest; and 5) Involve speech, occupational, and physical therapy to support developmental milestones.

Nursing Diagnosis 4

Knowledge deficit regarding pathophysiology of condition, management, and available community resources related to insufficient information; misconceptions evidenced by statements of concerns and questions by parents.

NIC:
1) Ascertain readiness, level of knowledge, and individual learning needs of parents; 2) Provide positive reinforcement; and 3) Validate the importance for infant follow-up with a pediatric cardiologist if discharged.

Condition:
Patent Ductus Arteriosus (PDA)

Age:

Link & Explain
• Nursing Interventions Classification (NIC)
• Laboratory and Diagnostic Procedures
• Medications

Nursing Diagnosis 5

NIC:

Medications

a. Indomethacin (Indocin)

b.

c.

d.

Laboratory & Diagnostic Procedures

a. EKG

b. Echocardiogram

c. Chest x-ray

d.

CONDITION: Preterm or Premature Infant

PHYSIOLOGY: Preterm or premature infant is an infant born any time before the completion of the 37th week of gestation. In the United States, approximately 7.1% of white infants and 13.4% of nonwhite infants are born prematurely. Chances of survival depend on the gestational age, maturity achieved, and quality of care. Premature birth is the leading cause of infant death related to pulmonary ventilation, infection, intracranial hemorrhage, and congenital anomalies. Frequently, premature infants are handicapped because of neurological deficits later in life. Risk factors include the mother having had a previous preterm delivery, being nonwhite, being younger than 17 years of age or older than 35 years of age when delivering, being unmarried, having low socioeconomic status, having children closely spaced, and living in an urban area. Physical limitations of the preterm infant include weak sucking and swallowing reflexes, impaired renal functions, incomplete capillary development in the lungs, immature lung alveoli, weak thoracic muscles, inability to regulate body temperature, incomplete or poorly developed enzyme systems, hepatic immaturity, and poor antenatal storage of minerals, vitamins, and immune compounds (*Taber's*, 2009).

HANDOFF COMMUNICATION

S Situation	Assess what is currently happening in a short statement.	Infant presents as _____
B Background	Summarize important past assessment data for your patient here. Place lab results and medications on the concept map.	**Age:** **Gender:** **Allergies:**
A Assessment	Use the assessment data to complete your concept map.	**Nursing Diagnosis:** Place the Nursing Diagnoses in prioritized order on the concept map and add any needed for your specific patient. **Plan:** Place any further Nursing Interventions Classifications (NIC) needed on the map.

Implement Your Plan of Care

R Recommendation	Evaluate your nursing care and make recommendations related to the achievement of your desired outcomes. Were they met, or do new goals need to be established?		**EVALUATE YOUR CARE**	

	Diag	**Nursing Outcomes Classification (NOC)**	**Outcome met**
	1	Demonstrates improved ventilation and adequate oxygenation of tissue demonstrated by appropriate skin color, arterial blood gases (ABGs), or pulse oximetry within normal limits (WNL) and is free of symptoms of respiratory distress.	☐ Yes ☐ No
	2	Establishes normal and effective respiratory pattern with ABGs WNL. Is free of cyanosis and other signs of hypoxia.	☐ Yes ☐ No
	3	Regains or maintains appropriate body temperature for age and size.	☐ Yes ☐ No
	4	Maintains and demonstrates fluid balance evidenced by adequate urine output, stable vital signs (VS), moist mucous membranes, and good skin turgor.	☐ Yes ☐ No
	5		☐ Yes ☐ No

Nursing Diagnosis 1

Impaired gas exchange related to alveolar-capillary membrane changes (inadequate surfactant levels), altered blood flow (immaturity of pulmonary arteriole musculature), altered O_2 supply (immaturity of central nervous system [CNS] and neuromuscular system), tracheobronchial obstruction, or altered O_2-carrying capacity of blood (anemia).

NIC:
1) Assess respiratory rate and depth; **2)** Maintain supine position; **3)** Assess oximetry reading and vital signs (VS) as well as arterial blood gases (ABGs) if ordered; **4)** Auscultate breath sounds; and **5)** Administer O_2 as prescribed.

Nursing Diagnosis 2

Ineffective breathing pattern related to immaturity of the respiratory center, poor positioning, drug-related depression, metabolic imbalances, decreased energy, fatigue, evidenced by dyspnea, tachypnea, periods of apnea, nasal flaring, use of accessory muscles, cyanosis, abnormal ABGs, or tachycardia.

NIC:
1) Evaluate respiratory function;
2) Auscultate; **3)** Monitor ABGs;
4) Maintain pulse oximetry; and
5) Maintain O_2.

Nursing Diagnosis 3

Risk for ineffective thermoregulation related to immature CNS development (temperature regulating center), decreased ratio of body mass to surface area, ↓ subcutaneous fat, limited brown fat stores, inability to shiver or sweat, poor metabolic reserves, muted response to hypothermia, or frequent interventions.

NIC:
1) Note conditions of infection or environment that would decrease body temperature; **2)** Measure temperature; **3)** Adjust linen into a nest to conserve energy; **4)** Decrease environmental drafts; and **5)** Keep dry.

Nursing Diagnosis 4

Risk for fluid volume deficit related to extremes of age and weight, excessive fluid losses (thin skin, lack of insulating fat, increased environmental temperature, immature kidney, and failure to concentrate urine).

NIC:
1) Monitor VS, capillary refill, status of mucus membranes and skin turgor;
2) Monitor fluid intake; and **3)** Review electrolytes and renal function tests.

Condition:
Preterm or Premature Infant

Age:

Link & Explain
• Nursing Interventions Classification (NIC)
• Laboratory and Diagnostic Procedures
• Medications

Nursing Diagnosis 5

NIC:

Medications

a. Synthetic lung surfactant related to RDS (respiratory distress syndrome)

b.

c.

d.

Laboratory & Diagnostic Procedures

a. Frequent glucose monitoring until stable

b. CBC with differential related to high risk for anemia and infection

c. Blood gases to monitor respiratory distress

d.

CONDITION: Respiratory Distress Syndrome (Neonatal)

PHYSIOLOGY: Respiratory distress syndrome (RDS) is due to severe impairment of the respiratory function in the newborn, usually related to prematurity, and is rarely seen in infants over 37 weeks gestation. It is the leading cause of infant death in the United States. Shortly after birth, the infant has a low Apgar score and develops signs of acute respiratory distress owing to atelectasis of the lung, impaired perfusion of the lung, and reduced pulmonary compliance. Tachypnea, tachycardia, retractions of the rib cage during inspiration, cyanosis, and grunting during expiration are present. Blood gases studies reflect the impaired ventilatory function. Radiographic examination of the lung reveals atelectasis. Infants with RDS require treatment in a NICU (neonatal intensive care unit). Therapy is supportive to ensure hydration and electrolyte control. Supplemental oxygen is given and, if necessary, assisted ventilation is used. Instillation of surfactant into the respiratory tract is essential in managing RDS (*Taber's*, 2009).

HANDOFF COMMUNICATION

S	Situation	Assess what is currently happening in a short statement.	Infant presents as _____
B	Background	Summarize important past assessment data for your patient here. Place lab results and medications on the concept map.	**Age:** **Gender:** **Allergies:**
A	Assessment	Use the assessment data to complete your concept map.	**Nursing Diagnosis:** Place the Nursing Diagnoses in prioritized order on the concept map and add any needed for your specific patient. **Plan:** Place any further Nursing Interventions Classifications (NIC) needed on the map.

Implement Your Plan of Care

			EVALUATE YOUR CARE	
R	Recommendation	Evaluate your nursing care and make recommendations related to the achievement of your desired outcomes. Were they met, or do new goals need to be established?	**Diag** / **Nursing Outcomes Classification (NOC)**	**Outcome met**
			1 — Demonstrates improved ventilation and oxygenation evidenced by blood gas levels within normal parameters for the neonatal patient.	☐ Yes ☐ No
			2 — Maintains urine output at 2–5 mL/hr.	☐ Yes ☐ No
			3 — Maintains white blood cell count and differential within normal limits; remains free from symptoms of infection.	☐ Yes ☐ No
			4 — Initiate appropriate measures to develop a safe, nurturing environment.	☐ Yes ☐ No
			5 —	☐ Yes ☐ No

Nursing Diagnosis 1

Impaired gas exchange related to immature or underdeveloped lungs evidenced by retractions, grunting, nasal flaring, and cyanosis.

NIC:
1) Assess respiratory status using the Silverman-Anderson index; 2) Auscultate breath sounds frequently; 3) Continuously monitor O_2 saturation; 4) Observe for circumoral or central cyanosis; 5) Minimize handling; 6) Monitor O_2 settings on equipment; and 7) Maintain appropriate temperature in the environment.

Nursing Diagnosis 2

Risk for fluid volume deficit related to respiratory energy expenditure.

NIC:
1) Weigh diapers; 2) Check urine specific gravity; 3) Monitor TPN (total parenteral nutrition) and IV (intravenous) fluids; and 4) Maintain environmental temperature.

Nursing Diagnosis 3

Risk for infection related to invasive procedures.

NIC:
1) Meticulous hand scrubbing; 2) Assess skin integrity frequently; 3) Assess temperature q3h; 4) Note and report abnormal lab values; 5) Bathe per protocol; 6) Maintain strict asepsis for central lines; 7) Cluster care to decrease frequency of contacts; 8) Use breast milk as soon as possible; and 9) Monitor for behavioral changes such as increased monitor violations.

Nursing Diagnosis 4

Impaired parenting related to NICU admission.

NIC:
1) Assess characteristic of parenting style and behaviors; 2) Appraise parent support systems; 3) Provide education about care; 4) Model appropriate handling; 5) Encourage parents to interact and participate in care; 6) Teach parents to take behavioral cues from infant; 7) Provide support groups for NICU parents; and 8) Primary nursing.

Condition:
Respiratory Distress Syndrome (Neonatal)

Age:

Link & Explain
• Nursing Interventions Classification (NIC)
• Laboratory and Diagnostic Procedures
• Medications

Nursing Diagnosis 5

NIC:

Medications

a. Surfactant therapy

b. O_2 therapy

c. TPN and IV therapy

d.

Laboratory & Diagnostic Procedures

a. Blood gases

b. Chest x-ray

c. CBC and differential

d.

CONDITION: TORCH

PHYSIOLOGY: TORCH is an acronym originally coined from the first letters of *t*oxoplasmosis, *r*ubella, *c*ytomegalovirus, and *h*erpes simplex. Contemporary revisions describe the *O* as standing for "other" transplacental infections (by human immunodeficiency virus, hepatitis B, human parvovirus, and syphilis). TORCH infections can attack a growing embryo or fetus and cause abnormal development, severe congenital anomalies, mental retardation, and fetal or neonatal death (*Taber's*, 2009).

HANDOFF COMMUNICATION

S	Situation	Assess what is currently happening in a short statement.	Infant presents as _____
B	Background	Summarize important past assessment data for your patient here. Place lab results and medications on the concept map.	**Age:** **Gender:** **Allergies:**
A	Assessment	Use the assessment data to complete your concept map.	**Nursing Diagnosis:** Place the Nursing Diagnoses in prioritized order on the concept map and add any needed for your specific patient. **Plan:** Place any further Nursing Interventions Classifications (NIC) needed on the map.

Implement Your Plan of Care

R	Recommendation	Evaluate your nursing care and make recommendations related to the achievement of your desired outcomes. Were they met, or do new goals need to be established?	*(see table below)*

EVALUATE YOUR CARE

Diag	Nursing Outcomes Classification (NOC)	Outcome met
1	Maintains current visual field and acuity.	☐ **Yes** ☐ **No**
2	Identify behaviors to prevent and reduce infection.	☐ **Yes** ☐ **No**
3	Communicate thoughts and feelings utilizing available support systems such as family, spiritual leaders, and other resources. Demonstrate coping behaviors that reduce anxiety.	☐ **Yes** ☐ **No**
4	Express feelings freely and effectively; begin to progress through recognized stages of grief, focusing on one day at a time.	☐ **Yes** ☐ **No**
5		☐ **Yes** ☐ **No**

Nursing Diagnosis 1

Risk for disturbed visual sensory perception related to inflammation of the retina.

NIC:
1) Assess type and degree of visual loss; 2) Recommend follow-up assessment as soon as possible; 3) Recommend environmental changes to assist patient to manage visual impairment if present; and 4) Instill eye medications as prescribed.

Nursing Diagnosis 2

Risk for infections related to exposure to, or contact with, blood or body fluids.

NIC:
1) Maintain aseptic techniques such as good hand washing; 2) Monitor maternal temperature; 3) Obtain body fluid specimen for culture and sensitivity; and 4) Monitor health and number of caregivers.

Nursing Diagnosis 3

Parental anxiety related to infant condition evidenced by increased tension, apprehension, feelings of helplessness, inadequacy, and worry.

NIC:
1) Ascertain what information the patient has about the diagnosis and expected course of the condition; 2) Provide an atmosphere of concern and anticipatory guidance; 3) Encourage questions; and 4) Explore spiritual support.

Nursing Diagnosis 4

Grieving related to loss of newborn well-being and chronic physiopsychological alterations evidenced by parental verbalization.

NIC:
1) Identify stages of grieving; 2) Assist parents to verbalize feelings; 3) Note comments of bargaining; 4) Accept expressions of anger; and 5) Assist and encourage parents to take control of infant care.

Condition:
TORCH
Age:

Link & Explain
• Nursing Interventions Classification (NIC)
• Laboratory and Diagnostic Procedures
• Medications

Nursing Diagnosis 5

NIC:

Medications

a. Antiviral drugs, such as ganciclovir and acyclovir, are used to decrease viral load.

b.

c.

d.

Laboratory & Diagnostic Procedures

a. IVIG (intravenous immunoglobulin), CytoGam titers

b.

c.

d.

Concept Maps for Pediatric Patients

2

This chapter provides care maps that describe health conditions experienced by children. As with the infant care maps, the parents or caregivers need to be included in order to maintain appropriate care after discharge. The nursing care of children always needs to be appropriate to the child's developmental stage because it affects all nursing interventions from pain assessment to diversional activities. Many health-care issues for children are now dealt with on an outpatient basis. Children who are hospitalized are usually acutely ill and need intensive nursing care. The care maps listed in this chapter are for both inpatient and outpatient pediatric care and provide a list of the more common conditions you will come across in both care settings.

The conditions included in this chapter are:
1. Anticipatory Guidance, Growth and Development—Newborn to Infant
2. Anticipatory Guidance, Growth and Development—Toddler to Preschool
3. Anticipatory Guidance, Growth and Development—School-Age Child to Adolescent
4. Appendectomy
5. Asthma
6. Autism Spectrum Disorder
7. Biliary Atresia
8. Candidiasis (Thrush)
9. Casts/Traction
10. Celiac Disease
11. Cerebral Palsy (CP)
12. Child Abuse/Neglect (Battered Child Syndrome)
13. Cleft Lip and Palate
14. Congenital Heart Defects (CHD)
15. Cystic Fibrosis (CF)
16. Deafness (Hearing Loss)
17. Developmental Dysplasia of Hip (DDH) or Congenital Hip Dysplasia
18. Duchenne Muscular Dystrophy
19. Encephalitis
20. Glomerulonephritis or Acute Nephrotic Syndrome
21. Hemophilia
22. Hirschsprung's Disease
23. Hydrocephalus
24. Hypertropic Pyloric Disorder (Pyloric Stenosis)
25. Immunizations, Anticipatory Guidance
26. Intussusception and Malrotation
27. Juvenile Rheumatoid Arthritis (Juvenile Idiopathic Arthritis)
28. Lead Poisoning
29. Leukemia
30. Nephroblastoma (Wilms' Tumor)
31. Nephrotic Syndrome (NS)
32. Neural Tube Defects (Spinal Bifida and Myelomeningocele)
33. Phenylketonuria (PKU)
34. Respiratory Croup or Laryngotracheobronchitis
35. Respiratory Syncytial Virus (RSV)
36. Scarlet Fever
37. Sepsis
38. Talipes Equinovarus (Clubfoot)
39. Varicella (Chickenpox)

CONDITION: Anticipatory Guidance, Growth and Development—Newborn to Infant

PHYSIOLOGY:

Stages: *Newborn—birth–1 month; infant—1–12 months.*

Physical: Primitive reflexes are adaptive reflexes (Moro, rooting, sucking, tonic neck, grasp, Babinski, etc.). At birth, most of the primitive reflexes are present because the lower portions of the nervous system (spinal cord and brainstem) are mature. Primitive reflexes are adaptive mechanisms that protect the developing brain and lay the groundwork for higher cognitive function. Most infant reflexes, except for Babinski, should disappear at 4 months of age. Primitive reflexes are a red flag of alteration in development if they persist beyond 6 months.

Sensory: Exploration through touch, smell, hearing, and vision (last sense to fully develop).

Motor (gross to fine): Cephalocaudal and proximodistal development.

Theories: *Psychosocial (Erikson)*—trust versus mistrust. *Psychosexual (Freud)*—oral stage. *Behavioral (Kohlberg)*—preconventional level (concrete/egocentric).

Physical: Infant should gain 1.5 lb a month, double birth weight by 6 months, and triple birth weight by 1 year. Length increases by 2.5 cm by first 6 months, then slows. The head circumference is plotted for brain growth and should equal chest circumference by 1 year.

Important developmental milestones: 1) Social smile occurs at 2 months; infant follows moving objects and responds to sound or noise at birth. **2)** Posterior fontanel closes by 2 months; anterior fontanel closes 12 months. **3)** No head lag by 4 months. **4)** *Gross motor:* turns over completely at 6–7 months; crawls and pulls to stand at 8–9 months; walks by 15 months. **5)** *Fine motor:* at 6–12 months, the infant should transfer objects, stack blocks, bang objects together, and scribble. **6)** *Language:* laughs at 4 months; babbles at 6 months and speaks at least one word by 1 year. **7)** Object permanence should be established by 7–8 months; the infant knows objects exist even though they are not present; develops attachment and stranger anxiety; plays peek-a-boo at 9 months (Doenges, Moorhouse, & Murr, 2009; Ward & Hisley, 2009).

HANDOFF COMMUNICATION

S Situation	Assess what is currently happening in a short statement.	Child presents as _____
B Background	Summarize important past assessment data for your patient here. Place lab results and medications on the concept map.	**Age:** **Gender:** **Allergies:** **Fall Risk:** **Isolation:** **Immunization status:** **PMH:** **PSH:**
A Assessment	Use the assessment data to complete your concept map.	**Nursing Diagnosis:** Place the Nursing Diagnoses in prioritized order on the concept map and add any needed for your specific patient. **Plan:** Place any further Nursing Interventions Classifications (NIC) needed on the map.

Implement Your Plan of Care

			EVALUATE YOUR CARE	
R Recommendation	Evaluate your nursing care and make recommendations related to the achievement of your desired outcomes. Were they met, or do new goals need to be established?	**Diag**	**Nursing Outcomes Classification (NOC)**	**Outcome met**
		1	Newborn/infant has adequate nutrition to meet body requirements evidenced by adequate weight gain and caloric intake.	☐ Yes ☐ No
		2	Child demonstrates optimal growth and development based on physical and cognitive abilities.	☐ Yes ☐ No
		3	Parents/caregivers demonstrate a safe environment for infant, and child has decreased incidence of injury.	☐ Yes ☐ No
		4	Parents/caregivers identify resources within themselves to deal with the situation.	☐ Yes ☐ No
		5		☐ Yes ☐ No

Nursing Diagnosis 1

Risk for imbalanced nutrition due to parental/caregiver knowledge deficit.

NIC:
1) Maintain accurate growth charts at scheduled primary care visit advised by the American Academy of Pediatrics (AAP); **2)** Plot weight, length, and head circumference; **3)** Use appropriate scale to chart infant's development; **4)** Instruct family that infant will require breast milk or formula to 1 year of age; **5)** Instruct parents/caregivers on proper infant cues for feeding and introduction of solid foods (4–6 months); **6)** Initial solid foods are rice cereal, then vegetables and fruits; introduce new foods one at a time, 5 days apart; introduce meats at 9 months; **7)** Introduce cup at 9 months, and wean from bottle by 1 year; **8)** Advise no bottle at bed time and never to put food in bottles or mix with formula; **9)** Assist with, observe, and document caregiver interaction during feeding; and **10)** Provide role modeling and education to caregiver on feeding skills, infant care, and positive feedback.

Nursing Diagnosis 2

Risk for altered growth and development due to parental/caregiver knowledge deficit.

NIC:
1) Assess and record developmental progress; **2)** Assess with models like Denver Developmental II assessment tool up to 6 years of age; **3)** Instruct family in nurturing sensory, physical, and cognitive development; **4)** Developmental toys include music box, bright colored mobiles (1 month); rattle or unbreakable mirror (4 months); soft dolls and fabric books (6 months); stacking toys, busy boxes, toy phone (7–12 months); **5)** Assist, observe, and document caregiver interaction; and **6)** Provide role modeling and education to caregiver on developmental skills, infant care, and positive feedback.

Nursing Diagnosis 3

Risk for alteration in safety based on parental/caregiver knowledge deficit.

NIC:
1) Assess parents'/caregivers' knowledge base of safety environment; **2)** Instruct them on safety measures such as hot water thermostat (120°F), easy access to poison control contact, crib standards; **3)** Instruct on sleep patterns, firm sleep surface, back to sleep, avoidance of overheating, and removal of small, soft objects and loose bedding from crib; **4)** Instruct on use of infant car seat and never to leave infant unattended; **5)** Assist with, observe, and document caregiver interaction on safety standards; and **6)** Provide role modeling and education to caregiver on infant safety and positive feedback.

Nursing Diagnosis 4

Risk for compromised family coping related to temporary family disorganization.

NIC:
1) Establish a rapport and acknowledge the difficulty of the situation; **2)** Assess level of anxiety; and **3)** Refer to appropriate resources.

Condition:
Anticipatory Guidance, Growth and Development— Newborn to Infant
Age:
Link & Explain
• Nursing Interventions Classification (NIC)
• Laboratory and Diagnostic Procedures
• Medications

Nursing Diagnosis 5

NIC:

Medications

a.

b.

c.

d.

Laboratory & Diagnostic Procedures

a. Newborn metabolic screen

b. Hemoglobin screen at 12 months

c. Newborn hearing screen prior to discharge

d. Lead screen, 12 months if high risk

CONDITION: Anticipatory Guidance, Growth and Development—Toddler to Preschool

PHYSIOLOGY:

Stages: *Toddler*—1–3 years; *preschooler*—3–5 years.

Physical: *Toddler*—growth slows, physiological anorexia, increased mobility. *Preschooler*—vertical growth, increasing muscle strength, agility, and fine motor skills.

Cognitive: *Toddler*—Piaget's fifth to sixth stage of cognitive development, which entails understanding a cause-and-effect relationship and ability to imitate others. *Preschooler*—Piaget's preoperational stage of development whereby the preschooler increases verbal skills and concrete and magical thinking.

Theories: *Psychosocial (Erikson): Toddler*—autonomy versus shame and doubt. *Preschooler*—initiative versus guilt. *Psychosexual (Freud): Toddler*—anal stage. *Preschooler*—phallic stage. *Behavioral (Kohlberg):* preconventional level (concrete/egocentric).

Physical: Slow growth and weight gain. Average weight gain, 4–6 lb/yr; average height gain, 3 in./yr. Physiological anorexia—decreased appetite due to decreased growth.

Developmental milestones: *Fine and gross motor skills:* **1)** Runs and jumps by age 2. **2)** Removes own clothes and walks unaided; **3)** Holds a spoon or large crayon. **4)** Goes up and down stairs with alternating feet, draws circle, and builds 9–10 block tower at age 3. **5)** Uses scissors, washes face, and skips/hops; hand dominance is apparent by age 4. **6)** Draws 3–4 part person, skips, copies diamond and triangle, and dresses self by age 5.

Language: **1)** Moves from single words to 2- to 3-word phrases. **2)** Toddler uses simple sentences such as "I do" or "I want." **3)** Preschooler's ability to verbalize increases, and vocabulary increases to 1,500–2,000 words by age 5. **4)** Preschooler uses sentences and can convey thoughts. *Sleep:* Toddlers and preschoolers need 11–14 hours a day with 1–2 naps a day; routines are important (Doenges, Moorhouse, & Murr, 2009; Ward & Hisley, 2009).

HANDOFF COMMUNICATION

S	Situation	Assess what is currently happening in a short statement.	Child presents as _____
B	Background	Summarize important past assessment data for your patient here. Place lab results and medications on the concept map.	Age: Gender: Allergies: Fall Risk: Isolation: Immunization status: PMH: PSH:
A	Assessment	Use the assessment data to complete your concept map.	**Nursing Diagnosis:** Place the Nursing Diagnoses in prioritized order on the concept map and add any needed for your specific patient. **Plan:** Place any further Nursing Interventions Classifications (NIC) needed on the map.

Implement Your Plan of Care

		Diag	EVALUATE YOUR CARE	
R	Recommendation — Evaluate your nursing care and make recommendations related to the achievement of your desired outcomes. Were they met, or do new goals need to be established?		Nursing Outcomes Classification (NOC)	Outcome met
		1	Child has adequate nutrition to meet body requirements evidenced by adequate weight gain and caloric intake.	☐ Yes ☐ No
		2	Child demonstrates optimal growth and development based on child's physical and cognitive ability.	☐ Yes ☐ No
		3	Parents/caregivers demonstrate a safe environment for child; child has decreased incidence of injury.	☐ Yes ☐ No
		4	Parents/caregivers identify resources within themselves to deal with the situation.	☐ Yes ☐ No
		5		☐ Yes ☐ No

Nursing Diagnosis 1

Risk for imbalanced nutrition due to parental/caregiver knowledge deficit.

NIC:
1) Maintain accurate growth charts at scheduled primary care visit advised by the American Academy of Pediatrics (AAP). Plot weight, length, and head circumference; record BMI starting at 2 years of age; **2)** Use appropriate scale for infant's development; standometer scale is most often used until 2 years of age; **3)** Instruct caregiver to encourage toddler to feed self, and review importance of establishing mealtime rituals and selection of nutritional foods; **4)** Instruct caregiver that a toddler should not drink more than 24 oz of milk a day and can have low-fat milk after 2 years of age; **5)** Instruct parents/caregivers to offer small portions and avoid foods that can easily aspirate (nuts, cereal, hot dogs, grapes, and hard candy), and explain to parents/caregivers about physiological anorexia; **6)** Assist with, observe, and document caregiver interaction during feeding; and **7)** Provide role modeling and education to caregiver on feeding skills, child care, and positive feedback.

Nursing Diagnosis 2

Risk for altered growth and development due to parental/caregiver knowledge deficit.

NIC:
1) Assess and record developmental process; **2)** Assess with models like Denver Developmental II assessment tool until 6 years of age; administer Modified Checklist for Autism in Toddlers (M-CHAT) screen at 18 and 24 months if indicated; **3)** Instruct family in nurturing sensory, physical, and cognitive development; **4)** Instruct caregivers that toddlers engage in parallel play and transition to associative play during preschool years; **5)** Instruct caregivers on toy selection to support development, such as sandbox, crayon and coloring book, clay, dress-up, finger paint, and encourage reading books; **6)** Instruct parents/caregivers on toilet training readiness when child is physiologically ready (2 years) and provides cues, such as feels discomfort with messy pants, identifies elimination, follows direction, removes clothes, walks unaided, and stoops; **7)** Instruct parents/caregivers on discipline and temper tantrums, such as being consistent in routines; avoiding threats, promises; providing safe environment; remaining calm; and disciplining with time out with reasonable limits; **8)** Assist with, observe, and document caregiver interaction; and **9)** Provide role modeling and education to caregiver on developmental skills and positive feedback.

Nursing Diagnosis 3

Risk for alteration in safety based on parental/caregiver knowledge deficit.

NIC:
1) Assess parents'/caregivers' knowledge base of safety environment; **2)** Instruct them on added safety measures needed as the toddler begins to explore: keeping toddler away from motor vehicles and protecting toddler from burns, sharp objects, drowning, and other dangers; **3)** Instruct parents/caregivers on sleep patterns and routines; **4)** Instruct them on use of car seat and to never leave child unattended; **5)** Assist with, observe, and document caregiver interaction on safety standards; and **6)** Provide role modeling and education to caregiver on child safety and positive feedback.

Nursing Diagnosis 4

Risk for compromised family coping related to temporary family disorganization.

NIC:
1) Establish a rapport and acknowledge the difficulty of the situation; **2)** Assess level of anxiety; and **3)** Refer to appropriate resources.

Condition:
Anticipatory Guidance, Growth and Development— Toddler to Preschool

Age:

Link & Explain
• Nursing Interventions Classification (NIC)
• Laboratory and Diagnostic Procedures
• Medications

Nursing Diagnosis 5

NIC:

Medications
a.
b.
c.
d.

Laboratory & Diagnostic Procedures
a. Hemoglobin screen, 12 and 24 months
b. Vision and hearing screens, 4–6 years; oral health screen starting at 2 years and continuing throughout lifespan
c. Lead screening if high risk by 12 and/or 24 months
d. Dyslipidemia screen starting at 2 years if high risk

CONDITION: Anticipatory Guidance, Growth and Development—School-Age Child to Adolescent

PHYSIOLOGY:

Stages: *School age*—6–12 years; *adolescent*—13–18 years.

Physical: Variations in growth based on cultural and familial genetics as well as environment. *School age*—average weight gain, 4–6 lb/yr; average height gain, 2–3 in./yr. *Adolescent*—dramatic growth rates.

Cognitive: *School age:* Piaget—concrete operation and improved memory and language; identifies theories of conservation. *Adolescent:* Piaget— formal operations; abstract thinking.

Theories: *Psychosocial (Erikson): School age*—industry versus inferiority. *Adolescent*—identity versus role confusion. ***Psychosexual (Freud):*** *School age*—latency stage. *Adolescent*—genital stage. ***Behavioral (Kohlberg):*** conventional level.

Physical: 1) Puberty begins in females, on average, between 8 and 14 years of age; note by thelarche (breast development). **2)** The average age of menarche is 8–14 years. **3)** Puberty in males begins with testicular enlargement at 10–12 years of age. **4)** Secondary characteristics such as breast development, testicular and penile enlargement, and pubic hair are documented by Tanner Stage of Development (Doenges, Moorhouse, & Murr, 2009; Ward & Hisley, 2009).

HANDOFF COMMUNICATION

S Situation	Assess what is currently happening in a short statement.	Child presents as _____
B Background	Summarize important past assessment data for your patient here. Place lab results and medications on the concept map.	**Age:** **Gender:** **Allergies:** **Fall Risk:** **Isolation:** **Immunization status:** **PMH:** **PSH:**
A Assessment	Use the assessment data to complete your concept map.	**Nursing Diagnosis:** Place the Nursing Diagnoses in prioritized order on the concept map and add any needed for your specific patient. **Plan:** Place any further Nursing Interventions Classifications (NIC) needed on the map.

Implement Your Plan of Care

			EVALUATE YOUR CARE	
R Recommendation	Evaluate your nursing care and make recommendations related to the achievement of your desired outcomes. Were they met, or do new goals need to be established?	**Diag**	**Nursing Outcomes Classification (NOC)**	**Outcome met**
		1	Child/adolescent has adequate nutrition to meet body requirements evidenced by adequate weight gain and caloric intake.	☐ Yes ☐ No
		2	Child/adolescent demonstrates optimal growth and development based on child's physical and cognitive ability.	☐ Yes ☐ No
		3	Parents/caregivers demonstrate a safe environment; child has decreased incidence of injury and high-risk behaviors.	☐ Yes ☐ No
		4	Parents/caregivers identify resources to deal with developmental situation.	☐ Yes ☐ No
		5		☐ Yes ☐ No

Nursing Diagnosis 1

Risk for imbalanced nutrition due to parental/caregiver/child knowledge deficit.

NIC:
1) Maintain accurate growth charts and Tanner staging with each scheduled primary care visit advised by the American Academy of Pediatrics (AAP); **2)** Calculate BMI with every primary care visit; **3)** Assess child's/adolescent's attitudes on weight and body image; **4)** Counsel on nutritional meals/snacks and the importance of 2–3 dairy products a day; discuss the importance of diet and physical exercise; and **5)** Provide role modeling and education on healthy lifestyle.

Nursing Diagnosis 2

Risk for altered growth and development due to knowledge deficit and loss of control.

NIC:
1) Assess and document child's/adolescent's success and/or struggles in school, friendships, and extracurricular activities (e.g., ask about bullying); **2)** Instruct parents/caregivers on need for cooperative play, team sports/activities, and growing independence during school age and adolescence; **3)** Instruct caregiver/child on the importance of balancing school, activities, and sleep; and **4)** Instruct caregiver on parenting techniques (e.g., the importance of establishing rules and maintaining natural consequences for illicit behavior).

Nursing Diagnosis 3

Risk for alteration in safety based on parental/caregiver knowledge deficit.

NIC:
1) Assess parents'/caregivers'/child's knowledge base of safety environment; **2)** Instruct parents/caregivers/child on helmet safety, fights, sport's protective equipment, seat belts, and motor vehicle accidents; **3)** Instruct on sleep patterns and routines; **4)** Instruct on emergency procedures and calling 911; **5)** Assess for high-risk behaviors such as smoking, alcohol and drug abuse, self mutilation, sexual activity and suicide/depression; **6)** Assist with, observe, document interaction on safety standards and response; provide counseling as needed; and **7)** Provide role modeling and education to caregiver/child and provide positive feedback.

Nursing Diagnosis 4

Risk for compromised family coping related to temporary family disorganization.

NIC:
1) Establish a rapport and acknowledge the difficulty of the situation; **2)** Assess level of anxiety; and **3)** Refer to appropriate resources.

Condition:
Anticipatory Guidance, Growth and Development— School-Age Child to Adolescent

Age:

Link & Explain
• Nursing Interventions Classification (NIC)
• Laboratory and Diagnostic Procedures
• Medications

Nursing Diagnosis 5

NIC:

Medications

a.

b.

c.

d.

Laboratory & Diagnostic Procedures

a. Urinalysis, adolescence

b. Hemoglobin in adolescent females

c. Dyslipidemia screen in high-risk patients

d. Vision screen and scoliosis assessment school age and adolescence

CONDITION: Appendectomy

PHYSIOLOGY: An appendectomy is a surgical removal of the vermiform appendix usually due to appendicitis or inflammation caused by blockage of the lumen of the appendix followed by infection. It may be acute or subacute, chronic, and occasionally may be difficult to diagnose because many other illnesses also produce acute abdominal pain (*Taber's*, 2009).

HANDOFF COMMUNICATION

S Situation	Assess what is currently happening in a short statement.	Child presents as _____	
B Background	Summarize important past assessment data for your patient here. Place lab results and medications on the concept map.	**Age:** **Allergies:** **Isolation:**	**Gender:** **Fall Risk:**
A Assessment	Use the assessment data to complete your concept map.	**Nursing Diagnosis:** Place the Nursing Diagnoses in prioritized order on the concept map and add any needed for your specific patient. **Plan:** Place any further Nursing Interventions Classifications (NIC) needed on the map.	

Implement Your Plan of Care

R Recommendation	Evaluate your nursing care and make recommendations related to the achievement of your desired outcomes. Were they met, or do new goals need to be established?	**EVALUATE YOUR CARE**		
		Diag	**Nursing Outcomes Classification (NOC)**	**Outcome met**
		1	Patient reports pain control or pain control is observed.	☐ Yes ☐ No
		2	Demonstrate adequate fluid balance as evidenced by stable vital signs (VS), palpable pulses of good quality, normal skin turgor, moist mucous membranes; individual appropriate output; lack of weight fluctuation—loss or gain; and absence of edema.	☐ Yes ☐ No
		3	Surgical site is clean and dry with no increase in white blood cell (WBC) count.	☐ Yes ☐ No
		4	Caregivers (family) verbalize understanding of postoperative care and signs of surgical complications.	☐ Yes ☐ No
		5		☐ Yes ☐ No

Nursing Diagnosis 1

Acute pain related to surgical incision evidenced by crying, grimaces, and distracted behavior.

NIC:
1) Perform routine comprehensive pain assessment; **2)** Accept child's description of pain; **3)** Investigate changes in or frequency of pain; **4)** Observe for rigidity, crying; **5)** Provide comfort measures, holding, repositioning; and **6)** Encourage sleep and rest periods.

Nursing Diagnosis 2

Deficient fluid volume related to fluid restriction, hypermetabolic state, nausea, and vomiting evidenced by low output.

NIC:
1) Monitor I&O; **2)** Promote postoperative diet by making fluid and food choices specific to patient; **3)** Medicate with antiemetic medication as needed; and **4)** Maintain IV fluid as ordered.

Nursing Diagnosis 3

Risk for infection related to surgical site.

NIC:
1) Monitor temperature; **2)** Assess surgical site and dressing frequently for drainage or redness; and **3)** Monitor WBC count and differential if ordered.

Nursing Diagnosis 4

Ineffective health maintenance related to deficit knowledge of parents/caregivers regarding surgical site and postoperative care evidenced by questions and repeated instructions to parents/caregivers.

NIC:
1) Teach parents/caregivers postoperative care; **2)** Model postoperative caregiving; **3)** Provide written discharge instructions; and **4)** Assess knowledge about when to call health-care provider for complications.

Condition:
Appendectomy
Age:

- - - - - - - - - -
Link & Explain
• Nursing Interventions Classification (NIC)
• Laboratory and Diagnostic Procedures
• Medications

Nursing Diagnosis 5

NIC:

Medications

a. Analgesics

b. Antiemetic: Reglan (metoclopramide)

c.

d.

Laboratory & Diagnostic Procedures

a. CBC with differential

b.

c.

d.

CONDITION: Asthma

PHYSIOLOGY: Asthma is a disease caused by increased responsiveness of the tracheobronchial tree to various stimuli, which results in episodic narrowing and inflammation of the airways. Clinically, most patients present with episodic wheezing, shortness of breath, and/or cough. Between attacks, the patient may or may not have normal respiratory functions. The reoccurrence and severity of the attacks are influenced by the triggers, of which exposure to tobacco smoke and viral illnesses are the most frequently identified factors. Other respiratory exposures, such as air pollution, allergens, dust, cold air, exercise, fumes, or medicines, may contribute to the attacks. Autonomic and inflammatory mediators play and important part (*Taber's*, 2009).

HANDOFF COMMUNICATION

S	**Situation**	Assess what is currently happening in a short statement.	Child presents as _____
B	**Background**	Summarize important past assessment data for your patient here. Place lab results and medications on the concept map.	**Age:** **Gender:** **Allergies:** **Fall Risk:** **Isolation:**
A	**Assessment**	Use the assessment data to complete your concept map.	**Nursing Diagnosis:** Place the Nursing Diagnoses in prioritized order on the concept map and add any needed for your specific patient. **Plan:** Place any further Nursing Interventions Classifications (NIC) needed on the map.

Implement Your Plan of Care

		EVALUATE YOUR CARE		
R	**Recommendation** — Evaluate your nursing care and make recommendations related to the achievement of your desired outcomes. Were they met, or do new goals need to be established?	**Diag**	**Nursing Outcomes Classification (NOC)**	**Outcome met**
		1	Patient's airway is maintained with breath sounds clear or clearing; patient demonstrates behaviors to improve airway clearance.	☐ Yes ☐ No
		2	Patient demonstrates improved ventilation and adequate oxygenation of tissues by arterial blood gases (ABGs) within patient's normal range, is free of symptoms of respiratory distress, and participates in treatment regimen within level of ability and situation.	☐ Yes ☐ No
		3	Patient appears relaxed and reports or demonstrates relief from somatic manifestations of anxiety.	☐ Yes ☐ No
		4	Family verbalizes understanding of condition, disease process, and treatment; initiates necessary lifestyle changes; and participates in treatment regimen.	☐ Yes ☐ No
		5		☐ Yes ☐ No

Nursing Diagnosis 1

Ineffective airway clearance related to increased production of and retained pulmonary secretions, bronchospasms, decreased energy, fatigue evidenced by wheezing, difficulty breathing and change in respiratory depth and rate, use of accessory muscles, and persistent cough with or without sputum production.

NIC:
1) Auscultate breath sounds; 2) Assess and monitor respiration rate; 3) Note presence and degree of dyspnea and air hunger; 4) Position patient for comfort; 5) Keep environment free from triggers or pollutants; 6) Assist with abdominal or pursed-lip breathing; 7) Observe for cough; 8) Hydrate; and 9) Medicate as ordered.

Nursing Diagnosis 2

Impaired gas exchange related to altered delivery of inspired oxygen and trapped air evidenced by dyspnea, restlessness, reduced tolerance for activity, cyanosis, and changes in ABGs and vital signs.

NIC:
1) Assess respiratory rate and depth; 2) Raise head of bed (HOB); 3) Encourage expectoration of sputum; 4) Auscultate breath sounds; 5) Palpate chest for fremitus; and 6) Monitor vital signs (VS), sleep patterns, and activity level.

Nursing Diagnosis 3

Anxiety related to perceived threat of death evidenced by apprehension, fearful expression, and extraneous movements.

NIC:
1) Establish an atmosphere of calmness; 2) Prepare patient for activities and procedures; 3) Ensure child of his/her safety; 4) Refrain from unnecessary conversation; 5) Promote family interactions; 6) Provide child with age-appropriate choices; 7) Do not separate child from peers; and 8) Schedule age-appropriate diversional activity.

Nursing Diagnosis 4

Knowledge deficit related to condition, self-care, and discharge needs related to lack of familiarity with information resources for family evidenced by request for information.

NIC:
1) Encourage family to ask questions; 2) Explain and reinforce explanations of disease process, including factors that lead to exacerbation episodes; 3) Review breathing exercises and coughing effectiveness; 4) Avoid people with URIs (upper respiratory infections); 5) Identify and avoid individual triggers; and 6) Review harmful effects of smoking and secondhand smoke.

Condition:
Asthma
Age:

Link & Explain
• Nursing Interventions Classification (NIC)
• Laboratory and Diagnostic Procedures
• Medications

Nursing Diagnosis 5

NIC:

Medications

a. Bronchodilators such as anticholinergic agents

b. Beta-agonists such as epinephrine or albuterol

c. Leukotriene antagonists such as Singulair

d. Anti-inflammatory drugs such as prednisone

Laboratory & Diagnostic Procedures

a. ABGs

b.

c.

d.

CONDITION: Autism Spectrum Disorder

PHYSIOLOGY: Autism spectrum disorder is a syndrome that appears in childhood with symptoms of self-absorption, inaccessibility, aloneness, avoidance of eye contact, inability to relate, highly repetitive play, rage reactions if interrupted, rhythmical body movements, and many language disturbances. The cause is unknown, but some research suggests anomalies in serotonin transport increase the likelihood of the disease (*Taber's*, 2009).

HANDOFF COMMUNICATION

S Situation	Assess what is currently happening in a short statement.	Child presents as _____
B Background	Summarize important past assessment data for your patient here. Place lab results and medications on the concept map.	**Age:** **Gender:** **Allergies:** **Fall Risk:** **Isolation:**
A Assessment	Use the assessment data to complete your concept map.	**Nursing Diagnosis:** Place the Nursing Diagnoses in prioritized order on the concept map and add any needed for your specific patient. **Plan:** Place any further Nursing Interventions Classifications (NIC) needed on the map.

Implement Your Plan of Care

R Recommendation	Evaluate your nursing care and make recommendations related to the achievement of your desired outcomes. Were they met, or do new goals need to be established?	**EVALUATE YOUR CARE**		
		Diag	**Nursing Outcomes Classification (NOC)**	**Outcome met**
		1	Promote reality-based thought processes.	☐ Yes ☐ No
		2	Monitor growth and development.	☐ Yes ☐ No
		3	Keep free of injury.	☐ Yes ☐ No
		4	Encourage positive parenting.	☐ Yes ☐ No
		5		☐ Yes ☐ No

Nursing Diagnosis 1

Disturbed thought processes related to syndrome evidenced by introversion.

NIC:
1) Orient to time, place, and person; **2)** Approach calmly; and **3)** Provide referrals for occupational, physical, and play therapy.

Nursing Diagnosis 2

Delayed growth and development related to syndrome evidenced by inappropriate responses to environmental stimuli.

NIC:
1) Assess current growth and developmental stage; **2)** Use age-appropriate tests; **3)** Determine cognitive and perceptual level; **4)** Encourage self-care activities; and **5)** Provide parents/caregivers with information.

Nursing Diagnosis 3

Risk for injury related to developmental difficulties.

NIC:
1) Identify individual risk factors; **2)** Handle gently and calmly; **3)** Provide appropriate level of supervision; **4)** Initiate safety precautions; **5)** Have age-appropriate equipment; and **6)** Review home situation for safety.

Nursing Diagnosis 4

Compromised family coping related to child's needs evidenced by verbalization from parents/caregivers.

NIC:
1) Review feelings of hopelessness, helplessness, and loss of control over life; level of anxiety; and perceptions of situation; **2)** Establish a therapeutic nurse-patient relationship; **3)** Assess presence of coping skills and inner strength; **4)** Encourage family to talk about situation; and **5)** Discuss feelings of self-blame.

Condition:
Autism Spectrum Disorder

Age:

Link & Explain
• Nursing Interventions Classification (NIC)
• Laboratory and Diagnostic Procedures
• Medications

Nursing Diagnosis 5

NIC:

Medications

a.

b.

c.

d.

Laboratory & Diagnostic Procedures

a.

b.

c.

d.

CONDITION: Biliary Atresia

PHYSIOLOGY: Biliary atresia, or extrahepatic biliary atresia (EHBA), is an idiopathic, progressive inflammatory process that causes both intrahepatic and extrahepatic bile duct fibrosis and obstruction. Biliary atresia is the second-most common liver disease diagnosed in infants with an incidence that ranges from 1 in 8,000 to 21,000 live births and is fatal within the first 2 years of life if not corrected. The disease is more common in girls and premature infants. In the United States, the incidence is twice as high in African American infants as in Caucasian infants. The exact cause of biliary atresia is unknown. EHBA has two distinct presentations, postnatal and fetal, with differing mechanisms of development suggested. Infections and immune-related mechanisms are implicated in postnatal EHBA, which represents 65% to 90% of cases. In the fetal form, there is a congenital absence of patent biliary ducts (Ward & Hisley, 2009).

HANDOFF COMMUNICATION

S Situation	Assess what is currently happening in a short statement.	Child presents as _____
B Background	Summarize important past assessment data for your patient here. Place lab results and medications on the concept map.	**Age:** **Gender:** **Allergies:** **Fall Risk:** **Isolation:**
A Assessment	Use the assessment data to complete your concept map.	**Nursing Diagnosis:** Place the Nursing Diagnoses in prioritized order on the concept map and add any needed for your specific patient. **Plan:** Place any further Nursing Interventions Classifications (NIC) needed on the map.

Implement Your Plan of Care

		EVALUATE YOUR CARE	
R Recommendation	Evaluate your nursing care and make recommendations related to the achievement of your desired outcomes. Were they met, or do new goals need to be established?	**Diag** / **Nursing Outcomes Classification (NOC)**	**Outcome met**
		1 Patient experiences no signs of malnutrition.	☐ Yes ☐ No
		2 Family participates in activities to reduce the risk of infection.	☐ Yes ☐ No
		3 Parents/caregivers follow prescribed therapeutic regimen.	☐ Yes ☐ No
		4 Family verbalizes understanding of condition, treatment, and complications.	☐ Yes ☐ No
		5	☐ Yes ☐ No

Nursing Diagnosis 1

Nutrition: less than body requirements related to blocked biliary duct evidenced by poor weight gain.

NIC:
1) Assess abdomen, noting circumference, bowel sounds, and distention; **2)** Observe color and consistency of stools; **3)** Maintain NPO and gastric suctioning in acute phase; **4)** Administer parenteral feedings as ordered; and **5)** Provide nonnutritive sucking.

Nursing Diagnosis 2

Risk for infection related to procedures or Kasai procedure (surgical procedure to connect the liver to the intestines to go around the abnormal ducts).

NIC:
1) Follow strict aseptic technique; **2)** Model and emphasize good hand washing; **3)** Observe for signs and symptoms of infection; **4)** Prepare for surgical intervention or postoperative care; **5)** Take vital signs (VS) frequently; and **6)** Note change in respirations or heart rate.

Nursing Diagnosis 3

Pain related to hunger and abdominal discomfort evidenced by crying.

NIC:
1) Hold child and provide therapeutic touch; **2)** Provide nonnutritive sucking; **3)** Administer analgesic as prescribed; **4)** Monitor with age-appropriate pain scale; and **5)** Maintain stress-free environment.

Nursing Diagnosis 4

Knowledge deficit related to condition, prognosis, and treatment evidenced by frequent family questions.

NIC:
1) Review condition and prognosis; **2)** Explore available treatments; **3)** Review importance of keeping child NPO and providing comfort to child; and **4)** Involve family in care of child.

Nursing Diagnosis 5

NIC:

Condition:
Biliary Atresia
Age:

Link & Explain
• Nursing Interventions Classification (NIC)
• Laboratory and Diagnostic Procedures
• Medications

Medications

a.

b.

c.

d.

Laboratory & Diagnostic Procedures

a. Abdominal x-ray and cholangiogram

b. Abdominal ultrasound

c. Bilirubin levels

d. Hepatobiliary iminodiacetic acid (HIDA) (cholescintigraphy)

CONDITION: Candidiasis (Thrush)

PHYSIOLOGY: Candidiasis is a fungal infection of the skin or mucous membranes with any species of *Candida* but chiefly *Candida albicans*. *Candida* species are part of the body's normal flora. *Candida* grows in warm, moist areas, causing superficial infections of the mouth, vagina, nails, and skinfolds in healthy people. In patients with immunodeficiencies, central venous lines, and burns or those receiving peritoneal dialysis, it can invade the bloodstream, causing disseminated infections. Children often get thrush or oral lesions (*Taber's*, 2009).

HANDOFF COMMUNICATION

S	Situation	Assess what is currently happening in a short statement.	Child presents as _____
B	Background	Summarize important past assessment data for your patient here. Place lab results and medications on the concept map.	**Age:** **Gender:** **Allergies:** **Fall Risk:** **Isolation:**
A	Assessment	Use the assessment data to complete your concept map.	**Nursing Diagnosis:** Place the Nursing Diagnoses in prioritized order on the concept map and add any needed for your specific patient. **Plan:** Place any further Nursing Interventions Classifications (NIC) needed on the map.

Implement Your Plan of Care

R	Recommendation	Evaluate your nursing care and make recommendations related to the achievement of your desired outcomes. Were they met, or do new goals need to be established?	**EVALUATE YOUR CARE**

Diag	Nursing Outcomes Classification (NOC)	Outcome met
1	Patient is free of, or displays improved healing of, infection.	☐ Yes ☐ No
2	Patient displays relieved pain level.	☐ Yes ☐ No
3	Parents/caregivers verbalize understanding of condition, treatment, prevention, and possible complications.	☐ Yes ☐ No
4	Patient experiences no signs of malnutrition.	☐ Yes ☐ No
5		☐ Yes ☐ No

Nursing Diagnosis 1

Impaired skin/tissue integrity related to infectious lesions, evidenced by disruption of skin surfaces and mucous membranes.

NIC:
1) Assess skin daily; **2)** Instruct parents/caregivers about good hygiene; **3)** Keep child's fingers away from mouth if possible; and **4)** Wash all feeding equipment well.

Nursing Diagnosis 2

Impaired comfort related to exposure of irritated skin and mucous membranes evidenced by restlessness.

NIC:
1) Assess for pain often; **2)** Provide diversionary activity; and **3)** Provide oral care.

Nursing Diagnosis 3

Risk for knowledge deficit of parents/caregivers related to infectious spread.

NIC:
1) Determine parents'/caregivers' perception of condition; **2)** Review disease process with parents/caregivers; **3)** Review medication, dose, frequency, and possible side effects; and **4)** Stress importance of good hand washing and aseptic techniques when feeding child.

Nursing Diagnosis 4

Nutrition: less than body requirements related to sore oral cavity evidenced by poor weight gain.

NIC:
1) Provide small, frequent meals; **2)** Serve child's favorite foods; and **3)** Increase fluids.

Condition:
Candidiasis (Thrush)

Age:

Link & Explain
- Nursing Interventions Classification (NIC)
- Laboratory and Diagnostic Procedures
- Medications

Nursing Diagnosis 5

NIC:

Medications

a. Fluconazole

b. Clotrimazole lozenges

c. Nystatin oral solution

d.

Laboratory & Diagnostic Procedures

a.

b.

c.

d.

CONDITION: Casts/Traction

PHYSIOLOGY: A cast is a solid mold of a body part, usually applied in situ for immobilization of fractures, dislocations, and other severe injuries. It is carefully applied to the immobilized part and allowed to dry and harden (over several to 48 hours depending on the type of material used). Care is taken not to apply any pressure to the cast until the cast is dried and hardened. Synthetic materials, such as fiberglass, are also used especially for non-weight-bearing parts of the body.

Traction is the process of drawing or pulling. Several types of traction are used in pediatric patients, including:

Bryant's—Traction applied to the lower leg with the force pulling vertically. It is used especially for treating fractures of the femur in children.

Buck's extension—A method of producing traction by applying regular flannel-backed adhesive tape to the skin and keeping it in close contact by circular bandaging of the part to which it is applied. The adhesive strips are aligned with the long axis of the arm or leg, the superior ends being about 1 inch from the fracture site. Weight sufficient to produce the required extension is fastened to the inferior end of the adhesive strips by a rope that is run over a pulley to permit free motion.

Cervical—Traction applied to the cervical spine by applying force to lift the head or mobilization techniques to distract individual joints of the vertebrae (*Taber's*, 2009).

HANDOFF COMMUNICATION

S	Situation	Assess what is currently happening in a short statement.	Child presents as _____
B	Background	Summarize important past assessment data for your patient here. Place lab results and medications on the concept map.	**Age:** **Gender:** **Allergies:** **Fall Risk:** **Isolation:**
A	Assessment	Use the assessment data to complete your concept map.	**Nursing Diagnosis:** Place the Nursing Diagnoses in prioritized order on the concept map and add any needed for your specific patient. **Plan:** Place any further Nursing Interventions Classifications (NIC) needed on the map.

Implement Your Plan of Care

			EVALUATE YOUR CARE	
R	Recommendation	Evaluate your nursing care and make recommendations related to the achievement of your desired outcomes. Were they met, or do new goals need to be established?	**Diag** / **Nursing Outcomes Classification (NOC)**	**Outcome met**
			1 Patient reports pain control or pain control is observed.	☐ Yes ☐ No
			2 Patient maintains function evidenced by sensation and movement within normal range for the individual.	☐ Yes ☐ No
			3 Patient demonstrates behavior and techniques to promote healing and prevent complications.	☐ Yes ☐ No
			4 Patient performs self-care activities within level of ability.	☐ Yes ☐ No
			5	☐ Yes ☐ No

Nursing Diagnosis 1

Acute pain related to fracture, trauma, bone fragments, injury to soft tissue, traction evidenced by verbal reports, guarding or distraction behaviors, self-focus, alteration in muscle tone, or changes in vital signs (VS).

NIC:
1) Assess pain frequently using age-appropriate pain scale; **2)** Medicate as ordered; **3)** Decrease environmental stimuli to promote rest; and **4)** Position and check cast and/or traction frequently.

Nursing Diagnosis 2

Risk for peripheral neurovascular dysfunction related to fracture, cast, traction, or immobilization**.**

NIC:
1) Assess presence, location, and degree of swelling or edema formation; **2)** Measure extremity and compare with unaffected extremity; **3)** Note position, location of casts and traction; **4)** Evaluate pulses, pain, color, paresthesia, paralysis, changes in motor and sensory function of extremity and compare to unaffected extremity; **5)** Assess capillary return; and **6)** Apply ice as appropriate.

Nursing Diagnosis 3

Risk for impaired skin integrity related to cast, traction, or altered sensation or circulation.

NIC:
1) Check tension on skin; **2)** Assess for any drainage; **3)** Teach patient not to touch repair or traction site; **4)** Maintain clean cast; and **5)** Clean skin that is exposed.

Nursing Diagnosis 4

Self-care deficit related to cast or traction evidenced by inability to complete activities of daily living (ADLs).

NIC:
1) Assess degree of functional impairment; **2)** Provide assistance with physical limitations; **3)** Allow sufficient time to perform tasks; and **4)** Schedule age-appropriate activities when energy level is highest to decrease fatigue.

Condition:
Casts/Traction
Age:

Link & Explain
• Nursing Interventions Classification (NIC)
• Laboratory and Diagnostic Procedures
• Medications

Nursing Diagnosis 5

NIC:

Medications

a. Analgesics

b.

c.

d.

Laboratory & Diagnostic Procedures

a.

b.

c.

d.

CONDITION: Celiac Disease

PHYSIOLOGY: Celiac disease causes malabsorption, weight loss, and diarrhea resulting from immunological intolerance to dietary wheat products, especially gluten and gliadin. Clinically, patients suffer bloating, flatulence, steatorrhea, anemia, weakness, malnutrition, vitamin and mineral deficiencies, rashes, bone loss, attenuated growth, delayed puberty, or failure to thrive. The disease is common, occurring in about 1 in 110 Americans (*Taber's*, 2009).

HANDOFF COMMUNICATION

S	Situation	Assess what is currently happening in a short statement.	Child presents as _____
B	Background	Summarize important past assessment data for your patient here. Place lab results and medications on the concept map.	**Age:** **Gender:** **Allergies:** **Fall Risk:** **Isolation:**
A	Assessment	Use the assessment data to complete your concept map.	**Nursing Diagnosis:** Place the Nursing Diagnoses in prioritized order on the concept map and add any needed for your specific patient. **Plan:** Place any further Nursing Interventions Classifications (NIC) needed on the map.

Implement Your Plan of Care

	Evaluate your nursing care and make recommendations related to the achievement of your desired outcomes. Were they met, or do new goals need to be established?	**EVALUATE YOUR CARE**		
		Diag	**Nursing Outcomes Classification (NOC)**	**Outcome met**
R Recommendation		1	Patient demonstrates progressive weight gain toward goal with normalization of laboratory values.	☐ Yes ☐ No
		2	Patient has reduction in frequency of stools, and stools return to more normal consistency.	☐ Yes ☐ No
		3	Patient maintains adequate hydration with stable vital signs, good skin turgor, capillary refill, strong peripheral pulses, and appropriate urine output.	☐ Yes ☐ No
		4	Parents acknowledge own coping abilities and demonstrate necessary lifestyle changes to limit or prevent recurrent episodes.	☐ Yes ☐ No
		5		☐ Yes ☐ No

Nursing Diagnosis 1

Imbalanced nutrition: less than body requirements related to malabsorption of nutrients evidenced by decreased subcutaneous fat and muscle mass, poor muscle tone, hyperactive bowel sounds, steatorrhea.

NIC:

1) Keep patient on gluten-free diet; **2)** Administer IV, TPN, or enteral feeding as indicated; **3)** Encourage well-rounded diet; **4)** Allow meals to be unhurried and calm; **5)** Assess abdomen, noting presence and character of bowel sounds, abdominal distention, and reports of nausea; **6)** Provide frequent mouth care to sooth dry mucous membranes; and **7)** Monitor laboratory values such as Hgb/Hct, electrolytes, and albumin levels.

Nursing Diagnosis 2

Diarrhea related to inflammation, irritation, or malabsorption of the bowel evidenced by increased bowel sounds; frequent, severe watery stools; abdominal cramping.

NIC:

1) Observe and record stool frequency, characteristics, and amount; **2)** Provide room deodorizers; **3)** Identify foods and fluids that precipitate diarrhea; and **4)** Offer clear liquids hourly and avoid cold fluids.

Nursing Diagnosis 3

Risk for deficient fluid volume related to excessive losses through diarrhea, nausea, fever, and anorexia.

NIC:

1) Monitor I&O; note number, character, and amount of stool; **2)** Assess BP, peripheral pulses, and mucous membranes; **3)** Monitor laboratory values such as Hgb/Hct and electrolytes to determine hydration status; and **4)** Weigh daily.

Nursing Diagnosis 4

Altered parenting due to inability of parents/caregivers to provide a nurturing environment related to impaired child-parent/caregiver attachment, feeding difficulties, and demands of interdisciplinary care evidenced by parental anxiety or verbalization.

NIC:

1) Assess and document parent/caregiver-child interactions; **2)** Teach appropriate stimulation activities, feeding, and daily care; **3)** Allow family time to express feelings of frustration and concerns; **4)** Assist in coordination of interdisciplinary services; **5)** Provide access information for contact person and identify available community resources and support groups; **6)** Prepare child for procedures in accordance with development; **7)** Encourage child and parent/caregiver to participate in care; and **8)** Document child's/parents' or caregivers' understanding of disorder and treatments.

Condition:
Celiac Disease
Age:

Link & Explain
• Nursing Interventions Classification (NIC)
• Laboratory and Diagnostic Procedures
• Medications

Nursing Diagnosis 5

NIC:

Medications
   a. Antidiarrheals: diphenoxylate (Lomotil), loperamide (Imodium)
   b. Anti-inflammatories: mesalamine (Pentasa, Asacol)
   c. Steroids: hydrocortisone (Cortenema), prednisolone (Delta-Cortef)
   d. Immune system suppressors: azathioprine (Imuran)

Laboratory & Diagnostic Procedures
   a. Serum electrolytes, CBC, serum iron, prealbumin/albumin/total proteins
   b. Esophagogastroduodenoscopy or colonoscopy
   c. MRI, CT scan
   d. Stool specimens, rectal biopsy

CONDITION: Cerebral Palsy (CP)

PHYSIOLOGY: Cerebral palsy is an umbrella term for a group of progressive, but often changing, motor impairments secondary to lesions or anomalies of the brain arising in early stages of development. CP is a symptom complex rather than a specific disease. For the vast majority of children born at term in whom CP later develops, the disorder cannot reasonably be ascribed to birth injury or hypoxic-ischemic insults during delivery. CP rarely occurs without associated defects such as mental retardation (60% of cases) or seizures (50% of cases). Risk factors have been divided into three groups: those occurring prior to pregnancy, such as an unusually short interval (less than 3 months) or unusually long interval since the previous pregnancy; those occurring during pregnancy, including physical malformation, twin gestation, abnormal fetal presentation, fetal growth retardation, or maternal hypothyroidism; and perinatal factors such as prematurity, premature separation of the placenta, or fetal encephalopathy. Nonetheless, among infants with one or more of these risk factors, 95% do have CP.

CP is classified by the extremity involved and the type of neurological dysfunction present, such as spastic (50%), hypotonic, dystonic, athetonic (20%), ataxic (10%), or a combination of these. It is not possible to diagnose CP in the neonatal period, and early diagnosis is complicated by the changing pattern of the disease in the first year of life. Many patients have impaired swallowing and/or drooling. Impaired speech is present in about 80% of these children, and many also have dental abnormalities, vision and/or hearing deficits, and reading disabilities (*Taber's*, 2009).

HANDOFF COMMUNICATION

S Situation	Assess what is currently happening in a short statement.	Child presents as _____	
B Background	Summarize important past assessment data for your patient here. Place lab results and medications on the concept map.	**Age:** **Allergies:** **Isolation:**	**Gender:** **Fall Risk:**
A Assessment	Use the assessment data to complete your concept map.	**Nursing Diagnosis:** Place the Nursing Diagnoses in prioritized order on the concept map and add any needed for your specific patient. **Plan:** Place any further Nursing Interventions Classifications (NIC) needed on the map.	

Implement Your Plan of Care

		EVALUATE YOUR CARE	
R Recommendation	Evaluate your nursing care and make recommendations related to the achievement of your desired outcomes. Were they met, or do new goals need to be established?	**Diag** / **Nursing Outcomes Classification (NOC)**	**Outcome met**
		1 Patient maintains position of function evidenced by absence of contractures and footdrop.	☐ Yes ☐ No
		2 Patient recognizes sensory impairments and identifies behaviors to compensate for deficits.	☐ Yes ☐ No
		3 Patient demonstrates progressive weight gain toward goal with normalization of laboratory values.	☐ Yes ☐ No
		4 Patient/family express feelings and progress through stages of grief focusing on one day at a time.	☐ Yes ☐ No
		5	☐ Yes ☐ No

Nursing Diagnosis 1

Impaired physical mobility related to neuromuscular impairment evidenced by inability to purposefully move or by un-coordinated movements.

NIC:
1) Monitor motor function continuously; **2)** Perform or assist with range of motion (ROM); **3)** Maintain ankles at 90 degrees with footboard; **4)** Assess for edema of an-kles and feet and raise lower extremities as indicated; **5)** Assess BP before and after activity until stable; **6)** Change positions slowly; **7)** Position periodically when sit-ting in chair; **8)** Prepare for weight-bearing activities such as the use of a tilt table; and **9)** Inspect all skin surfaces for reddened areas by use of a mirror if necessary.

Nursing Diagnosis 2

Disturbed sensory perception related to destruction of sensory tracts with altered sensory reception, transmission, and inte-gration evidenced by change in usual response to stimuli.

NIC:
1) Assess and document sensory function and deficit by means of touch, pinprick, heat, cold; **2)** Protect from bodily harm, such as falls, burns, and positioning; and **3)** Assist the patient to recognize and compensate for alterations in sensation.

Nursing Diagnosis 3

Imbalanced nutrition: less than body requirements related to difficulty swallowing of nutrients evidenced by decreased subcutaneous fat and muscle mass, or poor muscle tone.

NIC:
1) Keep patient on vitamins and offer foods that they like in puree form; **2)** Progress slowly from liquid to solids; **3)** Allow meals to be unhurried and calm; **4)** Provide frequent mouth care to sooth dry mucous membranes; and **5)** Teach parents CPR and Heimlich maneuver.

Nursing Diagnosis 4

Grieving related to perceived or actual loss of physio-psychosocial well-being of child evidenced by expressions of distress, denial, guilt, fear, sadness, altered affect.

NIC:
Identify signs of grieving such as shock, denial, anger, and depression. *Shock:* (a) Provide simple and accurate informa-tion to the patient without false reassur-ance. (b) Encourage expressions of sadness, grief, guilt, and fear. *Denial:* (a) Assist patient to verbalize feelings; avoid judgment. (b) Focus on present needs such as skin care, exercise, ROM. *Anger:* (a) Accept expressions of anger and hopelessness. Set limits on acting out with abusive language, sexually aggressive behavior. (b) Encourage patient to take control when able, such as food choices and diversional activities. *Depression:* (a) Note loss of interest in living, sleep disturbance, suicidal thoughts. (b) Offer support.

Condition:
Cerebral Palsy (CP)
Age:

Link & Explain
• Nursing Interventions Classification (NIC)
• Laboratory and Diagnostic Procedures
• Medications

Nursing Diagnosis 5

NIC:

Medications

a.

b.

c.

d.

Laboratory & Diagnostic Procedures

a.

b.

c.

d.

CONDITION: Child Abuse/Neglect (Battered Child Syndrome)

PHYSIOLOGY: Child abuse/neglect (battered child syndrome) is emotional, physical, or sexual injury to a child. It may be due to either an action or an omission by those responsible for the care of the child. In domestic situations in which a child is abused, it is important to examine other children and infants living in the home; about 20% will have signs of physical abuse. The examination should be done without delay. An infant or child must never be allowed to remain in an environment where abuse has occurred. All health-care providers, teachers, and others who work with children are responsible for identifying and reporting abusive situations as soon as possible (*Taber's*, 2009).

HANDOFF COMMUNICATION

S	Situation	Assess what is currently happening in a short statement.	Child presents as _____
B	Background	Summarize important past assessment data for your patient here. Place lab results and medications on the concept map.	**Age:** **Gender:** **Allergies:** **Fall Risk:** **Isolation:**
A	Assessment	Use the assessment data to complete your concept map.	**Nursing Diagnosis:** Place the Nursing Diagnoses in prioritized order on the concept map and add any needed for your specific patient. **Plan:** Place any further Nursing Interventions Classifications (NIC) needed on the map.

Implement Your Plan of Care

		EVALUATE YOUR CARE		
R	Recommendation — Evaluate your nursing care and make recommendations related to the achievement of your desired outcomes. Were they met, or do new goals need to be established?	**Diag**	**Nursing Outcomes Classification (NOC)**	**Outcome met**
		1	Modify environment as indicated to prevent trauma.	☐ Yes ☐ No
		2	Be involved in problem-solving solutions for current situation.	☐ Yes ☐ No
		3	Patient verbalizes or demonstrates acceptance of self and an increased sense of self-worth.	☐ Yes ☐ No
		4	Patient demonstrates ability to deal with emotional reactions in an individually appropriate manner.	☐ Yes ☐ No
		5		☐ Yes ☐ No

Nursing Diagnosis 1

Risk for trauma related to dependent position in relationship and vulnerability.

NIC:
1) Refer to appropriate authorities, social services, or case manager to remove child from the situation; observe parent/caregiver-child interactions; and 2) Promote counseling for child and family.

Nursing Diagnosis 2

Interrupted family processes/impaired parenting related to poor role model, unrealistic expectations, presence of stressors, and lack of support evidenced by verbalization on negative feelings, inappropriate caretaking behaviors, and evidence of physical or psychological trauma to the child.

NIC:
1) Determine existing situation and parents'/caregivers' perception of problem; 2) Observe parents with child; and 3) Refer to social services, case manager for counseling.

Nursing Diagnosis 3

Chronic low self-esteem related to deprivation and negative feedback of family members, personal vulnerability, feelings of abandonment, evidenced by lack of eye contact, withdrawal from social contacts, discounting own needs, nonassertiveness or passiveness, indecisive or overly conforming behavior.

NIC:
1) Provide opportunity for and encourage verbalization or acting out of individual situation; 2) Spend time with child; 3) Provide reinforcement for positive actions; 4) Encourage expressions of feelings of guilt, shame, and anger; and 5) Involve in play therapy or group therapy.

Nursing Diagnosis 4

Posttrauma syndrome related to sustained or reoccurring abuse evidenced by acting-out behavior.

NIC:
1) Assess physical trauma or use a sexual-assault nurse examiner (SANE) to collect evidence; 2) Evaluate behavior; 3) Assess signs or stages of grieving; 4) Identify support systems; and 5) Refer to counselor.

Condition:
Child Abuse (Battered Child Syndrome)

Age:

Link & Explain
• Nursing Interventions Classification (NIC)
• Laboratory and Diagnostic Procedures
• Medications

Nursing Diagnosis 5

NIC:

Medications

a.

b.

c.

d.

Laboratory & Diagnostic Procedures

a.

b.

c.

d.

CONDITION: Cleft Lip and Palate

PHYSIOLOGY: Cleft lip and palate present as an isolated defect, or both can occur. The disorder is considered a multifactorial defect that has a genetic predisposition that interacts with an environmental trigger at a vulnerable time of fetal development. The disorder is associated with maternal smoking, maternal ingestion of drugs such as phenytoin (Dilantin), and genetic disorders such as trisomy 18.

During fetal life, there is incomplete fusion of embryonic soft tissues and/or palatal arch. The disorder is often diagnosed on fetal ultrasound. A cleft lip is obvious, but cleft palate needs to be assessed in a newborn mouth via examination at the time of admission in the well-baby nursery.

Surgical correction is required. The cleft lip is often repaired at 3–6 months of age, and cleft palate is repaired before 18 months of age.

Complications of the defect can result in aspiration/pneumonia, speech difficulties, frequent incidence of otitis media, hearing loss, dental malposition, and dental decay (Doenges, Moorhouse, & Murr, 2009; Ward & Hisley, 2009).

HANDOFF COMMUNICATION

S Situation	Assess what is currently happening in a short statement.	Child presents as _____
B Background	Summarize important past assessment data for your patient here. Place lab results and medications on the concept map.	**Age:** **Gender:** **Allergies:** **Fall Risk:** **Isolation:** **Immunization status:** **PMH:** **PSH:**
A Assessment	Use the assessment data to complete your concept map.	**Nursing Diagnosis:** Place the Nursing Diagnoses in prioritized order on the concept map and add any needed for your specific patient. **Plan:** Place any further Nursing Interventions Classifications (NIC) needed on the map.

Implement Your Plan of Care

		EVALUATE YOUR CARE	
R Recommendation	Evaluate your nursing care and make recommendations related to the achievement of your desired outcomes. Were they met, or do new goals need to be established?	**Diag** / **Nursing Outcomes Classification (NOC)**	**Outcome met**
		1 Patient's airway remains patent without incidence of aspiration/pneumonia evidenced by normal vital signs and without symptoms of respiratory distress.	☐ Yes ☐ No
		2 Client demonstrates adequate nutrition evidenced by steady weight gain, sufficient calorie consumption, and decreased feeding difficulties.	☐ Yes ☐ No
		3 Client/caregiver demonstrates appropriate parenting behavior evidenced by appropriate parent-infant attachment behaviors, verbalization of positive feelings toward infant, demonstrating knowledge and competency in infant care.	☐ Yes ☐ No
		4 Infant is infection free, and incision will heal evidenced by lack of erythema, edema, and purulent drainage.	☐ Yes ☐ No
		5	☐ Yes ☐ No

Nursing Diagnosis 1

Risk of aspiration/pneumonia due to anatomical abnormality.

NIC:
1) Monitor vital signs (VS) every 2–4 hours; 2) Maintain infant position to support open airway before and after feeds to prevent regurgitation preoperatively; 3) Perform gentle oral or nasopharyngeal suctioning prn; and 4) Maintain supine or side-lying position postoperatively in cleft lip repair and prone or side-lying in postoperative cleft palate repair.

Nursing Diagnosis 2

Insufficient nutrition to meet body requirements related to abnormal sucking patterns due to craniofacial abnormalities evidenced by difficulty feeding or poor weight gain.

NIC:
1) Keep accurate I&O; 2) Assess and record episodes of feeding difficulties such as gagging, regurgitation via nares, and choking; 3) Weigh infant on same scale and at same time of day; 4) Position infant in an upright, side-lying, or semi-sitting position during feeding; 5) Use appropriate feeding instruments, such as Haberman nipple, Breck feeder, medicine dropper, cup, soft catheter-tip syringe; 6) Do not nipple feed longer than 30 minutes, and then substitute with nasogastric (NG) feedings; 7) Frequently burp with feeding and allow time for rest, remove nipple if coughing episodes ensue; 8) Utilize ESSR method (enlarge nipple, stimulate sucking, swallow, and rest) to feed; and 9) Instruct family; assess and document results.

Nursing Diagnosis 3

Altered parenting due to inability of parent/caregiver to provide a nurturing environment related to impaired infant-parent attachment, feeding difficulties, and demands of interdisciplinary care evidenced by parental anxiety or verbalization.

NIC:
1) Assess and document parent-infant interactions; 2) Teach appropriate stimulation activities, infant holding, feeding, and daily care; 3) Allow family time to express feelings of frustration and concerns; 4) Assist in coordination of interdisciplinary services; 5) Provide access information for contact person, and identify available community resources and support groups; 6) Prepare child for procedures in accordance with development; 7) Encourage child and parent/caregiver participation in care; and 8) Document parents'/caregivers' understanding of surgical correction and informed consent.

Nursing Diagnosis 4

Risk for postoperative impaired skin integrity and risk of infection due to surgical closure and trauma.

NIC:
1) Assess and document suture line characteristics; 2) Provide suture line care as indicated and apply antibiotic ointment; 3) Place elbow/arm restraints as indicated to prevent trauma to suture line; remove restraints q2h and provide movement; 4) Use special appliances to feed infant to avoid stress on suture line (e.g., dropper with cleft lip); and avoid pacifier, straw, spoon, fork; 5) Advance diet as tolerated, clear to soft, with cleft palate; 6) After feedings, rinse mouth to avoid milk residue; and 7) Position child to avoid trauma to suture line and drainage of copious secretions with postoperative repair with cleft palate.

Condition:
Cleft Lip and Palate
Age:

Link & Explain
• Nursing Interventions Classification (NIC)
• Laboratory and Diagnostic Procedures
• Medications

Nursing Diagnosis 5

NIC:

Medications
a. Antibiotics pre- and postoperatively
b. Analgesics and/or narcotics postoperatively
c. Ibuprofen and acetaminophen postoperatively
d.

Laboratory & Diagnostic Procedures
a. Pre- and postoperative labs as prescribed and indicated
b. Hearing screen due to high risk for hearing deficit
c.
d.

CONDITION: Congenital Heart Defects (CHD)

PHYSIOLOGY: Congenital heart defects can result in cyanosis, heart failure, shunting of blood through abnormal valves and structural defects, ventricular hypertrophy, arrhythmias, polycythemia, altered growth and development. Acyanotic defects usually have normal saturation and cause increased pulmonary blood flow.

Cyanotic defects can have an overall saturation of 85%–70% and often have an obstruction to the right side of the heart with decreased pulmonary blood flow. Some defects require the fetal shunts to remain open for the initial stabilization with emergency cardiac catheterization (foramen ovale) and/or prostaglandin E1 (PGE1) to maintain patency of the patent ductus arteriosus.

CHD can cause heart failure as well as alter growth and cognitive development.

1. Cyanotic CHD includes transposition of the great arteries, tetralogy of Fallot with severe pulmonary stenosis, total anomalous pulmonary venous return, tricuspid atresia, pulmonary atresia, Epstein's anomaly, truncus arteriosus, single ventricle.
2. Acyanotic CHD includes ventricle septal defect (VSD), atrial septal defect (ASD), patent ductus arteriosus (PDA), and AV canal.
3. Obstructive lesions include pulmonary stenosis, aortic stenosis, coarctation of aorta, and interrupted aortic arch.
4. Mixed lesions include hypoplastic left heart syndrome, transposition of the great arteries, and truncus arteriosus (Doenges, Moorhouse, & Murr, 2009; Ward & Hisley, 2009).

HANDOFF COMMUNICATION

S	Situation	Assess what is currently happening in a short statement.	Child presents as _____
B	Background	Summarize important past assessment data for your patient here. Place lab results and medications on the concept map.	**Age:** **Gender:** **Allergies:** **Fall Risk:** **Isolation:** **Immunization status:** **PMH:** **PSH:**
A	Assessment	Use the assessment data to complete your concept map.	**Nursing Diagnosis:** Place the Nursing Diagnoses in prioritized order on the concept map and add any needed for your specific patient. **Plan:** Place any further Nursing Interventions Classifications (NIC) needed on the map.

Implement Your Plan of Care

R	Recommendation	Evaluate your nursing care and make recommendations related to the achievement of your desired outcomes. Were they met, or do new goals need to be established?		**EVALUATE YOUR CARE**

	Diag	**Nursing Outcomes Classification (NOC)**	**Outcome met**
	1	Patient demonstrates cardiac pump effectiveness with adequate blood volume ejected from the heart to support pulmonary and systemic circulation. Vital signs (VS), oxygen saturations are within acceptable range according to defect	☐ Yes ☐ No
	2	Patient maintains fluid balance between intracellular and extracellular fluid compartments, normal electrolytes, and decreased complications from fluid overload.	☐ Yes ☐ No
	3	Patient receives nutrients to meet metabolic demands, normal weight gain, normal growth and development parameters.	☐ Yes ☐ No
	4	Patient maintains optimal growth and developmental milestones.	☐ Yes ☐ No
	5		☐ Yes ☐ No

Nursing Diagnosis 1

Decreased cardiac output related to alterations in structure, preload, afterload, and inotropic functions.

NIC:
1) Assess VS, quality of respirations, oxygen saturations, and temperature; **2)** Administer supplemental oxygen as ordered; **3)** Administer PGE1 continuous IV infusion for ductal-dependent lesions (monitor for apnea, hypotension, fever, and flushing); **4)** Administer cardiac medications and diuretics as ordered; **5)** Maintain normal hematocrit and prevent anemia and polycythemia in cyanotic cardiac lesions; **6)** Monitor for episodes of desaturation in patients with tetralogy of Fallot; and **7)** Maintain infant/child in semi-Fowler's position to enhance lung expansion.

Nursing Diagnosis 2

Impaired fluid and electrolyte balance related to metabolic demands and cardiac function and diuretics.

NIC:
1) Strict I&O; **2)** Monitor fluid and electrolytes as obtained; **3)** Measure every diaper in infants; **4)** Record daily weights at the same time with the same scale; **5)** Measure abdominal girth in patient with chronic heart failure (CHF) or ascites; **6)** Maintain fluid-restricted diet if prescribed, if patient is in CHF; and **7)** Administer diuretics as prescribed.

Nursing Diagnosis 3

Imbalanced nutrition: less than body requirements related to complexity of condition and chronic illness.

NIC:
1) Allow PO feeding via breastfeeding or bottle for only 20 minutes; provide gavage or tube feedings as necessary; feed infant at 45-degree angle; **2)** Conserve calories with normal thermal temperature, clustering nursing care, and allowing period for rest; **3)** Plot weight, height, and head circumference weekly on growth chart to provide adequate caloric intake; **4)** Use high-calorie formulas or diet; and **5)** Consult speech therapist and nutritionist to assist with dietary needs and caloric intake.

Nursing Diagnosis 4

Delays in growth and development due to hospitalization and chronic illness.

NIC:
1) Perform baseline developmental assessment, such as Denver Developmental Assessment; **2)** Monitor developmental milestones and provide appropriate developmental tasks; **3)** Involve play therapist with selection of activities; **4)** Plan for play periods with rest; and **5)** Involve speech, occupational, and physical therapy to support developmental milestones.

Condition:
Congenital Heart Defects (CHD)

Age:

Link & Explain
• Nursing Interventions Classification (NIC)
• Laboratory and Diagnostic Procedures
• Medications

Nursing Diagnosis 5

NIC:

Medications

a. Digoxin

b. Diuretics: Lasix, Diuril, Aldactone

c. PGE1

d. Captopril and aspirin

Laboratory & Diagnostic Procedures

a. Chest x-ray, EKG, Holter monitor

b. Basic metabolic panel and CBC with differential and platelets

c. Cardiac catheterization

d. Echocardiogram

CONDITION: Cystic Fibrosis (CF)

PHYSIOLOGY: Cystic fibrosis (CF) is an autosomal recessive disease that manifests itself in multiple body systems, including the lungs, pancreas, urogenital system, skeleton, and skin. It causes chronic obstructive pulmonary disease, frequent lung infections, deficient elaboration of pancreatic enzymes, osteoporosis, and an abnormally high electrolyte concentration in the sweat. The name is derived from the characteristic histological changes in the pancreas. CF usually begins in infancy and is the major cause of severe chronic lung disease in children. In the United States, CF occurs in 1 in 2,500 white live births and 1 in 17,000 black live births and is the most common fatal genetic disease in European-American children. A great variety of clinical manifestations may be present, including nasal polyposis; lung changes related to thick, tenacious secretions leading to bronchiectasis; bronchitis; pneumonia; atelectasis; emphysema; and respiratory failure; gallbladder diseases; intussusceptions; meconium ileus; salt depletion; pancreatic exocrine deficiency causing intestinal malabsorption of fats, proteins, and to a lesser extent, carbohydrates; pancreatitis; peptic ulcer; rectal prolapse; diabetes; nutritional deficiencies; arthritis; absent vas deferens with consequent aspermia and absence of fructose in the ejaculate; failure to thrive; and delayed puberty. The child exhibits a nonproductive paroxysmal cough, barrel chest, cyanosis, clubbed fingers and toes, malabsorption leading to poor weight gain and growth, fat-soluble vitamin deficiency (A, D, E, K) leading to clotting abnormalities, and excretion of frequent pale stools that are bulky, foul-smelling, and have a high fat content (*Taber's*, 2009).

HANDOFF COMMUNICATION

S Situation	Assess what is currently happening in a short statement.	Child presents as _____
B Background	Summarize important past assessment data for your patient here. Place lab results and medications on the concept map.	Age: Gender: Allergies: Fall Risk: Isolation:
A Assessment	Use the assessment data to complete your concept map.	**Nursing Diagnosis:** Place the Nursing Diagnoses in prioritized order on the concept map and add any needed for your specific patient. **Plan:** Place any further Nursing Interventions Classifications (NIC) needed on the map.

Implement Your Plan of Care

			EVALUATE YOUR CARE	
R Recommendation	Evaluate your nursing care and make recommendations related to the achievement of your desired outcomes. Were they met, or do new goals need to be established?	**Diag**	**Nursing Outcomes Classification (NOC)**	**Outcome met**
		1	Patient maintains patent airway with breath sounds clear or clearing; and demonstrates behaviors to improve airway clearance.	☐ Yes ☐ No
		2	Patient demonstrates improved ventilation and adequate oxygenation of tissues by arterial blood gases (ABGs) within normal range, is free of symptoms of respiratory distress, and participates in treatment regimen within level of ability and situation.	☐ Yes ☐ No
		3	Patient has adequate nutrition evidenced by gaining weight and sufficient caloric consumption.	☐ Yes ☐ No
		4	Patient/caregiver participates in learning process; identifies interferences to learning and specific actions to deal with them; verbalizes understanding of condition, disease process, and treatment; performs necessary procedures correctly, and explains reasons for the actions.	☐ Yes ☐ No
		5		☐ Yes ☐ No

Nursing Diagnosis 1

Ineffective airway clearance related to increased production and retained pulmonary secretions, bronchospasms, decreased energy, fatigue evidenced by wheezing, difficulty breathing and change in respiratory depth and rate, use of accessory muscles, and persistent cough with or without sputum production.

NIC:
1) Auscultate breath sounds; **2)** Assess and monitor respiration rate; **3)** Note presence and degree of dyspnea and air hunger; **4)** Position patient for comfort; **5)** Keep environment free from triggers or pollutants; **6)** Assist with abdominal or pursed-lip breathing; **7)** Observe for cough; **8)** Hydrate; **9)** Medicate as ordered; **10)** Arrange respiratory treatments as ordered; and **11)** Use flutter device.

Nursing Diagnosis 2

Impaired gas exchange related to altered delivery of inspired oxygen and trapped air evidenced by dyspnea, restlessness, reduced tolerance for activity, cyanosis, and changes in ABGs and vital signs (VS).

NIC:
1) Assess respiratory rate and depth; **2)** Raise HOB (head of bed); **3)** Encourage expectoration of sputum; **4)** Auscultate breath sounds; **5)** Palpate chest for fremitus; and **6)** Monitor VS, sleep patterns, and activity level.

Nursing Diagnosis 3

Altered nutrition less than body requirements related to malabsorption of nutrients.

NIC:
1) Weigh every day with the same scale and at the same time; **2)** Record daily caloric counts; **3)** Start enteral feeding as prescribed and monitor tolerance; and **4)** If child is on long-term parenteral nutrition, monitor complete metabolic panel weekly.

Nursing Diagnosis 4

Knowledge deficit regarding pathophysiology of condition, management, and available community resources related to insufficient information and misconceptions evidenced by statements of concerns and questions.

NIC:
1) Ascertain readiness, level of knowledge, and individual learning needs; **2)** Provide positive reinforcement; **3)** Provide access information for contact person and identify available community resources and support groups; **4)** Explain to the parents that CF is a hereditary trait and they did nothing wrong during the pregnancy. Also, inform them that because it is hereditary, CF can be passed down to another child; and **5)** Encourage fluids and a high-protein diet.

Condition:
Cystic Fibrosis (CF)
Age:

Link & Explain
• Nursing Interventions Classification (NIC)
• Laboratory and Diagnostic Procedures
• Medications

Nursing Diagnosis 5

NIC:

Medications

a. Antibiotics

b. Mucolytic agent

c. Aerosolized recombinant human DNase (rhDNase)

d. Pancreatic enzymes

Laboratory & Diagnostic Procedures

a. Bronchoalveolar lavage

b. Genetic testing

c. Nutritional panel

d.

CONDITION: Deafness (Hearing Loss)

PHYSIOLOGY: Deafness is a partial or complete loss of hearing. Hearing is the sense or perception of sound. The normal ear can detect sounds with frequencies ranging from 20 Hz to 20,000 Hz but is most sensitive to sounds in the 1,500 Hz to 3,000 Hz frequency range, which is the range most used in speech. Hearing deficits occur when sound waves are not conducted properly to the cochlea, when lesions interrupt the workings of the cochlear nerve, or when central nervous system pathways involved in the processing of auditory stimuli are injured (*Taber's*, 2009).

HANDOFF COMMUNICATION

S	Situation	Assess what is currently happening in a short statement.	Child presents as _____
B	Background	Summarize important past assessment data for your patient here. Place lab results and medications on the concept map.	**Age:** **Gender:** **Allergies:** **Fall Risk:** **Isolation:**
A	Assessment	Use the assessment data to complete your concept map.	**Nursing Diagnosis:** Place the Nursing Diagnoses in prioritized order on the concept map and add any needed for your specific patient. **Plan:** Place any further Nursing Interventions Classifications (NIC) needed on the map.

Implement Your Plan of Care

			EVALUATE YOUR CARE		
R	Recommendation	Evaluate your nursing care and make recommendations related to the achievement of your desired outcomes. Were they met, or do new goals need to be established?	**Diag**	**Nursing Outcomes Classification (NOC)**	**Outcome met**
			1	Patient demonstrates improved and appropriate response to stimuli.	☐ Yes ☐ No
			2	Patient demonstrates improved communication ability.	☐ Yes ☐ No
			3	Family expresses more realistic understanding and expectations of patient.	☐ Yes ☐ No
			4	Parents/caregivers use available resources appropriately.	☐ Yes ☐ No
			5		☐ Yes ☐ No

Nursing Diagnosis 1

Disturbed sensory perception (auditory) related to hearing deficit evidenced by lack of response to noise.

NIC:
1) Assess degree of impairment; **2)** Use visual clues to explain tests and procedures; and **3)** Refer to audiologist.

Nursing Diagnosis 2

Impaired verbal communication related to hearing loss evidenced by delayed speech.

NIC:
1) Take time with child; **2)** Assess child's usual form of communication; **3)** Use interpreter service such as signing; **4)** Prompt child to use speech as much as possible; and **5)** Refer to speech therapy.

Nursing Diagnosis 3

Compromised family coping related to needs of a child with sensory disorder evidenced by inability of a family to make appropriate adjustments.

NIC:
1) Establish a rapport and acknowledge the situation for the family; **2)** Determine their current knowledge and perception of the situation; **3)** Assess family's level of anxiety; and **4)** Assist family with problem-solving and care of the patient.

Nursing Diagnosis 4

Risk for caregiver role strain related to safeguarding child with hearing deficit.

NIC:
1) Determine parents'/caregivers' current knowledge and perception of the situation; **2)** Assess strengths of caregiver; and **3)** Determine available resources and supports.

Condition:
Deafness (Hearing Loss)
Age:

Link & Explain
• Nursing Interventions Classification (NIC)
• Laboratory and Diagnostic Procedures
• Medications

Nursing Diagnosis 5

NIC:

Medications

a.

b.

c.

d.

Laboratory & Diagnostic Procedures

a. Hearing screens

b.

c.

d.

CONDITION: Developmental Dysplasia of Hip (DDH) or Congenital Hip Dysplasia

PHYSIOLOGY: DDH refers to a number of conditions in which the femoral head and acetabulum are incorrectly aligned. The cause is unknown, but there are familial-genetic and prenatal risks. Prenatal risks include breech delivery, multiple gestation, large-sized infant, and maternal hormones causing laxity of the hip joint. Cultural factors are also involved: the condition occurs less in infants carried on caregiver's hip, a position that maintains the infant's hips in an abducted position. Diagnosis is made by physical exam with a positive Ortolani or Barlow sign (a palpable click or clunk) on abduction and adduction of hips. Other symptoms are unequal gluteal folds and positive Allis sign with uneven knee height with child in supine position and thigh flexed at a 90-degree angle. Manifestations in an older child include Trendelenburg sign, which is unequal pelvic tilt (pelvis tilts downward on unaffected side); delay in walking; and abnormal gait (Doenges, Moorhouse, & Murr, 2009).

HANDOFF COMMUNICATION

S Situation	Assess what is currently happening in a short statement.	Child presents as _____	
B Background	Summarize important past assessment data for your patient here. Place lab results and medications on the concept map.	**Age:** **Gender:** **Allergies:** **Fall Risk:** **Isolation:** **Immunization status:**	
A Assessment	Use the assessment data to complete your concept map.	**Nursing Diagnosis:** Place the Nursing Diagnoses in prioritized order on the concept map and add any needed for your specific patient. **Plan:** Place any further Nursing Interventions Classifications (NIC) needed on the map.	

Implement Your Plan of Care

		EVALUATE YOUR CARE	
R Recommendation	Evaluate your nursing care and make recommendations related to the achievement of your desired outcomes. Were they met, or do new goals need to be established?	**Diag** **Nursing Outcomes Classification (NOC)**	**Outcome met**
		1 Patient has adequate stimulation to promote physical mobility in upper extremities and promote growth and development.	☐ Yes ☐ No
		2 Patient has intact skin integrity and no symptoms of skin infection from harness or brace.	☐ Yes ☐ No
		3 Parents/caregivers participate in learning process; verbalize understanding of condition, disease process, and treatment; perform necessary procedures correctly and explain reasons for the action.	☐ Yes ☐ No
		4 Parents/caregivers identify risk factors, verbalize understanding of treatment/therapy regimen, and demonstrate behaviors and techniques to prevent skin breakdown.	☐ Yes ☐ No
		5	☐ Yes ☐ No

Nursing Diagnosis 1

Impaired physical mobility related to prescribed therapy and congenital disorder evidenced by apparatus that makes it difficult for the child to move.

NIC:
1) Assess degree of immobility produced by defect and/or treatment; **2)** Maintain a stimulating environment and child's normal development by playing and spending time with the child; infants/children need to develop upper extremities and to receive adequate stimulation with age-appropriate toys; **3)** Keep the cast or brace and surrounding area clean and dry and reposition child every 2 hours; **4)** Elevate an extremity and provide good hygiene to prevent skin breakdown; **5)** Notify the health-care provider if the child has a fever, signs and symptoms of infection, or unrelieved pain; **6)** Position hip into flexed and abducted position with Pavlik harness for infants under 6 months; and **7)** Children older than 6 months may require surgery and a spica cast.

Nursing Diagnosis 2

Risk of impaired skin integrity related to harness or brace.

NIC:
1) Assess skin routinely, noting moisture, color, abrasions, rubbing, blistering, and elasticity; **2)** Perform neurovascular checks if patient is in a cast or brace; **3)** Observe for symptoms of infection (temperature, drainage from cast or brace, or foul odor from beneath cast/brace); **4)** Ensure proper application and removal of Pavlik harness with sponge bath, and assess skin daily; **5)** Instruct parent/caregiver on proper application of harness and assessment of skin to prevent skin breakdown; sponge bath and diaper changes with harness off; and **6)** Instruct parent/caregiver to ensure child does not place small or sharp items down cast.

Nursing Diagnosis 3

Impaired parenting related to growth and development possibly evidenced by growth and/or development lag in child.

NIC:
1) Assess parenting skill level, considering intellectual, emotional, and physical strengths and limitations; **2)** Determine existing situation and parental perception of the problems, noting presence of specific factors such as physical illness and disabilities of the child; **3)** Note presence and effectiveness of extended family support; and **4)** Emphasize positive aspects of situation, maintaining a positive attitude toward parents'/caregivers' capabilities and potential for improving.

Nursing Diagnosis 4

Knowledge deficit related to treatment and home care evidenced by questions and apprehension of parents/caregivers.

NIC:
1) Assess readiness to learn and individual learning needs including level of knowledge, anticipatory needs, and support persons requiring information; modification of positioning child car seat; and feeding infant; **2)** Involve the parent/caregiver by using age-appropriate materials tailored to the family's literacy skills, questions, and dialogue; **3)** Provide access information for contact person to answer questions and validate information after discharge; **4)** Encourage compliance and follow-up care; and **5)** Instruct on safety measures with a child in brace, cast, or harness.

Condition:
Developmental Dysplasia of Hip (DDH) or Congenital Hip Dysplasia

Age:
- - - - - - - - - - - - - - - - - -
Link & Explain
• Nursing Interventions Classification (NIC)
• Laboratory and Diagnostic Procedures
• Medications

Nursing Diagnosis 5

NIC:

Medications
a. Ibuprofen prn for pain
b. Acetaminophen prn for pain
c.
d.

Laboratory & Diagnostic Procedures
a. Hip ultrasound in high-risk infants younger than 4 months of age
b. Radiographs older than 4 months of age
c.
d.

CONDITION: Duchenne Muscular Dystrophy

PHYSIOLOGY: Duchenne muscular dystrophy is pseudohypertrophic muscular dystrophy marked by weakness and pseudohypertrophy of the affected muscles. It is caused by mutation of the gene responsible for producing the protein dystrophin. The disease begins in childhood, is progressive, and affects the shoulder and girdle muscles. The disease, mostly in males, is transmitted as a sex-linked recessive trait (*Taber's*, 2009).

HANDOFF COMMUNICATION

S	Situation	Assess what is currently happening in a short statement.	Child presents as _____
B	Background	Summarize important past assessment data for your patient here. Place lab results and medications on the concept map.	Age: Gender: Allergies: Fall Risk: Isolation:
A	Assessment	Use the assessment data to complete your concept map.	**Nursing Diagnosis:** Place the Nursing Diagnoses in prioritized order on the concept map and add any needed for your specific patient. **Plan:** Place any further Nursing Interventions Classifications (NIC) needed on the map.

Implement Your Plan of Care

		EVALUATE YOUR CARE		
	Evaluate your nursing care and make recommendations related to the achievement of your desired outcomes. Were they met, or do new goals need to be established?	**Diag**	**Nursing Outcomes Classification (NOC)**	**Outcome met**
R	Recommendation	**1**	Patient maintains position of function evidenced by absence of contractures or foot drop.	☐ Yes ☐ No
		2	Patient demonstrates weight and growth stabilization or progresses toward age-appropriate size; performs motor, social, and/or expressive skills typical of age group within scope of present capabilities.	☐ Yes ☐ No
		3	Patient ingests nutritionally adequate diet for age, activity level, and metabolic demands and demonstrates stable weight or progressive weight gain toward goal.	☐ Yes ☐ No
		4	Parents/caregivers identify and verbalize resources within themselves to deal with the situation; express more realistic understanding and expectations of patient; interact appropriately with patient and health-care providers, providing support and assistance as indicated; and verbalize knowledge and understanding of disability, disease process, and community resources.	☐ Yes ☐ No
		5		☐ Yes ☐ No

Nursing Diagnosis 1

Impaired physical mobility related to musculoskeletal impairment or weakness evidenced by decreased muscle strength, control, and mass; limited ROM (range of motion); and impaired coordination.

NIC:
1) Continually assess motor function; 2) Provide means to summon help if needed; 3) Perform or assist with full ROM exercises on all extremities; 4) Space periods of rest and activities; 5) Reposition often; 6) Inspect skin; and 7) Consult with occupational and physical therapists.

Nursing Diagnosis 2

Delayed growth and development related to effects of physical disability evidenced by altered physical growth and altered ability to perform self-care or self-control activities appropriate to age.

NIC:
1) Measure weight and height; 2) Measure developmental level using age-appropriate tools; 3) Determine cognitive and perceptual levels; and 4) Provide parents with information about appropriate growth and development.

Nursing Diagnosis 3

Risk for imbalanced nutrition: more than body requirements related to sedentary lifestyle.

NIC:
1) Determine ability to chew, swallow, and taste; 2) Determine child's current nutritional status using age-appropriate tools; 3) Elicit typical food intake pattern; 4) Determine psychosocial, cultural, or religious factors; clarify parents'/caregivers' access to resources; and 5) Discuss importance of well-balanced nutritious intake.

Nursing Diagnosis 4

Compromised family coping related to situational crises evidenced by preoccupation around personal reactions and displaying protective behavior disproportionate to patient's ability or autonomy.

NIC:
1) Determine family's understanding of the disease process; 2) Discuss family's willingness to be involved in the child's care; 3) Assess other factors affecting family's ability to provide needed support, such as work; 4) Encourage free expression of feelings; and 5) Encourage family to strengthen problem-solving skills to deal with situation.

Condition:
Duchenne Muscular Dystrophy

Age:

Link & Explain
• Nursing Interventions Classification (NIC)
• Laboratory and Diagnostic Procedures
• Medications

Nursing Diagnosis 5

NIC:

Medications

a.

b.

c.

d.

Laboratory & Diagnostic Procedures

a.

b.

c.

d.

CONDITION: Encephalitis

PHYSIOLOGY: Encephalitis is inflammation of the white and gray matter of the brain. It is almost always associated with inflammation of the meninges (meningoencephalitis) and may involve the spinal cord (encephalomyelitis). In the United States, 20,000 cases are reported annually (*Taber's*, 2009).

HANDOFF COMMUNICATION

S	Situation	Assess what is currently happening in a short statement.	Child presents as _____
B	Background	Summarize important past assessment data for your patient here. Place lab results and medications on the concept map.	**Age:** **Gender:** **Allergies:** **Fall Risk:** **Isolation:**
A	Assessment	Use the assessment data to complete your concept map.	**Nursing Diagnosis:** Place the Nursing Diagnoses in prioritized order on the concept map and add any needed for your specific patient. **Plan:** Place any further Nursing Interventions Classifications (NIC) needed on the map.

Implement Your Plan of Care

				EVALUATE YOUR CARE	
R	Recommendation	Evaluate your nursing care and make recommendations related to the achievement of your desired outcomes. Were they met, or do new goals need to be established?	**Diag**	**Nursing Outcomes Classification (NOC)**	**Outcome met**
			1	Patient demonstrates stable vital signs (VS) and absence of signs of increased intracranial pressure (ICP).	☐ Yes ☐ No
			2	Patient regains or maintains appropriate body temperature for age and size.	☐ Yes ☐ No
			3	Patient manifests decreased restlessness or irritability.	☐ Yes ☐ No
			4	Patient is free of injury.	☐ Yes ☐ No
			5		☐ Yes ☐ No

Nursing Diagnosis 1

Risk for ineffective cerebral tissue perfusion related to cerebral edema altering or interrupting cerebral arterial or venous blood flow.

NIC:
1) Monitor and document age-appropriate neurological status frequently and compare to baseline assessment; **2)** Evaluate eye opening, response to environmental stimuli, and pupil reactivity; **3)** Assess verbal responses; **4)** Assess motor responses; **5)** Monitor VS; and **6)** Note presence of age-appropriate reflexes.

Nursing Diagnosis 2

Hyperthermia related to increased metabolic rate evidenced by increased body temperature, warm skin, and increased pulse and respiratory rate.

NIC:
1) Note conditions that promote fever; **2)** Measure temperature using properly functioning thermometer; **3)** Be aware of heat loss for body size and mass; **4)** Adjust bedclothes, linen, and environment; and **5)** Administer antipyretics.

Nursing Diagnosis 3

Acute pain related to inflammation or irritation of the brain and cerebral edema evidenced by changes in VS, restlessness, and crying.

NIC:
1) Perform routine comprehensive pain assessment; **2)** Accept child's description of pain; **3)** Investigate changes or frequency of pain; **4)** Observe for rigidity, crying; **5)** Provide comfort measures, holding, repositioning; and **6)** Encourage sleep and rest periods.

Nursing Diagnosis 4

Risk for trauma related to restlessness, altered sensorium, cognitive impairment, or vertigo.

NIC:
1) Handle gently; **2)** Identify risk factors such as confusion; **3)** Use age-appropriate equipment; **4)** Maintain side rail; **5)** Encourage parents/caregivers or family to stay; and **6)** Seizure precautions: low lighting and subdued environment.

Condition:
Encephalitis
Age:

Link & Explain
• Nursing Interventions Classification (NIC)
• Laboratory and Diagnostic Procedures
• Medications

Nursing Diagnosis 5

NIC:

Medications

a. Ibuprofen (Motrin) or acetaminophen (Tylenol)

b. Steroids (dexamathasone)

c. Antiviral medications, such as acyclovir (Zovirax) and foscarnet (Foscavir) or antibiotics

d. Antiseizure medications (phenytoin)

Laboratory & Diagnostic Procedures

a. Brain MRI

b. CT scan of head

c. Culture of cerebrospinal fluid (CSF) and serology tests

d. Electroencephalogram (EEG)

CONDITION: Glomerulonephritis or Acute Nephrotic Syndrome

PHYSIOLOGY: This condition is a form of nephritis in which the lesions involve primarily the glomeruli. It may be acute, subacute, or chronic. Acute glomerulonephritis, also known as acute nephritic syndrome, frequently follows infections, especially those of the upper respiratory tract caused by particular strains of streptococci. It may also be caused by systemic lupus erythematosus, subacute bacterial endocarditis, cryoglobulinemia, and various forms of vasculitis including polyarteritis nodosa, Henoch-Schönlein purpura, and visceral abscess. The condition is characterized by the presence of blood in the urine (hematuria), protein in the urine (proteinuria), and red cell casts; oliguria, edema, pruritus, nausea, constipation, and hypertension. Investigation of serum complement levels and renal biopsy facilitates diagnosis and helps to establish the prognosis (*Taber's*, 2009).

HANDOFF COMMUNICATION

S	Situation	Assess what is currently happening in a short statement.	Child presents as _____
B	Background	Summarize important past assessment data for your patient here. Place lab results and medications on the concept map.	Age: Gender: Allergies: Fall Risk: Isolation:
A	Assessment	Use the assessment data to complete your concept map.	**Nursing Diagnosis:** Place the Nursing Diagnoses in prioritized order on the concept map and add any needed for your specific patient. **Plan:** Place any further Nursing Interventions Classifications (NIC) needed on the map.

Implement Your Plan of Care

R	Recommendation	Evaluate your nursing care and make recommendations related to the achievement of your desired outcomes. Were they met, or do new goals need to be established?	**EVALUATE YOUR CARE**	
			Diag / **Nursing Outcomes Classification (NOC)**	**Outcome met**
			1 Patient demonstrates adequate fluid balance evidenced by stable vital signs (VS), palpable pulses of good quality, normal skin turgor, moist mucous membranes, individual-appropriate urinary output, lack of excessive weight fluctuations, and absence of edema.	☐ Yes ☐ No
			2 Patient manifests decreased restlessness or irritability.	☐ Yes ☐ No
			3 Patient experiences no signs of malnutrition.	☐ Yes ☐ No
			4 Patient's growth and development are monitored.	☐ Yes ☐ No
			5	☐ Yes ☐ No

Nursing Diagnosis 1

Excess fluid volume related to failure of regulatory mechanism (inflammation of glomerular membrane filtration) evidenced by weight gain, edema or anasarca, intake greater than output, and blood pressure changes.

NIC:
1) Monitor VS, mucous membranes, weight, skin turgor, breath sounds, urinary and gastric output; **2)** Review intake of fluids; and **3)** Administer IV using a control pump for pediatric patients.

Nursing Diagnosis 2

Acute pain related to circulation of toxins and edema and distention of renal capsule evidenced by verbal reports, guarding or distracted behavior, and changes in VS.

NIC:
1) Perform routine comprehensive pain assessment; **2)** Accept child's description of pain; **3)** Investigate changes in or frequency of pain; **4)** Observe for rigidity, crying; **5)** Provide comfort measures, holding, repositioning; **6)** Encourage sleep and rest periods; and **7)** Administer analgesics as ordered.

Nursing Diagnosis 3

Imbalanced nutrition: less than body requirements related to anorexia and dietary restrictions evidenced by aversion to eating, altered taste, weight loss, or decreased intake.

NIC:
1) Assess abdomen noting circumference, bowel sounds, and distention; **2)** Observe color and consistency of stools; **3)** Promote foods that are high in protein; **4)** Administer parenteral feedings as ordered; and **5)** Provide nonnutritive sucking.

Nursing Diagnosis 4

Risk for disproportionate growth related to chronic illness.

NIC:
1) Assess current growth and developmental stage; **2)** Use age-appropriate tests; **3)** Determine cognitive and perceptual levels; **4)** Encourage self-care activities; and **5)** Provide parents with information, support, and referrals.

Condition:
Glomerulonephritis or Acute Nephrotic Syndrome
Age:

Link & Explain
• Nursing Interventions Classification (NIC)
• Laboratory and Diagnostic Procedures
• Medications

Nursing Diagnosis 5

NIC:

Medications

a.

b.

c.

d.

Laboratory & Diagnostic Procedures

a. Abdominal CT scan and ultrasound; chest x-ray

b. Urinalysis for creatinine clearance, protein, uric acid, specific gravity

c. Blood for albumin, antiglomerular basement membrane antibodies, antineutrophil cytoplasmic antibodies (ANCAs), BUN and creatinine, and complement component 3 complement levels

d. IVP (intravenous pyelogram)

CONDITION: Hemophilia

PHYSIOLOGY: Hemophilia is a group of hereditary bleeding disorders marked by deficiencies of blood-clotting proteins. Hemophilias are rare. Hemophilia A affects 1 in 5,000 to 10,000 boys; hemophilia B is present in about 1 in 30,000 boys (*Taber's*, 2009).

HANDOFF COMMUNICATION

S	Situation	Assess what is currently happening in a short statement.	Child presents as _____
B	Background	Summarize important past assessment data for your patient here. Place lab results and medications on the concept map.	**Age:** **Gender:** **Allergies:** **Fall Risk:** **Isolation:**
A	Assessment	Use the assessment data to complete your concept map.	**Nursing Diagnosis:** Place the Nursing Diagnoses in prioritized order on the concept map and add any needed for your specific patient. **Plan:** Place any further Nursing Interventions Classifications (NIC) needed on the map.

Implement Your Plan of Care

		EVALUATE YOUR CARE		
R	Recommendation	Evaluate your nursing care and make recommendations related to the achievement of your desired outcomes. Were they met, or do new goals need to be established?	**Diag** / **Nursing Outcomes Classification (NOC)**	**Outcome met**
			1 Patient demonstrates improved tissue perfusion evidenced by stabilized vital signs (VS), strong and palpable peripheral pulses, adequate urinary output, absence of pain, usual mental status, normal capillary refill, warm and dry skin, natural pale pink nail beds and lips, and absence of paresthesia.	☐ Yes ☐ No
			2 Patient manifests decreased restlessness or irritability and reports of pain.	☐ Yes ☐ No
			3 Patient's strength and function in affected body parts are maintained or increased.	☐ Yes ☐ No
			4 Patient engages in satisfying activities within personal limitations.	☐ Yes ☐ No
			5	☐ Yes ☐ No

Nursing Diagnosis 1

Ineffective tissue perfusion related to bleeding into joints evidenced by swollen and painful joints.

NIC:
1) Monitor VS carefully; **2)** Assess joints or area of bleeding; **3)** Assess area peripheral to the bleed for circulation; **4)** Maintain adequate fluid intake; **5)** Evaluate for edema and swelling; and **6)** Administer clotting factor as prescribed.

Nursing Diagnosis 2

Acute pain related to inflammation and hematoma development in joints or soft tissue producing edema evidenced by changes in VS, restlessness, complaints, and crying.

NIC:
1) Perform routine comprehensive pain assessment; **2)** Accept child's description of pain; **3)** Investigate changes in or frequency of pain; **4)** Observe for areas of bleed; **5)** Provide comfort measures; **6)** Encourage sleep and rest periods; **7)** Splint and apply ice to area of bleed; and **8)** Medicate as indicated.

Nursing Diagnosis 3

Impaired mobility related to pain, swelling, and discomfort in joint evidenced by limited joint range of motion (ROM).

NIC:
1) Determine functional ability on a scale of 0–4; **2)** Note emotional responses to impaired mobility; **3)** Splint affected limb in acute phase; **4)** Ice joint to decrease bleeding; **5)** Plan appropriate activities and rest periods; and **6)** Refer to physical therapy.

Nursing Diagnosis 4

Deficit diversional activity related to physical limitations caused by "bleed" evidenced by statements of boredom or withdrawal behavior.

NIC:
1) Determine previous hobbies or activities; **2)** Encourage a mix of activities; **3)** Change scenery when possible; and **4)** Refer to occupational or recreational therapist.

Condition:
Hemophilia
Age:

Link & Explain
• Nursing Interventions Classification (NIC)
• Laboratory and Diagnostic Procedures
• Medications

Nursing Diagnosis 5

NIC:

Medications

a. Factor VIII or IX replacement

b.

c.

d.

Laboratory & Diagnostic Procedures

a. X-ray of affected limb

b.

c.

d.

CONDITION: Hirschsprung's Disease

PHYSIOLOGY: Hirschsprung's disease is the most common cause of lower gastrointestinal obstruction in neonates. It occurs in 1 in 5,000 children, with a male-to-female ratio of 4:1. About 15% of cases are diagnosed in the first month of life, 64% by the third month, and 80% by age 1 year. Patients with this disease exhibit signs of an extremely dilated colon and accompanying chronic constipation, fecal impaction, and overflow diarrhea. This condition is caused by congenital absence of some or all of the normal bowel parasympathetic ganglion cells. The aganglionic bowel segment contracts, but there is no reciprocal relaxation, so feces cannot be propelled onward through the bowel. Barium contrast enema is usually used for diagnosis, but rectal biopsy is the diagnostic standard. Treatment is surgical excision of the affected segment and reanastomosis of healthy bowel by any of several procedures. Unless diagnosed and treated quickly, the colonic obstruction of Hirschsprung's may result in fecal stagnation, bacterial overgrowth with toxin production, enterocolitis, hypovolemic shock, and infant death (*Taber's*, 2009).

HANDOFF COMMUNICATION

S Situation	Assess what is currently happening in a short statement.	Child presents as _____	
B Background	Summarize important past assessment data for your patient here. Place lab results and medications on the concept map.	**Age:** **Allergies:** **Isolation:**	**Gender:** **Fall Risk:**
A Assessment	Use the assessment data to complete your concept map.	**Nursing Diagnosis:** Place the Nursing Diagnoses in prioritized order on the concept map and add any needed for your specific patient. **Plan:** Place any further Nursing Interventions Classifications (NIC) needed on the map.	

Implement Your Plan of Care

		EVALUATE YOUR CARE		
R Recommendation	Evaluate your nursing care and make recommendations related to the achievement of your desired outcomes. Were they met, or do new goals need to be established?	**Diag**	**Nursing Outcomes Classification (NOC)**	**Outcome met**
		1	Patient demonstrates adequate fluid balance evidenced by stable vital signs (VS), normal skin turgor, moist mucous membranes, adequate urinary output, and lack of excessive weight loss.	☐ Yes ☐ No
		2	Patient indicates pain is relieved or controlled; manifests decreased restlessness and irritability; and demonstrates age-appropriate blood pressure, pulse, and respiratory rate. Patient/caregiver follows prescribed pharmacological regimen, verbalizes (if possible) nonpharmacological methods that provide relief, and demonstrates use of diversional activities as indicated.	☐ Yes ☐ No
		3	Patient/caregiver verbalizes understanding of individual causative factors or risk factors, identifies interventions to prevent or reduce risk of infection, and demonstrates techniques to promote a safe environment. Patient achieves timely wound healing, is free of purulent drainage or erythema, and is afebrile.	☐ Yes ☐ No
		4	Patient/caregiver identifies individual risk factors, verbalizes understanding of treatment/therapy regimen, and demonstrates behaviors and techniques to prevent skin breakdown.	☐ Yes ☐ No
		5		☐ Yes ☐ No

Nursing Diagnosis 1

Deficient fluid volume related to active fluid loss evidenced by decreased urine output, decreased skin turgor, dry mucous membranes, weight loss, and increased pulse rate.

NIC:
1) Monitor VS, mucous membranes, weight, skin turgor, and urinary output; **2)** Review child's intake of fluids; and **3)** Discuss individual risk factors, potential problems, and specific interventions (e.g., fluid replacement options).

Nursing Diagnosis 2

Acute pain/impaired comfort related to disease process and/or surgical intervention as possibly evidenced by changes in appetite, eating, sleep patterns, restlessness, and irritability.

NIC:
1) Assess etiology/precipitating contributory factors; **2)** Evaluate patient's response to pain (use pain rating scale appropriate for age and cognition); and **3)** Assist patient to explore methods for alleviation/control of pain (suggest parental presence during procedures to comfort child).

Nursing Diagnosis 3

Risk for infection may be related to inadequate primary defenses (altered peristalsis) and/or invasive and surgical procedures.

NIC:
1) Note risk factors for occurrence of infection (e.g., extremes of age, skin/tissue wounds, invasive/surgical procedures); **2)** Observe for signs of infection at insertion sites of invasive lines, sutures, surgical incisions; **3)** Note signs and symptoms of sepsis (systemic infection); and **4)** Administer medication regimen including antibiotics and immunizations as indicated and ordered.

Nursing Diagnosis 4

Risk for impaired skin integrity may be related to extremes of age, imbalanced nutritional status, impaired metabolic state, and mechanical factors.

NIC:
1) Assess skin routinely, noting moisture, color, and elasticity; **2)** Review pertinent lab results (e.g., Hb/Hct, glucose, presence of infectious agents, albumin, and protein) that may correlate with decreased wound healing; **3)** Handle patient gently (particularly infant), as epidermis is thin and prone to injury; **4)** Maintain meticulous skin hygiene using mild nondetergent soap, drying thoroughly and lubricating with emollient, as indicated; and **5)** Emphasize importance of adequate nutritional and fluid intake.

Condition:
Hirschsprung's Disease
Age:

Link & Explain
• Nursing Interventions Classification (NIC)
• Laboratory and Diagnostic Procedures
• Medications

Nursing Diagnosis 5

NIC:

Medications

a. Polyethylene glycol 3350

b. Metronidazole (Flagyl)

c. Normal saline rectal irrigations 3–4 times daily

d. Nutritional Supplement

Laboratory & Diagnostic Procedures

a. Abdominal radiographic studies

b. Barium enema

c. Rectal manometry

d. Rectal biopsy

CONDITION: Hydrocephalus

PHYSIOLOGY: Hydrocephalus is the accumulation of excessive amounts of cerebrospinal fluid (CSF) within the ventricles of the brain, resulting from blockage or destruction of the normal channels for CSF drainage. Common causes include congenital lesions (e.g., spinal bifida or aqueductal stenosis), traumatic lesions, neoplastic lesions, and infections such as meningoencephalitis. Sometimes the accumulated fluid leads to increased intracranial pressure (ICP) (*Taber's*, 2009).

HANDOFF COMMUNICATION

S Situation	Assess what is currently happening in a short statement.	Child presents as _____
B Background	Summarize important past assessment data for your patient here. Place lab results and medications on the concept map.	**Age:** **Gender:** **Allergies:** **Fall Risk:** **Isolation:**
A Assessment	Use the assessment data to complete your concept map.	**Nursing Diagnosis:** Place the Nursing Diagnoses in prioritized order on the concept map and add any needed for your specific patient. **Plan:** Place any further Nursing Interventions Classifications (NIC) needed on the map.

Implement Your Plan of Care

R Recommendation	Evaluate your nursing care and make recommendations related to the achievement of your desired outcomes. Were they met, or do new goals need to be established?	**Diag**	**EVALUATE YOUR CARE** **Nursing Outcomes Classification (NOC)**	**Outcome met**
		1	Patient maintains usual or improved level of consciousness (LOC), cognition, and motor and sensory function.	☐ Yes ☐ No
		2	Patient maintains current visual field and acuity without further loss.	☐ Yes ☐ No
		3	Patient maintains or increases strength and function in affected body parts.	☐ Yes ☐ No
		4	Parents/caregivers participate in learning process; identify interferences to learning and specific actions to deal with them; verbalize understanding of condition, disease process, and treatment; and perform necessary procedures correctly and explain reasons for the actions.	☐ Yes ☐ No
		5		☐ Yes ☐ No

Nursing Diagnosis 1

Ineffective cerebral tissue perfusion related to fluid accumulation evidenced by altered states of consciousness.

NIC:
1) Monitor and document age-appropriate neurological status frequently and compare to baseline assessment; **2)** Evaluate eye opening, response to environmental stimuli, and pupil reactivity; **3)** Assess verbal responses; **4)** Assess motor responses; **5)** Monitor vital signs (VS); and **6)** Note presence of age-appropriate reflexes.

Nursing Diagnosis 2

Disturbed visual sensory perception related to pressure on sensorimotor nerves evidenced by strabismus, nystagmus, papillary changes, and optic atrophy.

NIC:
1) Provide safety in environment: reduce clutter, use side rails or crib rails, arrange furniture, put objects so child can see if possible; **2)** Elevate head of bed (HOB); and **3)** Use correct lighting.

Nursing Diagnosis 3

Risk for impaired physical mobility related to neuromuscular impairment, decreased muscle strength, and impaired coordination.

NIC:
1) Determine functional ability on a scale of 0–4; **2)** Note emotional responses to impaired mobility; **3)** Plan appropriate activities and rest periods; and **4)** Refer to physical therapy.

Nursing Diagnosis 4

Knowledge deficit (caretakers) regarding pathophysiology of condition, management, and available community resources related to insufficient information, and misconceptions evidenced by statements of concerns and questions.

NIC:
1) Ascertain readiness, level of knowledge, and individual learning needs; **2)** Provide positive reinforcement; **3)** Provide access information for contact person and identify available community resources and support groups; **4)** Explain to family the process of the treatments; and **5)** Encourage verbalization.

Condition:
Hydrocephalus
Age:

Link & Explain
• Nursing Interventions Classification (NIC)
• Laboratory and Diagnostic Procedures
• Medications

Nursing Diagnosis 5

NIC:

Medications

a. Antibiotics may be ordered

b.

c.

d.

Laboratory & Diagnostic Procedures

a. Head CT

b. Arteriography, brain scan using radioisotopes; cranial ultrasound (an ultrasound of the brain)

c. Lumbar puncture and examination of the cerebrospinal fluid

d. Skull x-ray

CONDITION: Hypertropic Pyloric Disorder (Pyloric Stenosis)

PHYSIOLOGY: Pyloric stenosis is a narrowing of the pyloric orifice located at the lower portion of the stomach that opens into the duodenum. In infants, excessive thickening of the pyloric sphincter or hypertrophy of the mucosa of the pylorus is responsible for the condition. Infantile pyloric stenosis is usually diagnosed in the first 6 months of life when infants have trouble with vomiting after eating, sometimes with projectile vomiting and consequent dehydration. The disease occurs in 2 to 3 infants per 1,000 births and is more common in boys than girls. In infants, treatment may involve open or laparoscopic division of the muscles of the pylorus (*Taber's*, 2009).

HANDOFF COMMUNICATION

S	Situation	Assess what is currently happening in a short statement.	Child presents as _____
B	Background	Summarize important past assessment data for your patient here. Place lab results and medications on the concept map.	**Age:** **Gender:** **Allergies:** **Fall Risk:** **Isolation:** **Immunization status:** **PMH:** **PSH:**
A	Assessment	Use the assessment data to complete your concept map.	**Nursing Diagnosis:** Place the Nursing Diagnoses in prioritized order on the concept map and add any needed for your specific patient. **Plan:** Place any further Nursing Interventions Classifications (NIC) needed on the map.

Implement Your Plan of Care

		EVALUATE YOUR CARE		
R	Recommendation *Evaluate your nursing care and make recommendations related to the achievement of your desired outcomes. Were they met, or do new goals need to be established?*	**Diag**	**Nursing Outcomes Classification (NOC)**	**Outcome met**
		1	Patient demonstrates adequate fluid balance evidenced by stable vital signs (VS), normal skin turgor, moist mucous membranes, adequate urinary output, and lack of excessive weight loss.	☐ Yes ☐ No
		2	Patient indicates pain is relieved or controlled; manifests decreased restlessness and irritability; demonstrates age-appropriate blood pressure, pulse, and respiratory rate. Parents/patient follow prescribed pharmacological regimen, verbalize nonpharmacological methods that provide relief, and demonstrate use of diversional activities as indicated.	☐ Yes ☐ No
		3	Patient maintains stable weight, demonstrates progressive weight gain toward goal with normalization of laboratory values, and is free of signs of malnutrition.	☐ Yes ☐ No
		4	Improvement in sleep or rest pattern is observed or reported.	☐ Yes ☐ No
		5		☐ Yes ☐ No

Nursing Diagnosis 1

Fluid volume deficit related to the effects of frequent vomiting evidenced by decreased urine output, decreased skin turgor, dry mucous membranes, weight loss, and increased pulse rate.

NIC:
1) Monitor VS, laboratory values, mucous membranes, weight, skin turgor, and urinary output; **2)** Review child's intake of fluids and IV; and **3)** Discuss individual risk factors, potential problems, and specific interventions (e.g., fluid replacement options).

Nursing Diagnosis 2

Acute pain/impaired comfort may be related to disease process and/or surgical intervention as possibly evidenced by changes in appetite, eating, sleep patterns, restlessness, and irritability.

NIC:
1) Assess etiology/precipitating contributory factors; **2)** Evaluate client's response to pain (use pain rating scale appropriate for age and cognition); and **3)** Assist client to explore methods for alleviation/control of pain (suggest parental presence during procedures to comfort child).

Nursing Diagnosis 3

Nutrition imbalance: less than body requirements related to vomiting and gradual reintroduction of feeding evidenced by weight loss, lab tests reflecting nutritional deficiencies, and poor muscle tone.

NIC:
1) Note admission weight and compare with subsequent readings; **2)** Monitor tolerance to fluid and food intake when resumed; and **3)** Monitor laboratory studies: Hb/Hct, electrolytes, and total protein and albumin.

Nursing Diagnosis 4

Sleep pattern disturbed related to hunger and discomfort evidenced by wakefulness, disrupted sleep, irritability, and lethargy.

NIC:
1) Adhere to regular sleep schedule and rituals; **2)** Administer medications as ordered to reduce discomfort; **3)** Reduce environmental sounds that could interfere with restful sleep; **4)** Avoid or limit interruptions such as awakening for medications or therapies; and **5)** Position for comfort as needed.

Nursing Diagnosis 5

NIC:

Condition:
Hypertropic Pyloric Disorder (Pyloric Stenosis)
Age:
_____
Link & Explain
• Nursing Interventions Classification (NIC)
• Laboratory and Diagnostic Procedures
• Medications

Medications

a.

b.

c.

d.

Laboratory & Diagnostic Procedures

a. Abdominal ultrasound

b. Upper gastrointestinal (UGI) study

c. Labs: CBC, serum electrolytes, protein, albumin

d.

CONDITION: Immunizations, Anticipatory Guidance

PHYSIOLOGY: Immunizations protect against many devastating childhood diseases, including diphtheria, pertussis, tetanus (DTaP); polio virus (IPV); measles, mumps, rubella (MMR); *Haemophilus* influenzae type B (HIB); varicella; pneumococcus infection (Prevnar); rotavirus; hepatitis A and B; human papillomavirus (Gardasil); meningococcal infection (Menactra); and influenza. Immunizations are either passive or active. Active immunizations require administration of a weakened antigen, which stimulates the production of antibodies against the disease without causing clinical disease, such as a live virus (MMR or varicella). Passive immunizations may be provided with administration of antibodies in a vaccine form. The antibodies are produced in a human or animal host and given to the child to prevent the disease or reduce its severity from a single exposure. Examples of passive immunity are Iga antibodies in breastfeeding and hepatitis immunoglobulin given to an infant whose mother is hepatitis B positive (Doenges, Moorhouse, & Murr, 2009; Ward & Hisley, 2009).

HANDOFF COMMUNICATION

S Situation	Assess what is currently happening in a short statement.	Child presents as _____	
B Background	Summarize important past assessment data for your patient here. Place lab results and medications on the concept map.	**Age:** **Allergies:** **Isolation:** **Immunization status:**	**Gender:** **Fall Risk:**
A Assessment	Use the assessment data to complete your concept map.	**Nursing Diagnosis:** Place the Nursing Diagnoses in prioritized order on the concept map and add any needed for your specific patient. **Plan:** Place any further Nursing Interventions Classifications (NIC) needed on the map.	

Implement Your Plan of Care

		EVALUATE YOUR CARE		
R Recommendation	Evaluate your nursing care and make recommendations related to the achievement of your desired outcomes. Were they met, or do new goals need to be established?	**Diag**	**Nursing Outcomes Classification (NOC)**	**Outcome met**
		1	Patient has adequate immune protection from vaccine-preventable disease.	☐ Yes ☐ No
		2	Parents/caregivers sign consent for vaccine, confirm reason for vaccine, acknowledge common side effects and treatment.	☐ Yes ☐ No
		3	Parents'/caregivers' anxiety is reduced; patient has minimal adverse side effects from vaccines and is easily comforted.	☐ Yes ☐ No
		4	Patient has reduced severe reaction to an immunization; occurrences are managed efficiently and reported to the appropriate agencies.	☐ Yes ☐ No
		5		☐ Yes ☐ No

Nursing Diagnosis 1

Risk of infection due to immature immune function and opportunistic infections.

NIC:
1) Assess immunization record for each child's well visit and hospitalizations; 2) Review health history and contradictions to immunizations (e.g., immunocompromised child, child on chemotherapy or high-dose steroids); 3) Review allergies or adverse effects from prior immunizations; and 4) Identify vaccines that can be given simultaneously.

Nursing Diagnosis 2

Knowledge deficit of caregiver for effective therapeutic measures related to current myths evidenced by caregiver relating fears and untruths about immunizations.

NIC:
1) Document consent for immunizations; 2) Educate parents/caregivers and adolescent on the need for specific vaccines, risks of nonimmunization, and side effects; 3) Describe common side effects with each immunization, such as swelling, redness at injection site, fever, irritability, and rash; 4) Explain treatment for side effects such as administration of acetaminophen, ibuprofen, and cool pack to extremity; and 5) Document immunization administration and instruction to caregiver.

Nursing Diagnosis 3

Pain and discomfort due to pain associated with injection and fear/anxiety evidenced by child crying.

NIC:
1) Prepare immunizations prior to administration to be given without delay in order to decrease anxiety; 2) Provide distraction or immobilize child for safe administration; 3) Provide appropriate age/developmental preparation before administering immunization; 4) Provide praise, rewards, and comfort after injection; and 5) Consider EMLA cream 15–30 minutes prior to injection.

Nursing Diagnosis 4

Risk of injury related to adverse immunization reaction.

NIC:
1) Emergency equipment available in outpatient and inpatient facilities to prepare for severe anaphylaxis reaction; 2) Monitor child for at least 15 minutes after immunization; 3) Inform parents to report fever 104°F within 48 hours, inconsolable crying >3 hours, pale or limp within 48 hours, and seizure within 72 hours; and 4) Report all adverse side effects to VAERS (Vaccine Adverse Event Report System), a CDC website.

Condition:
Immunizations, Anticipatory Guidance
Age:

Link & Explain
• Nursing Interventions Classification (NIC)
• Laboratory and Diagnostic Procedures
• Medications

Nursing Diagnosis 5

NIC:

Medications

a. Acetaminophen

b. Ibuprofen

c. EMLA cream for injection site

d. Sucrose 12% or 24% po

Laboratory & Diagnostic Procedures

a.

b.

c.

d.

CONDITION: Intussusception and Malrotation

PHYSIOLOGY: Intussusception is a gastrointestinal obstruction disorder that occurs in the proximal section of the intestine and mesentery and telescopes into a distal section of the intestine. The common occurrence is between 3 months and 5 years of age and often occurs in children 5–9 months of age. The cause is often unknown, but predisposing factors include Meckel's diverticulum, constipation, parasites, rotavirus, adenovirus, Henoch-Schonlein purpura, lymphomas, and lipomas. The signs and symptoms include intermittent acute abdominal pain, screaming, drawing up legs with period of rest, a sausage shape mass in the upper right quadrant of the abdomen (Dance's sign) or other areas on palpation, fever, projectile bilious vomiting, abdominal distention, and currant jelly stools. The treatment includes a barium or air enema in which the pressure allows the bowel to unfold and return to its normal position. If radiological intervention is not successful, surgery is indicated.

Malrotation occurs when the small bowel fails to rotate into its normal position during fetal life at 5–10 weeks' gestation. Volvulus is a twisting of the bowel upon itself, causing obstruction and ischemia. The defect usually occurs at sigmoid and ileocecal areas of intestine. The disorder leads to necrosis (tissue death) of twisted portion of the intestine due to obstruction of the superior mesenteric artery (SMA) and is one of the common causes of short gut syndrome. The child usually presents in early in infancy with bilious vomiting, abdominal distention, and lethargy. Older children can present with cyclic vomiting and abdominal pain. Complication in both disorders can result in dehydration, shock, bowel necrosis, bowel perforation, and sepsis (Doenges, Moorhouse, & Murr, 2009; Ward & Hisley, 2009).

HANDOFF COMMUNICATION

S	Situation	Assess what is currently happening in a short statement.	Child presents as _____
B	Background	Summarize important past assessment data for your patient here. Place lab results and medications on the concept map.	**Age:**　　　　　　　　　　　　　**Gender:** **Allergies:**　　　　　　　　　**Fall Risk:** **Isolation:** **Immunization status:**
A	Assessment	Use the assessment data to complete your concept map.	**Nursing Diagnosis:** Place the Nursing Diagnoses in prioritized order on the concept map and add any needed for your specific patient. **Plan:** Place any further Nursing Interventions Classifications (NIC) needed on the map.

Implement Your Plan of Care

			EVALUATE YOUR CARE	
R	Recommendation	Evaluate your nursing care and make recommendations related to the achievement of your desired outcomes. Were they met, or do new goals need to be established?	**Diag** / **Nursing Outcomes Classification (NOC)**	**Outcome met**
			1 Patient has adequate circulating fluid volume evidenced by adequate fluid intake, age-appropriate vital signs, and adequate perfusion.	☐ Yes ☐ No
			2 Patient indicates pain is relieved or controlled; manifests decreased restlessness and irritability; demonstrates age-appropriate blood pressure, pulse, and respiratory rate. Parents/caregivers/patient follow prescribed pharmacological regimen, verbalize nonpharmacological methods that provide relief, and demonstrate use of diversional activities as indicated.	☐ Yes ☐ No
			3 Child has decreased symptoms or is free of an infection evidenced by normal temperature; age-appropriate vital signs; no abdominal tenderness or inflammation; CBC within normal limits (WNL); negative blood culture; and lack of lethargy, pallor, and vomiting.	☐ Yes ☐ No
			4 Patient has adequate nutrition evidenced by gaining weight and sufficient caloric consumption.	☐ Yes ☐ No
			5	☐ Yes ☐ No

Nursing Diagnosis 1

Deficient fluid volume related to decreased amount of circulating fluid volume related to vomiting evidenced by decreased urine output, decreased skin turgor, dry mucous membranes, weight loss, and increased pulse rate.

NIC:
1) Monitor vital signs, mucous membranes, weight, skin turgor, and urinary output; **2)** Review child's fluid intake; **3)** Discuss individual risk factors, potential problems, and specific interventions (e.g., fluid replacement options); **4)** Keep accurate I&O; **5)** Maintain NPO as ordered; and **6)** Ensure nasogastric (NG) tube is patent, record drainage, and replace fluid as appropriate.

Nursing Diagnosis 2

Acute pain/impaired comfort related to disease process and/or surgical intervention evidenced by changes in appetite, eating, sleep patterns, restlessness, and irritability.

NIC:
1) Assess etiology/precipitating contributory factors; **2)** Evaluate client's response to pain (use pain rating scale appropriate for age and cognition); and **3)** Assist client to explore methods for alleviation/control of pain (suggest parental presence during procedures to comfort child).

Nursing Diagnosis 3

Risk for infection may be related to necrotic bowel, risk of perforation, peritonitis evidenced by fever, abdominal distention, abdominal tenderness and erythema, lethargy, symptoms of septic shock.

NIC:
1) Assess and record VS q2h–q4h; **2)** Maintain good hand-washing technique; **3)** Note signs and symptoms of sepsis (systemic infection); **4)** Check and record results of CBC with differential, C-reactive protein (CRP), and blood cultures; notify primary care practitioner of abnormal results; **5)** Administer medication regimen, including antibiotics and antipyretics as prescribed; and **6)** Monitor surgical incision postoperatively.

Nursing Diagnosis 4

Altered nutrition less than body requirements related to nothing by mouth (NPO) status, potential bowel necrosis and resection and short bowel syndrome (especially with malrotation) evidenced by weight loss or lack of weight gain.

NIC:
1) Weigh infant every day with the same scale and at the same time; **2)** Record daily caloric counts; **3)** Administer total parenteral nutrition (TPN) via central or peripheral access as prescribed; **4)** Start enteral feedings as prescribed, and monitor tolerance; and **5)** If child is on long-term parenteral nutrition, monitor complete metabolic panel weekly.

Condition:
Intussusception and Malrotation

Age:

Link & Explain
• Nursing Interventions Classification (NIC)
• Laboratory and Diagnostic Procedures
• Medications

Nursing Diagnosis 5

NIC:

Medications

a. Antibiotics with gram-positive, gram-negative, and anaerobic coverage

b. Analgesics and or narcotics

c. Ibuprofen and acetaminophen

d. Total parenteral nutrition (TPN)

Laboratory & Diagnostic Procedures

a. Abdominal radiographic studies

b. Barium enema or air pressure enema

c. Surgical bowel resection

d. CBC with differential and platelets; C reactive protein (CRP); basic or complete metabolic panel; blood culture if indicated

CONDITION: Juvenile Rheumatoid Arthritis (Juvenile Idiopathic Arthritis)

PHYSIOLOGY: Juvenile rheumatoid arthritis (JRA) is a group of chronic, inflammatory diseases involving the joints and other organs in children under age 16. The age of onset is variable, as are the extra-articular manifestations. JRA affects about 1 in 1,000 children (150,000–250,000 in the United States alone) with overall incidence twice as high in females and is the most common form of arthritis in childhood. At least five subgroups are recognized (*Taber's*, 2009).

HANDOFF COMMUNICATION

S	Situation	Assess what is currently happening in a short statement.	Child presents as _____
B	Background	Summarize important past assessment data for your patient here. Place lab results and medications on the concept map.	Age: Gender: Allergies: Fall Risk: Isolation:
A	Assessment	Use the assessment data to complete your concept map.	**Nursing Diagnosis:** Place the Nursing Diagnoses in prioritized order on the concept map and add any needed for your specific patient. **Plan:** Place any further Nursing Interventions Classifications (NIC) needed on the map.

Implement Your Plan of Care

			EVALUATE YOUR CARE	
R	Recommendation	Evaluate your nursing care and make recommendations related to the achievement of your desired outcomes. Were they met, or do new goals need to be established?	**Diag** / **Nursing Outcomes Classification (NOC)**	**Outcome met**
			1 Patient manifests decreased restlessness or irritability and reports of pain.	☐ Yes ☐ No
			2 Patient maintains or increases strength and function in affected body parts.	☐ Yes ☐ No
			3 Patient's growth and development are monitored.	☐ Yes ☐ No
			4 Patient identifies stable support system and supportive individuals, uses resources for assistance as appropriate, and expresses increased self-esteem.	☐ Yes ☐ No
			5	☐ Yes ☐ No

Nursing Diagnosis 1

Acute or chronic pain related to accumulation of fluid, inflammation process, degeneration of joint, and deformity evidenced by verbal reports, behavior, and physical withdrawal.

NIC:
1) Perform routine comprehensive pain assessment; **2)** Accept child's description of pain; **3)** Investigate changes in or frequency of pain; **4)** Observe for area of edema; **5)** Provide comfort measures; **6)** Encourage sleep and rest periods; **7)** Apply ice to area; and **8)** Administer medication.

Nursing Diagnosis 2

Impaired physical mobility related to musculoskeletal deformities, pain, decreased muscle strength, limited range of motion (ROM) evidenced by reluctance to move.

NIC:
1) Determine functional ability on a scale of 0–4; **2)** Note emotional responses to impaired mobility; **3)** Splint affected limb in acute phase; **4)** Ice joint to decrease edema; **5)** Plan appropriate activities and rest periods; **6)** Use warm-up exercises before activities; and **7)** Refer to physical therapy.

Nursing Diagnosis 3

Risk for delayed development related to effects of physical disabilities and required therapies.

NIC:
1) Assess current growth and developmental stage; **2)** Use age-appropriate tests; **3)** Determine cognitive and perceptual levels; **4)** Encourage self-care activities; and **5)** Provide parents with information.

Nursing Diagnosis 4

Risk for social isolation related to altered state of wellness and changes in physical appearance.

NIC:
1) Determine child's response to condition; **2)** Assess coping mechanisms; **3)** Discuss concerns of child if the child is old enough; **4)** Identify available support systems; **5)** Assist child to problem-solve; and **6)** Be alert to verbal and nonverbal clues of withdrawal.

Condition:
Juvenile Rheumatoid Arthritis (Juvenile Idiopathic Arthritis)

Age:

Link & Explain
• Nursing Interventions Classification (NIC)
• Laboratory and Diagnostic Procedures
• Medications

Nursing Diagnosis 5

NIC:

Medications

a. Methotrexate; biologic drugs, such as etanercept and infliximab, block high levels of proteins that cause inflammation

b.

c.

d.

Laboratory & Diagnostic Procedures

a. Rheumatoid factor (not raised in all patients), CBC with differential

b. Erythrocyte sedimentation rate (ESR)

c. ANA (may be high); HLA antigens for HLA B27

d. Joint x-ray, eye exam, chest x-ray, ECG

CONDITION: Lead Poisoning

PHYSIOLOGY: Lead poisoning is caused by ingestion or inhalation of substances containing lead. Symptoms of acute lead poisoning include a metallic taste in the mouth, burns in the throat and pharynx, and later abdominal cramps and prostration. Chronic lead poisoning is characterized by anorexia, nausea, vomiting, excess salivation, anemia, a lead line on the gums, abdominal pains, muscle cramps, kidney failure, encephalopathy, seizures, learning disabilities, and pains in the joints (*Taber's*, 2009).

HANDOFF COMMUNICATION

S	Situation	Assess what is currently happening in a short statement.	Child presents as _____
B	Background	Summarize important past assessment data for your patient here. Place lab results and medications on the concept map.	**Age:** **Gender:** **Allergies:** **Fall Risk:** **Isolation:**
A	Assessment	Use the assessment data to complete your concept map.	**Nursing Diagnosis:** Place the Nursing Diagnoses in prioritized order on the concept map and add any needed for your specific patient. **Plan:** Place any further Nursing Interventions Classifications (NIC) needed on the map.

Implement Your Plan of Care

			EVALUATE YOUR CARE	
R	Recommendation	Evaluate your nursing care and make recommendations related to the achievement of your desired outcomes. Were they met, or do new goals need to be established?	**Diag** / **Nursing Outcomes Classification (NOC)**	**Outcome met**
			1 — Patient's prescribed drug regimen is maintained without untoward effects.	☐ Yes ☐ No
			2 — Patient is free of injury.	☐ Yes ☐ No
			3 — Patient maintains fluid volume at a functional level evidenced by individually adequate urinary output with normal specific gravity, stable vital signs (VS), moist mucous membranes, good skin turgor, and prompt capillary refill.	☐ Yes ☐ No
			4 — Parents/caregivers participate in learning process; verbalize understanding of condition, disease process, and treatment; identify relationship of signs/symptoms to the disease process and correlate symptoms with causative factors; initiate necessary lifestyle changes; and participate in treatment regimen.	☐ Yes ☐ No
			5 —	☐ Yes ☐ No

Nursing Diagnosis 1

Poisoning related to flaking or peeling paint, improperly lead-glazed ceramic pottery, unprotected contact with lead, imported herbal products or medicines evidenced by abdominal cramping, headache, irritability, decreased attentiveness, constipation, and/or tremors.

NIC:
1) Determine source of lead; **2)** Observe for changes in behavior and physiological signs and test results; **3)** Obtain serum level as ordered; and **4)** Administer medication as ordered.

Nursing Diagnosis 2

Risk for trauma related to loss of coordination, altered level of consciousness (LOC), clonic or tonic muscle activity, and/or neurological damage.

NIC:
1) Identify individual risk factors; **2)** Have age-appropriate equipment; **3)** Use side rails or crib rails; **4)** Assess LOC frequently; and **5)** Assist out of bed (OOB).

Nursing Diagnosis 3

Risk for fluid volume deficit related to excessive vomiting, diarrhea, or decreased intake.

NIC:
1) Monitor VS; **2)** Palpate peripheral pulses; **3)** Monitor I&O; **4)** Monitor daily weight; **5)** Ascertain child's beverage preference; and **6)** Administer IV as ordered.

Nursing Diagnosis 4

Knowledge deficit regarding pathophysiology of condition, management, and available community resources related to insufficient information and misconceptions evidenced by statements of concerns and questions.

NIC:
1) Ascertain readiness, level of knowledge, and individual learning needs; **2)** Provide positive reinforcement; **3)** Provide access information for contact person and identify available community resources and support groups; **4)** Explain preventative interventions needed; and **5)** Encourage fluids and a high-protein diet.

Condition:
Lead Poisoning
Age:

Link & Explain
• Nursing Interventions Classification (NIC)
• Laboratory and Diagnostic Procedures
• Medications

Nursing Diagnosis 5

NIC:

Medications

a. Chelation therapy

b. Treatment of iron, calcium, and zinc deficiencies

c. Anticonvulsives

d.

Laboratory & Diagnostic Procedures

a. Blood lead level (BLL)

b.

c.

d.

CONDITION: Leukemia

PHYSIOLOGY: Leukemia is any of a class of hematological malignancies of bone marrow cells in which there is a production of white blood cells (WBCs) that do not mature correctly but continue to reproduce. As normal blood cells are depleted from the body, anemia, infection, hemorrhage, or death may result. Acute lymphocytic leukemia (ALL) is the most common leukemia that affects children between the ages of 2 and 4 years. Acute myelogenous leukemia (AML) is the second-most common form of leukemia that affects children by the age of 2, and it is often seen in teenagers. Children with genetic syndromes such as Down syndrome, Bloom syndrome, and Kostmann syndrome are at a higher risk for developing AML than other children. In children, gene mutations and chromosome abnormalities in cells that cause leukemia occur by chance and are not inherited.

HANDOFF COMMUNICATION

S	Situation	Assess what is currently happening in a short statement.	Child presents as _____
B	Background	Summarize important past assessment data for your patient here. Place lab results and medications on the concept map.	**Age:** **Gender:** **Allergies:** **Fall Risk:** **Isolation:**
A	Assessment	Use the assessment data to complete your concept map.	**Nursing Diagnosis:** Place the Nursing Diagnoses in prioritized order on the concept map and add any needed for your specific patient. **Plan:** Place any further Nursing Interventions Classifications (NIC) needed on the map.

Implement Your Plan of Care

		EVALUATE YOUR CARE		
	Evaluate your nursing care and make recommendations related to the achievement of your desired outcomes. Were they met, or do new goals need to be established?	**Diag**	**Nursing Outcomes Classification (NOC)**	**Outcome met**
R (Recommendation)		1	Patient maintains or demonstrates improvement in laboratory values.	☐ Yes ☐ No
		2	Family participates in activities to reduce the risk of infection.	☐ Yes ☐ No
		3	Patient participates in customary activities at desired level; reports or displays absence of fatigue.	☐ Yes ☐ No
		4	Parents/caregivers/patient participate in learning process; identify interferences to learning and specific actions to deal with them; verbalize understanding of condition, disease process, and treatment; perform necessary procedures correctly and explain reasons for the actions.	☐ Yes ☐ No
		5		☐ Yes ☐ No

Nursing Diagnosis 1

Ineffective protection related to abnormal blood profiles, drug therapy (cytotoxic agents, steroids), radiation treatments evidenced by deficient immunity, impaired healing, altered clotting, or weakness.

NIC:
1) Note reports of increasing fatigue and weakness; 2) Monitor vital signs (VS); 3) Evaluate responses to activity; 4) Observe signs and symptoms of infection; 5) Monitor laboratory values; and 6) Administer medications as indicated.

Nursing Diagnosis 2

Risk for infection related to inadequate secondary defenses (alterations in mature WBCs), increased number of immune lymphocytes, immunosuppression and bone marrow suppression), invasive procedures, and/or malnutrition.

NIC:
1) Strict aseptic technique; 2) Model and emphasize good hand washing; 3) Observe for signs and symptoms of infection; 4) Prepare for surgical intervention or postoperative care; 5) Take VS frequently; and 6) Note change in respirations or heart rate.

Nursing Diagnosis 3

Activity intolerance related to reduced energy stores, increased metabolic rate, imbalance between O_2 supply and demand: anemia, hypoxia, therapeutic restrictions evidenced by general weakness and fatigue.

NIC:
1) Determine child's usual activity level; 2) Note emotional responses to impaired mobility; 3) Plan appropriate activities and rest periods; 4) Refer to physical therapy; and 5) Allow child to engage in usual play activities within tolerance.

Nursing Diagnosis 4

Knowledge deficit regarding pathophysiology of condition, management, and available community resources related to insufficient information and misconceptions evidenced by statements of concerns and questions.

NIC:
1) Ascertain readiness, level of knowledge, and individual learning needs; 2) Provide positive reinforcement; 3) Provide access information for contact person and identify available community resources and support groups; 4) Explain treatments, procedures, and prognosis; 5) Encourage fluids and a high-protein diet; and 6) Provide information to child related to age of understanding.

Condition:
Leukemia
Age:

- -
Link & Explain
• Nursing Interventions Classification (NIC)
• Laboratory and Diagnostic Procedures
• Medications

Nursing Diagnosis 5

NIC:

Medications

a. Chemotherapy, intrathecal medications/chemotherapy

b. Chlorambucil or cyclophosphamide

c. Prednisone

d. Radiation therapy

Laboratory & Diagnostic Procedures

a. Frequent CBCs with differential

b. Bone marrow examination

c.

d.

CONDITION: Nephroblastoma (Wilms' Tumor)

PHYSIOLOGY: A rapidly developing tumor of the kidney that usually occurs in children. It is the most common renal tumor of childhood. It is associated with chromosomal deletions, especially from chromosomes 11 and 16. In the past, the mortality from this type of cancer was extremely high; however, newer approaches to therapy have been very effective in controlling the tumor in about 90% of patients (*Taber's*, 2009).

HANDOFF COMMUNICATION

S Situation	Assess what is currently happening in a short statement.	Child presents as _____
B Background	Summarize important past assessment data for your patient here. Place lab results and medications on the concept map.	**Age:** **Gender:** **Allergies:** **Fall Risk:** **Isolation:**
A Assessment	Use the assessment data to complete your concept map.	**Nursing Diagnosis:** Place the Nursing Diagnoses in prioritized order on the concept map and add any needed for your specific patient. **Plan:** Place any further Nursing Interventions Classifications (NIC) needed on the map.

Implement Your Plan of Care

			EVALUATE YOUR CARE	
R Recommendation	Evaluate your nursing care and make recommendations related to the achievement of your desired outcomes. Were they met, or do new goals need to be established?	**Diag**	**Nursing Outcomes Classification (NOC)**	**Outcome met**
		1	Patient manifests decreased restlessness or irritability.	☐ Yes ☐ No
		2	Patient experiences no signs of malnutrition.	☐ Yes ☐ No
		3	Parents/caregivers/patient participate in learning process; identify interferences to learning and specific actions to deal with them; verbalize understanding of condition, disease process, and treatment; perform necessary procedures correctly and explain reasons for the actions.	☐ Yes ☐ No
		4	Patient's growth and development are monitored.	☐ Yes ☐ No
		5		☐ Yes ☐ No

Nursing Diagnosis 1

Acute pain related to tumor enlargement evidenced by verbal reports, guarding or distracted behavior, and changes in vital signs (VS).

NIC:
1) Perform routine comprehensive pain assessment; **2)** Accept child's description of pain; **3)** Investigate changes in or frequency of pain; **4)** Observe for rigidity, crying; **5)** Provide comfort measures, holding, repositioning; **6)** Encourage sleep and rest periods; **7)** Do not palpate tumor; and **8)** Administer analgesics as ordered.

Nursing Diagnosis 2

Imbalanced nutrition: less than body requirements related to anorexia and dietary restrictions evidenced by aversion to eating, altered taste, weight loss, or decreased intake.

NIC:
1) Assess abdomen noting circumference, bowel sounds, and distention; **2)** Observe color and consistency of stools; **3)** Promote foods that are high in protein; **4)** Administer parenteral feedings as ordered; and **5)** Provide nonnutritive sucking.

Nursing Diagnosis 3

Knowledge deficit regarding pathophysiology of condition, management, and available community resources related to insufficient information and misconceptions evidenced by statements of concerns and questions.

NIC:
1) Ascertain readiness, level of knowledge, and individual learning needs; **2)** Provide positive reinforcement; **3)** Provide access information for contact person and identify available community resources and support groups; and **4)** Explain treatments, procedures, and prognosis.

Nursing Diagnosis 4

Risk for disproportionate growth related to genetic factors and/or chemotherapy.

NIC:
1) Assess current growth and developmental stage; **2)** Use age-appropriate tests; **3)** Determine cognitive and perceptual levels; **4)** Encourage self-care activities; and **5)** Provide parents with information.

Condition:
Nephroblastoma (Wilms' Tumor)
Age:

Link & Explain
• Nursing Interventions Classification (NIC)
• Laboratory and Diagnostic Procedures
• Medications

Nursing Diagnosis 5

NIC:

Medications

a. Radiation and chemotherapy

b.

c.

d.

Laboratory & Diagnostic Procedures

a. Abdominal x-ray and ultrasound and CT scan

b. Chest x-ray

c. BUN, CBC, creatinine, creatinine clearance, urinalysis

d. Intravenous pyelogram (IVP)

CONDITION: Nephrotic Syndrome (NS)

PHYSIOLOGY: NS is a condition marked by increased renal glomerular permeability to proteins, resulting in massive loss of proteins in the urine, edema, hypoalbuminemia, hyperlipidemia, and hypercoagulability. Several different types of glomerular injury can cause the syndrome, including membranous glomerulopathy, minimal change disease (lipid nephrosis), focal segmental glomerulosclerosis, and glomerulonephritis. These pathological findings in the kidney result from a broad array of diseases such as diabetic injury to the glomerulus, amyloidosis, immune-complex deposition disease, vasculitis, systemic lupus erythematosus (SLE), allergic reactions, infections, and toxic injury to the kidneys by drugs or heavy metals. Idiopathic NS is diagnosed when the known causes of NS have been excluded. The prognosis depends on the causative factor. Renal biopsy usually is needed to determine the precise histological cause, treatment, and prognosis (*Taber's*, 2009).

HANDOFF COMMUNICATION

S	Situation	Assess what is currently happening in a short statement.	Child presents as _____
B	Background	Summarize important past assessment data for your patient here. Place lab results and medications on the concept map.	**Age:** **Gender:** **Allergies:** **Fall Risk:** **Isolation:** **Immunization status:**
A	Assessment	Use the assessment data to complete your concept map.	**Nursing Diagnosis:** Place the Nursing Diagnoses in prioritized order on the concept map and add any needed for your specific patient. **Plan:** Place any further Nursing Interventions Classifications (NIC) needed on the map.

Implement Your Plan of Care

			EVALUATE YOUR CARE	
	Evaluate your nursing care and make recommendations related to the achievement of your desired outcomes. Were they met, or do new goals need to be established?	**Diag**	**Nursing Outcomes Classification (NOC)**	**Outcome met**
R Recommendation		**1**	Patient stabilizes fluid volume evidenced by balanced I&O, VS within patient's normal limits, stable weight, and no signs of edema. Patient/parent/caregiver verbalizes understanding of individual dietary and fluid restrictions, demonstrates behaviors to monitor fluid status and reduce recurrence of fluid excess, and lists signs that require further evaluation.	☐ Yes ☐ No
		2	Patient displays normalization of laboratory values and is free of signs of malnutrition. Patient/parent/caregiver verbalizes understanding of causative factors (when known) and necessary interventions and demonstrates behaviors, lifestyle changes to regain and/or maintain appropriate weight.	☐ Yes ☐ No
		3	Patient/parent/caregiver verbalizes understanding of individual causative or risk factor(s); identifies interventions to prevent or reduce risk of infection; and demonstrates techniques, lifestyle changes to promote safe environment.	☐ Yes ☐ No
		4	Patient/caregiver identifies risk factors, verbalizes understanding of treatment/therapy regimen, and demonstrates behaviors and techniques to prevent skin breakdown.	☐ Yes ☐ No
		5		☐ Yes ☐ No

Nursing Diagnosis 1

Excess fluid volume related to compromised regulatory mechanism with changes in hydrostatic/oncotic vascular pressure and increased activation of the renin-angiotensin-aldosterone system evidenced by edema/anasarca, possibly effusions/ascites, weight gain, intake greater than output, and blood pressure changes.

NIC:
1) Record accurate I&O; **2)** Weigh daily at same time of day, on same scale, with same equipment and clothing; **3)** Assess skin, face, and dependent areas for edema; evaluate degree of edema (on scale of 1–4); **4)** Monitor VS; **5)** Monitor laboratory diagnostic tests such as BUN, creatinine, Hgb/Hct, electrolytes; and **6)** Administer medications, such as diuretics, as indicated.

Nursing Diagnosis 2

Imbalanced nutrition: less than body requirements may be related to excessive protein losses and inability to ingest adequate nutrients (anorexia) evidenced by weight loss/muscle wasting (may be difficult to assess due to edema), lack of interest in food, and observed inadequate intake.

NIC:
1) Identify child at risk for malnutrition and/or prior nutritional deficiencies; **2)** Determine child's current nutritional status using age-appropriate measurements, including weight and body build, strength, activity level, and sleep and rest cycles; **3)** Establish a nutritional plan that meets individual needs incorporating specific food restrictions and special dietary needs. Consult dietitian or nutritional team, as indicated; and **4)** Review laboratory studies, such as serum albumin, iron, BUN, nitrogen balance studies, glucose, liver function, electrolytes, and total lymphocyte count.

Nursing Diagnosis 3

Risk for infection related to chronic illness and steroidal suppression of inflammatory responses.

NIC:
1) Note risk factors for occurrence of infection (e.g., extremes of age; skin/tissue wounds); **2)** Observe for signs of infection at insertion sites of invasive lines, sutures, surgical incisions; **3)** Note signs and symptoms of sepsis (systemic infection); **4)** Monitor laboratory studies, such as WBC count with differential; and **5)** Administer medication regimen including antibiotics and immunizations as indicated.

Nursing Diagnosis 4

Risk for impaired skin integrity related to presence of edema and activity restrictions.

NIC:
1) Assess skin routinely, noting moisture, color, and elasticity; **2)** Review pertinent lab results (e.g., Hgb/Hct, glucose, presence of infectious agents, albumin, and protein) that may correlate with decreased wound healing; **3)** Handle client gently (particularly infant), as epidermis is thin and prone to injury; **4)** Maintain meticulous skin hygiene using mild non-detergent soap, drying thoroughly, and lubricating with emollient as indicated; and **5)** Emphasize importance of adequate nutritional and fluid intake.

Condition:
Nephrotic Syndrome (NS)
Age:

Link & Explain
• Nursing Interventions Classification (NIC)
• Laboratory and Diagnostic Procedures
• Medications

Nursing Diagnosis 5

NIC:

Medications
a. Angiotensin-converting enzyme (ACE) inhibitors to reduce the degree of protein loss
b. Diuretics to treat symptomatic edema
c. Antibiotics to treat infection
d. Corticosteroids and immunosuppressive drugs to manage nephrosis

Laboratory & Diagnostic Procedures
a. Renal biopsy
b. Hgb/Hct, BUN, creatinine
c. Glucose
d. Albumin and protein

CONDITION: Neural Tube Defects (Spina Bifida and Myelomeningocele)

PHYSIOLOGY: Neural tube defects (NTD) are associated with malformations in the brain and spinal cord during fetal development. The cause is unknown but associated with maternal conditions such as diabetes, maternal obesity, alcohol abuse, folic acid deficiency, seizure medications (valproic acid and carbamazepine), and genetic factors.

Anencephaly is little or no brain development and is not compatible with life.

Encephalocele is protrusion of the cranial contents in a midline defect of the skull due to defective closure during embryonic development.

Spina bifida results in a defect in the lower spinal column.

Spinal occulta is a less severe local defect in the vertebral arch and does not involve the spinal cord and meninges.

Spinal cystica or **myelomeningocele** is the incomplete fusion of one or more of the vertebral laminae, which results in protrusion of the meninges, spinal cord, and nerves covered by transparent membrane. The higher the level of defect, the more severe is loss of spinal cord function below the defect. The disorder is often associated with abnormal brain development, syndromes like Chiari II malformations, and hydrocephalus. The child is also at risk for orthopedic disorders such as hip dislocation, club foot abnormalities, scoliosis, and kyphosis.

Diagnosis is made often by fetal ultrasound or high levels of fetal alpha protein levels in quadruple screening during pregnancy. Supplementation of folic acid before and during pregnancy has reduced incidence.

Children are at high risk for latex allergies and need to be in latex-free environment at birth (Doenges, Moorhouse, & Murr, 2009; Ward and Hisley, 2009).

HANDOFF COMMUNICATION

S	Situation	Assess what is currently happening in a short statement.	Child presents as _____
B	Background	Summarize important past assessment data for your patient here. Place lab results and medications on the concept map.	Age: Gender: Allergies: Fall Risk: Isolation: Immunization status: PMH: PSH:
A	Assessment	Use the assessment data to complete your concept map.	**Nursing Diagnosis:** Place the Nursing Diagnoses in prioritized order on the concept map and add any needed for your specific patient. **Plan:** Place any further Nursing Interventions Classifications (NIC) needed on the map.

Implement Your Plan of Care

		EVALUATE YOUR CARE	
R	Recommendation — Evaluate your nursing care and make recommendations related to the achievement of your desired outcomes. Were they met, or do new goals need to be established?	**Diag** / **Nursing Outcomes Classification (NOC)**	**Outcome met**
		1 Patient has no further neurosensory injury and has optimal function of lower extremities and bowel and bladder.	☐ Yes ☐ No
		2 Patient does not develop infection from exposed defect evidenced by normal lab values, VS, no symptoms of meningitis, and decreased incidence of UTI due to neurogenic bladder.	☐ Yes ☐ No
		3 Patient has recognized signs and symptoms of hydrocephalus, etiology diagnosed, and no increased neurological sequelae.	☐ Yes ☐ No
		4 Patient maximizes ability of movement and self-care activities and has no skin breakdown.	☐ Yes ☐ No
		5	☐ Yes ☐ No

Nursing Diagnosis 1

Neurosensory injury due to anatomical defect and potential trauma.

NIC:
1) Upon delivery, assess defect for size and type of contents; CSF leakage from defect; **2)** Position infant prone to prevent injury and do not place diaper over defect; cover defect with sterile nonadherent dressing moistened with sterile saline; **3)** Examine lower extremities for movement and sensation; assess voiding and defecation patterns; **4)** Do not perform rectal temperature due to risk of rectal prolapse; and **5)** Institute bowel and bladder program to assist with elimination.

Nursing Diagnosis 2

Risk of infection due to interruption in skin integrity, exposed meninges, required ventriculoperitoneal shunt, frequent urinary catheterization, and neurogenic bladder.

NIC:
1) Monitor VS every 2–4 hours; **2)** Assess for presence of infection: redness, purulent drainage, bleeding, and necrosis; **3)** Position properly and with sterile nonadherent dressing; **4)** Change dressing when soiled with aseptic technique; **5)** Administer antibiotics as prescribed; **6)** Postoperatively monitor suture line for infection and CSF leakage; **7)** Monitor for symptoms of meningitis (lethargy or irritability, temperature instability or fever, and vomiting); **8)** Monitor symptoms of UTI and perform intermittent catheterization with clean technique; and **9)** Monitor CBC with differential and platelets, C-reactive protein (CRP), and notify primary care practitioner of abnormal values.

Nursing Diagnosis 3

Risk of hydrocephalus due to brain abnormalities such as Chiari II and postsurgical correction.

NIC:
1) Assess for signs and symptoms of increased cranial pressure such as bulging fontanel, widened sutures, vomiting, lethargy, irritability, high-pitched cry, sunsetting sign, and change in vital signs; older children will complain of visual changes, strabismus, headaches, nausea and vomiting early in morning; **2)** Monitor for change in vital signs and emergency symptoms of Cushing triad (bradycardia, wide pulse pressure, and hypertension); notify primary care practitioner immediately; **3)** Assess vital signs every 2–4 hours and head circumference as prescribed; **4)** Coordinate neuroimaging such as head ultrasound, brain MRI/CT scan; and **5)** Prepare for surgical ventriculoperitoneal shunt.

Nursing Diagnosis 4

Impaired physical mobility due to neuromuscular and sensory deficits.

NIC:
1) Assess and document child's activity level; **2)** Coordinate interdisciplinary therapy with physical therapy and occupation therapy; **3)** Perform active and passive range of motion exercises as prescribed; **4)** Encourage self-care activities; **5)** Maintain proper body alignment in bed, wheelchair, and assist with use of splints, braces, and other appliances; and **6)** Reposition child every 2 hours and monitor skin for breakdown.

Condition:
Neural Tube Defects (Spina Bifida and Myelomeningocele)

Age:

Link & Explain
• Nursing Interventions Classification (NIC)
• Laboratory and Diagnostic Procedures
• Medications

Nursing Diagnosis 5

NIC:

Medications

a. Antibiotics pre- and postoperative care

b. Anticholinergics for improved urinary continence

c. Laxatives for bowel maintenance and to prevent constipation

d.

Laboratory & Diagnostic Procedures

a. Brain and spinal MRI or CAT scan

b. Head ultrasound to rule out hydrocephalus

c. Renal ultrasound and voiding cystourethrogram (VCUG) for urological evaluation

d.

TION: Phenylketonuria (PKU)

PHYSIOLOGY: PKU is an inherited Mendelian recessive disorder that affects the body's protein utilization with abnormal metabolism of the amino acid phenylalanine. Phenylalanine is an essential amino acid found in natural protein foods. The disorder results in a deficiency in the liver enzyme phenylalanine hydroxylase, which is important in the metabolism of amino acid phenylalanine into tyrosine. The result is an accumulation phenylalanine metabolite levels in the blood, which has a toxic effect on the neurotransmitter, thereby affecting protein synthesis, myelinization, and degradation of white and gray matter in the brain. The infant will develop mental retardation.

Clinical manifestations are seizures; musty body and urine odor; irritability; vomiting; failure to thrive; eczema-type rash; blond hair, fair skin, and blue eyes due to decreased production of melanin. Many infants are normal at birth and diagnosed with the newborn screen drawn after protein ingestion at 24 hours of age for abnormal phenylalanine level (normal < 2mg/dl) (Doenges, Moorhouse, & Murr, 2009; Ward & Hisley, 2009).

HANDOFF COMMUNICATION

S	Situation	Assess what is currently happening in a short statement.	Child presents as _____
B	Background	Summarize important past assessment data for your patient here. Place lab results and medications on the concept map.	**Age:** **Gender:** **Allergies:** **Fall Risk:** **Isolation:** **Immunization status:** **PMH:** **PSH:**
A	Assessment	Use the assessment data to complete your concept map.	**Nursing Diagnosis:** Place the Nursing Diagnoses in prioritized order on the concept map and add any needed for your specific patient. **Plan:** Place any further Nursing Interventions Classifications (NIC) needed on the map.

Implement Your Plan of Care

		EVALUATE YOUR CARE		
	Evaluate your nursing care and make recommendations related to the achievement of your desired outcomes. Were they met, or do new goals need to be established?	**Diag**	**Nursing Outcomes Classification (NOC)**	**Outcome met**
R Recommendation		1	Infant with PKU disorder is recognized early with state-required newborn screening programs; infant/child experiences optimal growth and development.	☐ Yes ☐ No
		2	Parent/caregiver complies with diet, and patient has acceptable phenylalanine serum blood levels.	☐ Yes ☐ No
		3	Parents/caregivers identify dietary restrictions and requirements for infant child with PKU and comply with diet.	☐ Yes ☐ No
		4	Parents/caregivers participate in learning process; identify interferences to learning and specific actions to deal with them; verbalize understanding of condition, disease process, and treatment; perform necessary procedures correctly; and explain reasons for the actions.	☐ Yes ☐ No
		5		☐ Yes ☐ No

Nursing Diagnosis 1

Risk of injury due to impaired growth and development.

NIC:
1) Obtain newborn screen prior to discharge from well-baby nursery after ingestion of protein for 24 hours; additional tests are done if an abnormal newborn screen is documented; **2)** Assess newborn screen results; **3)** Genetic counseling for identified patients to reduce further risk; and **4)** Monitor symptoms in children for ADHD or poor school performance as increased protein is introduced into diet.

Nursing Diagnosis 2

Risk for imbalanced nutrition due to abnormal protein utilization and metabolism.

NIC:
1) Identify disorders; child will require specialized formula (protein hydrolysate formula with phenylalanine removed); **2)** Breastfeeding is allowed with monitoring of phenylalanine levels 2–6 mg/dl; **3)** Consult nutritionist for foods and sugar substitutes with phenylalanine; **4)** Place child on protein-restricted diet for life; **5)** Arrange dietary or nutritional consult, and monitor phenylalanine levels as prescribed; and **6)** Future pregnancy will need to maintain a phenylalanine diet to protect fetus.

Nursing Diagnosis 3

Ineffective family process related to knowledge deficit of hereditary disease.

NIC:
1) Assess parents'/caregivers' knowledge base of disease and symptoms; **2)** Instruct them on diet management and formula preparation; recommend dietary consultation; **3)** Counsel parents/caregivers on avoiding high-protein foods, foods with aspartame; and **4)** Offer support and refer to community resources.

Nursing Diagnosis 4

Knowledge deficit regarding pathophysiology of condition, management, and available community resources related to insufficient information and misconceptions evidenced by statements of concerns and questions.

NIC:
1) Ascertain family readiness, level of knowledge, and individual learning needs; **2)** Provide positive reinforcement; **3)** Provide access information for contact person and identify available community resources and support groups; and **4)** Explain treatments, procedures, and prognosis.

Condition:
Phenylketonuria (PKU)
Age:

Link & Explain
• Nursing Interventions Classification (NIC)
• Laboratory and Diagnostic Procedures
• Medications

Nursing Diagnosis 5

NIC:

Medications

a.

b.

c.

d.

Laboratory & Diagnostic Procedures

a. Newborn screen

b. Phenylalanine levels

c.

d.

CONDITION: Respiratory Croup or Laryngotracheobronchitis

PHYSIOLOGY: Croup is a generic term that encompasses a group of illnesses affecting the larynx, trachea, and bronchi. The most common age group is between 3 months and 5 years of age. The common pathogens are parainfluenza virus types I, II, and III and respiratory syncytial virus (RSV), which occur during the fall and winter months. The trachea and lower airways become inflamed and narrowed due to the tissue response to the invading pathogen and the small airway passages of a child. The common clinical manifestations are upper respiratory infection with copious secretions, low-grade fever, inflamed pharynx, and barking or seal cough. The symptoms are often worse in the evening than the daytime. Worsening inflammation of the airways include tachypnea, retractions, stridor, and low O_2 saturations.

Bacterial tracheitis and epiglottitis cause life-threatening airway obstruction by streptococcus, staphylococcus, or *Haemophilus influenzae* organisms. Clinical manifestations of epiglottitis are preceded by URI, high fever (>102°F), toxic appearance, drooling, tripod position, respiratory distress, dysphagia, cherry red epiglottis, and patient preference for upright position. Bacterial tracheitis presents with high fever, stridor, copious secretions, croup cough, and patient can lie flat.

The *Haemophilus influenzae* type B (HIB) vaccine protects against bacterial invasion of soft tissue of the epiglottic area (Doenges, Moorhouse, & Murr, 2009; Ward & Hisley, 2009).

HANDOFF COMMUNICATION

S	Situation	Assess what is currently happening in a short statement.	Child presents as _____
B	Background	Summarize important past assessment data for your patient here. Place lab results and medications on the concept map.	**Age:** **Gender:** **Allergies:** **Fall Risk:** **Isolation:** **Immunization status:** **PMH:** **PSH:**
A	Assessment	Use the assessment data to complete your concept map.	**Nursing Diagnosis:** Place the Nursing Diagnoses in prioritized order on the concept map and add any needed for your specific patient. **Plan:** Place any further Nursing Interventions Classifications (NIC) needed on the map.

Implement Your Plan of Care

	Evaluate your nursing care and make recommendations related to the achievement of your desired outcomes. Were they met, or do new goals need to be established?	**EVALUATE YOUR CARE**		
R Recommendation		Diag	Nursing Outcomes Classification (NOC)	Outcome met
		1	Patient's temperature, pulse, respiratory effort, blood pressure are in the expected range for the child's age.	☐ Yes ☐ No
		2	Patient's O_2 status returns to baseline or remains at least >95% via pulse oximetry. The child rests in position of comfort and tolerates therapeutic measures.	☐ Yes ☐ No
		3	Patient/caregiver verbalizes understanding of individual causative or risk factor(s); identifies interventions to prevent or reduce risk of infection; and demonstrates techniques, lifestyle changes to promote safe environment.	☐ Yes ☐ No
		4	Patient has adequate hydration with equilibrium between extracellular and intercellular fluid compartments. The child's hydration status provides adequate perfusion, urine output, and stabilized weight within 24–48 hours.	☐ Yes ☐ No
		5		☐ Yes ☐ No

Nursing Diagnosis 1

Ineffective breathing pattern related to increased work of breathing, airway obstruction, and decreased energy evidenced by shortness of breath (SOB) and abnormal lung sounds.

NIC:
1) Collect and analyze patient data to maintain patent airway and adequate gas exchange; **2)** Assess respiratory status every 1–4 hours based on patient's respiratory status; **3)** Place child on cardiorespiratory (C-R) monitor with pulse oximetry with alarms set; **4)** Record data and notify primary care practitioner of changes in patient's status; and **5)** Collect specimens and lab data as prescribed.

Nursing Diagnosis 2

Impaired gas exchange related to ventilation perfusion mismatch related to increased secretions, airway obstruction, and edema evidenced by poor O_2 saturation or cyanosis.

NIC:
1) Administer humidified O_2 as ordered via nasal cannula, oxygen tent, or mask; **2)** Position child for comfort and effective breathing pattern; **3)** Relieve child's anxiety and restlessness; and **4)** Administer medications as prescribed, and assess response.

Nursing Diagnosis 3

Risk of infection (viral or bacterial) related to immature immunity.

NIC:
1) Note signs and symptoms of sepsis (systemic infection); **2)** Monitor laboratory studies, such as WBC count with differential and cultures; and **3)** Administer medication regimen including antibiotics and immunizations as indicated.

Nursing Diagnosis 4

Risk for fluid volume related to inability to meet body requirements and increased metabolic demand.

NIC:
1) Evaluate the need for IV fluid or TPN or oral hydration fluids; **2)** Maintain strict I&O q8h and serum electrolytes if prescribed; **3)** Perform daily weights with the same scale; **4)** Assess perfusion and hydration status (vital signs, capillary refill, mucous membranes); and **5)** Report changes as indicated.

Condition:
Respiratory Croup or Laryngotracheo-bronchitis

Age:
_____
Link & Explain
• Nursing Interventions Classification (NIC)
• Laboratory and Diagnostic Procedures
• Medications

Nursing Diagnosis 5

NIC:

Medications

a. Humidified O_2 delivery

b. Albuterol for bronchodilation/wheezing or Racemic, epinephrine for airway edema/stridor

c. Antibiotics to treat infection

d. Corticosteroids to manage inflammation and edema nephrosis

Laboratory & Diagnostic Procedures

a. Chest x-ray AP/LAT

b. Lateral neck films (acute epiglottitis)

c. ABG, CBC with differential and platelets, CRP; basic metabolic panel

d. Nasal and pharyngeal cultures, rapid RSV; blood culture if suspected bacterial sepsis

CONDITION: Respiratory Syncytial Virus (RSV)

PHYSIOLOGY: RSV is a single-stranded RNA virus that is an important cause of upper and lower respiratory tract disease in infants, children, and the elderly. When limited to the upper respiratory tract, it causes bronchiolitis, pneumonia, or respiratory distress and can be life threatening. RSV is the most common cause of lower respiratory infections in infants and children under age 2. It is spread by physical contact, usually with infected nasal or oral secretions. In the United States, its season begins in the fall and peaks in winter, and about 90,000 young children are hospitalized with RSV infections each year (*Taber's*, 2009).

HANDOFF COMMUNICATION

S	Situation	Assess what is currently happening in a short statement.	Child presents as _____
B	Background	Summarize important past assessment data for your patient here. Place lab results and medications on the concept map.	**Age:** **Gender:** **Allergies:** **Fall Risk:** **Isolation:**
A	Assessment	Use the assessment data to complete your concept map.	**Nursing Diagnosis:** Place the Nursing Diagnoses in prioritized order on the concept map and add any needed for your specific patient. **Plan:** Place any further Nursing Interventions Classifications (NIC) needed on the map.

Implement Your Plan of Care

		EVALUATE YOUR CARE	
	Evaluate your nursing care and make recommendations related to the achievement of your desired outcomes. Were they met, or do new goals need to be established?	**Diag** / **Nursing Outcomes Classification (NOC)**	**Outcome met**
R Recommendation		**1** Patient demonstrates improved ventilation and adequate oxygenation of tissues by arterial blood gases (ABGs) within patient's normal range, is free of symptoms of respiratory distress, and participates in treatment regimen within level of ability and situation.	☐ Yes ☐ No
		2 Patient's airway is maintained with breath sounds clear or clearing; patient demonstrates behaviors to improve airway clearance.	☐ Yes ☐ No
		3 Patient experiences no signs of malnutrition.	☐ Yes ☐ No
		4 Family verbalizes understanding of condition, disease process, and treatment; initiates necessary lifestyle changes; and participates in treatment regimen.	☐ Yes ☐ No
		5	☐ Yes ☐ No

Nursing Diagnosis 1

Impaired gas exchange related to altered delivery of inspired O_2 and trapped air evidenced by dyspnea, restlessness, reduced tolerance for activity, cyanosis, and changes in ABGs and vital signs (VS).

NIC:
1) Assess respiratory rate and depth; 2) Raise head of bed (HOB); 3) Encourage expectoration of sputum; 4) Auscultate breath sounds; 5) Palpate chest for fremitus; and 6) Monitor VS, sleep patterns, and activity level.

Nursing Diagnosis 2

Risk for ineffective airway clearance related to increased production and retained pulmonary secretions, bronchospasms, decreased energy, and fatigue.

NIC:
1) Auscultate breath sounds; 2) Assess and monitor respiration rate; 3) Note presence and degree of dyspnea and air hunger; 4) Position patient for comfort; 5) Keep environment free from triggers or pollutants; 6) Assist with abdominal or pursed-lip breathing; 7) Observe for cough; 8) Hydrate; and 9) Medicate as prescribed.

Nursing Diagnosis 3

Nutrition: less than body requirements related to lack of appetite, difficulty maintaining oxygenation while expending energy to eat evidenced by poor weight gain.

NIC:
1) Assess pulse oximeter readings while feeding; 2) Maintain hydration; 3) Maintain high-protein diet; 4) Administer parenteral feeding as ordered; and 5) Provide nonnutritive sucking if on parenteral feeds.

Nursing Diagnosis 4

Knowledge deficit related to condition, self-care, and discharge needs related to lack of familiarity with information resources for family evidenced by request for information.

NIC:
1) Explain and reinforce explanations of individual disease process; 2) Review breathing exercises and coughing effectiveness; 3) Teach to percuss if needed; 4) Instruct to avoid people with upper respiratory infections (URI); and 5) Instruct in meticulous hand washing.

Condition:
Respiratory Syncytial Virus (RSV)

Age:

Link & Explain
• Nursing Interventions Classification (NIC)
• Laboratory and Diagnostic Procedures
• Medications

Nursing Diagnosis 5

NIC:

Medications

a.

b.

c.

d.

Laboratory & Diagnostic Procedures

a. ABGs

b. CBC with differential

c. Pulse oximetry

d.

CONDITION: Scarlet Fever

PHYSIOLOGY: Scarlet fever is an acute, contagious disease characterized by pharyngitis and a pimply red rash. It is caused by a group A beta-hemolytic streptococcus and usually affects children between the ages of 3 and 15. After an incubation period of 1–7 days, children develop a fever, chills, vomiting, abdominal pain, and malaise. The pharynx and tonsils are swollen and red, and an exudate is present. A red pinpoint rash that blanches on pressure with a sandpapery texture appears on the trunk within 12 hours after the onset of fever. Faint lines in the elbow creases, called Pastia lines, are characteristic findings in full-blown disease. Over several days, sloughing of the skin begins, which lasts approximately 3 weeks. Scarlet fever is treated with 10 days of penicillin (or erythromycin in cases with penicillin allergy). A full course of therapy is vital to decrease the risk of rheumatic fever or glomerulonephritis. In general, parents are taught to isolate the infected child from siblings until they have received penicillin for 24 hours (*Taber's*, 2009).

HANDOFF COMMUNICATION

S	Situation	Assess what is currently happening in a short statement.	Child presents as _____
B	Background	Summarize important past assessment data for your patient here. Place lab results and medications on the concept map.	Age: Gender: Allergies: Fall Risk: Isolation: Immunization status: PMH: PSH:
A	Assessment	Use the assessment data to complete your concept map.	**Nursing Diagnosis:** Place the Nursing Diagnoses in prioritized order on the concept map and add any needed for your specific patient. **Plan:** Place any further Nursing Interventions Classifications (NIC) needed on the map.

Implement Your Plan of Care

		Diag	EVALUATE YOUR CARE	
			Nursing Outcomes Classification (NOC)	Outcome met
R	Recommendation	Evaluate your nursing care and make recommendations related to the achievement of your desired outcomes. Were they met, or do new goals need to be established?	**1** Patient maintains core temperature within normal range; parents/caregivers identify underlying cause or contributing factors and importance of treatment, as well as signs/symptoms requiring further evaluation or intervention.	☐ Yes ☐ No
			2 Patient reports or demonstrates pain is relieved or controlled. Parents/caregivers follow prescribed pharmacological regimen, verbalize nonpharmacological methods that provide relief, and demonstrate use of diversional activities as indicated.	☐ Yes ☐ No
			3 Patient demonstrates adequate fluid balance evidenced by stable vital signs (VS), normal skin turgor, moist mucous membranes, adequate urinary output, and lack of excessive weight loss.	☐ Yes ☐ No
			4 Family verbalizes understanding of condition, disease process, and treatment; initiates necessary lifestyle changes; and participates in treatment regimen.	☐ Yes ☐ No
			5	☐ Yes ☐ No

Nursing Diagnosis 1

Hyperthermia related to presence of toxins evidenced by warm skin and elevated temperature.

NIC:
1) Assess causative/contributing factors; **2)** Evaluate effect/degree hyperthermia; **3)** Assist with measures to reduce body temperature/restore normal body/organ function; and **4)** Promote wellness (teaching/discharge consideration).

Nursing Diagnosis 2

Acute pain/impaired comfort related to inflammation of mucous membranes and effects of circulating toxins (malaise, fever), possibly evidenced by verbal reports, distraction behaviors, guarding (decreased swallowing), and/or self-focus.

NIC:
1) Assess etiology/precipitating contributory factors; **2)** Evaluate client's response to pain (use pain rating scale appropriate for age and cognition); and **3)** Assist client to explore methods for alleviation/control of pain (suggest parental presence during procedures to comfort child).

Nursing Diagnosis 3

Risk for deficient fluid volume related to risk factors that may include hypermetabolic state (hyperthermia) or reduced intake.

NIC:
1) Monitor VS, mucous membranes, weight, skin turgor, and urinary output; **2)** Review child's intake of fluids; and **3)** Discuss individual risk factors, potential problems, and specific interventions (e.g., fluid replacement options).

Nursing Diagnosis 4

Knowledge deficit related to condition, self-care, and discharge needs related to lack of familiarity with information resources for family evidenced by request for information.

NIC:
1) Explain and reinforce explanations of individual disease process; **2)** Review care to reduce temperature; **3)** Teach to recognize signs of disease; **4)** Instruct to avoid people with URI (upper respiratory infections); and **5)** Instruct in meticulous hand washing.

Condition:
Scarlet Fever
Age:

Link & Explain
• Nursing Interventions Classification (NIC)
• Laboratory and Diagnostic Procedures
• Medications

Nursing Diagnosis 5

NIC:

Medications

a. Penicillin (or erythromycin in cases with penicillin allergy) may be given one, two, or three times in a day for 10 days.

b. Acetaminophen prn

c.

d.

Laboratory & Diagnostic Procedures

a. Throat culture/rapid strep test kit

b.

c.

d.

CONDITION: Sepsis

PHYSIOLOGY: Sepsis is a systemic inflammatory response to infection in which there is fever or hypothermia, tachycardia, tachypnea, and evidence of inadequate blood flow to internal organs. The syndrome is a common cause of death in critically ill patients. Roughly 50% of patients with sepsis die; between 200,000 and 400,000 deaths due to sepsis occur annually in the United States. Pathogenic organisms, including bacteria, mycobacteria, fungi, protozoa, and viruses, may initiate the cascade of inflammatory reactions that constitute sepsis. The number of patients with sepsis has increased significantly in the last 25 years as a result of several factors, including the aging of the population; the increased number of patients living with immune-suppressing illnesses (e.g., organ transplants); the increased number of patients living with multiple diseases; and the increased use of invasive or indwelling devices in health care, which serve as portals of entry for infection. Complications of sepsis may include shock, organ failure (e.g., adult respiratory distress syndrome or acute renal failure), disseminated intravascular coagulation (DIC), altered mental status, jaundice, metastatic abscess formation, and multiple organ system failure (*Taber's*, 2009).

HANDOFF COMMUNICATION

S	Situation	Assess what is currently happening in a short statement.	Child presents as _____
B	Background	Summarize important past assessment data for your patient here. Place lab results and medications on the concept map.	**Age:** **Gender:** **Allergies:** **Fall Risk:** **Isolation:**
A	Assessment	Use the assessment data to complete your concept map.	**Nursing Diagnosis:** Place the Nursing Diagnoses in prioritized order on the concept map and add any needed for your specific patient. **Plan:** Place any further Nursing Interventions Classifications (NIC) needed on the map.

Implement Your Plan of Care

		EVALUATE YOUR CARE	
		Diag · **Nursing Outcomes Classification (NOC)**	**Outcome met**
R Recommendation	Evaluate your nursing care and make recommendations related to the achievement of your desired outcomes. Were they met, or do new goals need to be established?	**1** Patient regains or maintains appropriate body temperature for age and size.	☐ Yes ☐ No
		2 Patient manifests decreased restlessness or irritability.	☐ Yes ☐ No
		3 Patient's adequate circulating fluid volume is evidenced by adequate fluid intake, age-appropriate vital signs (VS), and adequate perfusion.	☐ Yes ☐ No
		4 Parents/caregivers participate in learning process; identify interferences to learning and specific actions to deal with them; verbalize understanding of condition, disease process, and treatment; perform necessary procedures correctly and explain reasons for the actions.	☐ Yes ☐ No
		5	☐ Yes ☐ No

Nursing Diagnosis 1

Hyperthermia related to increased metabolic rate evidenced by increased body temperature, warm skin, and increased pulse and respiratory rate.

NIC:
1) Note conditions that promote fever; **2)** Measure temperature using properly functioning thermometer; **3)** Be aware of heat loss for body size and mass; **4)** Adjust bedclothes, linen, and environment; and **5)** Administer antipyretics.

Nursing Diagnosis 2

Acute pain related to circulation of toxins and visceral edema and distention evidenced by verbal reports, guarding or distracted behavior, and changes in VS.

NIC:
1) Perform routine comprehensive pain assessment; **2)** Accept patient's description of pain; **3)** Investigate changes in or frequency of pain; **4)** Observe for rigidity, crying; **5)** Provide comfort measures, holding, repositioning; **6)** Encourage sleep and rest periods; and **7)** Administer analgesics as ordered.

Nursing Diagnosis 3

Deficient fluid volume related to decreased amount of circulating fluid volume evidenced by vomiting, decreased urine output, decreased skin turgor, dry mucous membranes, weight loss, and increased pulse rate.

NIC:
1) Monitor VS, mucous membranes, weight, skin turgor, and urinary output; **2)** Review child's intake of fluids; **3)** Discuss individual risk factors, potential problems, and specific interventions (e.g., fluid replacement options); **4)** Keep accurate I&O; **5)** Maintain NPO as ordered; and **6)** Ensure patent nasogastric (NG) tube, record drainage, and replace fluid as appropriate.

Nursing Diagnosis 4

Deficient knowledge of caregiver that may be related to lack of exposure or recall, information misinterpretation, unfamiliarity with information resources, cognitive limitation, or lack of interest in learning.

NIC:
1) Ascertain readiness, level of knowledge, and individual learning needs; **2)** Provide positive reinforcement; **3)** Provide access information for contact person and identify available community resources and support groups; **4)** Prepare child for procedures in accordance with development; **5)** Encourage child and caregiver participation in care; **6)** Document parents'/caregivers' understanding and informed consent; and **7)** Counsel parents/caregivers on the risk of reoccurrence of infection.

Condition:
Sepsis
Age:

Link & Explain
• Nursing Interventions Classification (NIC)
• Laboratory and Diagnostic Procedures
• Medications

Nursing Diagnosis 5

NIC:

Medications

a. Antibiotics and/or antiviral

b. Oxygen

c. Corticosteroids

d.

Laboratory & Diagnostic Procedures

a. ABGs, CBC with differential

b. Kidney function tests; white blood cell count; fibrin degradation products

c. Platelet count

d. Cultures

CONDITION: Talipes Equinovarus (Clubfoot)

PHYSIOLOGY: Talipes equinovarus (clubfoot) is a foot deformity diagnosed in newborns. In children who have not had effective treatment, the most severe form of this condition resembles a "club." There are about one dozen different types of clubfoot. The most severe form and most commonly known is talipes equinovarus. The foot defect can be unilateral (more common) or bilateral. Talipes equinovarus affects boys twice as often as girls. Clubfoot deformities tend to run in families and are associated with spina bifida. In clubfoot, the foot is plantar flexed with an inverted heel and adducted forefoot. The defect is rigid and cannot be manipulated into a neutral position. There is a possibility that the position of the fetus in utero influences the formation of the clubfoot (*Taber's*, 2009).

HANDOFF COMMUNICATION

S	Situation	Assess what is currently happening in a short statement.	Child presents as _____
B	Background	Summarize important past assessment data for your patient here. Place lab results and medications on the concept map.	**Age:** **Gender:** **Allergies:** **Fall Risk:** **Isolation:** **Immunization status:** **PMH:** **PSH:**
A	Assessment	Use the assessment data to complete your concept map.	**Nursing Diagnosis:** Place the Nursing Diagnoses in prioritized order on the concept map and add any needed for your specific patient. **Plan:** Place any further Nursing Interventions Classifications (NIC) needed on the map.

Implement Your Plan of Care

R	Recommendation	Evaluate your nursing care and make recommendations related to the achievement of your desired outcomes. Were they met, or do new goals need to be established?	**EVALUATE YOUR CARE**	
			Diag / **Nursing Outcomes Classification (NOC)**	**Outcome met**
			1 — Patient maintains or increases strength and function of affected and/or compensatory body parts.	☐ Yes ☐ No
			2 — Parent/caregiver verbalizes realistic information and expectations of parenting role and demonstrates appropriate attachment and parenting behaviors.	☐ Yes ☐ No
			3 — Parent/caregiver verbalizes understanding of treatment/therapy regimen, identifies individual risk factors, and demonstrates behaviors and techniques to prevent skin breakdown.	☐ Yes ☐ No
			4 — Parent/caregiver participates in learning process; verbalizes understanding of condition, disease process, and treatment; performs necessary procedures correctly and explains reasons for the action.	☐ Yes ☐ No
			5 —	☐ Yes ☐ No

Nursing Diagnosis 1

Impaired physical mobility related to external devices (casts) evidenced by immobility.

NIC:
1) Assess degree of immobility produced by defect and/or treatment; **2)** Maintain a stimulating environment and child's normal development by playing and spending time with the child; **3)** Keep the cast and surrounding area clean and dry, and reposition every 2 hours; **4)** Elevate an extremity and provide good hygiene to prevent skin breakdown; and **5)** Notify the health-care provider if the child has a fever, signs and symptoms of infection, or unrelieved pain.

Nursing Diagnosis 2

Impaired parenting related to growth and development possibly evidenced by growth and/or development lag in child.

NIC:
1) Assess parenting skill level, considering intellectual, emotional, and physical strengths and limitations; **2)** Determine existing situation and parental perception of the problems, noting presence of specific factors such as physical disabilities of the child; **3)** Note presence and effectiveness of extended family support; and **4)** Emphasize positive aspects of situation, maintaining a positive attitude toward parents' capabilities and potential for improving.

Nursing Diagnosis 3

Risk for impaired skin integrity related to external devices (casts).

NIC:
1) Assess skin routinely, noting moisture, color, and elasticity; **2)** Review pertinent lab results (e.g., Hgb/Hct, glucose, presence of infectious agents, albumin, and protein) that may correlate with decreased wound healing; **3)** Handle client gently (particularly infant), as epidermis is thin and prone to injury; **4)** Maintain meticulous skin hygiene using mild nondetergent soap, drying thoroughly, and lubricating with emollient, as indicated; and **5)** Emphasize importance of adequate nutritional and fluid intake.

Nursing Diagnosis 4

Knowledge deficit related to treatment and home care evidenced by questions or anxiety.

NIC:
1) Assess readiness to learn and individual learning needs, including level of knowledge, anticipatory needs, and support persons requiring information (e.g., parent, caregiver); **2)** Involve the patient/caregiver by using age-appropriate materials tailored to client's literacy skills, questions, and dialogue; **3)** Provide access information for contact person to answer questions and validate information after discharge; and **4)** Identify available community resources and support groups.

Condition:
Talipes Equinovarus (Clubfoot)

Age:

Link & Explain
• Nursing Interventions Classification (NIC)
• Laboratory and Diagnostic Procedures
• Medications

Nursing Diagnosis 5

NIC:

Medications

a. Ibuprofen/Children's Motrin (<6 months, give 5–10 mg/kg q6h)

b. Choline magnesium trisalicylate/Trilisate (<81.5 lb, give 50 mg/kg/day divided into two doses)

c.

d.

Laboratory & Diagnostic Procedures

a. Ultrasound done before birth to detect talipes equinovarus

b. X-ray

c. CT scan

d.

CONDITION: Varicella (Chickenpox)

PHYSIOLOGY: Varicella is an acute infectious disease, usually seen in children under age 15, caused by varicella zoster virus. Its hallmark is a rash, described clinically as having a "dewdrop on a rose petal" pattern, scattered in clusters (crops) over the trunk, face, scalp, upper extremities, and sometimes the thighs. It is transmitted mainly by respiratory droplets that contain infectious particles; direct contact with a lesion and contaminated equipment can also spread the virus. Reactivation of the virus in adults causes shingles (*Taber's*, 2009).

HANDOFF COMMUNICATION

S	Situation	Assess what is currently happening in a short statement.	Child presents as _____
B	Background	Summarize important past assessment data for your patient here. Place lab results and medications on the concept map.	**Age:** **Gender:** **Allergies:** **Fall Risk:** **Isolation:**
A	Assessment	Use the assessment data to complete your concept map.	**Nursing Diagnosis:** Place the Nursing Diagnoses in prioritized order on the concept map and add any needed for your specific patient. **Plan:** Place any further Nursing Interventions Classifications (NIC) needed on the map.

Implement Your Plan of Care

		EVALUATE YOUR CARE		
R	Recommendation	Evaluate your nursing care and make recommendations related to the achievement of your desired outcomes. Were they met, or do new goals need to be established?	**Diag**	**Nursing Outcomes Classification (NOC)**	**Outcome met**

Diag	Nursing Outcomes Classification (NOC)	Outcome met
1	Parents/caregivers/patient demonstrate techniques and initiate lifestyle changes to avoid transmission to others.	☐ Yes ☐ No
2	Patient regains or maintains appropriate body temperature for age and size.	☐ Yes ☐ No
3	Patient manifests decreased restlessness or irritability.	☐ Yes ☐ No
4	Patient reports or demonstrates absence of or decrease in pruritus and scratching.	☐ Yes ☐ No
5		☐ Yes ☐ No

Nursing Diagnosis 1

Infection due to lack of immune function evidenced by varicella rash.

NIC:
1) Assess immunization record for each child's well visit and hospitalizations; **2)** Place in separate room; **3)** Monitor for complications (respiratory); **4)** Assess immune status of visitors; and **5)** If child is home, keep secluded from other children and the elderly.

Nursing Diagnosis 2

Hyperthermia related to increased metabolic rate evidenced by increased body temperature, warm skin, and increased pulse and respiratory rate.

NIC:
1) Note conditions that promote fever; **2)** Measure temperature using properly functioning thermometer; **3)** Be aware of heat loss for body size and mass; **4)** Adjust bedclothes, linen, and environment; and **5)** Administer antipyretics.

Nursing Diagnosis 3

Acute pain related to inflammation or irritation of the brain and cerebral edema evidenced by changes in vital signs (VS), restlessness, and crying.

NIC:
1) Perform routine comprehensive pain assessment; **2)** Accept child's description of pain; **3)** Investigate changes in or frequency of pain; **4)** Observe for rigidity, crying; **5)** Provide comfort measures, holding, repositioning; and **6)** Encourage sleep and rest periods.

Nursing Diagnosis 4

Impaired skin integrity related to varicella rash evidenced by itching.

NIC:
1) Encourage use of cool bath, baking soda, or starch; **2)** Apply calamine lotion as indicated; **3)** Provide age-appropriate diversional activity; **4)** Administer medications as indicated; and **5)** Avoid comments regarding child's appearance.

Condition:
Varicella (Chickenpox)
Age:

Link & Explain
• Nursing Interventions Classification (NIC)
• Laboratory and Diagnostic Procedures
• Medications

Nursing Diagnosis 5

NIC:

Medications

a. Calamine lotion

b. Immunization of other children in family

c.

d.

Laboratory & Diagnostic Procedures

a.

b.

c.

d.

Concept Maps for Women's Health

This chapter provides care maps that describe health conditions experienced by women. It covers conditions a nurse may encounter when caring for female patients in both outpatient and acute settings. It includes conditions that occur throughout a woman's life span: preconceptual, conceptual, and postmenopausal. The conditions are listed in alphabetical order to make them easier to locate. There is also a mix of conditions that women normally experience in the childbearing process, such as first trimester changes and vaginal delivery. These maps will enhance health promotion and disease prevention.

As with all the concept maps presented in this book, these maps are guides for patient care that you can individualize for each patient entrusted to your care.

The conditions included in this chapter are:

1. Abortion (Spontaneous or Induced)
2. Abruptio Placentae
3. Adoption
4. Breast Cancer
5. Candidiasis
6. Cesarean Birth
7. Delivery of a Child With Down Syndrome or Genetic Disorder
8. Dysfunctional Uterine Bleeding (DUB)
9. Ectopic Pregnancy
10. Family Experiencing a Fetal Demise
11. First Trimester Gestation
12. Gestational Diabetes Mellitus (GDM)
13. HELLP Syndrome (Hemolysis, Elevated Liver enzymes, and Low Platelets)
14. Hyperemesis Gravidarum
15. Hysterectomy
16. Infertility
17. Labor (Naturally Occurring, Induced, or Augmented)
18. Mastitis
19. Pelvic Inflammatory Disease (PID)
20. Placenta Previa
21. Postpartum
22. Postpartum Depression (PPD)
23. Postpartum Hemorrhage (PPH)
24. Precipitous Delivery or Out-of-Hospital (Extramural) Delivery
25. Pregnancy Induced Hypertension (PIH)
26. Preterm Labor (PTL)
27. Second Trimester Gestation
28. Sexually Transmitted Infection (STI)
29. Third Trimester Gestation
30. Toxic Shock Syndrome
31. Uterine Rupture
32. Vaginal Delivery

CONDITION: Abortion (Spontaneous or Induced)

PHYSIOLOGY: An abortion (AB) is a spontaneous or induced termination of pregnancy before the fetus reaches a viable age. The legal definition of viability is from 20 to 24 weeks depending on the state. Some preterm infants fewer than 24 weeks or 500 g are now viable. Symptoms of spontaneous abortion include abdominal cramps and vaginal bleeding sometimes with the passage of clots or tissue. Among the most common causes of a spontaneous abortion (miscarriage) are genetic anomalies of the embryo. Other causes may be placental abnormalities, endocrine disturbances, acute infections, trauma, and shock. Immunological factors and use of drugs may also cause a spontaneous abortion. Induced abortion, or the intentional termination of a pregnancy, is done by cervical dilatation and evacuation (D&E) of the uterus. Methods used include Laminaria tent or cannula, vacuum aspiration, or dilation and curettage (D&C) (*Taber's*, 2009).

HANDOFF COMMUNICATION

S	Situation	Assess what is currently happening in a short statement.	Patient presents as _____
B	Background	Summarize important past assessment data for your patient here. Place lab results and medications on the concept map.	**Age:** **Gender:** Female **Allergies:** **Fall Risk:** **Isolation:** **LMP (last menstrual period):**_____ **EDB (expected date of birth):**_____ **IPV (intimate partner violence):**_____ **Gravida (number of times pregnant):**_____ **term:**_____; **preterm:**_____; **abortion:**_____; **living:**_____
A	Assessment	Use the assessment data to complete your concept map.	**Nursing Diagnosis:** Place the Nursing Diagnoses in prioritized order on the concept map and add any needed for your specific patient. **Plan:** Place any further Nursing Interventions Classifications (NIC) needed on the map.

Implement Your Plan of Care

			EVALUATE YOUR CARE	
R	Recommendation	Evaluate your nursing care and make recommendations related to the achievement of your desired outcomes. Were they met, or do new goals need to be established?	**Diag**	**Nursing Outcomes Classification (NOC)**	**Outcome met**
			1	Patient reports a decrease in pain on a 0–10 scale by the end of the shift.	☐ Yes ☐ No
			2	Patient demonstrates balanced I&O for 24 hours.	☐ Yes ☐ No
			3	Patient verbalizes understanding of danger signs, proper sexual health, and emotional process.	☐ Yes ☐ No
			4	Patient identifies a support system.	☐ Yes ☐ No
			5		☐ Yes ☐ No

Nursing Diagnosis 1

Acute pain related to threatened AB or postsurgical AB evidenced by verbalization and/or guarding of abdomen.

NIC:
1) Monitor for pain q2h on even or odd hour; 2) Instruct patient to report pain as soon as it starts; 3) Administer pain medication as prescribed; 4) Consider alternative methods of pain relief such as massage, biofeedback, progressive relaxation, or guided imagery; 5) Provide calm, quiet environment; 6) Monitor VS q4h; 7) Monitor sleep–rest pattern; and 8) Allow time for verbalizations.

Nursing Diagnosis 2

Fluid and electrolyte imbalance related to bleeding or NPO status evidenced by low output or thirst.

NIC:
1) VS q2h; 2) Carefully observe for bleeding and signs of shock (pulse and BP); 3) Measure and record I&O; 4) Monitor IV fluid intake; and 5) Monitor mental status q2h.

Nursing Diagnosis 3

Knowledge deficit: ready for enhanced learning related to discharge instructions evidenced by questions.

NIC:
1) Discuss danger signs: fever, increased bleeding, prolonged depressed state; 2) Discuss postabortion sexual health including waiting 6 weeks before resuming intercourse and birth control methods; and 3) Discuss stages of the grieving process and refer to a support group.

Nursing Diagnosis 4

Anticipatory grieving related to loss evidenced by verbalization, anger, or tearful behavior.

NIC:
1) Provide emotional support; 2) Provide comfort measures; 3) Provide family privacy; and 4) Ask patient if she has a faith community.

Condition:
Abortion (Spontaneous or Induced)

Age:

Link & Explain
• Nursing Interventions Classification (NIC)
• Laboratory and Diagnostic Procedures
• Medications

Nursing Diagnosis 5

NIC:

Medications

a. RhoGAM for Rh negative women

b. Ibuprofen (Motrin) as ordered for pain

c. Tylenol and codeine as ordered for more intense pain

d. Methergine to ensure the uterus contracts properly

Laboratory & Diagnostic Procedures

a. Type and screen

b. Quantitative level of human chorionic gonadotropin (HCG) for threatened abortions

c. Ultrasound for fetal heart tones may also be done for non-elective abortions

d.

CONDITION: Abruptio Placentae

PHYSIOLOGY: An abruptio placentae is a sudden, premature, partial, or complete detachment of the placenta from a normal uterine site of implantation. The incidence of abruptio placentae is 1 in 120 births, and the risk of recurrence in later pregnancies is much higher than for cohorts. The cause is unknown; however, the condition often is associated with pregnancy-induced hypertension (PIH), cocaine abuse, intimate partner violence, or trauma. Abruption is classified according to the type and severity.

- *Grade 1:* vaginal bleeding with possible uterine tenderness and mild tetany; neither mother nor baby is in distress; approximately 10% to 20% of the placenta surface is detached.
- *Grade 2:* uterine tenderness, tetany, with or without uterine bleeding; fetal distress; mother is not in shock. Approximately 20% to 50% of the total surface area of the placenta is detached.
- *Grade 3:* uterine tetany is severe; mother is in shock although bleeding may be covert, and the fetus is dead. Often the patient develops coagulopathy. More than 50% of the placental surface is detached (*Taber's*, 2009).

HANDOFF COMMUNICATION

S	*Situation*	Assess what is currently happening in a short statement.	Patient presents as _____
B	*Background*	Summarize important past assessment data for your patient here. Place lab results and medications on the concept map.	**Age:** **Gender:** Female **Allergies:** **Fall Risk:** **Isolation:** **LMP (last menstrual period):**_____ **EDB (expected date of birth):**_____ **IPV (intimate partner violence):**_____ **Gravida (number of times pregnant):**_____ **term:**_____; **preterm:**_____; **abortion:**_____; **living:**_____
A	*Assessment*	Use the assessment data to complete your concept map.	**Nursing Diagnosis:** Place the Nursing Diagnoses in prioritized order on the concept map and add any needed for your specific patient. **Plan:** Place any further Nursing Interventions Classifications (NIC) needed on the map.

Implement Your Plan of Care

			EVALUATE YOUR CARE		
R	*Recommendation*	Evaluate your nursing care and make recommendations related to the achievement of your desired outcomes. Were they met, or do new goals need to be established?	**Diag**	**Nursing Outcomes Classification (NOC)**	**Outcome met**
			1	Tissue perfusion is maintained and improved, evidenced by stabilized VS, warm skin, palpable peripheral pulses, ABGs within norms, and adequate urine output.	☐ Yes ☐ No
			2	Patient discusses fears and concerns, verbalizes appropriate range of feelings, appears relaxed and reports anxiety is reduced to a manageable level, and demonstrates problem-solving and effective use of resources.	☐ Yes ☐ No
			3	Patient reports pain is controlled.	☐ Yes ☐ No
			4	Patient demonstrates improved fetal gas exchange.	☐ Yes ☐ No
			5		☐ Yes ☐ No

Nursing Diagnosis 1

Risk for shock related to hypotension and hypovolemia related to excessive bleeding.

NIC:
1) Investigate changes in levels of consciousness; 2) Auscultate apical pulse; 3) Assess skin for coolness; 4) Note urinary output; 5) Note reports of abdominal pain; and 6) Observe skin for pallor or redness.

Nursing Diagnosis 2

Fear related to threat of death (perceived or actual) to fetus and self, possibly evidenced by verbalizations or expressions.

NIC:
1) Monitor physiological responses; 2) Encourage verbalization of concerns; 3) Acknowledge that this is a fearful situation; and 4) Provide accurate information.

Nursing Diagnosis 3

Acute pain related to collection of blood between uterine wall and placenta and contractions evidenced by verbalization, guarding, muscle tension, and change in VS.

NIC:
1) Assess degree and characteristic of pain; 2) Assess VS, noting tachycardia; 3) Reposition as indicated; 4) Administer medication as ordered; and 5) Encourage relaxation techniques.

Nursing Diagnosis 4

Impaired fetal gas exchange related to altered uteroplacental oxygen transfer evidenced by alterations in fetal heart rate and movement.

NIC:
1) Monitor fetal heart tones; 2) Provide maternal oxygen mask as ordered; 3) Monitor maternal VS; 4) Reposition patient on left side to promote uterine circulation; and 5) Note hydration status.

Condition:
Abruptio Placentae
Age:

Link & Explain
• Nursing Interventions Classification (NIC)
• Laboratory and Diagnostic Procedures
• Medications

Nursing Diagnosis 5

NIC:

Medications

a. Terbutaline, 0.25 mg subQ, stat and q 20 min x 3 doses to provide uterine relaxation

b.

c.

d.

Laboratory & Diagnostic Procedures

a. CBC

b. Platelet count

c. Type and crossmatch in case replacement blood is needed

d. Ultrasound of the abdomen to determine the extent of placental detachments

CONDITION: Adoption

PHYSIOLOGY: Adoption (choosing to give a child to an adoptive family) is a legal procedure that allows the biological parent to relinquish responsibility of a child and turn the child over to a person or persons who are willing to assume responsibility of the child (*Taber's*, 2009).

HANDOFF COMMUNICATION

S Situation	Assess what is currently happening in a short statement.	Patient presents as _____
B Background	Summarize important past assessment data for your patient here. Place lab results and medications on the concept map.	**Age:** **Gender:** Female **Allergies:** **Fall Risk:** **Isolation:** **LMP (last menstrual period):**_____ **EDB (expected date of birth):**_____ **IPV (intimate partner violence):**_____ **Gravida (number of times pregnant):**_____ **term:**_____; **preterm:**_____; **abortion:**_____; **living:**_____
A Assessment	Use the assessment data to complete your concept map.	**Nursing Diagnosis:** Place the Nursing Diagnoses in prioritized order on the concept map and add any needed for your specific patient. **Plan:** Place any further Nursing Interventions Classifications (NIC) needed on the map.

Implement Your Plan of Care

		EVALUATE YOUR CARE		
R Recommendation	Evaluate your nursing care and make recommendations related to the achievement of your desired outcomes. Were they met, or do new goals need to be established?	**Diag**	**Nursing Outcomes Classification (NOC)**	**Outcome met**
		1	Grief resolution: patient identifies and expresses feelings appropriately; continues normal life activities, looking toward and planning for the future, one day at a time; verbalizes understanding of the stages of grief and loss.	☐ Yes ☐ No
		2	Patient acknowledges feelings and healthy ways to deal with them; verbalizes some control over present situation; makes choices related to her care and is involved in self-care.	☐ Yes ☐ No
		3	Patient uses positive language about adoption: reinforces the decision as a healthy option.	☐ Yes ☐ No
		4	Patient expresses willingness to look at own role in family growth and undertakes tasks leading to change.	☐ Yes ☐ No
		5		☐ Yes ☐ No

Nursing Diagnosis 1

Complicated grieving related to actual loss of child evidenced by verbalizations and behaviors congruent with sadness.

NIC:
1) Facilitate development of a trusting relationship; **2)** Provide open, nonjudgmental environment; **3)** Use therapeutic communication skills; **4)** Encourage verbalization; **5)** Accept expressions of sadness and anger; **6)** Monitor for depression; and **7)** Be aware of mood swings.

Nursing Diagnosis 2

Risk for powerlessness possibly due to perceived lack of options, no input into decisional process, or no control over outcome.

NIC:
1) Identify factors that lead to patient's feeling of powerlessness; **2)** Encourage active role in planning future; and **3)** Encourage patient's control and responsibility.

Nursing Diagnosis 3

Risk of knowledge deficit related to adoption terms.

NIC:
1) Using positive language reinforces the message that adoption is a healthy option; and **2)** Encourage patient to verbalize feelings.

Nursing Diagnosis 4

Readiness for enhanced family coping related to adoption decision evidenced by patient attempting to describe growth impact of crises on her own values, priorities, goals, or relationships.

NIC:
1) Provide opportunity for patient to talk; **2)** Discuss importance of open family communication and role-play communication styles; and **3)** Refer to support groups.

Condition:
Adoption
Age:

Link & Explain
• Nursing Interventions Classification (NIC)
• Laboratory and Diagnostic Procedures
• Medications

Nursing Diagnosis 5

NIC:

Medications

a. Normal postpartum medications

b.

c.

d.

Laboratory & Diagnostic Procedures

a. Postpartum Hct

b.

c.

d.

CONDITION: Breast Cancer

PHYSIOLOGY: Breast cancer is predominantly a disease of women over 40 with the incidence increasing with age. Breast cancer is considered a complex multifactorial disorder caused by both genetic and nongenetic factors such as specific biologic and endocrine characteristics of the individual, environmental exposures that may precipitate mutation of cells to malignancy, and a family risk of breast cancer. Tumor suppressor genes, such as BRCA1, BRCA2, and CHEK2, have been linked to susceptibility. Other risk factors include, but are not limited to, European ancestry, age over 40, personal history of breast cancer or benign breast disease, nulliparity (or age >30 for first-time pregnancy), menarche before 12, menopause after 55, postmenopausal obesity, and diethylstilbestrol (DES) exposure. Recent studies support an association of breast cancer with moderate alcohol intake, high-fat diet, and prolonged hormonal therapy. Environmental factors include exposure to radiation during childhood and/or exposure to pesticides. Breast cancer is classified as either noninvasive or invasive depending on whether or not the cancer cells invade tissue beyond the ducts and lobules. If it is found in early states (in situ with no node involvement), the 10-year survival rate is 70%–75% compared to 20%–25% with node involvement. The rate of cell division of the cancerous growth varies, but it is estimated that the time it takes for a tumor to become palpable ranges from 5 to 9 years. As the tumor grows, fibrosis formation causes the Cooper's ligaments to shorten, resulting in dimpling of the skin. Advanced tumors interrupt lymphatic drainage, causing edema and "orange peel" (peau d'orange) appearance. Untreated cancer may also erupt on the skin as an ulceration. Like other malignancies, breast cancer can metastasize to other areas of the body, increasing morbidity and mortality. Treatment and prognosis of breast cancer is based on the TNM (T = tumor size, N = involvement of regional lymph nodes, and M = metastasis) classification stage of the of disease at diagnosis. Treatment involves surgery and radiation either alone or in combination. Chemotherapy and hormonal therapy are used to provide systemic control. Adjuvant therapy (pharmacologic treatment given to patients with no detectable cancer after surgery) may be recommended because cancer cells can break away from the primary breast tumor and spread throughout the body via the bloodstream (*Taber's*, 2009).

HANDOFF COMMUNICATION

S	Situation	Assess what is currently happening in a short statement.	Patient presents as _____
B	Background	Summarize important past assessment data for your patient here. Place lab results and medications on the concept map.	**Age:** **Gender:** Female **Allergies:** **Fall Risk:** **Isolation:** **LMP (last menstrual period):**_____ **EDB (expected date of birth) if pregnant:**_____ **IPV (intimate partner violence):**_____ **Gravida (number of times pregnant):**_____ **term:**_____; **preterm:**_____; **abortion:**_____; **living:**_____
A	Assessment	Use the assessment data to complete your concept map.	**Nursing Diagnosis:** Place the Nursing Diagnoses in prioritized order on the concept map and add any needed for your specific patient. **Plan:** Place any further Nursing Interventions Classifications (NIC) needed on the map.

Implement Your Plan of Care

			EVALUATE YOUR CARE		
R	Recommendation	Evaluate your nursing care and make recommendations related to the achievement of your desired outcomes. Were they met, or do new goals need to be established?	**Diag**	**Nursing Outcomes Classification (NOC)**	**Outcome met**
			1	Patient verbalizes understanding of disease, diagnosis, treatment options, and prognosis.	☐ Yes ☐ No
			2	Patient demonstrates reduced level of anxiety evidenced by use of positive coping strategies.	☐ Yes ☐ No
			3	Patient verbalizes feelings related to body image changes and accesses available resources to assist in related lifestyle adjustments.	☐ Yes ☐ No
			4	Patient verbalizes adequate pain control on a 0–10 pain scale and demonstrates effective use of pain management techniques.	☐ Yes ☐ No
			5		☐ Yes ☐ No

Nursing Diagnosis 1

Deficient knowledge related to lack of information regarding disease process, diagnostic testing, and treatment evidenced by questions and information gathering.

NIC:
1) Assess understanding of disease process and treatment; **2)** Identify and communicate community resources, Web sites, and additional sources of information and support; **3)** Discuss diagnostic evaluation procedures and staging classifications as indicated; **4)** Explain treatment regimen, treatment options, and provide related information; **5)** Include family/support systems in informational sessions; **6)** Explain the importance of adherence to follow-up visits and screening; and **7)** Provide education regarding normal health maintenance practices, SBE (self-breast exams).

Nursing Diagnosis 2

Fear and anxiety related to diagnosis of cancer, treatments, and uncertain prognosis evidenced by verbalizations, crying, or withdrawn behaviors.

NIC:
1) Encourage verbalization of fears and concerns; **2)** Provide thorough explanation of care routines, diagnostic tests, and treatments; **3)** Provide ongoing assessment and early intervention for pain/side effects of treatment; **4)** Assess patient's repertoire of coping mechanisms/relaxation techniques; offer to consult clergy or support services as indicated; and **5)** Include family members in all aspects of care.

Nursing Diagnosis 3

Risk for situational low self-esteem related to disturbed body image.

NIC:
1) Acknowledge feelings of anger, denial, or depression as normal part of grieving process related to unanticipated change in body image; **2)** Provide sources for prosthesis; **3)** Discuss possibility of reconstructive surgery; **4)** Encourage verbalization of feelings and concerns; and **5)** Provide referrals to support groups, health-care providers, cosmetologists, and so on.

Nursing Diagnosis 4

Pain/discomfort related to pathology and/or side effects of treatment evidenced by verbalization of pain.

NIC:
1) Assess for severity and defining characteristics of pain and administer analgesics as indicated; **2)** Assess patient's expectations related to pain relief; **3)** Monitor effectiveness/side effects of pain relief therapies; **4)** Assess fears and concerns related to pain medication; **5)** Teach nonpharmacologic interventions for pain relief; and **6)** Consult pain specialist as indicated.

Condition:
Breast Cancer
Age:

Link & Explain
• Nursing Interventions Classification (NIC)
• Laboratory and Diagnostic Procedures
• Medications

Nursing Diagnosis 5

NIC:

Medications

a. Chemotherapeutic agents

b. Antiemetics

c. NSAIDs

d. Opioid analgesics

Laboratory & Diagnostic Procedures

a. Screening for tumor-related genetic markers, hormone receptor assays, related DNA and protein markers

b. Mammography, digital imaging, CT/MRI scan, ultrasonography, bone scan, breast biopsy

c. Radio-guided cellular aspiration and/or surgical biopsy

d. Tumor tissue markers, liver function test

CONDITION: Candidiasis

PHYSIOLOGY: Candidiasis is a fungal infection of the skin or mucous membranes with any species of *Candida* but chiefly *Candida albicans*. *Candida* species are part of the body's normal flora but can proliferate and grow in warm, moist areas, causing infections. Vulvovaginal candidiasis is common during pregnancy, possibly due to increased estrogen levels or elevated glucose levels. Vaginal infections are characterized by itching and a thick, cheesy discharge (*Taber's*, 2009).

HANDOFF COMMUNICATION

S	Situation	Assess what is currently happening in a short statement.	Patient presents as _____
B	Background	Summarize important past assessment data for your patient here. Place lab results and medications on the concept map.	**Age:** **Gender:** Female **Allergies:** **Fall Risk:** **Isolation:** **LMP (last menstrual period):**_____ **EDB (expected date of birth) if pregnant:**_____ **IPV (intimate partner violence):**_____ **Gravida (number of times pregnant):**_____ **term:____; preterm:____; abortion:____; living:____**
A	Assessment	Use the assessment data to complete your concept map.	**Nursing Diagnosis:** Place the Nursing Diagnoses in prioritized order on the concept map and add any needed for your specific patient. **Plan:** Place any further Nursing Interventions Classifications (NIC) needed on the map.

Implement Your Plan of Care

R	Recommendation	Evaluate your nursing care and make recommendations related to the achievement of your desired outcomes. Were they met, or do new goals need to be established?	**EVALUATE YOUR CARE**	
			Diag / **Nursing Outcomes Classification (NOC)**	**Outcome met**
			1 Wound healing: patient demonstrates tissue regeneration, achieves timely healing of area.	☐ **Yes** ☐ **No**
			2 Pain control: patient participates in activities and sleeps and rests approximately.	☐ **Yes** ☐ **No**
			3 Sexual functioning: patient verbalizes understanding of relationship of physical condition to sexual problems, identifies satisfying and acceptable sexual practices, and explores alternative methods.	☐ **Yes** ☐ **No**
			4 Patient verbalizes understanding of disease, diagnosis, treatment options, and prognosis.	☐ **Yes** ☐ **No**
			5	☐ **Yes** ☐ **No**

Nursing Diagnosis 1

Impaired skin/tissue integrity related to infectious lesions evidenced by disruption of skin surfaces and mucous membranes or redness and edema.

NIC:
1) Assess and document size and area of skin irritation; **2)** Administer medication as ordered; **3)** Keep clean and free from bodily fluids; and **4)** Promote good hand washing to decrease contamination.

Nursing Diagnosis 2

Impaired comfort related to itching and exposure of irritated skin and mucous membranes to excretions (urine, feces) evidenced by verbal reports.

NIC:
1) Maintain comfortable environmental temperature with loose, appropriate clothing; **2)** Assess reports of discomfort; and **3)** Administer medication as prescribed.

Nursing Diagnosis 3

Risk for sexual dysfunction related to presence of infectious process and vaginal discomfort.

NIC:
1) Determine patient and significant other's (SO) relationship before the outbreak; **2)** Reinforce information provided by health-care practitioner; and **3)** Review with patient and SO restrictions on sexual functioning.

Nursing Diagnosis 4

Deficient knowledge related to lack of information regarding disease process, diagnostic testing, and treatment evidenced by questions and information gathering.

NIC:
1) Assess understanding of disease process and treatment; **2)** Identify and communicate community resources, Web sites, and additional sources of information and support; **3)** Explain treatment regimen, treatment options, and provide related information; **4)** Explain the importance of adherence to follow-up visits and screening; and **5)** Provide education regarding normal health maintenance practices.

Condition:
Candidiasis
Age:

Link & Explain
• Nursing Interventions Classification (NIC)
• Laboratory and Diagnostic Procedures
• Medications

Nursing Diagnosis 5

NIC:

Medications

a. Azoles are antifungal drugs that end in the suffix *-azole*, which block the manufacture of ergosterol, a crucial material of the yeast cell wall

b. Polyene antifungals include nystatin and amphotericin B

c.

d.

Laboratory & Diagnostic Procedures

a. Culture of discharge possibly, but usually diagnosed by clinical manifestations.

b.

c.

d.

CONDITION: Cesarean Birth

PHYSIOLOGY: A cesarean birth (cesarean section) is delivery of the fetus by means of an incision through the abdominal wall and into the uterus. Operative approaches and techniques vary. A horizontal incision through the lower uterine segment is most common; the classic vertical midline incision of the abdomen and uterus may be used in an emergency. Elective cesarean birth is indicated for known cephalopelvic disproportion, malpresentation, some patients with pregnancy-induced hypertension (PIH), and active genital herpes. The most common reason for a cesarean delivery is fetal distress (*Taber's*, 2009).

HANDOFF COMMUNICATION

S — Situation

Assess what is currently happening in a short statement.

Patient presents as _____

B — Background

Summarize important past assessment data for your patient here. Place lab results and medications on the concept map.

Age: **Gender:** Female

Allergies: **Fall Risk:**

Isolation:

Date of delivery:_____

IPV (intimate partner violence):_____

Gravida (number of times pregnant):_____

term:_____; **preterm:**_____; **abortion:**_____; **living:**_____

A — Assessment

Use the assessment data to complete your concept map.

Nursing Diagnosis: Place the Nursing Diagnoses in prioritized order on the concept map and add any needed for your specific patient.
Plan: Place any further Nursing Interventions Classifications (NIC) needed on the map.

Implement Your Plan of Care

R — Recommendation

Evaluate your nursing care and make recommendations related to the achievement of your desired outcomes. Were they met, or do new goals need to be established?

Diag	EVALUATE YOUR CARE — Nursing Outcomes Classification (NOC)	Outcome met
1	Patient demonstrates attachment by making positive statements about the infant; smiles and vocalizes to the infant; and responds appropriately to the infant's cues.	☐ Yes ☐ No
2	Pain level: patient verbalizes relief or absence of pain; demonstrates relaxed body posture and ability to rest and sleep appropriately.	☐ Yes ☐ No
3	Risk control: patient experiences no physical injury.	☐ Yes ☐ No
4	Risk control: patient identifies interventions to prevent and reduce risk of infection.	☐ Yes ☐ No
5		☐ Yes ☐ No

Nursing Diagnosis 1

Risk for impaired attachment related to developmental transition or gain of a family member or situational crisis.

NIC:
1) Encourage early and frequent contact with infant; **2)** Medicate as needed to hold infant comfortably; **3)** Corroboratively make a schedule that helps patient care for infant; and **4)** Allow patient to talk about anxiety of caring for her infant.

Nursing Diagnosis 2

Acute pain related to surgical trauma, effects of anesthesia, hormonal effects, bladder or abdominal distention, after-birth pains, spinal headache, evidenced by facial mask of pain, guarding, irritability, or distracted behavior.

NIC:
1) Encourage patient to report type, location, and intensity of pain, rating it on a scale; **2)** Medicate as indicated; **3)** Provide comfort measures; and **4)** Monitor VS.

Nursing Diagnosis 3

Risk for injury related to biochemical or regulatory functions (orthostatic hypotension), effects of anesthesia, thromboembolism, abnormal blood profile (anemia or excessive blood loss), and tissue trauma.

NIC:
1) Assist with ambulation and self-care activities; **2)** Provide safe environment; **3)** Place call bell within reach; **4)** Keep side rails up when patient is feeding infant; and **5)** Assist patient to dangle before ambulating.

Nursing Diagnosis 4

Risk for infection related to tissue trauma, broken skin, decreased Hgb/Hct, invasive procedures, and/or increased environmental exposure, prolonged rupture of amniotic membranes, malnutrition.

NIC:
1) Note risk for occurrence of infection: environmental, compromised host, traumatic injury, loss of skin integrity; **2)** Observe for signs and symptoms of systemic infection: fever, chills, diaphoresis; **3)** Practice and demonstrate proper hand washing; and **4)** Review nutritional needs.

Condition:
Cesarean Birth
Age:

Link & Explain
• Nursing Interventions Classification (NIC)
• Laboratory and Diagnostic Procedures
• Medications

Nursing Diagnosis 5

NIC:

Medications

a. Analgesia as ordered

b. Colace 100 mg bid as a stool softener

c.

d.

Laboratory & Diagnostic Procedures

a. Postpartum Hgb/Hct to monitor blood loss

b.

c.

d.

CONDITION: Delivering a Child With Down Syndrome or Genetic Disorder

PHYSIOLOGY: Down syndrome is the clinical consequences of having three copies of chromosome 21. The condition is marked by mild to moderate mental retardation and physical characteristics that include a sloping forehead; low-set ears with small canals; and short, broad hands with single palmer crease (simian crease). Cardiac valvular disease and a tendency to develop Alzheimer-like changes in the brain are common consequences of the syndrome. The syndrome is present in about 1 in 700 births in the United States and is more common in women over age 34 or when the father is over 42. If women conceive after the age of 45, the incidence rises dramatically (*Taber's*, 2009).

HANDOFF COMMUNICATION

S	Situation	Assess what is currently happening in a short statement.	Patient presents as _____
B	Background	Summarize important past assessment data for your patient here. Place lab results and medications on the concept map.	**Age:** **Gender:** Female **Allergies:** **Fall Risk:** **Isolation:** **LMP (last menstrual period):**_____ **EDB (expected date of birth):**_____ **IPV (intimate partner violence):**_____ **Gravida (number of times pregnant):**_____ **term:**_____; **preterm:**_____; **abortion:**_____; **living:**_____
A	Assessment	Use the assessment data to complete your concept map.	**Nursing Diagnosis:** Place the Nursing Diagnoses in prioritized order on the concept map and add any needed for your specific patient. **Plan:** Place any further Nursing Interventions Classifications (NIC) needed on the map.

Implement Your Plan of Care

		EVALUATE YOUR CARE		
R	Recommendation	Evaluate your nursing care and make recommendations related to the achievement of your desired outcomes. Were they met, or do new goals need to be established?	**Diag** / **Nursing Outcomes Classification (NOC)**	**Outcome met**
			1 Anxiety/self-control: patient verbalizes awareness of anxiety and healthy ways to deal with them, reports anxiety is reduced to a manageable level, expresses concerns about effect of child's condition on lifestyle and position in family and society, demonstrates effective coping strategies and problem-solving skills.	☐ Yes ☐ No
			2 Knowledge of genetic condition: patient verbalizes understanding of condition and possible complications, verbalizes understanding of any tests that will be performed on the infant, initiates necessary lifestyle changes for the family.	☐ Yes ☐ No
			3 Spiritual distress: patient verbalizes concerns and feelings, identifies people in whom she is comfortable confiding.	☐ Yes ☐ No
			4 Chronic sorrow: patient verbalizes less sadness as time moves forward, describes coping strategies, demonstrates coping behavior.	☐ Yes ☐ No
			5	☐ Yes ☐ No

Nursing Diagnosis 1

Anxiety related to presence of a specific risk factor, situational crisis, threat to self-concept evidenced by increased tension, apprehension, uncertainty, feelings of inadequacy, expressed concern.

NIC:
1) Promote expression of fears and feelings such as guilt, anger, denial, and depression; 2) Encourage family and friends to verbalize; and 3) Explain expected process for diagnosis or treatment of infant if needed.

Nursing Diagnosis 2

Knowledge deficit related to lack of awareness of ramifications of diagnosis, process needed for analyzing available options, information misinterpretation evidenced by verbalization of concerns, misconceptions, and requests for information.

NIC:
1) Discuss the physiology of the condition; 2) Review any significant findings on the infant; 3) Encourage questions; and 4) Refer to a support group.

Nursing Diagnosis 3

Spiritual distress related to intense inner conflict about the outcome, normal grieving for loss of "perfect" child, anger directed at God or a greater power, evidenced by verbalization of inner conflict, questioning beliefs and choices.

NIC:
1) Arrange for religious practices if desired; and 2) Encourage questions and verbalization.

Nursing Diagnosis 4

Chronic sorrow related to child with a genetic disorder evidenced by verbalizations or sad behavior.

NIC:
1) Assess patient's coping mechanisms; 2) Listen to, empathize with, and support the patient; 3) Encourage patient to join a support group; 4) Have patient participate in her own self-care and care of infant; and 5) Identify need for pediatric specialists with patient.

Condition:
Delivering a Child With Down Syndrome or Genetic Disorder

Age:
_____
Link & Explain
• Nursing Interventions Classification (NIC)
• Laboratory and Diagnostic Procedures
• Medications

Nursing Diagnosis 5

NIC:

Medications

a.

b.

c.

d.

Laboratory & Diagnostic Procedures

a. Genetic testing of family members

b.

c.

d.

CONDITION: Dysfunctional Uterine Bleeding (DUB)

PHYSIOLOGY: Dysfunctional uterine bleeding (DUB) is an abnormal uterine bleeding that cannot be directly contributed to a known disease process. It can occur during the childbearing years and is especially common in the perimenopausal period. It can produce anemia and affect a woman's quality of life by limiting her ability to function socially and emotionally (*Taber's*, 2009).

HANDOFF COMMUNICATION

S	Situation	Assess what is currently happening in a short statement.	Patient presents as _____
B	Background	Summarize important past assessment data for your patient here. Place lab results and medications on the concept map.	**Age:** **Gender:** Female **Allergies:** **Fall Risk:** **Isolation:** **LMP (last menstrual period):**_____ **EDB (expected date of birth) if pregnant:**_____ **IPV (intimate partner violence):**_____ **Gravida (number of times pregnant):**_____ **term:**_____; **preterm:**_____; **abortion:**_____; **living:**_____
A	Assessment	Use the assessment data to complete your concept map.	**Nursing Diagnosis:** Place the Nursing Diagnoses in prioritized order on the concept map and add any needed for your specific patient. **Plan:** Place any further Nursing Interventions Classifications (NIC) needed on the map.

Implement Your Plan of Care

		EVALUATE YOUR CARE		
R	Recommendation	Evaluate your nursing care and make recommendations related to the achievement of your desired outcomes. Were they met, or do new goals need to be established?	**Diag** / **Nursing Outcomes Classification (NOC)**	**Outcome met**
			1 — Patient communicates thoughts and feelings utilizing available support systems such as family, spiritual leaders, and other resources; demonstrates coping behaviors that reduce anxiety.	☐ Yes ☐ No
			2 — Patient displays laboratory values (Hgb/Hct) within normal range.	☐ Yes ☐ No
			3 — Patient verbalizes understanding of disease, diagnosis, treatment options, and prognosis.	☐ Yes ☐ No
			4 — Sexual functioning: patient verbalizes understanding of relationship of physical condition to sexual problems; identifies satisfying and acceptable sexual practices and explores alternative methods.	☐ Yes ☐ No
			5 —	☐ Yes ☐ No

Nursing Diagnosis 1

Anxiety related to perceived change in health status and unknown etiology evidenced by apprehension, uncertainty, fear of unspecified consequences, expressed concerns, focus on self.

NIC:
1) Ascertain what information the patient has about diagnosis; **2)** Explain purpose and preparation for diagnostic tests; and **3)** Provide an atmosphere for concern and anticipatory guidance.

Nursing Diagnosis 2

Activity intolerance related to imbalance between O_2 supply and demand/decreased O_2-carrying capacity of blood (anemia) evidenced by reports of fatigue or weakness.

NIC:
1) Assess patient's ability to perform normal tasks and ADL, noting any reports of weakness, fatigue, and difficulty accomplishing tasks; **2)** Note changes in balance or gait; and **3)** Monitor BP, pulse, and respirations during activity and note any adverse responses to activity.

Nursing Diagnosis 3

Deficient knowledge related to lack of information regarding disease process, diagnostic testing, and treatment evidenced by questions and information gathering.

NIC:
1) Assess understanding of disease process and treatment; **2)** Identify and communicate community resources, Web sites, and additional sources of information and support; **3)** Discuss diagnostic evaluation procedures as indicated; **4)** Explain treatment regimen, treatment options, and provide related information; **5)** Include family/support systems in informational sessions; **6)** Explain the importance of adherence to follow-up visits and screening; and **7)** Provide education regarding normal health maintenance practices.

Nursing Diagnosis 4

Risk for sexual dysfunction related to presence of vaginal bleeding or discomfort.

NIC:
1) Determine patient's and partner's relationship before situation; **2)** Reinforce information provided by primary care practitioner; **3)** Review with patient and partner restrictions on sexual functioning; and **4)** Discuss alternative ways to show affection.

Condition:
Dysfunctional Uterine Bleeding (DUB)
Age:

Link & Explain
• Nursing Interventions Classification (NIC)
• Laboratory and Diagnostic Procedures
• Medications

Nursing Diagnosis 5

NIC:

Medications

a.

b.

c.

d.

Laboratory & Diagnostic Procedures

a. Hgb/Hct

b.

c.

d.

CONDITION: Ectopic Pregnancy

PHYSIOLOGY: An ectopic pregnancy is an extrauterine implantation of a fertilized ovum, usually in the fallopian tubes but occasionally in the peritoneum, ovary, or other locations. Ectopic implantation occurs in about 1 in every 150 pregnancies. Symptoms usually occur between 6 and 12 weeks after conception. Early complaints are consistent with those of a normally implanted pregnancy and consist of nausea, amenorrhea, and breast tenderness. Pregnancy tests are positive due to the HCG (human chorionic gonadotropin) levels in the blood and urine. As the growing embryo dilates, the fallopian tube signs and symptoms of the ectopic pregnancy become apparent. These include intermittent, unilateral pelvic or abdominal pain; orthostatic vertigo; referred shoulder pain; abdominal bleeding; and hypovolemic shock. Complaints usually arise from a ruptured fallopian tube (*Taber's*, 2009).

HANDOFF COMMUNICATION

S	Situation	Assess what is currently happening in a short statement.	Patient presents as _____
B	Background	Summarize important past assessment data for your patient here. Place lab results and medications on the concept map.	**Age:** **Gender:** Female **Allergies:** **Fall Risk:** **Isolation:** **LMP (last menstrual period):**_____ **EDB (expected date of birth):**_____ **IPV (intimate partner violence):**_____ **Gravida (number of times pregnant):**_____ **term:**_____; **preterm:**_____; **abortion:**_____; **living:**_____
A	Assessment	Use the assessment data to complete your concept map.	**Nursing Diagnosis:** Place the Nursing Diagnoses in prioritized order on the concept map and add any needed for your specific patient. **Plan:** Place any further Nursing Interventions Classifications (NIC) needed on the map.

Implement Your Plan of Care

			EVALUATE YOUR CARE	
R	Recommendation	Evaluate your nursing care and make recommendations related to the achievement of your desired outcomes. Were they met, or do new goals need to be established?	**Diag** **Nursing Outcomes Classification (NOC)**	**Outcome met**
			1 Patient verbalizes relief of pain, demonstrates a relaxed body posture.	☐ Yes ☐ No
			2 Patient demonstrates adequate fluid balance evidenced by stable VS, palpable pulses and good skin turgor, moist mucous membranes, and appropriate urinary output.	☐ Yes ☐ No
			3 Patient appears relaxed and anxiety is reduced to a manageable level. Patient verbalizes awareness of feelings and uses resources and support systems effectively.	☐ Yes ☐ No
			4 Patient identifies and expresses feelings freely and effectively.	☐ Yes ☐ No
			5	☐ Yes ☐ No

Nursing Diagnosis 1

Acute pain related to distention or rupture of fallopian tube evidenced by verbalizations, guarding, distracted behavior, facial mask of pain, diaphoreses, or changes in VS.

NIC:
1) Note reports of pain and nonverbal pain cues such as restlessness, guarding, tachycardia, diaphoresis; **2)** Use pain scale; and **3)** Medicate as indicated.

Nursing Diagnosis 2

Risk for bleeding/deficit fluid volume related to hemorrhagic losses, restricted or deficient intake.

NIC:
1) Measure I&O accurately; **2)** Monitor VS; note changes in blood pressure (BP), heart rate and rhythm, and respirations; and **3)** Calculate pulse pressure.

Nursing Diagnosis 3

Anxiety related to threat of death and possible inability to conceive again in the future evidenced by increased tension, apprehension, sympathetic stimulation, restlessness, and focus on self.

NIC:
1) Discuss patient's expectations and fears; **2)** Answer questions; and **3)** Identify and encourage previously successful coping behaviors.

Nursing Diagnosis 4

Grieving related to death of fetus evidenced by verbal expression of distress, anger, loss, crying, alterations in eating and sleeping.

NIC:
1) Provide open environment for parents to discuss feelings; **2)** Determine parents' meaning and perception of loss based on experience, culture; and **3)** Identify stage of grieving.

Condition:
Ectopic Pregnancy
Age:

Link & Explain
• Nursing Interventions Classification (NIC)
• Laboratory and Diagnostic Procedures
• Medications

Nursing Diagnosis 5

NIC:

Medications

a. Methotrexate (Rheumatrex)

b.

c.

d.

Laboratory & Diagnostic Procedures

a. Serum HCG levels

b. Ultrasound

c. Culdocentesis may show free blood in the perineum

d. Laparoscopy may reveal pregnancy outside the uterus

CONDITION: Family Experiencing a Fetal Demise

PHYSIOLOGY: Fetal death or demise (stillbirth) is the birth of a dead fetus usually after 20 weeks' gestation (*Taber's*, 2009).

HANDOFF COMMUNICATION

S Situation	Assess what is currently happening in a short statement.	Patient presents as _____
B Background	Summarize important past assessment data for your patient here. Place lab results and medications on the concept map.	**Age:** **Gender:** Female **Allergies:** **Fall Risk:** **Isolation:** **LMP (last menstrual period):**_____ **EDB (expected date of birth):**_____ **IPV (intimate partner violence):**_____ **Gravida (number of times pregnant):**_____ **term:**_____; **preterm:**_____; **abortion:**_____; **living:**_____
A Assessment	Use the assessment data to complete your concept map.	**Nursing Diagnosis:** Place the Nursing Diagnoses in prioritized order on the concept map and add any needed for your specific patient. **Plan:** Place any further Nursing Interventions Classifications (NIC) needed on the map.

Implement Your Plan of Care

		EVALUATE YOUR CARE	
R Recommendation	Evaluate your nursing care and make recommendations related to the achievement of your desired outcomes. Were they met, or do new goals need to be established?	**Diag** **Nursing Outcomes Classification (NOC)**	**Outcome met**
		1 Parents identify and express feelings freely and effectively.	☐ Yes ☐ No
		2 Parents verbalize realistic view and acceptance of self in situation.	☐ Yes ☐ No
		3 Parents identify meaning and purpose in life that reinforce hope, peace, and contentment.	☐ Yes ☐ No
		4 Parents identify resources within themselves to deal with the situation.	☐ Yes ☐ No
		5	☐ Yes ☐ No

Nursing Diagnosis 1

Grieving related to death of fetus/infant evidenced by verbal expression of distress, anger, loss, crying, alterations in eating and sleeping.

NIC:
1) Provide open environment for parents to discuss feelings; **2)** Determine parents' meaning and perception of loss based on experience, culture; and **3)** Identify stage of grieving.

Nursing Diagnosis 2

Situational low self-esteem related to perceived failure at a life event evidenced by negative self-appraisal, verbalization of negative feelings about self, helplessness, difficulty making decisions.

NIC:
1) Actively listen to family's concerns and fears; **2)** Encourage verbalization; **3)** Observe nonverbal communication; and **4)** Observe and describe behavior in objective terms.

Nursing Diagnosis 3

Risk for spiritual distress related to loss of a loved one, low self-esteem, poor relationships, or challenge to belief system.

NIC:
1) Listen to family's reports of anger and concern; **2)** Determine family's religious orientation if any; and **3)** Establish an environment that promotes free expression.

Nursing Diagnosis 4

Risk for compromised family coping related to temporary family disorganization.

NIC:
1) Establish a rapport and acknowledge the difficulty of the situation; **2)** Assess level of anxiety; and **3)** Refer to appropriate resources.

Condition:
Family Experiencing a Fetal Demise

Age:

Link & Explain
• Nursing Interventions Classification (NIC)
• Laboratory and Diagnostic Procedures
• Medications

Nursing Diagnosis 5

NIC:

Medications

a.

b.

c.

d.

Laboratory & Diagnostic Procedures

a. Genetic counseling.

b. CBC and platelet count

c. Fibrinogen level

d.

CONDITION: First Trimester Gestation

PHYSIOLOGY: *Fetal:* During the first trimester (conception to 12 weeks' gestation), major organs are formed for the fetus. Organogenesis is the formation of organs, and it occurs primarily during the first 8 weeks. During the first 8 weeks, the fetus is called an embryo. The development of the embryo to fetus progresses in a head to foot pattern (cephalocaudal). During the fetal period 9 to 12 weeks, the organs are formed but differentiating. By the 10th week of gestation, the face is recognizable, the intestines are contained in the abdomen, and the external genitalia can be differentiated. Also during this time, blood formation is done primarily by the liver (erythropoiesis), and then at 12 weeks, that function is taken over by the spleen. The fetus passes urine between 9 and 12 weeks.

Maternal: The uterus rises out of the pelvis by 12 weeks. During the first 12 weeks of gestation, the changing body effects for the mother are due to estrogen and progesterone. Estrogen increases vascularity and proliferates tissue (hyperplasia and hypertrophy), and progesterone is a smooth-muscle relaxer. The cervix softens (Goodell's sign), becomes a vascular blue (Chadwick's sign), and is occluded by a mucous plug. The breasts enlarge, and the Montgomery tubercles become pronounced. The distending uterus produces frequency of urination. Many women are nauseous and theoretically this is due to the HCG (human chorionic gonadotropin), which peaks between the 60th and 70th day of pregnancy (*Taber's*, 2009).

HANDOFF COMMUNICATION

S	Situation	Assess what is currently happening in a short statement.	Patient presents as _____
B	Background	Summarize important past assessment data for your patient here. Place lab results and medications on the concept map.	**Age:** **Gender:** Female **Allergies:** **Fall Risk:** **Isolation:** **LMP (last menstrual period):**_____ **EDB (expected date of birth):**_____ **IPV (intimate partner violence):**_____ **Gravida (number of times pregnant):**_____ **term:**_____; **preterm:**_____; **abortion:**_____; **living:**_____
A	Assessment	Use the assessment data to complete your concept map.	**Nursing Diagnosis:** Place the Nursing Diagnoses in prioritized order on the concept map and add any needed for your specific patient. **Plan:** Place any further Nursing Interventions Classifications (NIC) needed on the map.

Implement Your Plan of Care

		EVALUATE YOUR CARE		
R	Recommendation — Evaluate your nursing care and make recommendations related to the achievement of your desired outcomes. Were they met, or do new goals need to be established?	**Diag**	**Nursing Outcomes Classification (NOC)**	**Outcome met**
		1	Patient displays weight gain toward desired goal.	☐ Yes ☐ No
		2	Patient incorporates changes into self-concept without negating self-esteem.	☐ Yes ☐ No
		3	Patient verbalizes understanding of fetal growth and development as well as maternal care needs.	☐ Yes ☐ No
		4	Patient initiates and plans for necessary lifestyle changes.	☐ Yes ☐ No
		5		☐ Yes ☐ No

Nursing Diagnosis 1

Nutrition: readiness for enhanced nutrition related to increase caloric and vitamin needs of pregnancy evidenced by information-seeking behavior about dietary habits.

NIC:
1) Instruct patient on prenatal vitamins: take with food; **2)** Instruct patient to increase calorie intake: increase protein; **3)** Monitor weight gain of 25–35 lb total if normal BMI preconceptually; and **4)** Discuss iron and folic acid intake.

Nursing Diagnosis 2

Body image: disturbed related to growing uterus evidenced by verbalization about weight gain.

NIC:
1) Discuss body image; **2)** Reflect on patient's perceptions of body changes; **3)** Monitor caloric intake; and **4)** Discuss appropriate clothing to prevent infections from overly tight clothes or injury from high heels.

Nursing Diagnosis 3

Knowledge deficit: ready for enhanced knowledge related to pregnancy evidenced by questions.

NIC:
1) Teach danger signs: excessive vomiting, vaginal bleeding, and infections; **2)** Discuss immunizations; **3)** Discuss teratogens; and **4)** Discuss alcohol, smoking, and over-the-counter medication.

Nursing Diagnosis 4

Family processes: readiness for enhanced family processes related to changing family structure evidenced by verbalization of plans to incorporate infant into family system.

NIC:
1) Discuss plans for infant; **2)** Discuss relationships; and **3)** Discuss childcare responsibilities and plans for work and family time.

Condition:
First Trimester Gestation
Age:

Link & Explain
• Nursing Interventions Classification (NIC)
• Laboratory and Diagnostic Procedures
• Medications

Nursing Diagnosis 5

NIC:

Medications

a. Prenatal vitamins (if nauseous, take with food)

b.

c.

d.

Laboratory & Diagnostic Procedures

a. Type and screen

b. Urinalysis (protein, glucose, leukocytes, nitrites, ketosis)

c. Transvaginal ultrasound; fetal heart tones

d. VDRL (venereal disease reaction level) or RPR (rapid plasma reagent) (screen for sexually transmitted infections)

CONDITION: Gestational Diabetes Mellitus (GDM)

PHYSIOLOGY: GDM begins during pregnancy as a result of changes in glucose metabolism and insulin resistance. It affects 7% of all pregnant women in the United States. Although GDM usually subsides after delivery, women with GDM have a 45% risk of reoccurrence with the next pregnancy and a significant risk of developing type 2 diabetes later in life. Women at risk for GDM (over the age of 25, overweight at the start of pregnancy, previous history of GDM, previous history of an infant weighing over 9 pounds, history of a poor pregnancy outcome, glycosuria, polycystic ovarian syndrome, family history, or of an ethnic group with a high incidence of type 2 diabetes) should undergo oral glucose tolerance testing as soon as possible to assess blood glucose levels while fasting and after meals. Testing should be repeated at 24 to 28 weeks' gestation if the first screening is negative. Caloric restriction, exercise, and metformin or insulin are used to treat GDM (*Taber's*, 2009).

HANDOFF COMMUNICATION

S	Situation	Assess what is currently happening in a short statement.	Patient presents as _____
B	Background	Summarize important past assessment data for your patient here. Place lab results and medications on the concept map.	**Age:** **Gender:** Female **Allergies:** **Fall Risk:** **Isolation:** **LMP (last menstrual period):**_____ **EDB (expected date of birth):**_____ **IPV (intimate partner violence):**_____ **Gravida (number of times pregnant):**_____ **term:**_____; **preterm:**_____; **abortion:**_____; **living:**_____
A	Assessment	Use the assessment data to complete your concept map.	**Nursing Diagnosis:** Place the Nursing Diagnoses in prioritized order on the concept map and add any needed for your specific patient. **Plan:** Place any further Nursing Interventions Classifications (NIC) needed on the map.

Implement Your Plan of Care

		EVALUATE YOUR CARE		
R	Recommendation	Evaluate your nursing care and make recommendations related to the achievement of your desired outcomes. Were they met, or do new goals need to be established?	**Diag**	**Nursing Outcomes Classification (NOC)**	**Outcome met**

Diag	Nursing Outcomes Classification (NOC)	Outcome met
1	Patient verbalizes understanding of the disease process and potential complications, identifies relationship of signs and symptoms to the disease process and then correlates symptoms with causative agents, correctly performs necessary procedures and explains reasons for the actions, initiates necessary lifestyle changes, and participates in treatment regimens.	☐ Yes ☐ No
2	Patient maintains glucose in satisfactory range.	☐ Yes ☐ No
3	Patient identifies interventions to prevent or reduce risk of infection.	☐ Yes ☐ No
4	Family identifies resources within themselves to deal with situation, visits regularly and participates positively in care of patient, and provides patient opportunity to deal with situation on her own.	☐ Yes ☐ No
5		☐ Yes ☐ No

Nursing Diagnosis 1

Knowledge deficit regarding disease process, treatment, and individual care needs related to unfamiliarity with information evidenced by request for information and statements of concern.

NIC:
1) Create an environment of trust by listening to concerns; **2)** Work with patient to set mutual goals for learning; **3)** Select a variety of teaching strategies; **4)** Discuss essential elements of the disease process; **5)** Demonstrate fingerstick testing; **6)** Discuss dietary plan; **7)** Review medication regimen; and **8)** Review target blood glucose levels.

Nursing Diagnosis 2

Risk for unstable blood glucose level related to changes in insulin resistance and glucose metabolism.

NIC:
1) Determine individual factors that lead to situation of uncontrolled blood glucose levels; **2)** Perform fingerstick; **3)** Review medication; **4)** Weigh daily; and **5)** Include partner in meal planning.

Nursing Diagnosis 3

Risk for infection related to increased circulating glucose.

NIC:
1) Observe for signs of infection and inflammation (cloudy urine); **2)** Teach perineal care; **3)** Encourage proper dietary and fluid intake; and **4)** Encourage good hand washing.

Nursing Diagnosis 4

Compromised family coping related to diagnosis of GDM evidenced by verbalization about lifestyle alteration and concern for fetus.

NIC:
1) Establish rapport and acknowledge that situation will be an adjustment for family; **2)** Determine current knowledge and perception of situation; **3)** Assess level of anxiety; **4)** Evaluate prediagnosis and current behaviors that will interfere with care of the patient; and **5)** Involve partner in information giving.

Condition:
Gestational Diabetes Mellitus (GDM)

Age:

Link & Explain
• Nursing Interventions Classification (NIC)
• Laboratory and Diagnostic Procedures
• Medications

Nursing Diagnosis 5

NIC:

Medications

a. Insulin

b. Metformin

c.

d.

Laboratory & Diagnostic Procedures

a. Fingersticks

b. Hgb A1c

c. FBS (fasting blood sugar)

d. Urinalysis or urine dipstick

CONDITION: HELLP Syndrome (Hemolysis, Elevated Liver enzymes, and Low Platelets)

PHYSIOLOGY: HELLP syndrome is a combination of events signaling a variation in severe pre-eclampsia marked by hemolysis anemia, elevated liver enzymes, and low platelet count. This syndrome usually arises in the last trimester of pregnancy. Initially patients may complain of nausea, vomiting, epigastric pain, headache, and vision problems. Complications may include acute renal failure, DIC (disseminated intravascular coagulation), liver failure, respiratory failure, or multiple organ system failure (*Taber's*, 2009).

HANDOFF COMMUNICATION

S	**Situation**	Assess what is currently happening in a short statement.	Patient presents as _____
B	**Background**	Summarize important past assessment data for your patient here. Place lab results and medications on the concept map.	**Age:**　　　　　　　　　　　　　　　　　　　**Gender:** Female **Allergies:**　　　　　　　　　　　　　　　　**Fall Risk:** **Isolation:** **LMP (last menstrual period):**_____ **EDB (expected date of birth):**_____ **IPV (intimate partner violence):**_____ **Gravida (number of times pregnant):**_____ **term:**_____; **preterm:**_____; **abortion:**_____; **living:**_____
A	**Assessment**	Use the assessment data to complete your concept map.	**Nursing Diagnosis:** Place the Nursing Diagnoses in prioritized order on the concept map and add any needed for your specific patient. **Plan:** Place any further Nursing Interventions Classifications (NIC) needed on the map.

Implement Your Plan of Care

R	**Recommendation**	Evaluate your nursing care and make recommendations related to the achievement of your desired outcomes. Were they met, or do new goals need to be established?		**EVALUATE YOUR CARE**	
			Diag	**Nursing Outcomes Classification (NOC)**	**Outcome met**
			1	Patient demonstrates tissue integrity and tissue perfusion.	☐ Yes ☐ No
			2	Patient demonstrates improved VS and pulse oximetry readings.	☐ Yes ☐ No
			3	Patient reports a decrease in pain on a 0–10 scale.	☐ Yes ☐ No
			4	Patient verbalizes concerns about condition.	☐ Yes ☐ No
			5		☐ Yes ☐ No

Nursing Diagnosis 1

Ineffective tissue perfusion related to alternation in arterial and venous flow due to hemolytic anemia evidenced by changes in respirations, changes in mental status, decreased urinary output, and peripheral cyanosis.

NIC:
1) Initiate DVT (deep vein thrombosis) prevention; **2)** Monitor VS; **3)** Decrease cardiac consumption; **4)** Monitor pulse oximetry; and **5)** Monitor I&O.

Nursing Diagnosis 2

Impaired gas exchange related to hemolytic anemia and poor respiratory profusion evidenced by shortness of breath, changes in respiratory pattern, and lower pulse oximetry readings.

NIC:
1) Decrease oxygen consumption; **2)** Monitor rate, rhythm, depth, and effort of respirations; **3)** Auscultate breath sounds; and **4)** Monitor pulse oximetry.

Nursing Diagnosis 3

Acute pain related to liver enlargement evidenced by complaints of epigastric discomfort.

NIC:
1) Assess pain for location, characteristic, onset/duration, frequency, and so on; **2)** Assure patient analgesic care; and **3)** Evaluate effectiveness of pain control using a 0–10 scale.

Nursing Diagnosis 4

Anxiety related to sudden change in health status of self and effect on fetus evidenced by apprehension, focus on self and fetus, and restlessness.

NIC:
1) Use a calm, reassuring approach; **2)** Explain all procedures; **3)** Provide factual information; **4)** Encourage family to stay with patient; **5)** Listen attentively; and **6)** Control stimuli.

Condition:
HELLP Syndrome (Hemolysis, Elevated Liver Enzymes, and Low Platelets)

Age:
_____
Link & Explain
• Nursing Interventions Classification (NIC)
• Laboratory and Diagnostic Procedures
• Medications

Nursing Diagnosis 5

NIC:

Medications

a. $MgSO_4$

b. Corticosteroids

c. Antihypertensives

d. Platelets

Laboratory & Diagnostic Procedures

a. CBC, fibrin degradation products (FDPs)

b. Liver enzymes: aspartate aminotransferase (AST) (serum glutamic oxaloacetic transaminase [SGOT]) and alanine aminotransferase (ALT) (serum glutamic pyruvic transaminase [SGPT]), electrolytes

c. Renal function tests, coagulation studies

d. Urine for protein, lactate dehydrogenases

CONDITION: Hyperemesis Gravidarum

PHYSIOLOGY: Hyperemesis gravidarum is a persistent, continuous, severe, pregnancy-related nausea and vomiting, often accompanied by dry retching. The condition can cause systemic effects such as dehydration, weight loss, fluid-electrolyte and acid-base imbalance leading to metabolic acidosis and, rarely, death. About 2 out of 1,000 pregnant women require hospitalization for medical management of the disorder (*Taber's*, 2009).

HANDOFF COMMUNICATION

S — **Situation**

Assess what is currently happening in a short statement.

Patient presents as _____

B — **Background**

Summarize important past assessment data for your patient here. Place lab results and medications on the concept map.

Age: **Gender:** Female

Allergies: **Fall Risk:**

Isolation:

LMP (last menstrual period):_____

EDB (expected date of birth):_____

IPV (intimate partner violence):_____

Gravida (number of times pregnant):_____

term:_____; **preterm:**_____; **abortion:**_____; **living:**_____

A — **Assessment**

Use the assessment data to complete your concept map.

Nursing Diagnosis: Place the Nursing Diagnoses in prioritized order on the concept map and add any needed for your specific patient.
Plan: Place any further Nursing Interventions Classifications (NIC) needed on the map.

Implement Your Plan of Care

R — **Recommendation**

Evaluate your nursing care and make recommendations related to the achievement of your desired outcomes. Were they met, or do new goals need to be established?

Diag	EVALUATE YOUR CARE — Nursing Outcomes Classification (NOC)	Outcome met
1	Patient establishes a dietary pattern with adequate caloric intake for pregnancy, maintains electrolyte balance.	☐ Yes ☐ No
2	Patient maintains balanced I&O; adequate urine output; normal BP, pulse, and body temperature.	☐ Yes ☐ No
3	Patient verbalizes understanding of condition, disease process, and potential complications.	☐ Yes ☐ No
4	Patient expresses realistic understanding of the situation.	☐ Yes ☐ No
5		☐ Yes ☐ No

Nursing Diagnosis 1

Nutritional: less than body requirements related to excessive vomiting evidenced by weight loss or electrolyte imbalance.

NIC:
1) Establish minimum weight goal and caloric needs; **2)** Provide small, frequent calorically dense meals if tolerated; **3)** Monitor electrolytes; and **4)** Ensure patient receives adequate amounts of folic acid by eating a balanced diet and taking folic acid as ordered.

Nursing Diagnosis 2

Risk for fluid volume deficit related to vomiting and dehydration evidenced by low urine output, thirst, dry mucous membranes.

NIC:
1) Assess VS to monitor any respiratory or cardiac effects; **2)** Provide replacement electrolytes as ordered; **3)** Maintain strict I&O; **4)** Monitor IV fluid replacement; and **5)** Check skin turgor.

Nursing Diagnosis 3

Knowledge deficit related to condition and prognosis, information misinterpretation evidenced by questions, statements of concern, and/or inaccurate follow-through of instructions.

NIC:
1) Review disease process, treatments, and implications; **2)** Stress importance of the goal to provide a well-balanced diet and fluid intake; **3)** Use therapeutic communication to encourage patient to ask questions and verbalize concerns; and **4)** Provide reliable resources from Internet or written material.

Nursing Diagnosis 4

Risk for ineffective coping related to change in health status evidenced by patient expressing despair about situation.

NIC:
1) Assess level of anxiety in patient and family members; **2)** Establish rapport and acknowledge the difficulty of the situation; **3)** Discuss with patient and family the current condition causing lifestyle and role disruption; **4)** Refer to support services if needed; and **5)** Maintain therapeutic relationship to encourage verbalization.

Condition:
Hyperemesis Gravidarum
Age:

Link & Explain
• Nursing Interventions Classification (NIC)
• Laboratory and Diagnostic Procedures
• Medications

Nursing Diagnosis 5

NIC:

Medications

a. Antiemetics

b. IV fluids (with electrolytes)

c.

d.

Laboratory & Diagnostic Procedures

a. Albumin

b. CBC and differential

c.

d.

CONDITION: Hysterectomy

PHYSIOLOGY: A hysterectomy is a surgical procedure to remove the uterus. Each year about 500,000 women undergo hysterectomies. Indications for the surgery include benign or malignant changes in the uterine wall or cavity, cervical abnormalities including endometrial cancer, cervical cancer, severe dysfunctional bleeding, large or bleeding fibroid tumors (leiomyomas), prolapse of the uterus, intractable post-partum hemorrhage due to placenta accreta or uterine rupture, or severe endometriosis. This approach to excision may be either abdominal or vaginal. The abdominal approach is used most commonly to remove large tumors; when the ovaries and the fallopian tubes are also re-moved; and when there is a need to examine adjacent pelvic structures, such as the regional lymph nodes. Vaginal hysterectomy is appropri-ate when the uterine size is less than that of a 12-week gestation; no other pathology is suspected; and surgical plans included cystocele, enterocele, or rectocele repair (*Taber's*, 2009).

HANDOFF COMMUNICATION

S	Situation	Assess what is currently happening in a short statement.	Patient presents as _____
B	Background	Summarize important past assessment data for your patient here. Place lab results and medications on the concept map.	**Age:** **Gender:** Female **Allergies:** **Fall Risk:** **Isolation:** **LMP (last menstrual period):**_____ **IPV (intimate partner violence):**_____ **Gravida (number of times pregnant):**_____ **term:**_____; **preterm:**_____; **abortion:**_____; **living:**_____
A	Assessment	Use the assessment data to complete your concept map.	**Nursing Diagnosis:** Place the Nursing Diagnoses in prioritized order on the concept map and add any needed for your specific patient. **Plan:** Place any further Nursing Interventions Classifications (NIC) needed on the map.

Implement Your Plan of Care

			EVALUATE YOUR CARE	
R	Recommendation	Evaluate your nursing care and make recommendations related to the achievement of your desired outcomes. Were they met, or do new goals need to be established?	**Diag** / **Nursing Outcomes Classification (NOC)**	**Outcome met**
			1 Patient verbalizes pain is relieved or controlled and appears relaxed and able to sleep or rest appropriately.	☐ Yes ☐ No
			2 Patient empties bladder regularly and completely.	☐ Yes ☐ No
			3 Patient verbalizes understanding of physical condition to sexual problems, resumes sexual relationships as appropriate.	☐ Yes ☐ No
			4 Patient verbalizes concerns and healthy ways of dealing with them, verbalizes acceptance of self in situation and adaptation to change in body and self-image.	☐ Yes ☐ No
			5	☐ Yes ☐ No

Nursing Diagnosis 1

Acute pain related to tissue trauma and possibly abdominal incision evidenced by verbal reports, guarding or distraction behaviors, or changes in VS.

NIC:
1) Assess pain, noting location, characteristics, and intensity (0–10 scale); **2)** Encourage patient to verbalize concerns, and give appropriate information; **3)** Administer medication, such as opioids, analgesics, and patient-controlled analgesia (PCA) as indicated; and **4)** Provide comfort measures, mouth care, back rub, and repositioning.

Nursing Diagnosis 2

Risk for impaired urinary elimination or retention related to surgical manipulation or bladder atony.

NIC:
1) Note voiding pattern and monitor urine output; **2)** Palpate bladder; **3)** Provide routine voiding measures such as running water, privacy, normal position, and running warm water over the perineum; **4)** Use bladder scanner postvoiding; and **5)** Catheterize if necessary.

Nursing Diagnosis 3

Risk for sexual dysfunction related to concerns of altered body function or structure or changes in hormone levels.

NIC:
1) Determine patient and partner's sexual history before surgery; **2)** Review with patient and partner functioning; **3)** Reinforce information provided by physician; **4)** Discuss likelihood of sexual activity in approximately 6 weeks after discharge; and **5)** Refer to counseling or sex therapist as appropriate.

Nursing Diagnosis 4

Situational low self-esteem related to changes in femininity, effects on sexual relationship, and inability to have children evidenced by specific concerns and vague comments about the results of surgery.

NIC:
1) Provide time to listen to concerns and fears; **2)** Provide accurate information; **3)** Ascertain individual strengths and identify previous positive coping behaviors; **4)** Provide an open environment for patient to discuss sexual concerns; and **5)** Refer to pastoral staff, psychiatric CNS (clinical nurse specialist), and other professionals for counseling if needed.

Condition:
Hysterectomy
Age:

Link & Explain
• Nursing Interventions Classification (NIC)
• Laboratory and Diagnostic Procedures
• Medications

Nursing Diagnosis 5

NIC:

Medications

a. Opioid, analgesics, and/or PCA

b.

c.

d.

Laboratory & Diagnostic Procedures

a. Bladder scan

b. Urinalysis

c.

d.

CONDITION: Infertility

PHYSIOLOGY: Infertility is the inability to achieve pregnancy during a year or more of unprotected intercourse. The condition may be present in either or both partners and may be reversible. In the United States, about 20% of all couples are infertile. In women, infertility may be primary (i.e., present in women who have never conceived) or secondary (i.e., occurring after previous conceptions or pregnancies). Causes of primary infertility in women include ovulatory failure, anatomical anomalies of the uterus, Turner's syndrome, and eating disorders, among many others. Common causes of secondary infertility in women include, but are not limited to, tubal scarring (e.g., after sexually transmitted infections), endometriosis, cancers, and chemotherapy. In men, infertility usually is caused by failure to manufacture adequate amounts of sperm (e.g., as a result of exposures to environmental toxins, viruses or bacteria, developmental or genetic diseases, varicoceles, or endocrine abnormalities) (*Taber's*, 2009).

HANDOFF COMMUNICATION

S Situation	Assess what is currently happening in a short statement.	Patient presents as _____
B Background	Summarize important past assessment data for your patient here. Place lab results and medications on the concept map.	**Age:** **Gender:** Female **Allergies:** **Fall Risk:** **Isolation:** **LMP (last menstrual period):**_____ **IPV (intimate partner violence):**_____ **Gravida (number of times pregnant):**_____ **term:**_____; **preterm:**_____; **abortion:**_____; **living:**_____
A Assessment	Use the assessment data to complete your concept map.	**Nursing Diagnosis:** Place the Nursing Diagnoses in prioritized order on the concept map and add any needed for your specific patient. **Plan:** Place any further Nursing Interventions Classifications (NIC) needed on the map.

Implement Your Plan of Care

		EVALUATE YOUR CARE	
R Recommendation	Evaluate your nursing care and make recommendations related to the achievement of your desired outcomes. Were they met, or do new goals need to be established?	**Diag** / **Nursing Outcomes Classification (NOC)**	**Outcome met**
		1 Patient acknowledges self as an individual, views self as a capable person, verbalizes realistic view and acceptance of body.	☐ Yes ☐ No
		2 Patient verbalizes feelings of sorrow and coping mechanisms to deal with feelings.	☐ Yes ☐ No
		3 Patient verbalizes increased sense of self-concept and hope for the future.	☐ Yes ☐ No
		4 Patient verbalizes understanding of diagnosis, treatment options, and prognosis.	☐ Yes ☐ No
		5	☐ Yes ☐ No

Nursing Diagnosis 1

Situational low self-esteem related to functional impairment (inability to conceive), unrealistic self-expectations, or sense of failure evidenced by self-negating verbalizations, expressions of helplessness, perceived inability to deal with situation.

NIC:
1) Establish a therapeutic relationship; **2)** Promote self-concept; **3)** Acknowledge reality of the grieving process; **4)** Review information about fertility; **5)** Assess interaction between patient and partner; and **6)** Mutually identify strengths, resources, and previously effective coping strategies.

Nursing Diagnosis 2

Chronic sorrow related to perceived physical disability (inability to conceive) evidenced by expressions of anger, disappointment, emptiness, self-blame, helplessness, sadness, feelings interfering with ability to achieve maximum well-being.

NIC:
1) Allow couple to express feelings and participate in needed decision-making; **2)** Contact faith-based or cultural leader if requested; **3)** Determine social supports of couple; and **4)** Encourage the use of positive coping techniques.

Nursing Diagnosis 3

Risk for spiritual distress related to energy-consuming anxiety, low self-esteem, deteriorating relationship with partner, viewing situation as deserved or punishment for past behavior.

NIC:
1) Determine patient's religious orientation; **2)** Establish an environment to promote free expression of feelings; and **3)** Discuss difference between grief and guilt.

Nursing Diagnosis 4

Deficient knowledge related to lack of information regarding condition, diagnostic testing, and treatment evidenced by questions and information gathering.

NIC:
1) Assess understanding of condition and treatment; **2)** Identify and communicate community resources, Web sites and additional sources of information and support; **3)** Discuss diagnostic evaluation procedures as indicated; **4)** Explain treatment regimen, treatment options, and provide related information; **5)** Include family/support systems in informational sessions; **6)** Explain the importance of adherence to follow-up visits and screening; and **7)** Provide education regarding normal health maintenance practices.

Condition:
Infertility
Age:

Link & Explain
• Nursing Interventions Classification (NIC)
• Laboratory and Diagnostic Procedures
• Medications

Nursing Diagnosis 5

NIC:

Medications

a. Depends on the origin of the condition

b.

c.

d.

Laboratory & Diagnostic Procedures

a. Follicle-stimulationg hormone (FSH) and clomide challenge test, progestin challenge, basal body temperature charting, thyroid function

b. Pelvic exam; pelvic ultrasound; laparoscopy; hysterosalpingography (HSG)

c. Blood hormone levels; serum progesterone; luteinizing hormone urine test

d. For partner: semen analysis, testicular biopsy (rarely done)

CONDITION: Labor (Naturally Occurring, Induced, or Augmented)

PHYSIOLOGY: Labor is the process that begins with the onset of repetitive and forceful uterine contractions sufficient to cause dilation of the cervix and ends with delivery of the products of conception. Traditionally, labor is divided into three stages. The first stage of labor, progressive cervical dilation and effacement, is completed when the cervix is fully dilated, usually 10 cm. This stage is subdivided into the latent phase and the active phase. Stage 2 is from fully dilated to birth of the baby, and stage 3 is from birth of the baby to delivery of the placenta. Induced labor is the use of pharmacological, mechanical, or operative interventions to initiate labor or to assist the progression of a previously dysfunctional labor (*Taber's*, 2009).

HANDOFF COMMUNICATION

S Situation	Assess what is currently happening in a short statement.	Patient presents as _____	
B Background	Summarize important past assessment data for your patient here. Place lab results and medications on the concept map.	**Age:** **Allergies:** **Isolation:** **LMP (last menstrual period):**_____ **EDB (expected date of birth):**_____ **IPV (intimate partner violence):**_____ **Gravida (number of times pregnant):**_____ **term:**_____; **preterm:**_____; **abortion:**_____; **living:**_____	**Gender:** Female **Fall Risk:**
A Assessment	Use the assessment data to complete your concept map.	**Nursing Diagnosis:** Place the Nursing Diagnoses in prioritized order on the concept map and add any needed for your specific patient. **Plan:** Place any further Nursing Interventions Classifications (NIC) needed on the map.	

Implement Your Plan of Care

		EVALUATE YOUR CARE		
R Recommendation	Evaluate your nursing care and make recommendations related to the achievement of your desired outcomes. Were they met, or do new goals need to be established?	**Diag**	**Nursing Outcomes Classification (NOC)**	**Outcome met**
		1	Patient verbalizes understanding of the process of labor and individual needs.	☐ Yes ☐ No
		2	Patient identifies interventions appropriate for the situation, demonstrates behaviors necessary to protect self from injury if possible.	☐ Yes ☐ No
		3	Patient demonstrates good gas exchange and VS.	☐ Yes ☐ No
		4	Patient reports pain or discomfort is relieved or controlled, verbalizes methods that provide relief, follows prescribed pharmacological regimen.	☐ Yes ☐ No
		5		☐ Yes ☐ No

Nursing Diagnosis 1

Knowledge deficit regarding procedure, treatment needs, and possible outcomes related to lack of exposure/recall, information misinterpretation, and unfamiliarity with information resources evidenced by questions, statements of concern/misconceptions, or exaggerated behavior.

NIC:

1) Assess patient's and partner's knowledge about the labor process; **2)** Discuss reasons for different interventions; and **3)** Provide time for questions and clarifications.

Nursing Diagnosis 2

Risk for maternal injury related to adverse effects or response to therapeutic interventions.

NIC:

1) Prepare area and equipment, check stock and supplies; **2)** Determine primary needs of patient and check health alerts; and **3)** Evaluate patient's response to the labor process.

Nursing Diagnosis 3

Risk for impaired fetal gas exchange related to altered placental perfusion or cord prolapsed.

NIC:

1) Avoid supine hypotension; **2)** Discuss effects of drugs; and **3)** Monitor BP.

Nursing Diagnosis 4

Acute pain related to altered characteristics of chemically stimulated contractions, psychological concerns evidenced by verbal reports, increased muscle tone, distraction or guarding behavior, or narrowed focus.

NIC:

1) Determine specifics of pain, location, and scale; **2)** Provide nonpharmacological measures for relief such as counterpressure, relaxation techniques, guided imagery, breathing techniques, and distraction; and **3)** Administer analgesics as needed.

Condition:
Labor (Naturally Occurring, Induced, or Augmented)
Age:

Link & Explain
• Nursing Interventions Classification (NIC)
• Laboratory and Diagnostic Procedures
• Medications

Nursing Diagnosis 5

NIC:

Medications

a. Pitocin for induction or augmentation (titrated)

b. Analgesics

c. Anesthetics

d.

Laboratory & Diagnostic Procedures

a. Fetal and uterine monitoring

b. CBC, type, and Rh if not known

c.

d.

CONDITION: Mastitis

PHYSIOLOGY: Mastitis, or parenchymatous inflammation of the mammary glands, can occur during breastfeeding, typically in the second or third postpartum week; however, it may occur at other times and at any age. It occurs in about 1% of postpartum women, primarily in breastfeeding primiparas, but can occur in nonlactating females and rarely in males. Infection may be due to entry of disease-producing germs through cracks in the nipple. Most commonly, the microorganism is *Staphylococcus aureus*. Other predisposing factors include blocked milk ducts (from a tight bra or prolonged intervals between breastfeeding) and an incomplete let-down reflex (possibly related to emotional trauma). Infection begins in one lobe but may extend to other areas. The woman complains of breast swelling and tenderness and shooting pains during and between feedings, in addition to fever, headache, and malaise. A triangular flush underneath the affected breast is an early sign. Abnormal VS include tachycardia and fever. Heat should be applied locally, and appropriate antibiotics and analgesics should be administered (*Taber's* 2009).

HANDOFF COMMUNICATION

S Situation	Assess what is currently happening in a short statement.	Patient presents as _____
B Background	Summarize important past assessment data for your patient here. Place lab results and medications on the concept map.	**Age:** **Gender:** Female **Allergies:** **Fall Risk:** **Isolation:** **LMP (last menstrual period):**_____ **EDB (expected date of birth) if pregnant:**_____ **IPV (intimate partner violence):**_____ **Gravida (number of times pregnant):**_____ **term:**_____; **preterm:**_____; **abortion:**_____; **living:**_____
A Assessment	Use the assessment data to complete your concept map.	**Nursing Diagnosis:** Place the Nursing Diagnoses in prioritized order on the concept map and add any needed for your specific patient. **Plan:** Place any further Nursing Interventions Classifications (NIC) needed on the map.

Implement Your Plan of Care

			EVALUATE YOUR CARE	
R Recommendation	Evaluate your nursing care and make recommendations related to the achievement of your desired outcomes. Were they met, or do new goals need to be established?	**Diag**	**Nursing Outcomes Classification (NOC)**	**Outcome met**
		1	Patient expresses reduction in pain and discomfort.	☐ Yes ☐ No
		2	Patient achieves active, timely healing and is free from signs of infection and inflammation, purulent drainage, and fever.	☐ Yes ☐ No
		3	Patient verbalizes understanding of disease process and possible complications.	☐ Yes ☐ No
		4	Patient verbalizes understanding of causative factors, demonstrates techniques to enhance breastfeeding, assumes responsibility for effective breastfeeding, achieves a mutually satisfactory breastfeeding regimen with infant content after feeding and gaining weight appropriately.	☐ Yes ☐ No
		5		☐ Yes ☐ No

Nursing Diagnosis 1

Acute pain related to erythema and edema of breast tissue evidenced by verbal reports, guarding or distraction behavior, self-focusing, and changes in VS.

NIC:
1) Assess pain (0–10 scale), noting location, duration, and intensity; **2)** Explain cause of pain to patient; **3)** Provide heat to area; **4)** Provide appropriate pain medication on schedule; and **5)** Advise patient to keep bra on with good, not tight, fit.

Nursing Diagnosis 2

Risk for infection spread or abscess formation related to traumatized tissue, stasis of fluid, and insufficient knowledge to prevent complications.

NIC:
1) Stress importance of finishing antibiotic regimen; **2)** Practice and instruct patient in good hand washing; **3)** Inspect site often; **4)** Monitor VS, note onset of fever, chills, diaphoresis, and increased pain; and **5)** Administer antibiotics as appropriate.

Nursing Diagnosis 3

Knowledge deficit related to pathophysiology, treatment, and prevention related to lack of information evidenced by statements of concern and misconceptions.

NIC:
1) Review disease process; **2)** Encourage continuation of breastfeeding; **3)** Discuss need for frequent feeds and properly fitting clothing; **4)** Instruct on signs and symptoms of complications; and **5)** Stress importance of finishing antibiotic regimen.

Nursing Diagnosis 4

Risk for ineffective breastfeeding related to soreness.

NIC:
1) Assess patient's knowledge about breastfeeding; **2)** Assist mother to develop skill of adequate breastfeeding; **3)** Note incorrect myths and misunderstandings about breastfeeding with mastitis; **4)** Encourage frequent feeds starting on the affected side first; and **5)** Provide emotional support.

Condition:
Mastitis
Age:

Link & Explain
• Nursing Interventions Classification (NIC)
• Laboratory and Diagnostic Procedures
• Medications

Nursing Diagnosis 5

NIC:

Medications

a. Analgesics

b. Antibiotics

c.

d.

Laboratory & Diagnostic Procedures

a. Culture of breast milk

b. CBC with differential

c.

d.

CONDITION: Pelvic Inflammatory Disease (PID)

PHYSIOLOGY: PID is infection of the uterus, fallopian tubes, and adjacent pelvic structures that is not associated with surgery or pregnancy. PID usually is caused by an ascending infection in which disease-producing germs spread from the vagina and cervix to the upper portions of the female reproductive tract. *Chlamydia trachomatis* and *Neisseria gonorrhea* are the most frequent causes of PID (*Taber's*, 2009).

HANDOFF COMMUNICATION

S — Situation — Assess what is currently happening in a short statement.

Patient presents as _____

B — Background — Summarize important past assessment data for your patient here. Place lab results and medications on the concept map.

Age: **Gender:** Female

Allergies: **Fall Risk:**

Isolation:

LMP (last menstrual period):_____

EDB (expected date of birth) if pregnant:_____

IPV (intimate partner violence):_____

Gravida (number of times pregnant):_____

term:_____; **preterm:**_____; **abortion:**_____; **living:**_____

A — Assessment — Use the assessment data to complete your concept map.

Nursing Diagnosis: Place the Nursing Diagnoses in prioritized order on the concept map and add any needed for your specific patient.
Plan: Place any further Nursing Interventions Classifications (NIC) needed on the map.

Implement Your Plan of Care

R — Recommendation — Evaluate your nursing care and make recommendations related to the achievement of your desired outcomes. Were they met, or do new goals need to be established?

Diag	EVALUATE YOUR CARE — Nursing Outcomes Classification (NOC)	Outcome met
1	Patient achieves timely healing, is free from purulent drainage, and is afebrile.	☐ Yes ☐ No
2	Patient reports pain is controlled.	☐ Yes ☐ No
3	Patient maintains body temperature within normal range.	☐ Yes ☐ No
4	Patient verbalizes understanding of condition and participates in treatment regimen.	☐ Yes ☐ No
5		☐ Yes ☐ No

Nursing Diagnosis 1

Infection related to presence of infectious process in highly vascular pelvic structures or delay in treatment, lack of proper hygiene or proper nutrition, or other health habits evidenced by abdominal pain and/or foul discharge.

NIC:
1) Note risk factors; **2)** Assess VS frequently; **3)** Maintain aseptic technique when providing care; **4)** Instruct patient to practice good hand washing and perineal hygiene; and **5)** Note any vaginal drainage.

Nursing Diagnosis 2

Acute pain related to inflammation, edema, and congestion of reproductive and pelvic tissues evidenced by verbal reports, guarding or distracted behavior, self-focus, and changes in VS.

NIC:
1) Assess degree and characteristic of pain; **2)** Assess VS, noting tachycardia; **3)** Reposition as indicated; **4)** Encourage relaxation techniques and other nonpharmacological approaches; and **5)** Medicate as indicated.

Nursing Diagnosis 3

Hyperthermia related to inflammatory process and hypermetabolic state evidenced by increased body temperature, warm flushed skin, or tachycardia.

NIC:
1) Note temperature; **2)** Assess environmental temperature and modify; and **3)** Provide medication as ordered.

Nursing Diagnosis 4

Knowledge deficit related to cause, complications of condition, therapy needs, and transmission of disease to others related to lack of information, misinterpretation, evidenced by statements of concern, questions, misconceptions, development of preventable complications.

NIC:
1) Review the condition; **2)** Teach side effects and treatment protocol; and **3)** Discuss alternative lifestyle practices if indicated.

Condition:
Pelvic Inflammatory Disease (PID)

Age:

Link & Explain
• Nursing Interventions Classification (NIC)
• Laboratory and Diagnostic Procedures
• Medications

Nursing Diagnosis 5

NIC:

Medications

a. Antibiotics

b. Analgesics

c.

d.

Laboratory & Diagnostic Procedures

a. Culture and sensitivity

b.

c.

d.

CONDITION: Placenta Previa

PHYSIOLOGY: Placenta previa is a placenta that is implanted in the lower uterine segment. There are three types: centralis, lateralis, and marginalis. Placenta previa centralis (total or complete placenta previa) is the condition in which the placenta has been implanted in the lower uterine segment and has grown to completely cover the internal cervical os. Placenta previa lateralis (low marginal implantation) is the condition in which the placenta lies just within the lower uterine segment. Placenta previa marginalis is the condition in which the placenta partially covers the internal cervical os (partial or incomplete placenta previa) (*Taber's*, 2009).

HANDOFF COMMUNICATION

S	Situation	Assess what is currently happening in a short statement.	Patient presents as _____
B	Background	Summarize important past assessment data for your patient here. Place lab results and medications on the concept map.	**Age:** **Gender:** Female **Allergies:** **Fall Risk:** **Isolation:** **LMP (last menstrual period):**_____ **EDB (expected date of birth):**_____ **IPV (intimate partner violence):**_____ **Gravida (number of times pregnant):**_____ **term:**_____; **preterm:**_____; **abortion:**_____; **living:**_____
A	Assessment	Use the assessment data to complete your concept map.	**Nursing Diagnosis:** Place the Nursing Diagnoses in prioritized order on the concept map and add any needed for your specific patient. **Plan:** Place any further Nursing Interventions Classifications (NIC) needed on the map.

Implement Your Plan of Care

Evaluate your nursing care and make recommendations related to the achievement of your desired outcomes. Were they met, or do new goals need to be established?

R — Recommendation

		EVALUATE YOUR CARE	
Diag	**Nursing Outcomes Classification (NOC)**		**Outcome met**
1	Patient maintains fluid volume at a functional level evidenced by individually adequate urinary output with normal specific gravity, stable VS, moist mucous membranes, good skin turgor, and prompt capillary refill.		☐ Yes ☐ No
2	Patient maintains and improves tissue perfusion evidenced by stabilized VS, warm skin, palpable peripheral pulses, ABGs within norms, and adequate urine output.		☐ Yes ☐ No
3	Patient discusses fears and concerns, verbalizes appropriate range of feelings, appears relaxed and reports anxiety is reduced to a manageable level, and demonstrates problem-solving and effective use of resources.		☐ Yes ☐ No
4	Patient engages in satisfying activities within personal limitations.		☐ Yes ☐ No
5			☐ Yes ☐ No

Nursing Diagnosis 1

Risk for fluid volume deficit related to excessive vascular losses.

NIC:
1) Monitor VS; **2)** Palpate peripheral pulses; and **3)** Monitor urinary output.

Nursing Diagnosis 2

Impaired fetal gas exchange related to altered blood flow, altered O_2-carrying capacity of blood (maternal anemia), and decreased surface area of gas exchange at the site of placental attachment evidenced by changes in fetal heart rate, activity, or release of meconium.

NIC:
1) Monitor fetal heart tones; **2)** Provide maternal oxygen mask as ordered; **3)** Monitor maternal VS; **4)** Reposition; and **5)** Note hydration status.

Nursing Diagnosis 3

Fear related to threat of death (perceived or actual) to self or fetus evidenced by verbalization of specific concerns, increased tension, or sympathetic stimulation.

NIC:
1) Monitor physiological responses; **2)** Encourage verbalization of concerns; **3)** Acknowledge that this is a fearful situation; and **4)** Provide accurate information.

Nursing Diagnosis 4

Risk for deficit divisional activities related to imposed bedrest restriction.

NIC:
1) Determine avocation and hobbies patient previously pursued; **2)** Encourage participation in mix of activities and stimuli; and **3)** Provide change of scenery when possible.

Nursing Diagnosis 5

NIC:

Condition:
Placenta Previa
Age:

Link & Explain
• Nursing Interventions Classification (NIC)
• Laboratory and Diagnostic Procedures
• Medications

Medications

a. RhoGAM if indicated by negative maternal blood type

b.

c.

d.

Laboratory & Diagnostic Procedures

a. CBC and differential

b. Type and crossmatch

c. Fetal monitoring

d.

CONDITION: Postpartum

PHYSIOLOGY: Postpartum is the 6-week period after childbirth during which progressive physiological changes restore uterine size and system functions to nonpregnant status (*Taber's*, 2009).

HANDOFF COMMUNICATION

S Situation	Assess what is currently happening in a short statement.	Patient presents as _____
B Background	Summarize important past assessment data for your patient here. Place lab results and medications on the concept map.	**Age:**　　　　　　　　　　　**Gender:** Female **Allergies:**　　　　　　　　**Fall Risk:** **Isolation:** **Date of delivery:**_____ **IPV (intimate partner violence):**_____ **Gravida (number of times pregnant):**_____ **term:**____; **preterm:**____; **abortion:**____; **living:**____
A Assessment	Use the assessment data to complete your concept map.	**Nursing Diagnosis:** Place the Nursing Diagnoses in prioritized order on the concept map and add any needed for your specific patient. **Plan:** Place any further Nursing Interventions Classifications (NIC) needed on the map.

Implement Your Plan of Care

R Recommendation — Evaluate your nursing care and make recommendations related to the achievement of your desired outcomes. Were they met, or do new goals need to be established?

EVALUATE YOUR CARE

Diag	Nursing Outcomes Classification (NOC)	Outcome met
1	Patient verbalizes increased satisfaction with family process by discharge.	☐ Yes ☐ No
2	Patient maintains fluid volume at functional level evidenced by adequate urinary output with normal specific gravity, stable VS, moist mucous membranes, good skin turgor, and prompt capillary refill.	☐ Yes ☐ No
3	Patient reports pain is controlled.	☐ Yes ☐ No
4	Patient empties bladder regularly and completely.	☐ Yes ☐ No
5		☐ Yes ☐ No

Nursing Diagnosis 1

Readiness for enhanced family processes related to developmental transition and gain of a family member evidenced by expression of willingness to enhance family dynamic.

NIC:
1) Assist patient and partner in establishing realistic goals; **2)** Provide positive reinforcement for parenting tasks; **3)** Assist parents in identifying infant behavior patterns and cues; **4)** Assist parents in understanding normal growth and development patterns; and **5)** Identify support systems.

Nursing Diagnosis 2

Risk for fluid volume deficit/bleeding related to excessive blood loss and delivery, reduced intake, inadequate replacement, nausea, vomiting, increased urine output, and insensible losses.

NIC:
1) Check fundus and lochia; **2)** Monitor VS; **3)** Palpate peripheral pulses; **4)** Monitor output; and **5)** Provide PO fluids.

Nursing Diagnosis 3

Acute pain or impaired discomfort related to tissue trauma and edema, muscle contractions, bladder fullness, and physical and psychological exhaustion or related to episiotomy, lacerations, bruising, breast engorgement, sore nipples, epidural or IV site, hemorrhoids evidenced by reports of cramping (after pains), self-focusing, alteration in muscle tone, distraction behavior, changes in VS.

NIC:
1) Assess degree and characteristic of pain; **2)** Assess VS, noting tachycardia; **3)** Reposition as indicated; **4)** Encourage relaxation techniques; and **5)** Medicate as indicated.

Nursing Diagnosis 4

Impaired urinary elimination related to hormonal effects (fluid shifts, continued elevation in renal plasma flow), mechanical trauma, tissue edema, effects of medication and anesthesia evidenced by frequency, dysuria, urgency, incontinence, or retention.

NIC:
1) Note voiding pattern and monitor output; **2)** Palpate bladder or use bladder scan postvoid; **3)** Provide privacy to void, running water, or warm water over perineum; and **4)** Assess characteristic of urine, color, clarity, and odor.

Condition:
Postpartum
Age:

Link & Explain
• Nursing Interventions Classification (NIC)
• Laboratory and Diagnostic Procedures
• Medications

Nursing Diagnosis 5

NIC:

Medications

a. Colace, 1 tab bid

b. Ibuprofen, 800 mg q6h

c. Hydrocortisone cream, 0.5% to perineum prn

d.

Laboratory & Diagnostic Procedures

a. Hgb/Hct

b.

c.

d.

CONDITION: Postpartum Depression (PPD)

PHYSIOLOGY: PPD is depression occurring up to 6 months after childbirth and not resolving in 1 to 2 weeks. The disease occurs in approximately 10%–20% of women who have delivered. Patients report insomnia, psychomotor agitation, changes in appetite, tearfulness, despondency, feelings of hopelessness, worthlessness or guilt, decreased concentration, suicidal ideology, inadequacy, mood swings, inability to cope with infant care needs, irritability, fatigue, and loss of interest and pleasure. Two screening tools are used the Edinburgh Postnatal Depression Scale and the Postpartum Depression Screening Scale (*Taber's*, 2009).

HANDOFF COMMUNICATION

S	Situation	Assess what is currently happening in a short statement.	Patient presents as _____
B	Background	Summarize important past assessment data for your patient here. Place lab results and medications on the concept map.	**Age:** **Gender:** Female **Allergies:** **Fall Risk:** **Isolation:** **Date of delivery:**_____ **IPV (intimate partner violence):**_____ **Gravida (number of times pregnant):**_____ **term:**_____; **preterm:**_____; **abortion:**_____; **living:**_____
A	Assessment	Use the assessment data to complete your concept map.	**Nursing Diagnosis:** Place the Nursing Diagnoses in prioritized order on the concept map and add any needed for your specific patient. **Plan:** Place any further Nursing Interventions Classifications (NIC) needed on the map.

Implement Your Plan of Care

			EVALUATE YOUR CARE	
R	Recommendation	Evaluate your nursing care and make recommendations related to the achievement of your desired outcomes. Were they met, or do new goals need to be established?	**Diag** / **Nursing Outcomes Classification (NOC)**	**Outcome met**
			1 Patient demonstrates signs of positive attachment by responding appropriately to infant's cues.	☐ Yes ☐ No
			2 Patient demonstrates self-control evidenced by relaxed posture and nonviolent behavior.	☐ Yes ☐ No
			3 Family identifies resources within themselves to deal with the situation.	☐ Yes ☐ No
			4 Patient identifies resources within herself to deal with the situation.	☐ Yes ☐ No
			5	☐ Yes ☐ No

Nursing Diagnosis 1

Risk for impaired attachment related to anxiety associated with parent role, inability to meet personal needs, perceived guilt regarding relationship with infant.

NIC:
1) Role model infant care for patient; **2)** Educate patient on normal infant behavior, growth, and development; **3)** Involve family and partner in infant care; **4)** Refer to appropriate support services; and **5)** Encourage verbalization of feelings using therapeutic communication techniques.

Nursing Diagnosis 2

Risk for other-directed violence related to hopelessness, increased anxiety, mood swings, despondency, or severe depression.

NIC:
1) Observe for early signs of distress; **2)** Assist patient to identify adequate solutions and behaviors; and **3)** Monitor for suicidal or homicidal ideations.

Nursing Diagnosis 3

Risk for compromised family coping related to temporary family disorganization.

NIC:
1) Establish a rapport and acknowledge the difficulty of the situation; **2)** Assess level of anxiety; and **3)** Refer to appropriate resources.

Nursing Diagnosis 4

Disturbed sleep pattern related to inability to self-comfort evidenced by insomnia or disrupted sleeping patterns.

NIC:
1) Ascertain usual sleep patterns and changes that are occurring; **2)** Provide comfortable bedding and some of own possessions such as a pillow or an afghan; **3)** Establish new sleep routine incorporating old pattern and new environment; **4)** Encourage light physical activity during the day; **5)** Promote bedtime comfort regimens and avoid caffeine; and **6)** Provide an area with low external stimuli.

Condition:
Postpartum Depression (PPD)

Age:

Link & Explain
• Nursing Interventions Classification (NIC)
• Laboratory and Diagnostic Procedures
• Medications

Nursing Diagnosis 5

NIC:

Medications

a. Antidepressant medication

b.

c.

d.

Laboratory & Diagnostic Procedures

a. Thyroid studies to rule out thyroid dysfunction

b. PPD screening tool

c.

d.

CONDITION: Postpartum Hemorrhage (PPH)

PHYSIOLOGY: PPH occurs after childbirth. It is a major cause of maternal morbidity and mortality in childbirth. Early PPH is defined as a blood loss of more than 500 mL of blood during the first 24 hours after delivery. The most common cause is loss of uterine tone caused by overdistention. Other causes include prolonged or precipitate labor, uterine overestimation, trauma, rupture, inversion, lacerations of the lower genital tract, or blood coagulation disorder. Late postpartum hemorrhage occurs after 24 hours and is usually caused by retained placenta (*Taber's*, 2009).

HANDOFF COMMUNICATION

S	Situation	Assess what is currently happening in a short statement.	Patient presents as _____
B	Background	Summarize important past assessment data for your patient here. Place lab results and medications on the concept map.	**Age:** **Gender:** Female **Allergies:** **Fall Risk:** **Isolation:** **Date of delivery:**_____ **IPV (intimate partner violence):**_____ **Gravida (number of times pregnant):**_____ **term:**_____; **preterm:**_____; **abortion:**_____; **living:**_____
A	Assessment	Use the assessment data to complete your concept map.	**Nursing Diagnosis:** Place the Nursing Diagnoses in prioritized order on the concept map and add any needed for your specific patient. **Plan:** Place any further Nursing Interventions Classifications (NIC) needed on the map.

Implement Your Plan of Care

			EVALUATE YOUR CARE	
	Evaluate your nursing care and make recommendations related to the achievement of your desired outcomes. Were they met, or do new goals need to be established?	**Diag**	**Nursing Outcomes Classification (NOC)**	**Outcome met**
R Recommendation		**1**	Patient maintains fluid volume at a functional level evidenced by individually adequate urinary output with normal specific gravity, stable VS, moist mucous membranes, good skin turgor, and prompt capillary refill.	☐ Yes ☐ No
		2	Patient maintains and improves tissue perfusion evidenced by stabilized VS, warm skin, palpable peripheral pulses, ABGs within norms, and adequate urine output.	☐ Yes ☐ No
		3	Patient reports pain is controlled.	☐ Yes ☐ No
		4	Patient discusses fears and concerns, verbalizes appropriate range of feelings, appears relaxed and reports anxiety is reduced to a manageable level, and demonstrates problem-solving and effective use of resources.	☐ Yes ☐ No
		5		☐ Yes ☐ No

Nursing Diagnosis 1

Fluid volume deficit related to excessive vascular losses evidenced by hypotension, increased pulse rate, decreased venous filling, and decreased urine output.

NIC:
1) Monitor VS; 2) Palpate peripheral pulses; 3) Monitor urinary output; 4) Increase parenteral intake as ordered; 5) Massage fundus; and 6) Pad count.

Nursing Diagnosis 2

Risk for shock related to hypotension and hypovolemia.

NIC:
1) Investigate changes in levels of consciousness; 2) Auscultate apical pulse; 3) Assess skin for coolness; 4) Note urinary output; 5) Observe skin for pallor or redness; 6) Increase intake of IV fluids; 7) Administer medications as appropriate; 8) Massage fundus continuously; and 9) Pad count.

Nursing Diagnosis 3

Risk for acute pain related to tissue trauma and irritation of accumulating blood or manipulation of fundus.

NIC:
1) Assess degree of pain; 2) Assess VS, noting tachycardia; 3) Reposition as indicated; 4) Encourage relaxation techniques during exams; and 5) Medicate as appropriate.

Nursing Diagnosis 4

Fear related to threat of death (perceived or actual) to self evidenced by verbalization of specific concerns, increased tension, and sympathetic stimulation.

NIC:
1) Monitor physiological responses; 2) Encourage verbalization of concerns; 3) Acknowledge that this is a fearful situation; and 4) Provide accurate information.

Condition:
Postpartum Hemorrhage (PPH)
Age:

- - - - - - - - - - - - - - -
Link & Explain
• Nursing Interventions Classification (NIC)
• Laboratory and Diagnostic Procedures
• Medications

Nursing Diagnosis 5

NIC:

Medications

a. Oxytocin

b. Misoprostol

c. Methylergonovine

d. Prostoglandin F2 analogs

Laboratory & Diagnostic Procedures

a. Type and crossmatch

b.

c.

d.

CONDITION: Precipitous Delivery or Out-of-Hospital (Extramural) Delivery

PHYSIOLOGY: Precipitous delivery is an unexpected birth caused by swift progression through the second stage of labor with rapid fetal descent and expulsion. Labor is marked by sudden onset, rapid cervical effacement and dilation, and delivery within 3 hours of onset.
   Extramural delivery is a delivery that takes place outside the hospital walls (*Taber's*, 2009).

HANDOFF COMMUNICATION

S Situation	Assess what is currently happening in a short statement.	Patient presents as _____
B Background	Summarize important past assessment data for your patient here. Place lab results and medications on the concept map.	**Age:** **Gender:** Female **Allergies:** **Fall Risk:** **Isolation:** **Date of delivery:**_____ **IPV (intimate partner violence):**_____ **Gravida (number of times pregnant):**_____ **term:**_____; **preterm:**_____; **abortion:**_____; **living:**_____
A Assessment	Use the assessment data to complete your concept map.	**Nursing Diagnosis:** Place the Nursing Diagnoses in prioritized order on the concept map and add any needed for your specific patient. **Plan:** Place any further Nursing Interventions Classifications (NIC) needed on the map.

Implement Your Plan of Care

	EVALUATE YOUR CARE		
Evaluate your nursing care and make recommendations related to the achievement of your desired outcomes. Were they met, or do new goals need to be established?	**Diag**	**Nursing Outcomes Classification (NOC)**	**Outcome met**
R Recommendation	1	Patient maintains fluid volume at functional level evidenced by adequate urinary output with normal specific gravity, stable VS, moist mucous membranes, good skin turgor, and prompt capillary refill.	☐ Yes ☐ No
	2	Patient achieves timely healing, is free from purulent drainage, and is afebrile.	☐ Yes ☐ No
	3	Patient is free of injury.	☐ Yes ☐ No
	4	Patient demonstrates signs of positive attachment by responding appropriately to infant's cues.	☐ Yes ☐ No
	5		☐ Yes ☐ No

Nursing Diagnosis 1

Risk for fluid volume deficit related to nausea, vomiting, lack of intake, or excessive vascular loss.

NIC:
1) Check fundus and lochia frequently; **2)** Monitor VS; **3)** Palpate peripheral pulses; **4)** Monitor output; **5)** Provide PO or IV fluids; and **6)** Monitor for signs of hematoma development or injury to sulcus tissue.

Nursing Diagnosis 2

Risk for infection related to broken or traumatized tissue, increased environmental exposure, or prolonged rupture of amniotic membranes.

NIC:
1) Note risk factors; **2)** Assess VS frequently; **3)** Maintain aseptic technique when providing care; **4)** Practice good hand washing; and **5)** Note any abnormal vaginal drainage.

Nursing Diagnosis 3

Risk for fetal injury related to rapid descent and pressure changes, compromised circulation, or environmental exposure.

NIC:
1) Resuscitate if needed: suction, oxygen; **2)** Prevent against cold stress; **3)** Complete physical assessment to monitor for injuries (brachial plexus, fractures, hematomas); **4)** Maintain mother and baby in same space until properly identified; and **5)** Check blood glucose within 30 minutes.

Nursing Diagnosis 4

Risk for impaired attachment related to developmental transition (gain a family member), anxiety associated with the parent role, or lack of privacy.

NIC:
1) Role model infant care for parents; **2)** Educate on normal infant behavior, growth, and development; **3)** Encourage family to verbalize about incident; **4)** Use therapeutic communication techniques; and **5)** Involve appropriate support services.

Condition:
Precipitous Delivery or Out of Hospital (Extramural) Delivery

Age:

Link & Explain
• Nursing Interventions Classification (NIC)
• Laboratory and Diagnostic Procedures
• Medications

Nursing Diagnosis 5

NIC:

Medications

a. Pitocin for uterine contraction postdelivery

b.

c.

d.

Laboratory & Diagnostic Procedures

a. Hgb/Hct

b. Type and Rh if unknown

c.

d.

CONDITION: Pregnancy Induced Hypertension (PIH)

PHYSIOLOGY: PIH is a hypertensive condition that develops after the 20th week of pregnancy to the end of the first postpartum week. It is a complication that occurs in 3%–5% of pregnancies and is characterized by hypertension, edema, and proteinuria. The condition may progress rapidly from mild (pre-eclampsia) to severe (eclampsia). The cause is unknown, but the incidence is increased in adolescence; in first pregnancies; and in women who smoke, have diabetes, or are overweight. There are generalized vasospasms, damage to the glomerular membranes, hypovolemia, and hemoconcentration due to fluid shifting from intravascular to interstitial. Patients complain of headaches, sudden weight gain, and visual disturbances. Later signs include epigastric or abdominal pain, presacral and facial edema, oliguria, and hyperreflexia (*Taber's*, 2009).

HANDOFF COMMUNICATION

S Situation | Assess what is currently happening in a short statement. | Patient presents as _____

B Background | Summarize important past assessment data for your patient here. Place lab results and medications on the concept map. |
Age: **Gender:** Female

Allergies: **Fall Risk:**

Isolation:

LMP (last menstrual period):_____

EDB (expected date of birth):_____

IPV (intimate partner violence):_____

Gravida (number of times pregnant):_____

term:_____; **preterm:**_____; **abortion:**_____; **living:**_____

A Assessment | Use the assessment data to complete your concept map. |
Nursing Diagnosis: Place the Nursing Diagnoses in prioritized order on the concept map and add any needed for your specific patient.
Plan: Place any further Nursing Interventions Classifications (NIC) needed on the map.

Implement Your Plan of Care

R Recommendation | Evaluate your nursing care and make recommendations related to the achievement of your desired outcomes. Were they met, or do new goals need to be established?

		EVALUATE YOUR CARE	
	Diag	Nursing Outcomes Classification (NOC)	Outcome met
	1	Patient appears relaxed and anxiety is reduced to a manageable level; patient verbalizes awareness of feelings, uses resources and support systems effectively.	☐ Yes ☐ No
	2	Patient identifies interventions appropriate for the situation, demonstrates behaviors necessary to protect self from injury if possible.	☐ Yes ☐ No
	3	Patient maintains position and function evidenced by maintained muscle strength.	☐ Yes ☐ No
	4	Circulation status: patient participates in activities that reduce BP and cardiac workload, maintains BP and fetal heart rate in acceptable range.	☐ Yes ☐ No
	5		☐ Yes ☐ No

Nursing Diagnosis 1

Anxiety related to situational crisis, threat of change in health status or death (self/fetus), separation from support system evidenced by expression of concerns, apprehension, increased tension, decreased self-assurance, or difficulty concentrating.

NIC:
1) Discuss patient's expectations and fears; **2)** Use therapeutic communication; **3)** Answer questions; and **4)** Identify and encourage previously successful coping behaviors.

Nursing Diagnosis 2

Risk for maternal injury related to tissue edema, hypoxia, possible seizures, abnormal blood profile and/or clotting factors evidenced by high blood pressure and proteinuria.

NIC:
1) Prepare area and equipment, check stock and supplies; **2)** Determine primary needs of patient and check health alerts; **3)** Evaluate patient's response to medication regimen; if on magnesium sulfate, check reflexes q1h, BP, and reactivity every hour. Have calcium gluconate as an antidote if needed; **4)** Keep side rails up and secure; and **5)** Maintain quiet environment.

Nursing Diagnosis 3

Impaired physical mobility related to prescribed bedrest, discomfort, anxiety evidenced by difficulty turning, postural instability.

NIC:
1) Assess motor function; **2)** Provide full ROM; **3)** Monitor BP before and after any ambulation; **4)** Check reflexes; and **5)** Inspect skin regularly.

Nursing Diagnosis 4

Risk for decreased cardiac output related to increased vascular resistance, vasoconstriction.

NIC:
1) Measure BP in both arms; **2)** Note presence and quality of central and peripheral pulses; **3)** Monitor fetal heart rate if undelivered; **4)** Monitor dependent or generalized edema and proteinuria; and **5)** Strict I&O.

Condition:
Pregnancy Induced Hypertension (PIH)

Age:

Link & Explain
• Nursing Interventions Classification (NIC)
• Laboratory and Diagnostic Procedures
• Medications

Nursing Diagnosis 5

NIC:

Medications

a. Magnesium sulfate IV at 2–4 gm/h after a loading dose

b.

c.

d.

Laboratory & Diagnostic Procedures

a. Hgb/Hct

b. Magnesium levels

c. Platelet count

d. Liver enzymes

CONDITION: Preterm Labor (PTL)

PHYSIOLOGY: PTL is labor that begins before completion of 37 weeks from the last menstrual period. The condition affects 7%–10% of all live births, is one of the most important risk factors for preterm birth, and the primary cause of perinatal and neonatal mortality. Although associated risk factors do exist, in most cases the cause is unknown (*Taber's*, 2009).

HANDOFF COMMUNICATION

S	Situation	Assess what is currently happening in a short statement.	Patient presents as _____
B	Background	Summarize important past assessment data for your patient here. Place lab results and medications on the concept map.	**Age:** **Gender:** Female **Allergies:** **Fall Risk:** **Isolation:** **LMP (last menstrual period):**_____ **EDB (expected date of birth):**_____ **IPV (intimate partner violence):**_____ **Gravida (number of times pregnant):**_____ **term:**_____; **preterm:**_____; **abortion:**_____; **living:**_____
A	Assessment	Use the assessment data to complete your concept map.	**Nursing Diagnosis:** Place the Nursing Diagnoses in prioritized order on the concept map and add any needed for your specific patient. **Plan:** Place any further Nursing Interventions Classifications (NIC) needed on the map.

Implement Your Plan of Care

		EVALUATE YOUR CARE		
R	Recommendation	Evaluate your nursing care and make recommendations related to the achievement of your desired outcomes. Were they met, or do new goals need to be established?	**Diag**	**Nursing Outcomes Classification (NOC)**	**Outcome met**
			1	Patient communicates thoughts and feelings utilizing available support systems such as family, spiritual leaders, and other resources; demonstrates coping behaviors that reduce anxiety.	☐ Yes ☐ No
			2	Patient demonstrates appropriate attachment behaviors.	☐ Yes ☐ No
			3	Patient identifies interventions appropriate for the situation; demonstrates behaviors necessary to protect from injury if possible.	☐ Yes ☐ No
			4	Patient identifies and expresses feelings freely and effectively.	☐ Yes ☐ No
			5		☐ Yes ☐ No

Nursing Diagnosis 1

Anxiety related to situational crisis, threat of death or fetal loss evidenced by increased tension, apprehension, feelings of inadequacy, sympathetic stimulation, and repetitive questioning.

NIC:
1) Ascertain what information the patient has about PTL; **2)** Explain purpose and preparation for diagnostic tests and fetal surveillance tests; **3)** Provide an atmosphere for concern and anticipatory guidance; and **4)** Tour the NICU with the parents so they understand the care their preterm infant would receive if needed.

Nursing Diagnosis 2

Risk for disrupted maternal/fetal dyad related to possible surgical intervention or tocolytic drugs.

NIC:
1) Evaluate family's current emotional status; **2)** Encourage parents to express feelings; and **3)** Remain nonjudgmental.

Nursing Diagnosis 3

Risk for fetal injury related to preterm delivery.

NIC:
1) Prepare area and equipment, check stock and supplies; **2)** Determine primary needs of patient and check health alerts; **3)** Evaluate patient's and fetal response to the labor process; **4)** Have preterm infant resuscitation equipment ready; and **5)** Have NICU on standby.

Nursing Diagnosis 4

Grieving related to perceived potential fetal loss, evidence by expression of distress, guilt, anger, or choked feeling.

NIC:
1) Provide open environment for parents to discuss feelings; **2)** Determine parents' meaning and perception of loss based on experience, culture; and **3)** Identify stage of grieving.

Condition:
Preterm Labor (PTL)
Age:

Link & Explain
• Nursing Interventions Classification (NIC)
• Laboratory and Diagnostic Procedures
• Medications

Nursing Diagnosis 5

NIC:

Medications

a. Terbutaline (Brethine), 0.25 mg subQ q 20 min x 3 doses

b. Magnesium sulfate IV

c. Calcium channel blockers

d.

Laboratory & Diagnostic Procedures

a. Intravenous fluids

b. Continuous fetal monitoring

c.

d.

CONDITION: Second Trimester Gestation

PHYSIOLOGY: *Fetal:* During the second trimester (13–26 weeks' gestation), the fetus is rapidly growing in size and complexity. Vernix caseosa covers the fetal skin, and by 20 weeks, the fetus has lanugo. By 24 weeks, the fetal lungs have begun to secrete surfactant.
   Maternal: The uterus continues to rise out of the pelvis and at 20 weeks is at the level of the umbilicus. Quickening, or fetal movements, are felt usually between 18 and 20 weeks' gestation (*Taber's*, 2009).

HANDOFF COMMUNICATION

S | **Situation** | Assess what is currently happening in a short statement. | Patient presents as _____

B | **Background** | Summarize important past assessment data for your patient here. Place lab results and medications on the concept map. |
Age: **Gender:** Female
Allergies: **Fall Risk:**
Isolation:
LMP (last menstrual period):_____
EDB (expected date of birth):_____
IPV (intimate partner violence):_____
Gravida (number of times pregnant):_____
term:_____; **preterm:**_____; **abortion:**_____; **living:**_____

A | **Assessment** | Use the assessment data to complete your concept map. |
Nursing Diagnosis: Place the Nursing Diagnoses in prioritized order on the concept map and add any needed for your specific patient.
Plan: Place any further Nursing Interventions Classifications (NIC) needed on the map.

Implement Your Plan of Care

Evaluate your nursing care and make recommendations related to the achievement of your desired outcomes. Were they met, or do new goals need to be established?

R | **Recommendation**

	EVALUATE YOUR CARE	
Diag	Nursing Outcomes Classification (NOC)	Outcome met
1	Patient incorporates changes into self-concept without negating self-esteem.	☐ Yes ☐ No
2	Patient maintains effective respiratory pattern free of cyanosis, other signs of hypoxia, with breath sounds equal bilaterally and with clear lung fields.	☐ Yes ☐ No
3	Patient displays hemodynamic stability, such as stable cardiac output and BP.	☐ Yes ☐ No
4	Patient demonstrates stability of fluid volume with balanced I&O, stable weight gain, and absence of edema.	☐ Yes ☐ No
5		☐ Yes ☐ No

Nursing Diagnosis 1

Risk for disturbed body image related to perception of biophysical changes or response to others.

NIC:
1) Discuss body image; **2)** Reflect on patient's perceptions of body changes; and **3)** Monitor caloric intake.

Nursing Diagnosis 2

Ineffective breathing pattern related to impingement of the diaphragm by enlarging uterus, evidenced by reports of shortness of breath, dyspnea, and changes in respiratory rate.

NIC:
1) Evaluate respiratory status and rate; **2)** Auscultate lung fields; **3)** Observe chest excursion; **4)** Inspect skin and mucous membranes; **5)** Instruct patient to elevate head when sleeping; and **6)** Instruct patient to sit up straight when working at a desk.

Nursing Diagnosis 3

Risk for decompensated cardiac output related to increased cardiac demand, changes in preload and afterload, and ventricular hypertrophy.

NIC:
1) Monitor and document trends in heart rate and BP; **2)** Monitor and document any murmurs or abnormal heart sounds; **3)** Schedule rest periods; **4)** Monitor for edema; and **5)** Monitor for episodes of hypotension.

Nursing Diagnosis 4

Risk for excess fluid volume related to changes in regulatory mechanisms, sodium, and water.

NIC:
1) Monitor 24-hour I&O balance if indicated; **2)** Weigh daily; and **3)** Assess edema in dependent parts.

Condition:
Second Trimester Gestation

Age:

Link & Explain
• Nursing Interventions Classification (NIC)
• Laboratory and Diagnostic Procedures
• Medications

Nursing Diagnosis 5

NIC:

Medications

a. Prenatal vitamins

b.

c.

d.

Laboratory & Diagnostic Procedures

a. Hgb/Hct

b.

c.

d.

CONDITION: Sexually Transmitted Infection (STI)

PHYSIOLOGY: STI or sexually transmitted disease (STD) is any infection that may be acquired as a result of sexual intercourse or other intimate contact with an infected individual.

Transmitted bacteria include *Klebsiella granulomatis*, *Campylobacter* species, *Chlamydia trachomatis*, *Gardnerella vaginalis*, group B streptococcus, *Haemophilus ducreyi*, *Mycoplasma hominis*, *Neisseria gonorrhea*, *Shigella* species, *Treponema pallidum*, and *Ureaplasma urealyticum*.

Viruses include cytomegalovirus; hepatitis A, B, C; herpes simplex; human herpesvirus type 8; human immunodeficiency virus types 1 and 2; human papilloma viruses; human T-lymphotrophic retrovirus type 1; and a pox virus.

Protozoa include *Entamoeba histolytica*, *Giardia lamblia*, and *Trichomonas vaginalis*.

Ectoparasites include *Phthirus pubis* and *Sarcoptes scabiei* (*Taber's*, 2009).

HANDOFF COMMUNICATION

S	Situation	Assess what is currently happening in a short statement.	Patient presents as _____
B	**Background**	Summarize important past assessment data for your patient here. Place lab results and medications on the concept map.	**Age:** **Gender:** Female **Allergies:** **Fall Risk:** **Isolation:** **LMP (last menstrual period):**_____ **EDB (expected date of birth) if pregnant:**_____ **IPV (intimate partner violence):**_____ **Gravida (number of times pregnant):**_____ **term:**_____; **preterm:**_____; **abortion:**_____; **living:**_____
A	**Assessment**	Use the assessment data to complete your concept map.	**Nursing Diagnosis:** Place the Nursing Diagnoses in prioritized order on the concept map and add any needed for your specific patient. **Plan:** Place any further Nursing Interventions Classifications (NIC) needed on the map.

Implement Your Plan of Care

R	Recommendation	Evaluate your nursing care and make recommendations related to the achievement of your desired outcomes. Were they met, or do new goals need to be established?	Diag	Nursing Outcomes Classification (NOC)	Outcome met
				EVALUATE YOUR CARE	
			1	Patient is free of signs of infection and inflammation, purulent drainage, erythema, lesions, or fever.	☐ Yes ☐ No
			2	Patient demonstrates tissue regeneration.	☐ Yes ☐ No
			3	Patient verbalizes knowledge acquisition about safe sex.	☐ Yes ☐ No
			4	Sexual functioning: Patient verbalizes understanding of relationship of physical condition to sexual problems, identifies satisfying and acceptable sexual practices, and explores alternative methods.	☐ Yes ☐ No
			5		☐ Yes ☐ No

Nursing Diagnosis 1

Infection transmission related to contagious nature of infecting agent and insufficient knowledge to avoid exposure to or transmission of pathogens evidenced by positive cultures.

NIC:
1) Practice and instruct patient on good hand washing; **2)** Monitor VS; **3)** Review medication schedule; **4)** Administer antibiotics or antifungals as ordered; and **5)** Review safe sex practices.

Nursing Diagnosis 2

Impaired skin/tissue integrity related to invasive or irritation of pathogen organism evidenced by disruptions of skin or inflammation of mucous membranes.

NIC:
1) Assess and document color, depth, and characteristics of lesions or impaired skin integrity; **2)** Provide and teach appropriate skin care with aseptic technique to prevent secondary infections; **3)** Administer and teach to administer topical ointment if ordered; and **4)** Instruct to wear loose clothing.

Nursing Diagnosis 3

Knowledge deficit regarding condition or prognosis, complications, therapy needs, and transmission related to lack of information, misinterpretation, or lack of interest in learning evidenced by statements of concern, questions, misconceptions, inaccurate follow-through of instructions, development of preventable complications.

NIC:
1) Review the condition and transmission; **2)** Teach side effects and treatment protocol; and **3)** Discuss alternative sexual patterns to decrease reinfection.

Nursing Diagnosis 4

Risk for sexual dysfunction related to presence of infectious process and vaginal discomfort.

NIC:
1) Determine patient's and partner's relationship before the outbreak; **2)** Reinforce information provided by primary care practitioner; and **3)** Review with patient and partner restrictions on sexual functioning and partner treatment.

Condition:
Sexually Transmitted Infection (STI)

Age:

- - - - - - - - - - - - - -
Link & Explain
• Nursing Interventions Classification (NIC)
• Laboratory and Diagnostic Procedures
• Medications

Nursing Diagnosis 5

NIC:

Medications

a. Antibiotics, antiviral medications to treat specific infection

b.

c.

d.

Laboratory & Diagnostic Procedures

a. Culture and sensitivity of the cervix

b. RPR or VDRL blood test for syphilis

c.

d.

CONDITION: Third Trimester Gestation

PHYSIOLOGY: *Fetal:* During the third trimester (27–40 weeks' gestation), there is rapid fetal growth. The fetus practices breathing movements in utero. Subcutaneous fat deposits are laid to enhance extrauterine temperature regulation. At 28 weeks, the bone marrow takes over erythropoiesis from the spleen. By 35 weeks' gestation, the fetus is oriented to light and reflexes such as grasp are evident. Fetal heart rate should be 110–160 BPM. Nonstress tests may be ordered to assess fetal heart rate in relation to fetal movement.

    Maternal: The uterus continues to grow at 1 cm per week from 20 to 36 weeks' gestation. The patient should be advised to do daily fetal movement count (DFMC). Leopold's maneuvers can be done for fetal position. Engagement of the largest fetal part moving to the pelvic inlet occurs at 37 weeks for primigravidas and later for multigravidas (*Taber's*, 2009).

HANDOFF COMMUNICATION

S — Situation

Assess what is currently happening in a short statement.

Patient presents as _____

B — Background

Summarize important past assessment data for your patient here. Place lab results and medications on the concept map.

Age: **Gender:** Female

Allergies: **Fall Risk:**

Isolation:

LMP (last menstrual period):_____

EDB (expected date of birth):_____

IPV (intimate partner violence):_____

Gravida (number of times pregnant):_____

term:_____; **preterm:**_____; **abortion:**_____; **living:**_____

A — Assessment

Use the assessment data to complete your concept map.

Nursing Diagnosis: Place the Nursing Diagnoses in prioritized order on the concept map and add any needed for your specific patient.
Plan: Place any further Nursing Interventions Classifications (NIC) needed on the map.

Implement Your Plan of Care

R — Recommendation

Evaluate your nursing care and make recommendations related to the achievement of your desired outcomes. Were they met, or do new goals need to be established?

Diag	EVALUATE YOUR CARE Nursing Outcomes Classification (NOC)	Outcome met
1	Patient establishes a dietary pattern with caloric intake adequate to maintain appropriate weight gain.	☐ Yes ☐ No
2	Patient incorporates changes into self-concept without negating self-esteem.	☐ Yes ☐ No
3	Patient verbalizes understanding of condition, processes, and possible complications.	☐ Yes ☐ No
4	Patient and partner verbalize increased satisfaction with changing family process.	☐ Yes ☐ No
5		☐ Yes ☐ No

Nursing Diagnosis 1

Nutrition: readiness for enhanced nutrition related to increased demands of pregnancy evidenced by verbalization about weight and caloric intake.

NIC:
1) Establish weight goal and daily nutritional requirements; **2)** Use a diet history or 24-hour intake if needed; **3)** Monitor exercise program that is appropriate; and **4)** Provide smaller, frequent meals to keep steady glycemic levels.

Nursing Diagnosis 2

Body image: disturbed related to enlarging uterus evidenced by comments regarding size and shape.

NIC:
1) Discuss body image; **2)** Reflect on patient's perceptions of body changes; and **3)** Monitor caloric intake.

Nursing Diagnosis 3

Knowledge deficit: ready for enhanced knowledge related to labor and delivery needs evidenced by inquiries about labor and delivery.

NIC:
1) Assess readiness and baseline knowledge of patient and partner; **2)** Encourage prenatal classes for labor; **3)** Teach when to call primary care provider (PCP); and **4)** Review danger signs of third trimester each visit.

Nursing Diagnosis 4

Family processes: readiness for enhanced family processes related to imminence of changing family structure evidenced by behaviors to prepare for infant.

NIC:
1) Assist patient and partner in establishing realistic goals; **2)** Provide positive reinforcement for parenting tasks; **3)** Assist parents in identifying how lifestyle patterns will change; **4)** Assist parents in understanding normal growth and development patterns; and **5)** Identify support systems.

Condition:
Third Trimester Gestation
Age:

Link & Explain
• Nursing Interventions Classification (NIC)
• Laboratory and Diagnostic Procedures
• Medications

Nursing Diagnosis 5

NIC:

Medications

a. Prenatal vitamins

b.

c.

d.

Laboratory & Diagnostic Procedures

a. Fetal and uterine monitoring

b.

c.

d.

CONDITION: Toxic Shock Syndrome

PHYSIOLOGY: Toxic shock syndrome is a rare disorder similar to septic shock caused by an exotoxin produced by certain strains of *Staphylococcus aureus* and group A streptococci. It was originally discovered in young women using tampons but has been reported in users of contraceptive sponges, diaphragms, and after surgical packing. The diagnosis is made when the following criteria are met: fever of 102°F or greater; diffuse macular erythematous rash followed by 1–2 weeks of peeling skin, particularly the palms and soles; hypotension, and involvement of three or more of the following organ systems: gastrointestinal (vomiting and diarrhea), muscular (severe myalgia), mucous membranes (vaginal, oropharyngeal, or conjunctival), hyperemia, renal, hepatic, hematological (platelets <100,000/mm³), and central nervous system (disorientation). The disease can be fatal in 5%–15% of cases (*Taber's*, 2009).

HANDOFF COMMUNICATION

S	Situation	Assess what is currently happening in a short statement.	Patient presents as _____
B	Background	Summarize important past assessment data for your patient here. Place lab results and medications on the concept map.	**Age:** **Gender:** Female **Allergies:** **Fall Risk:** **Isolation:** **LMP (last menstrual period):**_____ **EDB (expected date of birth) if pregnant:**_____ **IPV (intimate partner violence):**_____ **Gravida (number of times pregnant):**_____ **term:**_____; **preterm:**_____; **abortion:**_____; **living:**_____
A	Assessment	Use the assessment data to complete your concept map.	**Nursing Diagnosis:** Place the Nursing Diagnoses in prioritized order on the concept map and add any needed for your specific patient. **Plan:** Place any further Nursing Interventions Classifications (NIC) needed on the map.

Implement Your Plan of Care

		EVALUATE YOUR CARE		
R	Recommendation Evaluate your nursing care and make recommendations related to the achievement of your desired outcomes. Were they met, or do new goals need to be established?	**Diag**	**Nursing Outcomes Classification (NOC)**	**Outcome met**
		1	Patient maintains body temperature between 97°F and 99°F.	☐ Yes ☐ No
		2	Patient maintains fluid volume at functional level evidenced by individually adequate urinary output with normal specific gravity, stable VS, moist mucous membranes, good skin turgor, and prompt capillary refill.	☐ Yes ☐ No
		3	Patient reports pain is controlled.	☐ Yes ☐ No
		4	Patient verbalizes understanding of disease, diagnosis, treatment options, and prognosis.	☐ Yes ☐ No
		5		☐ Yes ☐ No

Nursing Diagnosis 1

Hyperthermia related to inflammatory process, hypermetabolic state, and dehydration evidenced by increased body temperature, warm flushed skin, or tachycardia.

NIC:
1) Monitor VS; **2)** Maintain room temperature at 72°F; **3)** Medicate as ordered; **4)** Decrease bed covers; and **5)** Provide hypothermia blanket if needed.

Nursing Diagnosis 2

Fluid volume deficit related to increased gastric losses (diarrhea, vomiting), fever, hypermetabolic state, and decreased intake evidenced by dry mucous membranes; increased pulse; hypotension; delayed venous filling; decreased, concentrated urine; or hemoconcentration.

NIC:
1) Monitor VS; **2)** Palpate peripheral pulses; **3)** Monitor output; **4)** Weigh daily; **5)** Encourage fluids; and **6)** Assess skin turgor and capillary refill <3 seconds.

Nursing Diagnosis 3

Acute pain related to inflammatory process, effects of circulating toxins, and skin disruptions evidenced by verbal reports, guarding or distractive behaviors, self-focus, or changes in VS.

NIC:
1) Assess degree and characteristic of pain using a verified pain scale; **2)** Assess VS, noting tachycardia; **3)** Reposition as indicated; **4)** Encourage relaxation techniques; and **5)** Medicate as indicated.

Nursing Diagnosis 4

Deficient knowledge related to lack of information regarding disease process, diagnostic testing, and treatment evidenced by questions and information gathering.

NIC:
1) Assess understanding of disease process and treatment; **2)** Identify and communicate community resources, Web sites, and additional sources of information and support; **3)** Discuss diagnostic evaluation procedures as indicated; **4)** Explain treatment regimen, treatment options, and provide related information; **5)** Include family/support systems in informational sessions; **6)** Explain the importance of adherence to follow-up visits and screening; and **7)** Provide education regarding normal health maintenance practices.

Condition:
Toxic Shock Syndrome
Age:

Link & Explain
• Nursing Interventions Classification (NIC)
• Laboratory and Diagnostic Procedures
• Medications

Nursing Diagnosis 5

NIC:

Medications

a. Antibiotics

b.

c.

d.

Laboratory & Diagnostic Procedures

a. Blood cultures

b. CBC with differential

c.

d.

CONDITION: Uterine Rupture

PHYSIOLOGY: Uterine rupture is a rare condition in which the uterine muscles are torn apart by the stresses of unrelieved obstructed labor, the parting of an old cesarean scar, or aggressive induction or augmentation of labor (*Taber's*, 2009).

HANDOFF COMMUNICATION

S	Situation	Assess what is currently happening in a short statement.	Patient presents as _____
B	Background	Summarize important past assessment data for your patient here. Place lab results and medications on the concept map.	**Age:** **Gender:** Female **Allergies:** **Fall Risk:** **Isolation:** **LMP (last menstrual period):**_____ **EDB (expected date of birth) if pregnant:**_____ **IPV (intimate partner violence):**_____ **Gravida (number of times pregnant):**_____ **term:**_____; **preterm:**_____; **abortion:**_____; **living:**_____
A	Assessment	Use the assessment data to complete your concept map.	**Nursing Diagnosis:** Place the Nursing Diagnoses in prioritized order on the concept map and add any needed for your specific patient. **Plan:** Place any further Nursing Interventions Classifications (NIC) needed on the map.

Implement Your Plan of Care

			EVALUATE YOUR CARE	
R	Recommendation	Evaluate your nursing care and make recommendations related to the achievement of your desired outcomes. Were they met, or do new goals need to be established?	**Diag** / **Nursing Outcomes Classification (NOC)**	**Outcome met**
			1 Patient maintains fluid volume at a functional level evidenced by individually adequate urinary output with normal specific gravity, stable VS, moist mucous membranes, good skin turgor, and prompt capillary refill.	☐ Yes ☐ No
			2 Patient maintains and improves tissue perfusion evidenced by stabilized VS, warm skin, palpable peripheral pulses, ABGs within norms, and adequate urine output.	☐ Yes ☐ No
			3 Patient reports pain is controlled.	☐ Yes ☐ No
			4 Patient discusses fears and concerns, verbalizes appropriate range of feelings, appears relaxed and reports anxiety is reduced to a manageable level, and demonstrates problem-solving and effective use of resources.	☐ Yes ☐ No
			5	☐ Yes ☐ No

Nursing Diagnosis 1

Fluid volume deficit related to excessive vascular losses evidenced by hypotension, increased pulse rate, decreased venous filling, or decreased urine output.

NIC:
1) Monitor VS; 2) Palpate peripheral pulses; 3) Monitor urinary output; and 4) Administer isotonic IV fluid replacement.

Nursing Diagnosis 2

Risk for shock related to hypotension and hypovolemia.

NIC:
1) Investigate changes in level of consciousness; 2) Auscultate apical pulse; 3) Assess skin for coolness; 4) Note urinary output; 5) Note reports of abdominal pain; and 6) Observe skin for pallor or redness.

Nursing Diagnosis 3

Acute pain related to tissue trauma and irritation of accumulating blood evidenced by verbal reports, guarding or distracted behaviors, self-focus, or changes in VS.

NIC:
1) Assess degree and characteristic of pain; 2) Assess VS, noting tachycardia; 3) Reposition as indicated; 4) Encourage relaxation techniques; and 5) Medicate as indicated.

Nursing Diagnosis 4

Fear related to threat of death (perceived or actual) to fetus and self, possibly evidenced by verbalization of specific concerns, increased tension, and sympathetic stimulation.

NIC:
1) Monitor physiological responses; 2) Encourage verbalization of concerns; 3) Acknowledge that this is a fearful situation; 4) Provide accurate information; and 5) Provide spiritual referral if needed.

Condition:
Uterine Rupture
Age:

Link & Explain
• Nursing Interventions Classification (NIC)
• Laboratory and Diagnostic Procedures
• Medications

Nursing Diagnosis 5

NIC:

Medications

a. Isotonic IV

b. Volume expanders

c. Platelets

d.

Laboratory & Diagnostic Procedures

a. Type and crossmatch

b.

c.

d.

CONDITION: Vaginal Delivery

PHYSIOLOGY: Vaginal delivery is giving birth to a child by expulsion of the infant(s), placenta, and membranes through the birth canal (*Taber's*, 2009).

HANDOFF COMMUNICATION

S	Situation	Assess what is currently happening in a short statement.	Patient presents as _____
B	Background	Summarize important past assessment data for your patient here. Place lab results and medications on the concept map.	**Age:**　　　　　　　　　　　　　　　　　**Gender:** Female **Allergies:**　　　　　　　　　　　　　　**Fall Risk:** **Isolation:** **Date of delivery:**_____ **IPV (intimate partner violence):**_____ **Gravida (number of times pregnant):**_____ **preterm:**_____; **abortion:**_____; **living:**_____
A	Assessment	Use the assessment data to complete your concept map.	**Nursing Diagnosis:** Place the Nursing Diagnoses in prioritized order on the concept map and add any needed for your specific patient. **Plan:** Place any further Nursing Interventions Classifications (NIC) needed on the map.

Implement Your Plan of Care

			EVALUATE YOUR CARE	
R	Recommendation	Evaluate your nursing care and make recommendations related to the achievement of your desired outcomes. Were they met, or do new goals need to be established?	**Diag** / **Nursing Outcomes Classification (NOC)**	**Outcome met**
			1 Patient and partner verbalize increased satisfaction with family process by discharge.	☐ Yes ☐ No
			2 Patient maintains fluid volume at functional level evidenced by adequate urinary output with normal specific gravity, stable VS, moist mucous membranes, good skin turgor, and prompt capillary refill.	☐ Yes ☐ No
			3 Patient reports pain is controlled.	☐ Yes ☐ No
			4 Patient empties bladder regularly and completely.	☐ Yes ☐ No
			5	☐ Yes ☐ No

Nursing Diagnosis 1

Readiness for enhanced family process related to developmental transition of a family member evidenced by expressing willingness to enhance family dynamics.

NIC:
1) Assist patient and partner in establishing realistic goals; **2)** Provide positive reinforcement for parenting tasks; **3)** Assist parents in identifying infant behavior patterns and cues; **4)** Assist parents in understanding normal growth and development patterns; and **5)** Identify support systems.

Nursing Diagnosis 2

Risk for fluid volume deficit or bleeding related to reduced intake, inadequate replacement fluids, nausea, vomiting, increased urine output, and insensible losses.

NIC:
1) Check fundus and lochia; **2)** Monitor VS; **3)** Palpate peripheral pulses; **4)** Monitor output; **5)** Provide PO fluids or ice chips; and **6)** Assess skin turgor and capillary refill < 3 seconds.

Nursing Diagnosis 3

Acute pain or impaired comfort related to tissue trauma and edema, muscle contractions, bladder fullness, and physical or psychological exhaustion evidenced by reports of cramping, self-focusing, alteration in muscle tone, distraction behavior, or changes in VS.

NIC:
1) Assess degree and characteristic of pain; **2)** Assess VS, noting tachycardia; **3)** Reposition as indicated; **4)** Encourage relaxation techniques; and **5)** Medicate as ordered.

Nursing Diagnosis 4

Impaired urinary elimination related to hormonal effects (fluid shifts, continued elevation in renal plasma flow), mechanical trauma, tissue edema, and effects of medication and anesthesia evidenced by frequency, dysuria, urgency, incontinence, or retention.

NIC:
1) Note voiding pattern and monitor output; **2)** Palpate bladder or use bladder scan postvoid; **3)** Provide privacy to void, running water, or warm water over perineum; **4)** Assess characteristic of urine, color, clarity, and odor; and **5)** Straight catheterize if needed.

Condition:
Vaginal Delivery
Age:

Link & Explain
• Nursing Interventions Classification (NIC)
• Laboratory and Diagnostic Procedures
• Medications

Nursing Diagnosis 5

NIC:

Medications

a. Oxytocin (Pitocin)

b. Analgesics

c.

d.

Laboratory & Diagnostic Procedures

a. Postpartum hematocrit

b.

c.

d.

Concept Maps for Men's Health

This chapter provides care maps that describe health conditions experienced only by men. In recent years, prostate cancer has become a major health-care concern in the United States, and research is still being done to determine the difference between hyperplasia and abnormal growth due to cellular changes. These care maps will help the nurse care for men dealing with serious health issues specific to them.

The conditions included in this chapter are:

1. Benign Prostatic Hyperplasia (BPH)

2. Prostatectomy (Radical/Transurethral)

3. Testicular Cancer

CONDITION: Benign Prostatic Hyperplasia (BPH)

PHYSIOLOGY: BPH is excessive proliferation of normal cells in normal organs or hypertrophy (an increase in size of an organ) and is one of the most common disorders of older men. It is a nonmalignant enlargement of the prostate gland. It is the most common cause of obstruction of urine flow in men and results in more than 4.5 million visits to health-care providers annually in the United States. The degree of enlargement determines whether or not bladder outflow obstruction occurs. As the urethra becomes obstructed, the muscle inside the bladder hypertrophies in an attempt to assist the bladder to force out the urine. BPH may also cause the formation of a bladder diverticulum that remains full of urine when the patient empties the bladder. As the obstruction progresses, the bladder wall becomes thickened and irritable, and as it hypertrophies, it increases its own contractile force, leading to sensitivity even with small volumes of urine. The bladder gradually weakens and loses the ability to empty completely, leading to increased residual urine volume and urinary retention. With marked bladder distention, overflow incontinence may occur with any increase in intra-abdominal pressure such as that which occurs with coughing and sneezing. Complications of BPH include urinary stasis, urinary tract infection, renal calculi, overflow incontinence, hypertrophy of the bladder muscle, acute renal failure, hydronephrosis, and even chronic renal failure. Severity of symptoms is categorized by the American Urological Association's Symptom Score for BPH: mild: 0–7 points; moderate: 8–9 points; severe: 20–35 points (*Taber's*, 2009).

HANDOFF COMMUNICATION

S Situation	Assess what is currently happening in a short statement.	Patient presents as _____	
B Background	Summarize important past assessment data for your patient here. Place lab results and Medications on the concept map.	**Age:** **Allergies:** **Isolation:**	**Gender:** Male **Fall Risk:**
A Assessment	Use the assessment data to complete your concept map.	**Nursing Diagnosis:** Place the Nursing Diagnoses in prioritized order on the concept map and add any needed for your specific patient. **Plan:** Place any further Nursing Interventions Classifications (NIC) needed on the map.	

Implement Your Plan of Care

		EVALUATE YOUR CARE	
Evaluate your nursing care and make recommendations related to the achievement of your desired outcomes. Were they met, or do new goals need to be established?	**Diag**	**Nursing Outcomes Classification (NOC)**	**Outcome met**
R Recommendation	1	Patient voids in normal amounts with absence of symptoms related to urethral blockage.	☐ Yes ☐ No
	2	Patient appears relaxed and verbalizes that pain is relieved/controlled.	☐ Yes ☐ No
	3	Patient appears relaxed, reports decreased anxiety, and articulates personal coping strategies.	☐ Yes ☐ No
	4	Patient verbalizes knowledge of disease process, treatment regimen, and self-care needs.	☐ Yes ☐ No
	5		☐ Yes ☐ No

Nursing Diagnosis 1

Urinary retention related to urethral blockage evidenced by inability to void.

NIC:
1) Assess urinary elimination pattern and symptoms of urinary retention; **2)** Assess severity of symptoms using BHP scoring; **3)** Evaluate for need of urethral catheter; **4)** Administer medications to reduce prostate size and improve urinary flow; **5)** Monitor results of laboratory and diagnostic tests; and **6)** Prepare for more invasive medical management if indicated.

Nursing Diagnosis 2

Acute pain related to mucosal irritation and spasms evidenced by verbalization about discomfort.

NIC:
1) Perform comprehensive pain assessment; **2)** Provide comfort measures; **3)** Insert indwelling catheter; secure drainage tube to minimize catheter movement/pulling; and **4)** Administer medications as prescribed.

Nursing Diagnosis 3

Fear/anxiety related to change in health status evidenced by verbalization and/or withdrawn behavior.

NIC:
1) Establish trusting relationship; **2)** Encourage client and significant other to verbalize concerns/feelings; **3)** Provide information about tests/procedures and related effects; and **4)** Communicate accepting attitude to reduce client embarrassment.

Nursing Diagnosis 4

Deficient knowledge related to diagnosis and treatment and self-care needs evidenced by questions.

NIC:
1) Review disease process, treatment plan, and client expectations; **2)** Address embarrassment/sexual concerns; **3)** Reinforce need for routine medical follow-up; and **4)** Teach strategies to reduce symptom severity, recurrence, or aggravation of symptoms (including interactions with herbal and/or over-the-counter medications).

Condition:
Benign Prostatic Hyperplasia (BPH)

Age:

Link & Explain
• Nursing Interventions Classification (NIC)
• Laboratory and Diagnostic Procedures
• Medications

Nursing Diagnosis 5

NIC:

Medications

a. 5-alpha-reductase inhibitors (Proscar, Avodart)

b. Alpha-adrenergic antagonists (Uroxatral, Hytrin, Cardura, Flomax)

c. Antispasmodics (Ditropan); B&O suppositories

d. Antibiotics and antibacterials

Laboratory & Diagnostic Procedures

a. Electrolytes, BUN, creatinine, prostate-specific antigen (PSA)

b. Urinalysis/culture, postvoid residual urine, uroflowmetry

c. Digital rectal exam, transrectal prostatic ultrasound (TRUS)

d. Intravenous pyelography (IVP), cystourethrography, cystoscopy

CONDITION: Prostatectomy (Radical/Transurethral)

PHYSIOLOGY: Radical prostatectomy has been the recommended treatment option for men with middle-stage prostate cancer because of high cure rates. This procedure removes the entire prostate gland, including the prostatic capsule, the seminal vesicles, and a portion of the bladder neck. Two common side effects of prostatectomy are urinary incontinence and impotence. The urinary incontinence usually resolves with time and after performing Kegel exercises, although 10% to 15% of men continue to experience incontinence 6 months after surgery. Impotence occurs in 85% to 90% of patients. All men who undergo radical prostatectomy lack emission and ejaculation because of the removal of the seminal vesicles and transection of the vas deferens. Newer surgical techniques (nerve-sparing prostatectomy) preserves continence in most men and erectile function in selected cases.

Transurethral resection of the prostate (TURP) may be recommended for men with more advanced disease, especially if it is accompanied by symptoms of bladder outlet obstruction. This procedure is not a curative surgical technique for prostate cancer but does remove excess prostatic tissue that is obstructing the flow of urine through the urethra. The incidence of impotence following TURP is rare, although retrograde ejaculation (passage of seminal fluid back into the bladder) almost always occurs because of the destruction of the internal bladder sphincter during the procedure. Many men equate ejaculation with normal sexual functioning, and to some men, the loss of the ejaculatory sensation may be confused with the loss of sexual interest or potency. Also, a bilateral orchiectomy may be done to eliminate the source of the androgens because 85% of prostatic cancer is related to androgens (*Taber's*, 2009).

HANDOFF COMMUNICATION

S	Situation	Assess what is currently happening in a short statement.	Patient presents as _____
B	Background	Summarize important past assessment data for your patient here. Place lab results and Medications on the concept map.	**Age:** **Gender:** Male **Allergies:** **Fall Risk:** **Isolation:**
A	Assessment	Use the assessment data to complete your concept map.	**Nursing Diagnosis:** Place the Nursing Diagnoses in prioritized order on the concept map and add any needed for your specific patient. **Plan:** Place any further Nursing Interventions Classifications (NIC) needed on the map.

Implement Your Plan of Care

		EVALUATE YOUR CARE	
	Diag	**Nursing Outcomes Classification (NOC)**	**Outcome met**
R Recommendation Evaluate your nursing care and make recommendations related to the achievement of your desired outcomes. Were they met, or do new goals need to be established?	**1**	Patient voids normal amounts without retention and demonstrates behaviors to regain bladder urinary control.	☐ Yes ☐ No
	2	Patient maintains adequate hydration and circulation without excessive bleeding.	☐ Yes ☐ No
	3	Patient achieves timely healing and demonstrates no signs of infection.	☐ Yes ☐ No
	4	Patient appears relaxed and reports that pain is relieved or controlled.	☐ Yes ☐ No
	5		☐ Yes ☐ No

Nursing Diagnosis 1

Impaired urinary elimination related to mechanical obstruction, irritation, or loss of bladder tone evidenced by patient report.

NIC:
1) Monitor urinary output and catheter drainage system (especially during bladder irrigation); **2)** Record time, amount of void, size of urinary stream after catheter removal; **3)** Establish urinary training program; **4)** Teach client perineal exercises; and **5)** Instruct "dribbling" is normal and should subside (provide incontinence pads).

Nursing Diagnosis 2

Risk for deficient fluid volume/bleeding related to vascular nature of surgical area/postobstructive diuresis.

NIC:
1) Monitor I&O, vital signs (VS), capillary refill; **2)** Assess for pallor, restlessness, confusion, and dry mucous membranes; **3)** Anchor urethral catheter to avoid excessive manipulation; **4)** Observe urinary drainage and monitor for excess bleeding, clots; **5)** Monitor labs (Hgb/Hct, RBCs, coagulation studies, platelet count); **6)** Administer IV therapy as indicated; and **7)** Administer stool softeners or laxatives as indicated.

Nursing Diagnosis 3

Risk for infection related to invasive procedures.

NIC:
1) Maintain asepsis and good hygiene as indicated; **2)** Keep drainage bag in dependent position; **3)** Monitor incisions and dressings for signs and symptoms of infection; and **4)** Administer antibiotics as ordered.

Nursing Diagnosis 4

Acute pain related to irritation of bladder mucosa, reflex muscle spasm associated with surgical procedure or pressure from urinary catheter evidenced by patient report.

NIC:
1) Assess for amount, location, characteristics of pain; **2)** Maintain patency of catheter and drainage system; **3)** Provide comfort measures; and **4)** Administer antispasmodics.

Condition:
Prostatectomy (Radical/ Transurethral)

Age:

Link & Explain
• Nursing Interventions Classification (NIC)
• Laboratory and Diagnostic Procedures
• Medications

Nursing Diagnosis 5

NIC:

Medications

a. Antispasmodics

b. Antibiotics

c. Blood products

d. Stool softeners/laxatives

Laboratory & Diagnostic Procedures

a. Urinalysis/culture, CBC, coagulation studies

b. Ultrasound, CAT scan, MRI, chest x-ray, bone scan

c. Continuous bladder irrigation (CBI)

d.

CONDITION: Testicular Cancer

PHYSIOLOGY: Testicular cancer is a rare tumor that arises from the germinal cells (cells that produce sperm) of the embryonal tissues and causes less than 1% of all cancer deaths in men. Testicular tumors are classified as seminomas or nonseminomas. Seminomas are composed of uniform, undifferentiated cells that resemble primitive gonadal cells. This type of tumor represents 40% of all testicular cancer and is usually confined to the testes and retroperitoneal nodes. There are two types of seminomas: classical (occur between the late 30s and early 50s) and spermatocytic seminomas (occur around age 55, grow slowly, and do not metastasize). Nonseminomas show varying degrees of cell differentiation and include embryonal carcinoma (occur most often in 20- to 30-year-olds, grows rapidly, and metastasizes), teratoma (can occur in children and adults), choriocarcinoma (rare and highly malignant), and yolk cell carcinoma derivatives (most common in children up to 3 years of age and have a very good prognosis). Sometimes, testicular tumors are "mixed," containing elements distinctive to both groups. Staging is categorized typically as follows: stage I (confined to testes), stage II (regional lymph node spread), and stage III (spread beyond the retroperitoneal lymph nodes). The initial treatment for testicular cancer is surgical resection of the involved testicle (orchiectomy). A testicular prosthesis can be placed if the patient so desires. If a bilateral orchiectomy is performed, the patient may need hormonal replacement. It is controversial whether or not the retroperitoneal nodes should be resected or treated with chemotherapy. Surgical resection carries with it the likelihood of impotence. To preserve fertility, nerve-sparing retroperitoneal lymph node surgery protects the nerves and allows for normal ejaculation. Postoperatively, edema and intrascrotal hemorrhage are the two most common problems. Monitor the patient closely for swelling and bleeding. Elevate the scrotum on a rolled towel, and apply ice to assist with discomfort and decrease swelling. Observe for signs of infection. Encourage the patient to wear an athletic supporter during ambulation to minimize discomfort. Usually, the patient is encouraged to do so within 12 hours of surgery.

Depending on staging of the disease, radiation or chemotherapy may also be used. Tumors classified as seminomas are especially radiosensitive. External beam radiation is usually given after surgery if the peritoneal lymph system is disease-positive or if the pelvis and mediastinal and supraclavicular lymph nodes are involved. Inform the patient that, although the unaffected testicle is shielded during radiation, it does receive some radiation that is scattered, which may decrease spermatogenesis. Nonseminomatous tumors are not radiosensitive, and chemotherapy is the preferred treatment (*Taber's*, 2009).

HANDOFF COMMUNICATION

S	Situation	Assess what is currently happening in a short statement.	Patient presents as _____
B	Background	Summarize important past assessment data for your patient here. Place lab results and Medications on the concept map.	**Age:** **Gender:** Male **Allergies:** **Fall Risk:** **Isolation:**
A	Assessment	Use the assessment data to complete your concept map.	**Nursing Diagnosis:** Place the Nursing Diagnoses in prioritized order on the concept map and add any needed for your specific patient. **Plan:** Place any further Nursing Interventions Classifications (NIC) needed on the map.

Implement Your Plan of Care

		EVALUATE YOUR CARE		
R	Recommendation Evaluate your nursing care and make recommendations related to the achievement of your desired outcomes. Were they met, or do new goals need to be established?	**Diag**	**Nursing Outcomes Classification (NOC)**	**Outcome met**
		1	Patient verbalizes understanding of disease process, diagnostic procedures, treatment options, and available resources.	☐ Yes ☐ No
		2	Patient appears relaxed and verbalizes decreased/absent pain.	☐ Yes ☐ No
		3	Patient demonstrates ability to cope with bodily changes through open discussion and participation in care.	☐ Yes ☐ No
		4	Patient shares feelings/concerns related to sexual activity and reports satisfaction with physical intimacy.	☐ Yes ☐ No
		5		☐ Yes ☐ No

Nursing Diagnosis 1

Deficient knowledge of disease process, diagnostic/treatment regimen, and prognosis evidenced by questions.

NIC:
1) Provide information on disease process. Encourage questions related to diagnosis and treatment options and prognosis; **2)** Explain lab tests/procedures; **3)** Provide preop/postop teaching; and **4)** Provide referrals to reputable informational resources and support groups.

Nursing Diagnosis 2

Pain (acute) related to inflammation, tissue damage, tissue compression, or nerve irritation from tumor metastasis in the perineum, groin, or abdomen evidenced by complaint of pain.

NIC:
1) Assess pain level systematically and often; **2)** Administer analgesics as prescribed; **3)** Provide relaxation techniques/medication; and **4)** Provide transcutaneous electric nerve stimulation (TENS), information on hypnosis, heat/cold application.

Nursing Diagnosis 3

Disturbed body image related to orchiectomy evidenced by verbalizations.

NIC:
1) Assess feelings and perceived impact on body image; **2)** Acknowledge patient's feelings, fears, and frustrations; **3)** Assess prior coping strategies; **4)** Include patient in self-care activities and treatments; and **5)** Provide information/referral to resources/support groups for testicular cancer and prosthesis care.

Nursing Diagnosis 4

Risk for sexual dysfunction related to disease process, pain, hormonal changes, and infertility.

NIC:
1) Provide private time for the patient and his partner to ask questions, express concerns, and clarify information; and **2)** Offer the opportunity for sexuality and fertility counseling after discussing the impact of the surgery on anatomy and function.

Condition:
Testicular Cancer

Age:

Link & Explain
• Nursing Interventions Classification (NIC)
• Laboratory and Diagnostic Procedures
• Medications

Nursing Diagnosis 5

NIC:

Medications

a. Chemotherapy

b. NSAIDs/acetaminophen

c. Opioids/opioid-NSAID combination drugs

d. Hormone replacement

Laboratory & Diagnostic Procedures

a. Testicular self-exam

b. Diagnostic ultrasound, CAT scan, MRI, chest x-ray, bone scan

c. Laboratory tumor markers (alpha-fetoprotein, human chorionic gonadotropin)

d. Sperm banking

Concept Maps for Your Medical or Surgical Patients

This chapter provides care maps that describe health conditions experienced by adult patients with medical or surgical conditions. The majority of patients who are hospitalized today are experiencing one or more of these conditions, but it is easy to draw information from one map to add to another. Besides having multiple conditions, medical-surgical patients are becoming increasingly acute in the hospital, so we have tried to include many of the acute conditions, such as brain trauma, along with the chronic conditions that may have been preexisting. We know that medical-surgical nursing is becoming a specialty unto itself and that many nursing care units specialize in patients with a specific type of condition, such as cardiac. We have included a multitude of care maps on each body system to try to ensure you have an applicable care map. All of the care maps provide a wonderful foundation on which you, the student nurse, can individualize care!

The conditions included in this chapter are:

1. Abdominal Aortic Aneurysm (Postoperative)
2. Acute Respiratory Failure
3. Adrenal Insufficiency/Addisonian Crisis
4. Amputation
5. Amyotrophic Lateral Sclerosis (ALS)/Lou Gehrig's Disease
6. Anemia
7. Angina (Coronary Artery Disease, Acute Coronary Syndrome)
8. Arthroplasty/Joint Replacement: Total Hip, Knee, Shoulder
9. Burns
10. Cancer
11. Cellulitis
12. Cholecystectomy
13. Cholecystitis With Cholelithiasis
14. Chronic Obstructive Pulmonary Disease (COPD)
15. Chronic Renal Failure
16. Cirrhosis of the Liver
17. Colorectal Cancer
18. Cushing's Syndrome
19. Diabetes Mellitus: Diabetic Ketoacidosis (DKA)
20. Diabetes Mellitus: Type I & Type II
21. Disk Surgery
22. Endocarditis—Infective
23. Eye Trauma
24. Fecal Diversions: Postoperative Care of Ileostomy and Colostomy
25. Fractures
26. Gastric Partitioning, Gastroplasty, and Gastric Bypass
27. Glaucoma
28. Heart Failure (HF)—Chronic
29. Hepatitis
30. Herniated Nucleus Pulposus (Ruptured Intervertebral Disk)

31. Hiatal Hernia
32. Hip Fracture
33. Hospice Care/Death and Dying
34. Human Immunodeficiency Virus (HIV)
35. Hypertension
36. Hyperthyroidism (Graves' Disease, Thyrotoxicosis)
37. Inflammatory Bowel Disease
38. Intestinal Obstruction
39. Leukemia
40. Lung Cancer
41. Lymphoma
42. Multiple Sclerosis
43. Myasthenia Gravis
44. Obstructive Sleep Apnea
45. Osteoarthritis (Degenerative Joint Disease)
46. Osteoporosis
47. Paget's Disease of the Bone (Osteitis Deformans)
48. Pancreatitis
49. Parkinson's Disease
50. Peptic Ulcer
51. Peritonitis

52. Pneumonia
53. Radical Neck Surgery—Laryngectomy
54. Renal Dialysis—General Considerations
55. Rheumatoid Arthritis (RA)
56. Risk for Falls
57. Seizure Disorders
58. Sickle Cell Crisis (Vaso-Occlusive Crisis)
59. Systemic Lupus Erythematosus (SLE)
60. Thrombophlebitis and Pulmonary Emboli
61. Thyroidectomy
62. Total Nutritional Support: Parenteral/Enteral
63. Transplant Considerations—Postoperative and Lifelong
64. Tuberculosis (TB)
65. Upper Gastrointestinal Bleeding/Esophageal Bleeding
66. Urinary Diversion/Urostomy/Nephrostomy
67. Urinary Incontinence
68. Urolithiasis/Renal Calculi
69. Venous Stasis Ulcer
70. Ventilation Assistance (Mechanical)

CONDITION: Abdominal Aortic Aneurysm (Postoperative)

PHYSIOLOGY: Abdominal aortic aneurysm (AAA) is a localized abnormal dilation or outpouching of an artery due to a congenital defect or weakness in the wall of the vessel (*Taber's*, 2009). It is most common in the abdominal aorta between the renal arteries and the bifurcation. The middle layer of the artery weakens and produces stretching of the inner layer. Hypertension produces an increased enlargement because of the stress on the artery. The patient is at risk for arterial rupture and hemorrhage as the aneurysm enlarges.

Risk factors are male gender, over 65 years of age, tobacco use, coronary or peripheral disease, high cholesterol, and hypertension.

Clinical manifestations of AAA include back pain from compression of lumbar nerve, epigastric discomfort, altered bowel elimination, and bluish color of feet and toes with + pulses.

Repair for aneurysms that meet the criteria include:
1. Surgical intervention through an abdomen incision with placement of a synthetic graft.
2. Endovascular aneurysm repair (EVAR), which is the placement of a graft through the femoral artery.

HANDOFF COMMUNICATION

S	Situation	Assess what is currently happening in a short statement.	Patient presents as _____
B	Background	Summarize important past assessment data for your patient here. Place lab results and medications on the concept map.	Age: Gender: Allergies: Fall Risk: Isolation:
A	Assessment	Use the assessment data to complete your concept map.	**Nursing Diagnosis:** Place the Nursing Diagnoses in prioritized order on the concept map and add any needed for your specific patient. **Plan:** Place any further Nursing Interventions Classifications (NIC) needed on the map.

Implement Your Plan of Care

R	Recommendation	Evaluate your nursing care and make recommendations related to the achievement of your desired outcomes. Were they met, or do new goals need to be established?		

		EVALUATE YOUR CARE	
	Diag	**Nursing Outcomes Classification (NOC)**	**Outcome met**
	1	Patient demonstrates adequate perfusion with skin warm and dry, peripheral pulses present, color good, VS within normal limits, balanced I&O, and absence of edema.	☐ Yes ☐ No
	2	Patient reports pain is relieved or controlled.	☐ Yes ☐ No
	3	Patient demonstrates adequate fluid balance with stable VS and adequate urinary output.	☐ Yes ☐ No
	4	Patient achieves timely wound healing, free of signs of infection and inflammation such as purulent drainage, erythema, and fever.	☐ Yes ☐ No
	5	Patient verbalizes understanding of disease process and potential complications. Patient participates in treatment regimen.	☐ Yes ☐ No

Nursing Diagnosis 1

Ineffective tissue perfusion (cardiopulmonary, renal) related to interruption of blood flow—hemorrhage, thromboembolic evidenced by tachycardia, decreased BP, and decreased urine output.

NIC:
1) Inspect for pallor, cyanosis, mottling, cool and clammy skin. Note color of lower extremities and strength of peripheral pulses and capillary refill; **2)** Monitor for complications such as acute myocardial infarction, dysrhythmias, thromboembolism, pneumonia; **3)** Encourage active or assist with passive range of motion exercises; **4)** Apply antiemboli stockings or intermittent pneumatic compression devices to lower extremities; **5)** Monitor BP closely; prolonged hypotension may result in graft thrombosis; severe hypertension may result in rupture of sutures; **6)** Administer diuretics, vasodilators, or antihypertensives per protocol if hypertension develops; and **7)** Administer fluids and vasoconstrictors per protocol to prevent organ ischemia if hypotension develops.

Nursing Diagnosis 2

Acute pain related to abdominal incision evidenced by reports of pain, preoccupation with self, changes in sleep pattern.

NIC:
1) Assess patient's perception of pain, attitude toward pain, effect of medications to decrease pain; **2)** Perform comprehensive assessment of pain, noting location, duration, severity, using a 0–10 scale; **3)** Assess VS, noting tachycardia, hypertension, and increased respiration, even if patient denies pain; **4)** Note presence of behaviors associated with pain—changes in VS, crying, grimacing, sleep disturbance, withdrawal; **5)** Differentiate incisional pain from gas pain. Auscultate bowel sounds. Note passing of flatus; and **6)** Review intraoperative and recovery room record for type of anesthesia and medications administered for pain.

Nursing Diagnosis 3

Risk for deficient fluid volume related to hemorrhage evidenced by hypotension and tachycardia.

NIC:
1) Measure and record I&O, including drains and nasogastric tube. Review intraoperative record for potential imbalance; **2)** Monitor VS, noting decrease in BP, increase in heart rate, and changes in rhythm. Inspect mucous membranes and skin turgor; **3)** Administer IV solutions, packed RBC, volume expanders as prescribed; monitor Hgb/Hct, electrolytes, BUN; **4)** Assess for heart failure caused by fluid overload; and **5)** Inspect drainage devices and abdominal dressings at regular intervals; assess wound for swelling.

Nursing Diagnosis 4

Risk for infection related to invasive procedure, surgical incision.

NIC:
1) Practice and instruct in good hand washing and aseptic wound care; **2)** Inspect incision and drains and presence of erythema; **3)** Monitor VS and note onset of fever, chills, diaphoresis, changes in mentation, reports of increasing abdominal pain; **4)** Obtain drainage specimens for culture if prescribed; and **5)** Administer antibiotics as prescribed.

Condition:
Abdominal Aortic Aneurysm (Postoperative)

Age:

Link & Explain
• Nursing Interventions Classification (NIC)
• Laboratory and Diagnostic Procedures
• Medications

Nursing Diagnosis 5

Deficient knowledge regarding condition, prognosis, treatment, self-care, discharge needs related to unfamiliarity with information resources evidenced by questions, request for information.

NIC:
Counsel patient to **1)** increase activity slowly and take rest periods between activities; **2)** avoid lifting for 6 weeks after surgery; **3)** report any redness, swelling, increased pain, or drainage from incision site; **4)** report fever above 100°F (37.8°C); **5)** assess lower extremities and report a decrease in pulses, coolness to touch, or cyanosis; and **6)** Counsel male patient about possible sexual dysfunction after surgery.

Medications
a. Simvastatin (Zocor)
b. Doxycycline (Doryx)
c. Diuretics
d. Antihypertensives, vasodilators, vasoconstrictors

Laboratory & Diagnostic Procedures
a. Chest x-ray
b. Electrocardiogram (EKG)
c. Ultrasound, CT scan (3-D), magnetic resonance imaging (MRI)
d. Angiography

CONDITION: Acute Respiratory Failure

PHYSIOLOGY: Acute respiratory failure is a life-threatening emergency associated with the inability to maintain adequate amounts of oxygen in the arterial blood supply and/or removal of CO_2 from mixed venous blood. Critical values include a Pao_2 below 60 mm Hg and/or the Pco_2 above 50 mm Hg with a corresponding drop in pH below 7.35. Acute respiratory failure is further defined as ventilatory failure, oxygenation failure, or a combination of both ventilatory and oxygenation failure. Whatever the underlying problem, the patient in acute respiratory failure is always hypoxemic (low arterial blood oxygen levels).

Acute respiratory failure is often the result of three problems: a physical problem of the lungs or chest wall, a defect in the respiratory control center in the brain, or poor function of the respiratory muscles, especially the diaphragm.

Combined ventilatory and oxygenation failure involves hypoventilation (poor respiratory movements). Gas exchange at the alveolar-capillary membrane is poor so that too little oxygen reaches the blood and carbon dioxide is retained. This type of respiratory failure leads to more profound hypoxemia than either ventilatory failure or oxygenation failure alone (Ignatavicius & Workman, 2010).

HANDOFF COMMUNICATION

S	Situation	Assess what is currently happening in a short statement.	Patient presents as _____ *Identify possible contributing causes, current status, and respiratory support mechanisms in use.*
B	Background	Summarize important past assessment data for your patient here. Place lab results and medications on the concept map.	**Age:** **Gender:** **Allergies:** **Fall Risk:** **Isolation:**
A	Assessment	Use the assessment data to complete your concept map.	**Nursing Diagnosis:** Place the Nursing Diagnoses in prioritized order on the concept map and add any needed for your specific patient. **Plan:** Place any further Nursing Interventions Classifications (NIC) needed on the map.

Implement Your Plan of Care

			EVALUATE YOUR CARE	
R	Recommendation Evaluate your nursing care and make recommendations related to the achievement of your desired outcomes. Were they met, or do new goals need to be established?	**Diag**	**Nursing Outcomes Classification (NOC)**	**Outcome met**
		1	Patient demonstrates improved oxygenation/ventilation, pulmonary gas exchange is improved as evidenced by eupnea, no use of accessory muscles, and arterial blood gases consistent with patient's normal baseline.	☐ Yes ☐ No
		2	Patient's airway remains patent evidenced by airway free of secretions and clear lung sounds.	☐ Yes ☐ No
		3	Patient remains afebrile.	☐ Yes ☐ No
		4	Patient experiences absence or decreased anxiety, demonstrating a calm demeanor.	☐ Yes ☐ No
		5	Patient/family verbalize understanding of disease process, procedures, and treatment.	☐ Yes ☐ No

Nursing Diagnosis 1

Impaired spontaneous ventilation related to alteration in usual oxygen/carbon dioxide ratio evidenced by tachypnea and bradypnea.

NIC:
1) Assess work and effectiveness of breathing; observe for changes in respiratory status, signs of hypoxia; **2)** Monitor VS, pulse oximetry, and ABGs; assess for advance directive/medical power of attorney; and **3)** Assist with ventilatory support measures as appropriate.

Nursing Diagnosis 2

Risk for ineffective airway clearance related to inability to cough effectively.

NIC:
1) Assess for significant alterations in lung sounds (rhonchi, wheezes); **2)** Assess for changes in ventilation (rate, depth, or use of accessory muscles); **3)** Assess secretions: color, consistency, amount; **4)** Assess patient's ability to cough, deep breathe, and use incentive spirometer; **5)** Change patient position every 2 hours; and **6)** Suction airway as needed and provide humidified oxygen therapy when indicated.

Nursing Diagnosis 3

Risk for infection related to invasive procedures.

NIC:
1) Monitor temperature and notify care provider of temperature over 38.5°C (101.3°F); **2)** Monitor white blood cell (WBC) count; **3)** Observe secretions for color, consistency, quantity, and odor; **4)** Monitor sputum cultures and sensitivity; **5)** Practice conscientious bronchial hygiene, good hand-washing techniques, and sterile suctioning; **6)** Provide frequent mouth care; **7)** Keep head of bed elevated >30 degrees; and **8)** Maintain patients' personal hygiene, nutrition, and rest.

Nursing Diagnosis 4

Anxiety related to situational crisis; threat to self-concept evidenced by insomnia and restlessness.

NIC:
1) Assess for signs of increased anxiety; **2)** Provide means of communication if patient is unable to speak due to respiratory status; **3)** Anticipate questions and provide explanations as needed; **4)** Display confident, calm manner and understanding attitude; **5)** Involve family/significant others in care; **6)** Ensure close, continuous monitoring and prompt interventions; and **7)** Utilize supportive measures (medications, clergy, social services, etc.) as indicated.

Condition:
Acute Respiratory Failure

Age:

Link & Explain
• Nursing Interventions Classification (NIC)
• Laboratory and Diagnostic Procedures
• Medications

Nursing Diagnosis 5

Deficient knowledge related to lack of exposure or recall evidenced by questions about care.

NIC:
1) Encourage patient/family to verbalize feelings/concerns; **2)** Explain the disease process to patient/family; **3)** Include patient/family in plan of care; **4)** Explain equipment, tests, procedures, and other therapies; **5)** Instruct on preventative measures, including avoiding respiratory irritants and allergens; and **6)** Provide guidelines for health maintenance and promotion, including the need for home oxygen and follow-up visits with healthcare provider.

Medications

a. Oxygen therapy

b. Bronchodilators (systemic or metered dose inhaler [MDI])

c. Anti-anxiety medications, sedatives, paralytics (if mechanically ventilated)

d. Pain medications if functional limitations due to pain from surgery/trauma, etc.

Laboratory & Diagnostic Procedures

a. ABGs

b. Ventilation/perfusion studies (VQ scan)

c. Radiologic studies

d. CBC, blood chemistry

CONDITION: Adrenal Insufficiency/Addisonian Crisis

PHYSIOLOGY: Adrenal insufficiency is insufficient secretion of the adrenal corticosteroids. The clinical manifestations have a slow onset and include weight loss, hyperpigmented skin, alopecia, hypotension, gastrointestinal symptoms, fatigue, anemia, hyponatremia, hypovolemia, hyperkalemia, decreased libido in women, decreased pubic and axillary hair, depression, delusions. The clinical manifestations of secondary adrenal insufficiency are the same as primary except there is no hyperpigmentation of the skin.

Cause

1. *Primary adrenal insufficiency* (Addison's disease) results from hypofunction of the adrenal cortex in which there is a decrease in all three adrenal corticosteroids: glucocorticoids, mineralocorticoids, and androgens. It can be caused by an autoimmune response whereby adrenal tissue is destroyed by antibodies. It can also be the result of tuberculosis, AIDS, fungal infection, and chemotherapy.
2. *Secondary adrenal insufficiency* results from lack of pituitary adrenocorticotrophic hormone (ACTH) secretion in which there is a decrease in two adrenal corticosteroids—glucocorticoids and androgens—but mineralocorticoids are usually normal.
   It can be caused by pituitary tumors, pituitary radiation, and hypophysectomy.
   Acute adrenal insufficiency is a life-threatening emergency caused by a sharp, sudden decrease in adrenocorticoid hormones. It can be triggered by stress, sudden withdrawal of corticosteroid hormone replacement therapy, postadrenal surgery, or sudden destruction of the pituitary gland. Symptoms include hypotension, tachycardia, hyponatremia, hyperkalemia, hypoglycemia, weakness, and confusion. Patients also have gastrointestinal symptoms such as nausea, vomiting, diarrhea, and abdominal pain.

HANDOFF COMMUNICATION

S	Situation	Assess what is currently happening in a short statement.	Patient presents as _____
B	Background	Summarize important past assessment data for your patient here. Place lab results and medications on the concept map.	Age: Gender: Allergies: Fall Risk: Isolation:
A	Assessment	Use the assessment data to complete your concept map.	**Nursing Diagnosis:** Place the Nursing Diagnoses in prioritized order on the concept map and add any needed for your specific patient. **Plan:** Place any further Nursing Interventions Classifications (NIC) needed on the map.

Implement Your Plan of Care

				EVALUATE YOUR CARE	
R	Recommendation	Evaluate your nursing care and make recommendations related to the achievement of your desired outcomes. Were they met, or do new goals need to be established?	**Diag**	**Nursing Outcomes Classification (NOC)**	**Outcome met**
			1	Patient demonstrates weight gain toward individually expected range and verbalizes nutritional needs.	☐ Yes ☐ No
			2	Patient's VS, heart rate, and urine output are within normal limits.	☐ Yes ☐ No
			3	Patient has normal laboratory values with an absence of muscle weakness and neurological irritability.	☐ Yes ☐ No
			4	Patient has normal laboratory values and EKG within normal limits for patient.	☐ Yes ☐ No
			5	Patient verbalizes understanding of therapeutic need and initiates necessary lifestyle changes.	☐ Yes ☐ No

Nursing Diagnosis 1

Imbalanced nutrition: less than body requirements related to inadequate food intake, gastrointestinal symptoms evidenced by body weight 15% less than ideal for height and frame.

NIC:
1) Maintain nasogastric tube for gastric decompression as needed. Document accurate I&O; **2)** Assess patient understanding of disease process and effect on gastrointestinal symptoms; **3)** Monitor electrolyte levels if patient has vomiting or diarrhea; **4)** Provide small, frequent meals when refeeding is initiated; and **5)** Encourage patient to drink supplements between meals as needed.

Nursing Diagnosis 2

Deficient fluid volume related to regulatory failure—adrenal disease evidenced by decreased blood pressure, tachycardia, decreased urine output.

NIC:
1) Monitor laboratory studies such as hemoglobin, hematocrit, BUN, creatinine; **2)** Monitor BP standing, sitting, and lying; monitor respirations, heart rate, and urine output; **3)** Palpate peripheral pulses; note capillary refill, skin color, and temperature; **4)** Weigh daily and compare with 24-hour fluid balance; **5)** Evaluate patient's ability to manage own hydration; and **6)** Administer high-dose hydrocortisone replacement and 0.9% saline solution for hypotension as ordered.

Nursing Diagnosis 3

Risk for electrolyte imbalance (hyponatremia) related to glucocorticoid and mineralocorticoid deficiency.

NIC:
1) Monitor electrolytes, report a decrease in sodium levels below normal range; **2)** Monitor I&O and calculate 24-hour fluid balance; **3)** Assess level of consciousness, behavior, and neuromuscular response; **4)** Monitor VS and pulse oximetry. Check the effectiveness of respiratory status if muscle weakness exists; **5)** Maintain a quiet environment, provide safety and seizure precautions; and **6)** Encourage foods and fluids that are high in sodium, such as bouillon, fruit juices, celery, tomatoes.

Nursing Diagnosis 4

Risk for electrolyte imbalance (hyperkalemia) related to glucocorticoid and mineralocorticoid deficiency.

NIC:
1) Monitor electrolytes, report an increase in potassium levels above normal range; **2)** Assess VS and report changes as needed; **3)** Auscultate heart sounds, noting rate, rhythm, presence of extra heartbeats, and dropped beats; **4)** Observe EKG monitor and obtain rhythm strip to document dysrhythmia; and **5)** Administer 0.9% saline solution with insulin and dextrose or Kayexalate for hyperkalemia as prescribed.

Condition:
Adrenal Insufficiency/ Addisonian Crisis

Age:

- - - - - - - - - - - - - - - - - -

Link & Explain
- Nursing Interventions Classification (NIC)
- Laboratory and Diagnostic Procedures
- Medications

Nursing Diagnosis 5

Deficient knowledge regarding condition, prognosis, treatment, self-care, and discharge needs related to lack of exposure to recall evidenced by inaccurate follow-through of instructions.

NIC:
1) Encourage patient to administer medication as prescribed; **2)** Utilize stress management techniques and increase medications as directed during physical or emotional stress such as influenza, running a marathon, surgery; **3)** Teach the patient to report symptoms of corticoid deficiency or excess (Cushing's); **4)** Teach patient taking mineralocorticoid therapy to take BP and increase salt intake; **5)** Encourage patient to wear a medical alert bracelet in case an unexpected event occurs; **6)** Instruct patient to carry an emergency kit containing hydrocortisone 100 mg injectable; and **7)** Teach patient and family members how to administer an intramuscular injection.

Medications
a. Corticosteroids
b. Mineralocorticoids
c.
d.

Laboratory & Diagnostic Procedures
a. Plasma cortisol levels, ACTH-stimulation test, urine cortisol and aldosterone levels, CT scan, MRI
b. Electrolytes, CBC, blood glucose, BUN
c. Removal of pituitary tumor via transsphenoidal approach, radiation therapy
d.

CONDITION: Amputation

PHYSIOLOGY: An amputation is the removal of a part of the body. The two different types of amputation are surgical amputation and traumatic amputation. A surgical amputation is often referred to as an "elective" surgery because it is ultimately the patient's choice to consent to removal of the body part. During surgical amputation, the surgeon attempts to preserve as much of the body part as possible, allowing for maximal postoperative mobility. Traumatic amputation occurs when the body part is severed unexpectedly. In these cases, the amputated body part may be healthy enough to attempt reattachment to the patient. Amputations most commonly involve the lower extremities, with only 10% of amputations being upper extremity removal. There are five types of lower extremity amputations: above the knee amputation (AKA), below the knee amputation (BKA), Syme amputation, midfoot amputation, and toe amputation. The higher the amputation, the more energy is required for ambulation postoperatively (*Taber's*, 2009).

There are many conditions that might cause the need for an amputation. Some of the more common causes are peripheral vascular disease (prominent among diabetic patients), infection such as necrotizing fasciitis (a bacterial infection that can destroy the skin, muscles, and underlying tissue), severe burns, and bone tumors.

Amputations are becoming less common due to success rates of modern revascularization and limb salvage techniques. Over 100,000 amputations are performed annually in the United States, with about 50% of them being performed on diabetic patients. Middle-aged or older diabetic men with a long history of smoking are the most commonly affected group for surgical amputations, while traumatic amputations are most common among young men who experience vehicular accidents or injuries by industrial work equipment.

Complications of amputation include hemorrhage, infection, phantom limb pain (PLP), problems associated with immobility, neuroma, and flexion contractures.

HANDOFF COMMUNICATION

S	Situation	Assess what is currently happening in a short statement.	Patient presents as _____ *Identify associated risk factors, length of identified symptoms, chronic diseases or infection, assessment of the affected area compared to the unaffected extremity.*
B	Background	Summarize important past assessment data for your patient here. Place lab results and medications on the concept map.	**Age:**　　　　　　　　　　　　　　　　**Gender:** **Allergies:**　　　　　　　　　　　　　　**Fall Risk:** **Isolation:**
A	Assessment	Use the assessment data to complete your concept map.	**Nursing Diagnosis:** Place the Nursing Diagnoses in prioritized order on the concept map and add any needed for your specific patient. **Plan:** Place any further Nursing Interventions Classifications (NIC) needed on the map.

Implement Your Plan of Care

			EVALUATE YOUR CARE		
R	Recommendation	Evaluate your nursing care and make recommendations related to the achievement of your desired outcomes. Were they met, or do new goals need to be established?	**Diag**	**Nursing Outcomes Classification (NOC)**	**Outcome met**
			1	Patient reports a decreased level of pain on a 0–10 numeric scale following implementation of medication or nonpharmacologic treatments.	☐ Yes ☐ No
			2	Patient reports an understanding of phantom limb pain (PLP) and methods used to resolve the pain.	☐ Yes ☐ No
			3	Patient demonstrates adaptation to changes in physical appearance with a positive adjustment to lifestyle change.	☐ Yes ☐ No
			4	Patient has increased mobility, uses assistive devices and participates in ADLs.	☐ Yes ☐ No
			5	Patient's wound heals without complications during hospitalization.	☐ Yes ☐ No

Nursing Diagnosis 1

Acute pain related to tissue and nerve trauma evidenced by guarding, reports of pain.

NIC:
1) Assess the pain to determine the onset, location, duration, characteristics, and aggravating and alleviating factors; 2) Determine the patient's current medication use; 3) Explore the need for opioid and nonopioid analgesics; 4) Administer pain medications when the patient reports pain, and assess pain relief 1 hour following administration; 5) Discuss alternative therapies for pain relief, such as distraction, massage, and meditation; 6) Describe the adverse effects of untreated pain; 7) Discuss the patient's fears of undertreated pain, addiction, and overdose; and 8) Plan nursing care when the patient is most comfortable, administering pain medication at least 30 minutes prior to activities that may increase pain.

Nursing Diagnosis 2

Chronic pain related to phantom limb sensation evidenced by verbalization of understanding of methods to relieve the pain.

NIC:
1) Assess the pain to determine the pain level on a 0–10 numeric scale, relieve pressure on remaining limb, which may cause neuropathic pain; 2) Administer Miacalin (Calcitonin-Salmon) IV to reduce PLP; 3) Administer tricyclic antidepressants, antiepileptics, or lidocaine topical patches depending on the character of the pain as described by the patient; 4) Discuss and teach alternative therapies for PLP, including transcutaneous electrical nerve stimulation, hypnosis, and biofeedback; 5) Check the prosthesis for correct fit; 6) Ask the patient to keep a record of pain, including pain rating, timing, treatments, and steps taken to relieve pain.

Nursing Diagnosis 3

Disturbed body image related to loss of body part evidenced by fear of rejection.

NIC:
1) Assess the extent of the patient's body image disturbance by asking questions related to body image during nursing assessment; 2) Assist the patient in voicing concerns related to his/her body changes; 3) Encourage the patient to discuss interpersonal and social conflicts that may arise; 4) Assess the patient's readiness to look at his/her wound; 5) Arrange for the patient to meet with a rehabilitated amputee; and 6) Provide the patient with appropriate resources, such as prosthesis companies.

Nursing Diagnosis 4

Impaired physical mobility related to loss of limb evidenced by decreased muscle strength.

NIC:
1) Assess the patient's level of mobility and need for assistive devices; 2) Reposition the patient frequently to prevent skin breakdown; 3) Consult physical and occupational therapy to work with the patient in attaining mobility needs; 4) Treat pain prior to beginning activities of increased mobility; 5) Promote early ambulation and muscle-strengthening activities; 6) Teach range of motion (ROM) exercises to prevent contractures; 7) Provide a trapeze and overhead frame to increase independence for a patient with a lower extremity amputation; 8) Discuss the options for physical therapy for prosthetic training; and 9) Refer the patient to social worker for help obtaining mobility assistance devices such as walker, cane, crutches, or wheelchair.

Condition:
Amputation
Age:

Link & Explain
• Nursing Interventions Classification (NIC)
• Laboratory and Diagnostic Procedures
• Medications

Nursing Diagnosis 5

Impaired skin integrity related to impaired circulation evidenced by slow wound healing.

NIC:
1) Assess the wound site for signs of inflammation. Document initial findings and daily changes; 2) Change soft dressing daily until sutures are removed; 3) Reposition the patient frequently to prevent breakdown; 4) Evaluate the need for a specialty bed or mattress; 5) Consult wound care team for detailed instructions on dressing changes; 6) Assess the patient's nutritional status, consulting the dietitian if needed; and 7) Teach the patient about wound care and signs and symptoms of infection.

Medications
a. IV calcitonin (reduces incidence of PLP)
b. Beta-blockers, anticonvulsants, antispasmodics (for PLP)
c. Broad spectrum antibiotics (infection prevention)
d. Analgesics (postoperative stump pain)

Laboratory & Diagnostic Procedures
a. Preoperative x-rays
b. Segmental limb blood pressures
c. Doppler ultrasonography for blood flow detection
d.

CONDITION: Amyotrophic Lateral Sclerosis (ALS)/Lou Gehrig's Disease

PHYSIOLOGY: ALS is a progressive neurological disorder that occurs more commonly in males and is characterized by degeneration of anterior horn cells of the spinal cord, the motor cranial nerve nuclei, and the corticospinal tracts. The clinical manifestations include the loss of motor function in the upper extremities, dysarthria, and dysphagia. Muscle wasting and fasciculations result from degeneration of the muscles. Pain, spasticity, drooling, emotional lability, and depression are common. The patient has physical limitations, but cognitive ability remains intact during this wasting disease. ALS usually leads to death within 6 years, which is usually the result of respiratory infection secondary to respiratory compromise (*Taber's*, 2009).

HANDOFF COMMUNICATION

S	Situation	Assess what is currently happening in a short statement.	Patient presents as _____
B	Background	Summarize important past assessment data for your patient here. Place lab results and medications on the concept map.	**Age:** **Gender:** **Allergies:** **Fall Risk:** **Isolation:**
A	Assessment	Use the assessment data to complete your concept map.	**Nursing Diagnosis:** Place the Nursing Diagnoses in prioritized order on the concept map and add any needed for your specific patient. **Plan:** Place any further Nursing Interventions Classifications (NIC) needed on the map.

Implement Your Plan of Care

		EVALUATE YOUR CARE		
R	Recommendation Evaluate your nursing care and make recommendations related to the achievement of your desired outcomes. Were they met, or do new goals need to be established?	**Diag**	**Nursing Outcomes Classification (NOC)**	**Outcome met**
		1	Patient performs self-care activities within level of ability and identifies community resources that will provide assistance.	☐ Yes ☐ No
		2	Patient identifies individual actions causing spasticity, muscular pain, and weakness and participates in recommended treatment plan.	☐ Yes ☐ No
		3	Patient verbalizes realistic view and acceptance of body and assumes the responsibility for meeting own needs.	☐ Yes ☐ No
		4	Patient participates in activities that stimulate cognitive function.	☐ Yes ☐ No
		5	Patient demonstrates feeding methods appropriate to individual situation, with aspiration prevention.	☐ Yes ☐ No

Nursing Diagnosis 1

Self-care deficit related to neuromuscular impairment evidenced by inability to perform tasks of self-care.

NIC:
1) Assess degree of functional impairment; 2) Provide assistive devices such as shower chair, elevated toilet seat with arm supports, specialized feeding utensils and drinking cups as indicated; 3) Provide strategies to assist with dressing, such as elastic waistbands, shoes and shirts that fasten with Velcro; 4) Allow sufficient time to perform tasks; 5) Provide active or passive range of motion exercises; and 6) Encourage the use of medications, cold packs, splints, and footboards as indicated.

Nursing Diagnosis 2

Muscle weakness related to physiological and emotional demands evidenced by inability to maintain usual routines; decreased performance.

NIC:
1) Determine need for mobility aids such as walker, cane, wheelchair, scooter; 2) Reinforce plan of care from speech pathologist; 3) Plan activities around scheduled rest periods during the day; 4) Provide moderate exercise to decrease spasticity of muscles; and 5) Bilevel positive airways pressure (BIPAP) may be used to aid breathing during sleep.

Nursing Diagnosis 3

Low self-esteem related to dependence and disruption in how patient perceives own body evidenced by denial, withdrawal, anger.

NIC:
1) Note behaviors indicating denial or anger; 2) Allow time for the patient to accept information; 3) Provide an open environment for the patient and significant other to discuss concerns; and 4) Acknowledge the grieving process related to actual or perceived changes.

Nursing Diagnosis 4

Reactive depression related to physical deterioration evidenced by isolation.

NIC:
1) Provide activities to stimulate cognitive function and enhance communication; 2) Interview patient about interests and read poems, articles, books to the patient as requested; 3) Include patient in discussions of his/her interests such as sports, current events; and 4) Provide gaming such as crossword puzzles.

Condition:
Amyotrophic Lateral Sclerosis (ALS)/Lou Gehrig's Disease

Age:
_____

Link & Explain
• Nursing Interventions Classification (NIC)
• Laboratory and Diagnostic Procedures
• Medications

Nursing Diagnosis 5

Risk for impaired swallowing related to neuromuscular impairment.

NIC:
1) Schedule activities to provide 30 minutes of rest before eating; 2) Assist patient with head control or support needed during meals; 3) Feed slowly, including 30–45 minutes for meals; 4) Incorporate favorite foods into meals; 5) Maintain upright for 45–60 minutes after eating; and 6) Record calorie count.

Medications

a. Riluzole (Rilutek)

b. Vitamin supplements

c. Opioids, benzodiazepines

d. Chlorpromazine (Thorazine)

Laboratory & Diagnostic Procedures

a. Creatine kinase (CK)

b. Electromyogram (EMG)

c.

d.

CONDITION: Anemia

PHYSIOLOGY: Decreased number of circulating red blood cells (RBCs), reduction of hemoglobin (Hgb) in the RBCs, or a combination of both, resulting in diminished oxygen-carrying capacity of the blood.

Types of Anemia

1. *Iron deficiency anemia:* inadequate iron stores, which result in insufficient hemoglobin. This anemia may be related to blood loss from gastric or duodenal ulcers, hemorrhoids, ulcerative colitis, inadequate diet, aspirin or NSAIDs.
2. *Anemia of chronic disease:* caused by chronic inflammatory, infectious, or neoplastic disorders. This anemia develops slowly and is primarily due to the slowed production of RBCs.
3. *Pernicious anemia:* lack of intrinsic factor in the stomach, possibly from Crohn's disease, gastrectomy, or gastric bypass, resulting in the inability to absorb vitamin B_{12}.
4. *Aplastic anemia:* failure of bone marrow to produce RBCs, WBCs, and platelets. It is caused by certain cancers, renal disease, hepatic disease, and some autoimmune conditions.
5. *Hemolytic anemia:* premature destruction of RBCs, which is caused by sickle cell disease, acute viral infections, or certain drugs.

HANDOFF COMMUNICATION

S	Situation	Assess what is currently happening in a short statement.	Patient presents as _____
B	Background	Summarize important past assessment data for your patient here. Place lab results and medications on the concept map.	Age: Gender: Allergies: Fall Risk: Isolation:
A	Assessment	Use the assessment data to complete your concept map.	**Nursing Diagnosis:** Place the Nursing Diagnoses in prioritized order on the concept map and add any needed for your specific patient. **Plan:** Place any further Nursing Interventions Classifications (NIC) needed on the map.

Implement Your Plan of Care

			EVALUATE YOUR CARE	
R	Recommendation	Evaluate your nursing care and make recommendations related to the achievement of your desired outcomes. Were they met, or do new goals need to be established?	**Diag** / **Nursing Outcomes Classification (NOC)**	**Outcome met**
			1 Patient demonstrates a decrease in physiological signs of intolerance: pulse, respirations, BP remain within patient's normal range.	☐ Yes ☐ No
			2 Patient demonstrates progressive weight gain or stable weight, with normalization of laboratory values.	☐ Yes ☐ No
			3 Patient establishes return-to-normal patterns of bowel function.	☐ Yes ☐ No
			4 Patient is free of signs of infection; achieves timely wound healing if present.	☐ Yes ☐ No
			5 Patient identifies causative factors and verbalizes understanding of therapeutic needs.	☐ Yes ☐ No

Nursing Diagnosis 1

Activity intolerance related to imbalance between oxygen supply and demand evidenced by weakness and fatigue.

NIC:
1) Assess patient's ability to perform ADLs, noting reports of weakness and fatigue; 2) Note changes in balance, gait disturbance, and muscle weakness; 3) Monitor BP, pulse, and respirations after activity. Note adverse response such as dysrhythmia, dizziness, dyspnea, tachypnea, and cyanosis of mucous membranes; 4) Encourage the patient to change positions slowly; and 5) Identify energy-saving techniques such as shower chair and sitting to perform tasks.

Nursing Diagnosis 2

Imbalanced nutrition related to failure to ingest food or absorb nutrients necessary for formation of RBCs evidenced by changes in gums, oral mucous membranes.

NIC:
1) Observe and record patient's food intake; 2) Weigh weekly and note decreases from previous weight; 3) Recommend small, frequent meals with between-meal nourishment; 4) Encourage patient to report nausea, vomiting, or increased flatus; and 5) Instruct patient to use good oral hygiene with a soft-bristle toothbrush and alcohol-free mouthwash.

Nursing Diagnosis 3

Constipation/diarrhea related to decreased dietary intake, changes in digestive process evidenced by reports of abdominal pain, urgency, cramping.

NIC:
1) Determine color, frequency, and amount of stool; 2) Avoid gas-forming foods; 3) Discuss use of stool softeners, mild stimulants, bulk-forming laxatives as needed for constipation; 4) Administer antidiarrheal medication such as diphenoxylate hydrochloride with atropine (Lomotil) as needed; and 5) Assess perianal skin condition frequently, noting changes or beginning of breakdown.

Nursing Diagnosis 4

Risk for infection related to inadequate primary defenses: broken skin, stasis of body fluids, invasive procedures, chronic disease, malnutrition.

NIC:
1) Promote meticulous hand washing by patient, visitors, and caregivers; 2) Maintain strict aseptic techniques for procedures; 3) Monitor temperature and note the presence of chills and tachycardia; 4) Provide meticulous skin, oral, and perineal care; and 5) Encourage frequent position changes and ambulation with coughing and deep-breathing exercises.

Condition:
Anemia
Age:

Link & Explain
• Nursing Interventions Classification (NIC)
• Laboratory and Diagnostic Procedures
• Medications

Nursing Diagnosis 5

Deficient knowledge regarding condition, prognosis, treatment, self-care, prevention of crisis, and discharge needs related to unfamiliarity with information resources evidenced by inaccurate follow-through of instructions, development of preventable complications.

NIC:
1) Provide information about anemia and explain the therapy depending on the type and severity of the anemia; 2) Explain that foods such as coffee, tea, egg yolks, and milk taken at the same time as iron-rich foods (meat) block the absorption of the iron from the meat; 3) Encourage cessation of smoking; 4) Stress importance of reporting symptoms such as weakness, paresthesias, irritability, or impaired memory; and 5) Instruct patient to avoid the use of aspirin. All other OTC medications should be discussed with the health-care provider before use.

Medications
a. Erythropoietin exogenous: darbepoetin alfa (Aranesp) (used in treatment of anemia to increase erythrocytes and hemoglobin levels)
b. Vitamin and mineral supplements: cyanocobalamin (vitamin B_{12}), folic acid (Folvite), and ascorbic acid (vitamin C) (replacement needed depending on the deficiencies identified)
c. Oral iron supplements: ferrous sulfate (Feosol), ferrous gluconate (Fergon), ferrous fumarate (Ircon) (used to enhance iron absorption and replace iron stores after several months)
d. IM/IV iron therapy: iron dextran (InFeD) (blood loss is too rapid for oral replacement to be effective or patient cannot absorb oral iron therapy)

Laboratory & Diagnostic Procedures
a. CBC: evaluates hemoglobin, hematocrit, RBC count, WBC count, platelets
b. Total iron-binding capacity: measures the amount of iron that can be carried through blood by transferrin
c. Guaiac: tests for hidden or occult blood, which may be in the stool or gastric content reflecting acute or chronic bleeding
d. Bone marrow aspiration/biopsy: determines the changes of number, size, and shape of blood cells to diagnose the type of anemia

CONDITION: Angina (Coronary Artery Disease, Acute Coronary Syndrome)

PHYSIOLOGY: Angina is a disorder resulting from an inadequate blood flow and oxygenation to the heart muscle causing transient myocardial ischemia and pain. The disorder is usually the result of narrowing of the coronary arteries (atherosclerosis) but may also occur as a result of coronary artery spasm or embolism. Angina typically accompanies activities resulting in increased myocardial oxygen demand such as increased physical exertion, consuming a large meal, or increased psychological stress. However, it can also be precipitated by limited myocardial oxygen supply resulting from hypoxia or severe anemia.

Patients generally complain of substernal pain/pressure with burning or squeezing qualities that radiates to the neck, jaw, shoulders, or arms and is often accompanied by shortness of breath, nausea/vomiting, diaphoresis, anxiety, and fear. Women, diabetics, and the elderly may present with atypical symptoms such as shortness of breath without pain.

Angina is classified as either *stable*, *unstable*, or *variant* (Prinzmetal's). Stable angina is the most common type and is usually precipitated by activities resulting in increased oxygen demand, typically lasts 3–5 minutes, and is relieved by rest and nitroglycerine. Unstable angina has no predictable pattern, usually lasts more than 30 minutes, is not relieved with rest or medications. Variant (Prinzmetal's) is a rare form of the condition that usually occurs at rest (midnight to early morning) with EKG changes associated with coronary artery spasm.

Severity of symptoms and resulting patient level of functional limitations are used as a basis for classification: *Class I*—no limitation of normal physical activity; *Class II*—minor limitation in normal physical activity; *Class III*—moderate limitation of activity (comfortable at rest but minimal activities precipitate symptoms); *Class IV*—unable to perform any physical activity without discomfort and may be symptomatic at rest.

HANDOFF COMMUNICATION

S	Situation	Assess what is currently happening in a short statement.	Patient presents as _____ *Type and classification of angina; frequency/onset/duration of signs and symptoms; history of heart disease (or related factors); interventions that relieve symptoms.*
B	Background	Summarize important past assessment data for your patient here. Place lab results and medications on the concept map.	**Age:** **Gender:** **Allergies:** **Fall Risk:** **Isolation:**
A	Assessment	Use the assessment data to complete your concept map.	**Nursing Diagnosis:** Place the Nursing Diagnoses in prioritized order on the concept map and add any needed for your specific patient. **Plan:** Place any further Nursing Interventions Classifications (NIC) needed on the map.

Implement Your Plan of Care

		EVALUATE YOUR CARE		
R	Recommendation Evaluate your nursing care and make recommendations related to the achievement of your desired outcomes. Were they met, or do new goals need to be established?	**Diag**	**Nursing Outcomes Classification (NOC)**	**Outcome met**
		1	Patient verbalizes relief of chest discomfort and appears relaxed and comfortable.	☐ Yes ☐ No
		2	Patient maintains adequate cardiac output, VS within normal limits; reports decreased anginal episodes; and demonstrates behaviors that reduce workload of the heart.	☐ Yes ☐ No
		3	Patient reports that anxiety is reduced to a manageable level, verbalizes awareness of healthy ways to recognize and deal with anxiety, demonstrates normal sleep patterns and stable VS.	☐ Yes ☐ No
		4	Patient performs activity within limits of cardiac disease without recurrence of chest discomfort/pain or EKG changes.	☐ Yes ☐ No
		5	Patient verbalizes understanding of disease process, therapeutic plan of care, and initiates necessary lifestyle changes.	☐ Yes ☐ No

Nursing Diagnosis 1

Acute pain related to imbalance between myocardial oxygen supply and demand and related tissue ischemia.

NIC:
1) Assess patient's description of pain, associated characteristics, and exacerbating factors; **2)** Monitor EKG, administer oxygen, provide anti-anginal medications as ordered; **3)** Monitor VS; elevate head of bed if patient is short of breath; and **4)** Provide emotional support and explanation of treatments/procedures.

Nursing Diagnosis 2

Risk for decreased cardiac output related to decreased cardiac contractility resulting from recurring episodes of myocardial ischemia.

NIC:
1) Assess VS, oxygenation, and hemodynamic status frequently; monitor EKG; **2)** Provide for frequent/adequate rest periods; assist with ADL as needed; **3)** Encourage prompt reports of pain; administer medications/oxygen accordingly; **4)** Monitor laboratory studies and diagnostic tests; and **5)** Anticipate transfer to higher level of care as needed.

Nursing Diagnosis 3

Fear/anxiety related to worsening symptoms/disease process, situational crises, inability to perform ADL independently, changes in life/situational status.

NIC:
1) Encourage patient to verbalize feelings; **2)** Assess for fear, anxiety, insomnia, changes in VS; **3)** Implement measures to reduce anxiety; **4)** Explain all aspects of treatment regimen; **5)** Avoid factors that may precipitate angina; and **6)** Discuss impact of condition on present lifestyle.

Nursing Diagnosis 4

Activity intolerance related to anginal symptoms, fear, side effects of prescribed medications.

NIC:
1) Assess patient level of activity before onset of angina; **2)** Assess defining characteristics of angina before, during, and after activity; **3)** Assist patient in developing plan to achieve ADL, and pace activities with frequent rest periods; and **4)** Assist in discharge planning and identification of needed supports.

Condition:
Angina (Coronary Artery Disease, Acute Coronary Syndrome)

Age: _____

Link & Explain
• Nursing Interventions Classification (NIC)
• Laboratory and Diagnostic Procedures
• Medications

Nursing Diagnosis 5

Deficient knowledge regarding condition, treatment needs, self-care, and discharge needs.

NIC:
1) Discuss pathology of condition and means of preventing/managing anginal attacks; **2)** Encourage avoidance of factors that precipitate episodes; **3)** Encourage patient to follow prescribed treatment regimen and follow-up care; **4)** Discuss impact of condition on lifestyle and needed modifications/supports; and **5)** Arrange home care and support services as indicated.

Medications

a. Oxygen, nitroglycerine, morphine

b. Beta blockers (decreases cardiac workload, peripheral vasodilation)

c. Aspirin (anti-platelet properties)

d.

Laboratory & Diagnostic Procedures

a. Cardiac enzymes, serum lipids, homocysteine, C-reactive protein; Hgb/Hct; coagulation studies; markers for metabolic activity (Pco_2, potassium, and myocardial lactate)

b. EKG, stress test, 24-hour cardiac monitoring (Holter)

c. Echocardiography, CT scans; coronary CT; coronary MRI; myocardial perfusion imaging angiography

d. Coronary computed tomography angiography (CTA); cardiac catheterization with angiography

CONDITION: Arthroplasty/Joint Replacement: Total Hip, Knee, Shoulder

PHYSIOLOGY: Arthroplasty is the replacement of a total joint through surgical removal of the affected joint and replacement with a prosthetic joint. Rheumatoid arthritis, osteoarthritis, congenital deformity, and injury place a patient at risk for the need for a joint replacement. Replacement arthroplasty is available for the hip, knee, ankle, elbow, shoulder, and phalangeal joints of the fingers. Surgery is followed by physical and occupational therapy. Full recovery usually takes a few months.

Infection is a serious complication of joint surgery with staphylococci and streptococci being the most common causative organisms.

HANDOFF COMMUNICATION

S Situation	Assess what is currently happening in a short statement.	Patient presents as _____	
B Background	Summarize important past assessment data for your patient here. Place lab results and medications on the concept map.	**Age:** **Allergies:** **Isolation:**	**Gender:** **Fall Risk:**
A Assessment	Use the assessment data to complete your concept map.	**Nursing Diagnosis:** Place the Nursing Diagnoses in prioritized order on the concept map and add any needed for your specific patient. **Plan:** Place any further Nursing Interventions Classifications (NIC) needed on the map.	

Implement Your Plan of Care

		EVALUATE YOUR CARE	
R Recommendation	Evaluate your nursing care and make recommendations related to the achievement of your desired outcomes. Were they met, or do new goals need to be established?	**Diag** / **Nursing Outcomes Classification (NOC)**	**Outcome met**
		1 Patient verbalizes relief from pain and is able to sleep.	☐ Yes ☐ No
		2 Patient adheres to restrictions regarding mobility; unaffected extremities are strong.	☐ Yes ☐ No
		3 Patient's extremities are warm, pulses good, capillary refill normal.	☐ Yes ☐ No
		4 Patient discusses understanding of follow-up care and rehabilitation.	☐ Yes ☐ No
		5	☐ Yes ☐ No

Nursing Diagnosis 1

Acute pain related to bone and soft tissue trauma evidenced by restlessness and facial grimacing.

NIC:
1) Observe and document location, severity (0–10 scale), characteristics of pain (steady, intermittent, colicky); **2)** Assess ability of the patient to utilize a patient-controlled analgesia (PCA) control, or administer narcotic analgesics every 3–4 hours as prescribed; **3)** Inform the patient to request pain medication before it increases in severity; **4)** Maintain position changes with joint precautions every 2 hours; **5)** Provide comfort measures such as back rub, guided imagery, diversional activities, and repositioning; and **6)** Note response to medication; report if pain is not relieved.

Nursing Diagnosis 2

Impaired physical mobility related to surgery evidenced by participation in rehabilitation program.

NIC:
1) Assess the patient's perception of immobility related to postoperative restrictions; **2)** Instruct patient while assisting with passive or active ROM exercises; **3)** Administer analgesics before repositioning or rehabilitation; **4)** Instruct the patient about precautions and guidelines during repositioning; **5)** Assist with mobility with the use of wheelchair, walker, crutches, and cane as needed. Maintain weight-bearing as prescribed (hip/knee); **6)** Apply the continuous passive motion (CPM) to affected leg including the degrees as prescribed (knee); **7)** Maintain an immobilizer and then provide a sling (shoulder); and **8)** Monitor BP when resuming activity; note reports of dizziness.

Nursing Diagnosis 3

Risk for ineffective tissue perfusion related to surgery.

NIC:
1) Evaluate presence and quality of peripheral pulse distal to surgical area via palpation or Doppler. Compare with non-surgical limb; **2)** Assess capillary return, skin color, and warmth distal to the surgical site; **3)** Report severe unrelieved pain, paresthesia, change in pulse quality distal to injury, decreased skin temperature, pallor; **4)** Apply sequential compression device and thromboembolic deterrent (TED) stockings; **5)** Monitor VS, note general pallor, cyanosis, cool skin, or changes in mentation; and **6)** Administer enoxaparin (Lovenox) as prescribed; monitor coagulation status.

Nursing Diagnosis 4

Deficient knowledge related to unfamiliarity with discharge plan evidenced by asking multiple questions about care.

NIC:
1) Maintain hip abductor device in place; **2)** Avoid extreme internal rotation and 90-degree hip flexion for 4–6 weeks postoperatively; **3)** Report sharp pain or popping sound in the hip; **4)** Use walker or crutches with prescribed weight-bearing (knee/hip); **5)** Report excessive pain or swelling of the knee; **6)** Perform ROM exercises of shoulder and arm and increase exercise as prescribed; **7)** Avoid external rotation and abduction of shoulder; and **8)** Monitor for signs of infection such as purulent or foul-smelling drainage from incision site, elevated temperature, chills.

Condition:
Arthroplasty/ Joint Replacement: Total Hip, Knee, Shoulder

Age:

Link & Explain
• Nursing Interventions Classification (NIC)
• Laboratory and Diagnostic Procedures
• Medications

Nursing Diagnosis 5

NIC:

Medications
a. Opioids
b. NSAIDs
c. Enoxaparin (Lovenox)
d.

Laboratory & Diagnostic Procedures
a. X-rays, bone scans, CT scan, MRI
b. CBC, coagulation profile
c.
d.

CONDITION: Burns

PHYSIOLOGY: Burns include local and systemic responses that affect skin and other tissue depending on the burn injury and physiologic response. Systemic response can cause cardiovascular, respiratory, and metabolic problems.

Types of Burns

Thermal burns occur from flame, hot fluid or gas, exposure to cold objects such as nitrogen or dry ice. These burns are often associated with smoke and inhalation injury. Smoke or inhalation injury results in redness and swelling in the airway and is a predictor of mortality.
Chemical burns occur from acid or alkaline substance. The degree of injury depends on the type and concentration of the substance.
Electrical burns occur when a current travels through the body. The degree of injury is related to the voltage.

Classification of Wound

Superficial partial thickness (first degree)—superficial epidermis, red and painful with mild edema (sunburn).
Deep (second degree)—epidermis and dermis, fluid-filled vesicles, painful, moderate edema (flame, chemical, electric current).
Full thickness (third and fourth degree)—destruction of nerves, muscle, tendons, bones, and skin is waxy, leathery, hard; painless because nerves are damaged (flame, chemical, electric current).

HANDOFF COMMUNICATION

S Situation	Assess what is currently happening in a short statement.	Patient presents as _____ VS: LOC:
B Background	Summarize important past assessment data for your patient here. Place lab results and medications on the concept map.	**Age:** **Gender:** **Allergies:** **Fall Risk:** **Isolation:**
A Assessment	Use the assessment data to complete your concept map.	**Nursing Diagnosis:** Place the Nursing Diagnoses in prioritized order on the concept map and add any needed for your specific patient. **Plan:** Place any further Nursing Interventions Classifications (NIC) needed on the map.

Implement Your Plan of Care

			EVALUATE YOUR CARE	
R Recommendation	Evaluate your nursing care and make recommendations related to the achievement of your desired outcomes. Were they met, or do new goals need to be established?	**Diag**	**Nursing Outcomes Classification (NOC)**	**Outcome met**
		1	Patient demonstrates clear breath sounds, respiratory rate is within normal range and free of dyspnea and cyanosis.	☐ Yes ☐ No
		2	Patient demonstrates improved fluid balance by adequate urinary output with normal specific gravity, stable VS, and moist mucous membranes.	☐ Yes ☐ No
		3	Patient displays relaxed facial expressions and body posture, adequate sleep and rest.	☐ Yes ☐ No
		4	Patient achieves timely wound healing free of purulent exudate; maintains afebrile status.	☐ Yes ☐ No
		5	Patient demonstrates stable weight and muscle mass measurements, intake adequate to meet nutritional needs, tissue regeneration, positive nitrogen balance.	☐ Yes ☐ No

Nursing Diagnosis 1

Risk for ineffective airway related to tracheobronchial obstruction from mucosal edema; circumferential full-thickness burns of the neck, thorax, and chest.

NIC:
1) Obtain history of injury and note presence of preexisting respiratory conditions and history of smoking; 2) Assess gag reflex, note upper airway burns, drooling, hoarseness, wheezy cough; 3) Auscultate lungs, noting stridor, wheezing, crackles, diminished breath sounds, brassy cough; 4) Note presence of pallor or cherry-red skin of unburned skin. Monitor carbon monoxide levels; 5) Assess for changes in behavior, mentation such as restlessness, agitation, confusion; 6) Administer humidified oxygen; and 7) Prepare for intubation or tracheostomy with mechanical ventilation.

Nursing Diagnosis 2

Risk for deficient fluid volume related to increased need from metabolic state and loss of fluid through burn wounds.

NIC:
1) Monitor VS, capillary refill, and strength of peripheral pulses; 2) Monitor urinary output and specific gravity. Observe urine color, and Hematest as needed for release of myoglobin; 3) Estimate wound drainage and insensible water loss; 4) Insert and maintain indwelling urinary catheter; 5) Insert and maintain large-bore IV catheters for replacement of fluids, electrolytes, albumin, plasma; and 6) Elevate extremities as needed to decrease edema.

Nursing Diagnosis 3

Acute pain related to destruction of skin and tissues, edema evidenced by reports of pain, guarding behavior, facial expressions, crying.

NIC:
1) Wrap digits and extremities in position of function, avoid flexed positions of affected joints. Use splints and footboards as needed; 2) Change position frequently, assist with active or passive ROM exercises; 3) Assess reports of pain, note location and intensity (1–10 scale). Medicate as indicated prior to dressing change; and 4) Provide emotional support as needed.

Nursing Diagnosis 4

Risk for infection related to inadequate primary defenses such as destruction of skin barrier.

NIC:
1) Maintain isolation techniques as indicated and provide hand-washing instructions for patient and family; 2) Use gowns, gloves, mask, and aseptic technique during direct wound care; 3) Monitor VS for fever and increased respiratory rate in association with changes in mentation; 4) Administer topical antimicrobial agents as indicated; 5) Remove dressings and cleanse burned areas in hydrotherapy if indicated; and 6) Examine wounds daily; note and document changes in appearance, odor, or quality of drainage.

Condition:
Burns
Age:

Link & Explain
- Nursing Interventions Classification (NIC)
- Laboratory and Diagnostic Procedures
- Medications

Nursing Diagnosis 5

Imbalanced nutrition: less than body requirements related to hypermetabolic state, protein catabolism, anorexia, restricted oral intake evidenced by decrease in total body weight, loss of muscle/subcutaneous fat, and development of negative nitrogen balance.

NIC:
1) Auscultate bowel sounds; note evidence of hypoactive or absent bowel sounds; 2) Maintain strict calorie count. Weigh daily. Reassess percentage of open body surface area and wounds weekly to calculate prescribed dietary calorie needs; 3) Encourage patient to make dietary choices high in calories and protein. Encourage family to bring food from home if appropriate; 4) Perform fingerstick glucose to assess for hyperglycemia if patient is receiving hyperalimentation to meet caloric needs; and 5) Monitor laboratory studies such as serum albumin, prealbumin, electrolytes, BUN, creatinine.

Medications
a. Analgesic: morphine (Avinza), sustained-release morphine (MS Contin), hydromorphone (Dilaudid)
b. Sedation: lorazepam (Ativan)
c. Anticoagulant therapy: enoxaparin (Lovenox)
d. Gastric acid prevention: esomeprazole (Nexium), lansoprazole (Prevacid)

Laboratory & Diagnostic Procedures
a. ABGs: reduced Pao_2 levels and increased $Paco_2$ levels
b. CBC, BUN, creatinine
c. Serum glucose, serum electrolytes, albumin, globulin, albumin/globulin ratio
d. Chest x-ray, bronchoscopy, pulmonary function studies

CONDITION: Cancer

PHYSIOLOGY: Malignant neoplasia marked by the disturbance of cellular growth, often with invasion of healthy tissues locally or throughout the body.

Classifications

Lymphomas originate in the infection-fighting organs.
Leukemias originate in the blood-forming organs.
Sarcomas originate in bones, muscle, or connective tissue.
Carcinomas originate in the epithelial cells.

Cancer cells can invade the lymphatic system and bloodstream and find places to grow in other tissues (metastasis).

Usually, as cancer cells proliferate, they become increasingly abnormal and require more of the body's metabolic output for their growth and development. Damage caused by their invasion of healthy tissues results in organ malfunction, pain, and often death.

HANDOFF COMMUNICATION

S	Situation	Assess what is currently happening in a short statement.	Patient presents as _____
B	Background	Summarize important past assessment data for your patient here. Place lab results and medications on the concept map.	Age: ⟶ Gender: Allergies: ⟶ Fall Risk: Isolation:
A	Assessment	Use the assessment data to complete your concept map.	**Nursing Diagnosis:** Place the Nursing Diagnoses in prioritized order on the concept map and add any needed for your specific patient. **Plan:** Place any further Nursing Interventions Classifications (NIC) needed on the map.

Implement Your Plan of Care

			EVALUATE YOUR CARE	
R	Recommendation	Evaluate your nursing care and make recommendations related to the achievement of your desired outcomes. Were they met, or do new goals need to be established?	**Diag** / **Nursing Outcomes Classification (NOC)**	**Outcome met**
			1 Patient reports maximum pain relief or control with minimal interference with ADL.	☐ Yes ☐ No
			2 Patient maintains adequate muscle mass and stable weight.	☐ Yes ☐ No
			3 Patient maintains adequate hydration with stable VS, good skin turgor, capillary refill, strong peripheral pulses, and appropriate urine output.	☐ Yes ☐ No
			4 Patient identifies actions to prevent or reduce risk of infection.	☐ Yes ☐ No
			5 Patient initiates lifestyle changes and participates in treatment regimen.	☐ Yes ☐ No

Nursing Diagnosis 1

Acute/chronic pain related to disease process: compression or destruction of nerve tissue, obstruction of nerve pathway, inflammation, metastasis to bones evidenced by reports of pain, distraction, guarding.

NIC:
1) Determine location, frequency, duration, and intensity of pain using a 0–10 rating scale; 2) Determine timing and "breakthrough" pain when using around-the-clock agents, whether oral, IV, topical, or epidural; 3) Discuss painful effects of specific therapies such as surgery, radiation, chemotherapy, or biotherapy; 4) Provide nonpharmacological comfort measures such as massage, repositioning, and back rubs and diversional activities such as music, reading, television; and 5) Administer analgesics as indicated for discomfort.

Nursing Diagnosis 2

Imbalanced nutrition: less than body requirements related to altered ability to digest or metabolize nutrients: nausea, vomiting evidenced by weight loss, lack of interest in food.

NIC:
1) Weigh regularly and establish current anthropometric measurements; 2) Determine the patient's dietary pattern, intake, and knowledge of nutrition; 3) Assess for nausea and vomiting and provide antiemetic as prescribed; 4) Discuss and document nutritional side effects of medications; 5) Provide information about foods and supplements that are high in calories, protein, vitamins, and minerals; 6) Monitor laboratory tests such as Hgb, albumin, prealbumin, potassium, and sodium; and 7) Adjust diet before and after chemotherapy to include cool, clear liquids, bland foods, crackers, toast, and carbonated drinks.

Nursing Diagnosis 3

Risk for deficient fluid volume related to excessive losses through normal routes (vomiting, diarrhea) and abnormal routes (indwelling tubes, wounds, fistulas).

NIC:
1) Monitor I&O, note all output sources such as emesis, diarrhea, draining wounds; 2) Assess VS, capillary refill, skin turgor, peripheral pulses, and mucous membranes; 3) Administer antiemetic therapy; 4) Monitor laboratory values such as CBC, electrolytes, and serum albumin; and 5) Administer IV fluids as prescribed.

Nursing Diagnosis 4

Risk for infection related to inadequate secondary defenses: alterations in mature WBCs with low granulocyte and abnormal lymphocyte count, increased number of immature lymphocytes, immunosuppression, bone marrow suppression.

NIC:
1) Require good hand-washing techniques for all personnel and visitors; 2) Implement neutropenic precautions, monitor absolute neutrophil count (ANC); 3) Monitor temperature and observe for tachycardia, hypotension, and subtle mental changes; 4) Stress importance of good oral hygiene; 5) Auscultate breath sounds, noting crackles and rhonchi. Observe for changes in sputum; and 6) Observe urine for cloudy color or foul smell, note presence of urgency and burning.

Condition:
Cancer
Age:

Link & Explain
• Nursing Interventions Classification (NIC)
• Laboratory and Diagnostic Procedures
• Medications

Nursing Diagnosis 5

Deficient knowledge regarding illness, prognosis, treatment, self-care, prevention of crisis, and discharge needs related to information misinterpretation, lack of recall evidenced by statement of misconception.

NIC:
1) Review specific diagnosis, treatment alternatives, and future expectations; 2) Provide anticipatory guidance regarding treatment protocol, length of therapy, expected results, and possible side effects; 3) Provide written materials about cancer, treatment, and available support systems; 4) Refer to community resources, such as social services, home health agencies, local chapter of American Cancer Society; and 5) Provide advice regarding avoidance of harsh shampoos, hair dye, exposure to wind and extreme heat or cold.

Medications
a. Chemotherapy
b. Radiation
c. Opioids, acetaminophen (Tylenol), NSAIDs
d.

Laboratory & Diagnostic Procedures
a. CBC, metabolic panel
b. MRI, CT scan, ultrasound
c. Biopsy
d. Tumor markers

CONDITION: Cellulitis

PHYSIOLOGY: A spreading bacterial infection of the skin and subcutaneous tissues, cellulitis is usually caused by streptococcal or staphylococcal infections in adults and occasionally by *Haemophilus* species in children. It may occur following damage to skin from an insect bite, an excoriation, or other injury. The extremities, especially the lower legs, are the most common sites. Adjacent soft tissue may be involved. Affected skin becomes inflamed: red, swollen, warm to the touch, and tender. Spread of infection up lymphatic channels may occur. Risk factors for cellulitis include diabetes mellitus, lymphedema, venous insufficiency, immune suppression, injection drug use, malnutrition, peripheral vascular disease, and previous skin diseases (*Taber's*, 2009).

HANDOFF COMMUNICATION

S — Situation

Assess what is currently happening in a short statement.

Patient presents as _____

B — Background

Summarize important past assessment data for your patient here. Place lab results and medications on the concept map.

Age: Gender:

Allergies: Fall Risk:

Isolation:

A — Assessment

Use the assessment data to complete your concept map.

Nursing Diagnosis: Place the Nursing Diagnoses in prioritized order on the concept map and add any needed for your specific patient.
Plan: Place any further Nursing Interventions Classifications (NIC) needed on the map.

Implement Your Plan of Care

R — Recommendation

Evaluate your nursing care and make recommendations related to the achievement of your desired outcomes. Were they met, or do new goals need to be established?

	EVALUATE YOUR CARE	
Diag	Nursing Outcomes Classification (NOC)	Outcome met
1	Patient demonstrates behaviors or techniques to facilitate healing.	☐ Yes ☐ No
2	Patient is free of chills and temperature returns to baseline.	☐ Yes ☐ No
3	Patient has adequate tissue perfusion evidenced by stable VS.	☐ Yes ☐ No
4	Patient reports pain is relieved or controlled.	☐ Yes ☐ No
5	Patient verbalizes understanding of disease process, prognosis, and potential complications.	☐ Yes ☐ No

Nursing Diagnosis 1

Impaired skin/tissue integrity related to altered sensation, circulation evidenced by itching, pain, numbness, pressure in affected area.

NIC:
1) Examine the skin for foreign bodies, open wounds, rashes, discoloration; 2) Keep area clean and dry. Encourage patient to eliminate touching and scratching of the infected area to decrease the chance of spreading the organism; 3) Elevate affected extremity to reduce edema; 4) Apply dry, sterile dressing if indicated; 5) Administer tetanus if prescribed; and 6) Administer antibiotics as prescribed.

Nursing Diagnosis 2

Hyperthermia related to increased metabolic rate, illness evidenced by elevated temperature higher than normal range.

NIC:
1) Assess patient for chills, diaphoresis, elevation of temperature; 2) Administer antipyretic such as acetaminophen (Tylenol) for temperature elevation above 100.9°F (38.3°C); 3) Monitor environmental temperature. Limit bed linens to maintain near body temperature; and 4) Increase PO fluid intake to prevent dehydration from temperature elevation.

Nursing Diagnosis 3

Risk for shock related to possible progression to a systemic infection.

NIC:
1) Review CBC results for elevated WBCs with differential having increased immature neutrophils (left shift); 2) Assess VS, noting tachycardia, progressive hypotension, widening pulse pressure, tachypnea; 3) Assess for altered mental status: confusion, agitation, restlessness, personality changes, stupor; 4) Maintain sequential compression devices (SCDs) as indicated; and 5) Administer antibiotics and IV fluids as indicated.

Nursing Diagnosis 4

Acute pain related to wound infection evidenced by reports of pain, preoccupation with self, changes in sleep pattern.

NIC:
1) Assess patient's perception of pain, attitude toward pain, effect of medications to decrease pain; 2) Perform comprehensive assessment of pain, noting location, duration, severity using a 0–10 scale; 3) Assess VS, noting tachycardia, hypertension, and increased respiration, even if patient denies pain; 4) Note presence of behaviors associated with pain: changes in VS, crying, grimacing, sleep disturbance, withdrawal; 5) Encourage patient to request pain medication before pain becomes severe; and 6) Administer pain medication as prescribed and evaluate effectiveness.

Condition:
Cellulitis
Age:

Link & Explain
• Nursing Interventions Classification (NIC)
• Laboratory and Diagnostic Procedures
• Medications

Nursing Diagnosis 5

Deficient knowledge regarding illness, prognosis, treatment, self-care, and discharge needs related to lack of exposure or recall evidenced by inaccurate follow-through of instructions.

NIC:
1) Counsel patient to eliminate the spread of infection to other areas of the body by frequent hand washing; 2) Counsel patient not to share towels, washcloths, clothing with other members of the family; 3) Encourage adequate rest periods with scheduled activities; 4) Discuss the need for good nutritional intake and balanced meals; 5) Encourage patient to report any signs of recurrent infection or temperature elevation; 6) Have patient demonstrate dressing change.

Medications
a. Antibiotics
b. Antipyretics
c.
d.

Laboratory & Diagnostic Procedures
a. CBC
b. Wound cultures
c.
d.

CONDITION: Cholecystectomy

PHYSIOLOGY: Cholecystectomy is indicated for the treatment of symptomatic gallstones, infection of the gallbladder or biliary ducts, calcified gallbladder, cancer, or trauma.

Procedure

Laparoscopic cholecystectomy—removal of small gallstones with use of a video endoscopy through a small abdominal incision.
Open cholecystectomy—removal of multiple large gallstones, common bile duct stones.

HANDOFF COMMUNICATION

S	Situation	Assess what is currently happening in a short statement.	Patient presents as _____
B	Background	Summarize important past assessment data for your patient here. Place lab results and medications on the concept map.	Age: Gender: Allergies: Fall Risk: Isolation:
A	Assessment	Use the assessment data to complete your concept map.	**Nursing Diagnosis:** Place the Nursing Diagnoses in prioritized order on the concept map and add any needed for your specific patient. **Plan:** Place any further Nursing Interventions Classifications (NIC) needed on the map.

Implement Your Plan of Care

R	Recommendation	Evaluate your nursing care and make recommendations related to the achievement of your desired outcomes. Were they met, or do new goals need to be established?	**EVALUATE YOUR CARE**	
			Diag / **Nursing Outcomes Classification (NOC)**	**Outcome met**
			1 Patient experiences no signs of respiratory compromise or complications.	☐ Yes ☐ No
			2 Patient demonstrates adequate fluid balance evidenced by stable VS, moist mucous membranes, good skin turgor, appropriate urinary output.	☐ Yes ☐ No
			3 Patient achieves wound healing without complications in a timely manner.	☐ Yes ☐ No
			4 Patient verbalizes understanding of disease process, prognosis, and potential complications. Patient initiates necessary lifestyle changes and participates in treatment regimen.	☐ Yes ☐ No
			5 Patient reports that pain is relieved or controlled. Patient demonstrates use of relaxation skills and diversional activities.	☐ Yes ☐ No

Nursing Diagnosis 1

Ineffective breathing pattern related to pain evidenced by tachypnea, respiratory depth changes, reduced vital capacity.

NIC:
1) Observe respiratory rate and depth; **2)** Auscultate breath sounds; **3)** Assist patient to turn, deep breathe, and cough. Teach the use of incentive spirometry. Demonstrate splinting of incision; and **4)** Elevate head of bed to low-Fowler's position.

Nursing Diagnosis 2

Risk for deficient fluid volume related to losses from nasogastric (NG) aspiration and vomiting.

NIC:
1) Maintain accurate I&O, noting output less than intake and increased urine-specific gravity. Assess skin, mucous membranes, peripheral pulses, and capillary refill. Weigh patient periodically; **2)** Monitor drainage from NG tube, T-tube, and wound; **3)** Monitor laboratory studies, such as CBC, electrolytes, prothrombin and clotting times, and amylase; **4)** Perform frequent oral hygiene with alcohol-free mouthwash; **5)** Assess for unusual bleeding, oozing from injections, epistaxis, bleeding gums, ecchymosis, hematemesis, melena; and **6)** Administer IV fluids and blood products as prescribed.

Nursing Diagnosis 3

Impaired skin/tissue integrity related to invasion of body structure: T-tube and incision evidenced by disruption of skin or subcutaneous tissues.

NIC:
1) Maintain T-tube in closed collection system and ensure that it is free flowing; **2)** Clean the skin with soap and water, use a protective barrier around tube site; **3)** Monitor puncture sites if endoscopic procedure is done; and **4)** Change dressing as needed.

Nursing Diagnosis 4

Deficient knowledge regarding condition, prognosis, treatment, self-care, and discharge needs related to information misinterpretation evidenced by inaccurate follow-through of instruction.

NIC:
1) Review disease process, surgical procedure, and prognosis; **2)** Demonstrate care of incisions, dressings and drains; **3)** Instruct in drainage of T-tube collection bag and recording of output; **4)** Emphasize importance of low-fat diet, eating small, frequent meals; **5)** Inform patient that loose stools may occur for several months, and it is necessary to avoid foods that aggravate it; and **6)** Report symptoms such as dark urine, jaundiced sclera and skin, clay-colored stools, recurrent heartburn or bloating.

Condition:
Cholecystectomy
Age:

Link & Explain
• Nursing Interventions Classification (NIC)
• Laboratory and Diagnostic Procedures
• Medications

Nursing Diagnosis 5

Acute pain related to physical factors: disruption of skin or tissues evidenced by reports of pain.

NIC:
1) Observe and document location, severity (0–10 scale), characteristics of pain (steady, intermittent, colicky); **2)** Observe for abdominal distention, rigid abdomen, severe right upper quadrant (RUQ) abdominal pain, fever, tachycardia; **3)** Provide comfort measures such as back rub and repositioning; **4)** Encourage use of relaxation techniques such as guided imagery and visualization. Provide diversional activities; **5)** Assist with ambulation; and **6)** Note response to medication, report if pain is not relieved.

Medications

a. Ondansetron (Zofran), promethazine (Phenergan)

b. Meperidine (Demerol), hydrocodone with acetaminophen (Vicodin), morphine, NSAIDs

c. Laxatives, dehydrocholic acid (Decholin)

d.

Laboratory & Diagnostic Procedures

a. CBC, amylase, prothrombin levels, clotting time, electrolytes

b. Abdominal ultrasound

c. Magnetic resonance cholangiopancreatography (MRCP)

d.

CONDITION: Cholecystitis With Cholelithiasis

PHYSIOLOGY: Cholecystitis is inflammation of the gallbladder, usually caused by obstruction of the biliary ducts by gallstones. It is more common in women, the obese, and those who have been dieting, and it can also occur following pregnancy. Its acute form is more common during middle age, the chronic form occurring more frequently in the elderly. The disease is marked by colicky pain developing shortly after a meal in the right upper quadrant of the abdomen.

Cholelithiasis are stones in the gallbladder. They are made up of cholesterol, calcium bilirubinate, or a mixture caused by changes in the bile composition. Failure to remove the impacted stone can lead to bile stasis or bacteremia and septicemia.

HANDOFF COMMUNICATION

S Situation	Assess what is currently happening in a short statement.	Patient presents as _____
B Background	Summarize important past assessment data for your patient here. Place lab results and medications on the concept map.	**Age:** **Gender:** **Allergies:** **Fall Risk:** **Isolation:**
A Assessment	Use the assessment data to complete your concept map.	**Nursing Diagnosis:** Place the Nursing Diagnoses in prioritized order on the concept map and add any needed for your specific patient. **Plan:** Place any further Nursing Interventions Classifications (NIC) needed on the map.

Implement Your Plan of Care

			EVALUATE YOUR CARE	
R Recommendation	Evaluate your nursing care and make recommendations related to the achievement of your desired outcomes. Were they met, or do new goals need to be established?	**Diag**	**Nursing Outcomes Classification (NOC)**	**Outcome met**
		1	Patient reports pain is relieved or controlled. Patient demonstrates use of relaxation skills and diversional activities.	☐ Yes ☐ No
		2	Patient demonstrates adequate fluid balance evidenced by stable VS, moist mucous membranes, good skin turgor, appropriate urinary output.	☐ Yes ☐ No
		3	Patient reports relief of nausea and vomiting and demonstrates progression toward desired weight as individually appropriate.	☐ Yes ☐ No
		4	Patient verbalizes understanding of disease process, prognosis, and potential complications. Patient initiates necessary lifestyle changes and participates in treatment regimen.	☐ Yes ☐ No
		5		☐ Yes ☐ No

Nursing Diagnosis 1

Acute pain related to obstruction or ductal spasm, inflammatory process, tissue ischemia and necrosis evidenced by reports of biliary colic and pain, guarding behavior.

NIC:
1) Observe and document location, severity (0–10 scale), characteristics of pain (steady, intermittent, colicky); **2)** Encourage patient to report pain before it becomes severe; **3)** Note response to medication, report if pain is not relieved; **4)** Promote bedrest, allowing patient to assume a position of comfort; and **5)** Encourage relaxation exercises, guided imagery, visualization, deep-breathing exercises.

Nursing Diagnosis 2

Risk for deficient fluid volume related to excessive loss through gastric suction, vomiting, and distention.

NIC:
1) Maintain accurate I&O, noting output less than intake and increased urine-specific gravity. Assess skin, mucous membranes, peripheral pulses, and capillary refill; **2)** Monitor for increased or continued nausea or vomiting, abdominal cramps, weakness, hypoactive or absent bowel sounds; **3)** Eliminate noxious smells from environment; **4)** Perform frequent oral hygiene with alcohol-free mouthwash; and **5)** Assess for unusual bleeding, oozing from injections, epistaxis, bleeding gums, ecchymosis, hematemesis, melena.

Nursing Diagnosis 3

Risk for imbalanced nutrition: less than body requirements related to loss of nutrients; impaired fat digestion due to obstruction of bile flow.

NIC:
1) Calculate caloric intake; **2)** Consult with the patient about likes and dislikes, foods that cause distress, and preferred meal schedule; **3)** Provide a pleasant atmosphere at mealtime; **4)** Provide oral hygiene before meals; **5)** Assess for abdominal distention, frequent belching, guarding, and reluctance to ambulate; **6)** Begin low-fat liquid diet after nasogastric tube is removed; **7)** Advance diet as prescribed, usually low fat, nonspicy, high fiber. Discuss restriction of gas-producing and fried foods; and **8)** Consult with dietitian for nutritional education.

Nursing Diagnosis 4

Deficient knowledge regarding condition, prognosis, treatment, self-care, and discharge needs related to information misinterpretation evidenced by inaccurate follow-through of instruction.

NIC:
1) Provide explanations of and reasons for test procedures and preparation needed; **2)** Review disease process and prognosis. Discuss treatment as indicated and encourage questions; **3)** Discuss weight reduction programs if indicated; **4)** Instruct patient to avoid diet high in fats such as whole milk, ice cream, fried foods, gravies, spicy foods; and **5)** Discuss the need to avoid aspirin-containing products, forceful blowing of nose, straining for bowel movement.

Condition:
Cholecystitis With Cholelithiasis
Age:

- - - - - - - - - - - - - - -
Link & Explain
• Nursing Interventions Classification (NIC)
• Laboratory and Diagnostic Procedures
• Medications

Nursing Diagnosis 5

NIC:

Medications

a. Dicyclomine (Bentyl), glycopyrrolate (Robinul), propantheline (Pro-Banthine)

b. Meperidine (Demerol), hydrocodone with acetaminophen (Vicodin)

c. Ondansetron (Zofran), promethazine (Phenergan)

d.

Laboratory & Diagnostic Procedures

a. CBC, alkaline phosphatase (ALP), alanine aminotransferase (ALT), bilirubin, amylase, prothrombin levels

b. Abdominal ultrasound

c. Magnetic resonance cholangiopancreatography (MRCP)

d. Endoscopic retrograde cholangiopancreatography (ERCP), extracorporeal shock wave lithotripsy (ESWL)

CONDITION: Chronic Obstructive Pulmonary Disease (COPD)

PHYSIOLOGY: COPD is a slowly progressive disease of airways characterized by gradual, irreversible loss of lung function. Commonly associated diagnoses include chronic bronchitis and emphysema. COPD is associated with a history of smoking (or exposure to secondhand smoke), air pollution, chemical irritants, and heredity (alpha-1-antitrypsin deficiency). The related pathology includes chronic airflow limitation (from excess tracheobronchial mucus production due to chronic inflammation of the bronchioles) and airway inflammation resulting in structural narrowing of the airway lumina, loss of recoil in lung parenchyma, and reduced expiratory outflow. The alveolar walls are destroyed by abnormal levels of enzymes (proteases). Gas exchange is further compromised by the reduced surface area that results from the destruction of alveolar walls. The chronic, progressive airflow obstruction may also be accompanied by airway hyperactivity. Clinical findings include dyspnea, productive cough, chest tightness, and wheezing with periodic exacerbations increasing in frequency and duration as the disease progresses.

Complications from COPD include recurrent respiratory infections, pneumothorax, cor pulmonale, and eventual respiratory failure. The chronic alveolar hypoventilation results in a chronic metabolic state associated with prolonged hypoxemia and hypercapnia. COPD affects approximately 15 million people annually and is the most common cause of death from respiratory disease in the United States.

Severity and progression of the disease is classified according to level of airflow obstruction, resulting functional limitation of activity, frequency of exacerbations, and degree of respiratory failure.

HANDOFF COMMUNICATION

S	Situation	Assess what is currently happening in a short statement.	Patient presents as _____ *Stage and progression of respiratory condition/other complicating factors (comorbidities/infection, etc.).*
B	Background	Summarize important past assessment data for your patient here. Place lab results and medications on the concept map.	**Age:** **Gender:** **Allergies:** **Fall Risk:** **Isolation:**
A	Assessment	Use the assessment data to complete your concept map.	**Nursing Diagnosis:** Place the Nursing Diagnoses in prioritized order on the concept map and add any needed for your specific patient. **Plan:** Place any further Nursing Interventions Classifications (NIC) needed on the map.

Implement Your Plan of Care

			EVALUATE YOUR CARE	
R	Recommendation	Evaluate your nursing care and make recommendations related to the achievement of your desired outcomes. Were they met, or do new goals need to be established?	**Diag** / **Nursing Outcomes Classification (NOC)**	**Outcome met**
			1 Patient maintains patent airway with clearing breath sounds, decreased work of breathing consistent with baseline respiratory parameters.	☐ Yes ☐ No
			2 Patient demonstrates improved ventilation and oxygenation of tissues by absence of respiratory distress, with ABGs and mentation consistent patient's baseline parameters.	☐ Yes ☐ No
			3 Patient maintains optimal nutritional status with stable body weight, adequate caloric intake, normal hemoglobin and albumin levels.	☐ Yes ☐ No
			4 Patient maintains normal body temperature with normal WBC count.	☐ Yes ☐ No
			5 Patient verbalizes an understanding of disease process and treatment including home care and follow-up with health-care provider.	☐ Yes ☐ No

Nursing Diagnosis 1

Ineffective airway clearance related to excess secretions, bronchospasm evidenced by changes in rate and depth of respiration, use of accessory muscles.

NIC:

1) Auscultate breath sounds. Note wheezes, rhonchi, or crackles; **2)** Assist with effective coughing techniques (splinting, use of abdominal muscles, specialized cough techniques); **3)** Administer oxygen as prescribed and perform suctioning as needed; **4)** Encourage fluid intake 3,000 ml per day unless contraindicated; **5)** Encourage activity and frequent position changes; and **6)** Minimize environmental respiratory irritants.

Nursing Diagnosis 2

Impaired gas exchange related to alveoli destruction evidenced by dyspnea, confusion, hypoxemia, and hypercapnia.

NIC:

1) Assess for altered breathing patterns/ dyspnea generalized appearance, restlessness, headache, confusion, dizziness, and reduced ability to follow instructions; **2)** Monitor ABGs and oxygen saturation; **3)** Instruct in optimal positioning and breathing techniques, incentive spirometry; **4)** Administer prescribed short-acting inhaled beta agonist, inhaled anticholinergic agents, leukotrienes, prednisone, antimicrobials; and **5)** Anticipate need for intubation and mechanical ventilation if needed.

Nursing Diagnosis 3

Imbalanced nutrition: less than body requirements related to dyspnea evidenced by weight loss and aversion to eating.

NIC:

1) Obtain diet history and assess impact of dyspnea/fatigue with adequate caloric intake; **2)** Assess for and report signs or symptoms of malnutrition, including BMI and weight; **3)** Refer to nutritional support team as needed; **4)** Implement measures to maintain adequate intake (including calorie count, supplements); and **5)** Stress importance of frequent oral hygiene.

Nursing Diagnosis 4

Risk for infection related to stasis of secretions evidenced by increased WBC count and fever.

NIC:

1) Auscultate lungs to monitor for significant alterations in breath sounds; **2)** Assess for significant changes in sputum such as yellow/green color, smell; **3)** Monitor for hyperthermia, chills, tachycardia; **4)** Encourage increased fluid intake (unless contraindicated); **5)** Minimize retained secretions by encouraging patient to cough/expectorate secretions frequently and suction as needed; and **6)** Follow universal precautions including proper hand-washing techniques to minimize microorganism transmission.

Condition:
Chronic Obstructive Pulmonary Disease (COPD)

Age:

Link & Explain
• Nursing Interventions Classification (NIC)
• Laboratory and Diagnostic Procedures
• Medications

Nursing Diagnosis 5

Deficient knowledge related to lack of information or unfamiliarity with resources evidenced by development of preventable complications.

NIC:

1) Assess knowledge of COPD and related disease processes; **2)** Assess patient's readiness to learn and encourage active participation in planning for health promotion and disease management; **3)** Discuss nutritional habits, energy conservation, and needed lifestyle adaptations; **4)** Discuss common factors that lead to exacerbation of respiratory condition; **5)** Instruct patient in therapeutic respiratory measures, breathing techniques, and home oxygen therapy; **6)** Refer to home care and support services as indicated; and **7)** Reinforce need for ongoing medical re-evaluation and health promotion practices such as pneumococcal pneumonia and influenza vaccines.

Medications

a. Anticholinergic expectorants, anticholinergic agents, beta agonists

b. Anti-inflammatories (systemic steroids)

c. Antibiotics

d. Vitamins/minerals

Laboratory & Diagnostic Procedures

a. Pulmonary function tests: forced vital capacity (FVC), forced expiratory volume in first second (FEV1), and peak expiratory flow (PEF)

b. ABGs

c. Chest x-ray

d. Serum albumin, total protein, ferritin, transferrin, Hgb/Hct

CONDITION: Chronic Renal Failure

PHYSIOLOGY: Chronic renal failure is the end result of progressive destruction of nephrons and decreased glomerular filtration rate (GFR), which causes loss kidney function and major changes in all body systems.

The stages are categorized according to the loss of nephron function.

Diabetes mellitus and hypertension are responsible for 70% of all cases of end-stage renal disease (ESRD).

There are multiple causes of renal failure, such as acute tubular necrosis from unresolved acute renal failure, chronic infections, vascular disease, obstructive processes, cystic disorders, tumors, and collagen diseases.

HANDOFF COMMUNICATION

S	Situation	Assess what is currently happening in a short statement.	Patient presents as _____ VS: LOC:
B	Background	Summarize important past assessment data for your patient here. Place lab results and medications on the concept map.	**Age:** **Gender:** **Allergies:** **Fall Risk:** **Isolation:**
A	Assessment	Use the assessment data to complete your concept map.	**Nursing Diagnosis:** Place the Nursing Diagnoses in prioritized order on the concept map and add any needed for your specific patient. **Plan:** Place any further Nursing Interventions Classifications (NIC) needed on the map.

Implement Your Plan of Care

		EVALUATE YOUR CARE		
R	Recommendation Evaluate your nursing care and make recommendations related to the achievement of your desired outcomes. Were they met, or do new goals need to be established?	**Diag**	**Nursing Outcomes Classification (NOC)**	**Outcome met**
		1	Patient experiences no signs of bleeding or hemorrhage; maintains improvement in laboratory values.	☐ Yes ☐ No
		2	Patient maintains blood pressure, heart rate and rhythm within normal range for patient. Patient has strong and equal peripheral pulses, prompt capillary refill time.	☐ Yes ☐ No
		3	Patient maintains optimal level of mentation.	☐ Yes ☐ No
		4	Patient maintains intact skin.	☐ Yes ☐ No
		5	Patient verbalizes understanding of therapeutic needs and correctly performs necessary procedures.	☐ Yes ☐ No

Nursing Diagnosis 1

Risk for ineffective protection related to abnormal blood profile: decreased RBC production and altered clotting factors.

NIC:
1) Observe for tachycardia, pallor, dyspnea, chest pain; **2)** Hematest gastrointestinal secretions and stool for blood; **3)** Evaluate response to activity and ability to perform tasks; **4)** Provide soft toothbrush and electric razor to reduce risk for bleeding and hematoma formation; **5)** Observe for oozing from venipuncture sites, petechiae, joint swelling, epistaxis, blood in urine; **6)** Monitor Hgb/Hct, prothrombin time (PT); and **7)** Administer erythropoietin, iron preparations, packed red blood cells (PRBCs) as prescribed.

Nursing Diagnosis 2

Risk for decreased cardiac output related to fluid imbalances affecting circulating volume and myocardial workload.

NIC:
1) Assess presence of hypertension, note BP with postural changes; **2)** Auscultate lung sounds, assess for dyspnea and peripheral edema; **3)** Auscultate heart sounds for development of S3 and S4; **4)** Assess color of skin, mucous membranes, and nailbeds. Note capillary refill; **5)** Provide supplemental oxygen as needed, monitor pulse oximetry; and **6)** Monitor I&O, electrolytes, BUN, creatinine.

Nursing Diagnosis 3

Disturbed thought processes related to accumulation of toxins, such as urea, ammonia, metabolic acidosis, electrolyte imbalance evidenced by memory deficit, altered attention span, decreased ability to grasp ideas.

NIC:
1) Assess extent of impairment in thinking ability, memory, and orientation; **2)** Provide calendars, clocks, windows to view outside; **3)** Provide a quiet, calm environment; TV and radio programs should be selected carefully; **4)** Present reality concisely and briefly without challenging illogical thinking; **5)** Communicate information in simple, short sentences and repeat as needed; and **6)** Provide patient with written information.

Nursing Diagnosis 4

Risk for impaired skin integrity related to altered metabolic state, circulation (anemia with tissue ischemia), and sensation (peripheral neuropathy).

NIC:
1) Inspect skin for changes in color, turgor, and vascularity. Note redness, excoriation, ecchymosis, purpura; **2)** Provide soothing skin care with ointments containing lanolin; restrict use of soap; **3)** Elevate legs as needed to decrease edema; **4)** Encourage frequent position change, pad bony prominences, use elbow and heel protectors; and **5)** Keep fingernails short; apply cool, moist compresses to pruritic areas.

Condition:
Chronic Renal Failure

Age:

Link & Explain
- Nursing Interventions Classification (NIC)
- Laboratory and Diagnostic Procedures
- Medications

Nursing Diagnosis 5

Deficient knowledge regarding condition, prognosis, treatment, self-care, and discharge needs related to unfamiliarity with information resources evidenced by questions, request for information, statement of misconception.

NIC:
1) Provide education regarding disease progression, dialysis modalities, renal transplant; **2)** Provide dietary information regarding the restriction of protein, phosphorus, sodium, and potassium as needed; **3)** Review fluid allowances and the use of hard candy or gum to keep mucous membranes moist; **4)** Encourage observation of urine amount, frequency, and characteristics; and **5)** Review medications and encourage the patient to discuss any OTC and herbal medications with health-care provider.

Medications
a. Erythropoietin exogenous: darbepoetin alfa (Aranesp) (for treatment of anemia resulting from renal failure)
b. Antihypertensives: clonidine (Catapres), prazosin (Minipress) (for treatment of hypertension; counteracts effects of decreased renal blood flow and volume overload)
c. ACE inhibitors: dopamine (Intropin) (protects kidneys from further damage)
d. Phosphate binders: calcium acetate (PhosLo), sevelamer (Renagel) (binds phosphate in the bowel and excretes it in the stool)

Laboratory & Diagnostic Procedures
a. BUN/creatinine ratio: normal ratio is 10:1; in late stages of failure, the ratio decreases because of impaired filtration
b. CBC: hemoglobin may be as low as 7–8 g/dl; bone marrow stimulation for RBC production is depressed because of decreased synthesis of erythropoietin
c. Proteins (especially albumin): decreased serum level indicates protein loss from urine, fluid shifts, or malnutrition; predicts mortality in patients receiving dialysis
d. Renal biopsy: indicated when renal impairment or proteinuria is present.

CONDITION: Cirrhosis of the Liver

PHYSIOLOGY: Cirrhosis of the liver is a progressive disease with extensive destruction of the liver parenchymal cells. The liver attempts to regenerate, which results in disorganized fibrotic connective tissue causing destruction of hepatic cells with impaired liver function and blood flow. Metabolic abnormalities, coagulation defects, malnutrition can occur. It can progress to liver failure with portal hypertension, bleeding varices, ascites, peritonitis, and encephalopathy.

Risk factors include excessive alcohol ingestion, chronic hepatitis B and chronic hepatitis C, biliary obstruction, and long-term right-sided heart failure.

HANDOFF COMMUNICATION

S	Situation	Assess what is currently happening in a short statement.	Patient presents as _____ VS: LOC:
B	Background	Summarize important past assessment data for your patient here. Place lab results and medications on the concept map.	**Age:** **Gender:** **Allergies:** **Fall Risk:** **Isolation:**
A	Assessment	Use the assessment data to complete your concept map.	**Nursing Diagnosis:** Place the Nursing Diagnoses in prioritized order on the concept map and add any needed for your specific patient. **Plan:** Place any further Nursing Interventions Classifications (NIC) needed on the map.

Implement Your Plan of Care

			EVALUATE YOUR CARE		
R	Recommendation	Evaluate your nursing care and make recommendations related to the achievement of your desired outcomes. Were they met, or do new goals need to be established?	**Diag**	**Nursing Outcomes Classification (NOC)**	**Outcome met**
			1	Patient maintains effective respiratory pattern and is free of dyspnea and cyanosis, with ABGs and vital capacity within acceptable range.	☐ Yes ☐ No
			2	Patient demonstrates behaviors to reduce risk of bleeding.	☐ Yes ☐ No
			3	Patient demonstrates stabilization of fluid volume, balanced I&O, absence of edema.	☐ Yes ☐ No
			4	Patient maintains food and fluid intake to meet nutritional status.	☐ Yes ☐ No
			5	Patient maintains usual level of mentation and reality orientation.	☐ Yes ☐ No

Nursing Diagnosis 1

Risk for ineffective breathing pattern related to intra-abdominal fluid collection.

NIC:
1) Monitor respiratory rate, depth, and effort; **2)** Auscultate breath sounds, noting crackles, wheezes, and rhonchi; **3)** Restrict sodium, administer diuretics and salt-poor albumin as ordered; **4)** Encourage coughing and deep-breathing exercises; note changes in color of sputum; **5)** Monitor ABGs, pulse oximetry, vital capacity, chest x-ray; and **6)** Prepare patient for paracentesis or shunt procedure.

Nursing Diagnosis 2

Risk for bleeding related to abnormal blood profile; altered clotting factors: decreased production of prothrombin, fibrinogen, and factors VIII, IX, and X; impaired vitamin K absorption.

NIC:
1) Assess for symptoms of gastric bleeding, frank or occult blood; observe color of stool, nasogastric drainage, and vomitus; **2)** Observe skin for presence of petechiae, ecchymosis, and bleeding from one or more sites; **3)** Monitor BP and pulse rate; **4)** Encourage the use of a soft toothbrush, electric razor; counsel to avoid straining for stool; **5)** Recommend avoidance of aspirin-containing products; **6)** Administer vasopressin (Pitressin), propranolol (Inderal) as prescribed for esophageal varices; and **7)** Administer vitamin K (Mephyton) as prescribed for clotting abnormalities.

Nursing Diagnosis 3

Fluid volume excess related to compromised regulatory system: decreased plasma proteins evidenced by weight gain, ascites, and dependent edema.

NIC:
1) Monitor I&O, note positive balance, weigh daily, note gain more than 2 lb/day; **2)** Assess BP, note jugular vein distention; **3)** Measure abdominal girth; **4)** Monitor laboratory values such as Hgb/Hct, sodium, serum albumin, electrolytes; and **5)** Assess respiratory status, noting increased respiratory rate and dyspnea.

Nursing Diagnosis 4

Imbalanced nutrition: less than body requirements related to insufficient intake to meet metabolic demands of anorexia, nausea and vomiting evidenced by changes in bowel sounds and function.

NIC:
1) Determine ability to chew, swallow, and taste as well as food preferences; **2)** Compare changes in fluid status and recent weight history; **3)** Limit foods with high salt content such as canned soups and vegetables and condiments; **4)** Monitor nutritional laboratory studies: serum glucose, prealbumin, albumin, total protein, ammonia; **5)** Restrict intake of caffeine and spicy foods to reduce gastric irritation; **6)** Encourage diet high in calories (1,500–2,000) and carbohydrates, low in fat; and **7)** Administer glucose polymer (Polycose) orally or via NG tube to increase protein-free calories.

Condition:
Cirrhosis of the Liver

Age:

_____

Link & Explain
• Nursing Interventions Classification (NIC)
• Laboratory and Diagnostic Procedures
• Medications

Nursing Diagnosis 5

Risk for acute confusion related to inability of liver to detoxify certain enzymes and drugs.

NIC:
1) Observe for changes in behavior and mentation: lethargy, confusion, drowsiness, slurred speech, and irritability; **2)** Evaluate sleep and rest schedule; **3)** Note development of asterixis, fetor hepaticus, and seizures; **4)** Monitor laboratory studies such as ammonia, electrolytes, BUN, and glucose; **5)** Recommend avoidance of narcotics, sedatives, and anti-anxiety medications; limit medications metabolized by the liver; and **6)** Administer lactulose (Cephulac) to decrease ammonia levels.

Medications
a. Diuretics: spironolactone (Aldactone) (blocks action of aldosterone, potassium sparing)
b. Vasopressor: vasopressin (Pitressin) (controls of bleeding in esophageal varices)
c. Laxative: lactulose (Cephulac) (promotes elimination of ammonia in feces)
d. Fat-soluble vitamin: vitamin K (Mephyton) (corrects clotting abnormalities)

Laboratory & Diagnostic Procedures
a. Serum bilirubin: elevation indicates blockage of bile ducts or liver disease; jaundice is evident when levels are high
b. Prothrombin time (PT)/activated partial prothromboplastin time (aPTT): determines bleeding and clotting time
c. Serum ammonia: product of breakdown of protein, which is normally converted to urea and excreted
d. Liver enzymes/isoenzymes: detect hepatitis, obstruction

CONDITION: Colorectal Cancer

PHYSIOLOGY: Colorectal cancer accounts for about 15% of all malignancies and for about 11% of cancer mortality in both men and women in the United States. It is the third-most common cause of death from cancer among men and women combined. In recent years, both the incidence and the mortality rates have shown a decline, which is attributed to early identification and improved treatment measures.

Of cancers of the colon, 65% occur in the rectum and in the sigmoid and descending colon, 25% occur in the cecum and ascending colon, and 10% occur in the transverse colon. Most colorectal tumors (95%) are adenocarcinomas and develop from an adenomatous polyp. Once malignant transformation occurs within the polyp, the tumor usually grows into the lumen of the bowel, causing obstruction, and invades the deeper layers of the bowel wall. After penetrating the serosa and the mesenteric fat, the tumor may spread by direct extension to nearby organs and the omentum. Metastatic spread through the lymphatic and circulatory systems occurs most frequently to the liver as well as the lung, bones, and brain.

The cause of colorectal cancer is largely unknown; however, there is much evidence to suggest that incidence increases with age. Risk factors include a family history of colorectal cancer and a personal history of past colorectal cancer, ulcerative colitis, Crohn's disease, or adenomatous colon polyps. Persons with familial polyposis coli, an inherited disease characterized by multiple (>100) adenomatous polyps, possess a risk for colorectal cancer that approaches 100% by age 40. Other risk factors include obesity, diabetes mellitus, alcohol usage, night-shift work, and physical inactivity.

It has been strongly suggested that diets high in fat and refined carbohydrates play a role in the development of colorectal cancer. High-fat content results in increased amounts of fecal bile acid. It is hypothesized that intestinal bacteria react with the bile salts and facilitate carcinogenic changes. In addition, fat and refined carbohydrates decrease the transit of food through the gastrointestinal (GI) tract and increase the exposure of the GI mucosa to carcinogenic substances that may be present.

HANDOFF COMMUNICATION

S	*Situation*	Assess what is currently happening in a short statement.	Patient presents as _____ *Note type/location and stage of cancer.*
B	*Background*	Summarize important past assessment data for your patient here. Place lab results and medications on the concept map.	**Age:** **Gender:** **Allergies:** **Fall Risk:** **Isolation:**
A	*Assessment*	Use the assessment data to complete your concept map.	**Nursing Diagnosis:** Place the Nursing Diagnoses in prioritized order on the concept map and add any needed for your specific patient. **Plan:** Place any further Nursing Interventions Classifications (NIC) needed on the map.

Implement Your Plan of Care

			EVALUATE YOUR CARE	
	Evaluate your nursing care and make recommendations related to the achievement of your desired outcomes. Were they met, or do new goals need to be established?	**Diag**	**Nursing Outcomes Classification (NOC)**	**Outcome met**
R *Recommendation*		**1**	Patient reports pain is relieved or controlled.	☐ Yes ☐ No
		2	Patient verbalizes accurate information about diagnosis, prognosis/treatment plan and identifies available resources.	☐ Yes ☐ No
		3	Patient remains free from infection and participates in interventions to reduce risk of infection.	☐ Yes ☐ No
		4	Patient demonstrates adaptation to situation evidenced by realistic goals, participation in treatment regimen, and involvement in personal relationships.	☐ Yes ☐ No
		5	Patient and family members express feelings freely and demonstrate appropriate problem-solving processes.	☐ Yes ☐ No

Nursing Diagnosis 1

Pain related to tissue invasion from tumor evidenced by reports of pain, self-focusing.

NIC:
1) Administer analgesics: opioids, NSAIDs, anticonvulsants, antidepressants as prescribed; evaluate effectiveness and adjust accordingly; **2)** Anticipate painful effects of therapies and invasive procedures and intervene to minimize discomfort; **3)** Provide nonpharmacological comfort measures, relaxation techniques, therapeutic touch; and **4)** Encourage patient to exercise daily.

Nursing Diagnosis 2

Deficient knowledge regarding illness, prognosis, treatment, self-care, and discharge needs related to lack of exposure evidenced by statement of misconception.

NIC:
1) Review understanding and expectations of patient/family regarding diagnosis, treatment, alternatives, and future expectations; **2)** Provide clear, accurate information in factual but sensitive manner; **3)** Refer to home care/hospice/community support groups as indicated; **4)** Provide information regarding advance directives; and **5)** Provide written information about disease process and treatments.

Nursing Diagnosis 3

Risk for infection related to side effects of chemotherapy, radiation, and/or surgical intervention.

NIC:
1) Assess for risk/early signs of infection; **2)** Maintain universal precautions/aseptic technique; implement protective isolation measures as indicated; **3)** Promote optimal nutrition and oral hygiene; promote adequate rest periods; **4)** Obtain cultures and administer antibiotics as indicated; and **5)** Monitor for hyperthermia and chills.

Nursing Diagnosis 4

Situational low-self-esteem related to disruption in how patient perceives own body evidenced by use of ineffective coping.

NIC:
1) Discuss how diagnosis/treatment are affecting personal, home, and work activities; **2)** Encourage problem-solving related to role; **3)** Include patient/family members in individualizing treatment plan; and **4)** Refer patient/family to support group programs.

Condition:
Colorectal Cancer
Age:

Link & Explain
• Nursing Interventions Classification (NIC)
• Laboratory and Diagnostic Procedures
• Medications

Nursing Diagnosis 5

Risk for interrupted family processes related to situational crisis.

NIC:
1) Identify patient support systems; **2)** Evaluate patterns of communication and interaction of family members; **3)** Support cultural/religious beliefs; **4)** Stress the importance of an ongoing open dialogue; **5)** Acknowledge difficulties of diagnosis and treatment of cancer with the possibility of death; and **6)** Refer to counseling, clergy, and family therapy as indicated.

Medications

a. Pain medications: analgesics/opioids

b. Antineoplastic drugs

c. Antiemetics

d. Antibiotics/anti-infectives as indicated

Laboratory & Diagnostic Procedures

a. Hematest stool, CBC with differential WBS/granulocyte count and platelets as indicated

b. Endoscopy, barium enema

c. Serum carcinoembryonic antigen (CEA)

d. CT scan, MRI, and abdominal x-rays to determine abdominal obstruction

CONDITION: Cushing's Syndrome

PHYSIOLOGY: Cushing's syndrome is an abnormality signified by an increase in corticosteroid levels, especially glucocorticoids. The clinical manifestations include truncal obesity, thin extremities, moon face, thin fragile skin, purplish striae, bruises, acne, poor wound healing, buffalo hump, hypervolemia, hypertension, edema of lower extremities, hypokalemia, hypercalciuria, muscle wasting, osteoporosis, hyperglycemia, euphoria, hypomania, depression, emotional lability, gynecomastia in men.

Causes

1. Administration of corticosteroids over a prolonged time period.
2. A pituitary tumor secreting an adrenocorticotrophic hormone (ACTH).
3. A neoplasm in the adrenal gland secreting cortisol.
4. A malignant growth outside the pituitary gland or the adrenal glands, usually in the lung, which secretes ACTH.

HANDOFF COMMUNICATION

S	Situation	Assess what is currently happening in a short statement.	Patient presents as _____
B	Background	Summarize important past assessment data for your patient here. Place lab results and medications on the concept map.	**Age:** **Gender:** **Allergies:** **Fall Risk:** **Isolation:**
A	Assessment	Use the assessment data to complete your concept map.	**Nursing Diagnosis:** Place the Nursing Diagnoses in prioritized order on the concept map and add any needed for your specific patient. **Plan:** Place any further Nursing Interventions Classifications (NIC) needed on the map.

Implement Your Plan of Care

			EVALUATE YOUR CARE	
R	Recommendation	Evaluate your nursing care and make recommendations related to the achievement of your desired outcomes. Were they met, or do new goals need to be established?	**Diag** / **Nursing Outcomes Classification (NOC)**	**Outcome met**
			1 Patient demonstrates change in eating patterns, such as food choices and quantity, to attain desirable body weight and optimal maintenance of health.	☐ Yes ☐ No
			2 Patient demonstrates behaviors and techniques to prevent skin breakdown and promote healing.	☐ Yes ☐ No
			3 Patient verbalizes a realistic view and acceptance of own body.	☐ Yes ☐ No
			4 Patient demonstrates techniques or lifestyle changes to reduce risk of infection. Patient verbalizes understanding of causative factors.	☐ Yes ☐ No
			5 Patient verbalizes understanding of therapeutic needs and plans to make changes in lifestyle.	☐ Yes ☐ No

Nursing Diagnosis 1

Imbalanced nutrition: more than body requirements related to excessive intake in relation to metabolic need and sedentary lifestyle evidenced by weight that is 10%–20% more than ideal for height and frame.

NIC:

1) Assess patient's understanding of difference between disease process and obesity; **2)** Discuss necessity for decreased caloric intake and limitation of saturated fats, salt, and sugar; **3)** Determine patient's desire to decrease weight; **4)** Discuss risk factors related to increased weight such as heart disease, hypertension, diabetes; **5)** Review dietary choices; encourage patient to increase fruits and vegetables; assist patient to identify foods that should be avoided; and **6)** Encourage patient to keep a diary of food intake.

Nursing Diagnosis 2

Risk for impaired skin integrity related to increased corticosteroids and fragile skin.

NIC:

1) Clean skin area gently and pat dry. Assess for purplish red striae, petechial hemorrhages, bruises, acne; **2)** Advise patient to wear cotton clothing that is non-irritating; **3)** Check skinfolds in groin, chest, abdomen, and perineum daily for breakdown because of truncal obesity; and **4)** Utilize frequent position changes and ambulation as tolerated, since wound healing is delayed.

Nursing Diagnosis 3

Low self-esteem related to disruption in how patient perceives own body evidenced by confusion about sense of self, purpose, direction in life.

NIC:

1) Note behaviors of withdrawal, increased dependency, manipulation, or decreased involvement in care; **2)** Acknowledge feelings of anger, depression, grief related to truncal obesity, bruising, hirsutism (women), gynecomastia (men). Help patient deal realistically with feelings; **3)** Note presence of depression or impaired thought processes; **4)** Explain that labile emotions are not unusual; and **5)** Assist with problem-solving to deal with these issues.

Nursing Diagnosis 4

Risk for infection related to suppression of immune system.

NIC:

1) Monitor VS and report any elevation in temperature; **2)** Document urine characteristics and note changes indicating urinary tract infection; **3)** Auscultate lungs for adventitious sounds; encourage coughing and deep-breathing exercises; and **4)** Encourage patient to stay out of crowds and away from those who are ill while resistance to infection is low.

Condition:
Cushing's Syndrome
Age:

Link & Explain
• Nursing Interventions Classification (NIC)
• Laboratory and Diagnostic Procedures
• Medications

Nursing Diagnosis 5

Deficient knowledge regarding condition, prognosis, treatment, self-care, and discharge needs related to lack of exposure or recall evidenced by inaccurate follow-through of instructions.

NIC:

1) Encourage patient to report symptoms of fever, purulent drainage, and inflammation; **2)** Encourage patient to report signs of chest pain, palpitations, dyspnea, tachycardia; **3)** Monitor weight daily and glucose as ordered; **4)** Discuss plan of treatment, which may include medication, radiation, or surgical intervention; and **5)** Monitor VS and symptoms of sodium and water retention.

Medications
a. Ketoconazole (Nizoral)
b. Aminoglutethimide (Cytadren)
c.
d.

Laboratory & Diagnostic Procedures
a. Plasma cortisol, urine for free cortisol, low-dose dexamethasone suppression test
b. Electrolytes, blood glucose, urine levels of 17-ketosteroids, CT scan, MRI: adrenals and pituitary
c. Removal of pituitary tumor via transsphenoidal approach, radiation therapy
d. Adrenalectomy, surgical removal of tumor causing increased ACTH

CONDITION: Diabetes Mellitus: Diabetic Ketoacidosis (DKA)

PHYSIOLOGY: DKA is a life-threatening emergency caused by a deficiency of insulin. Patients with diabetes type I are prone to DKA. The precipitating factors include illness, infection, inadequate insulin administration, undiagnosed type I diabetes, poor self-management. Symptoms of DKA include dehydration, poor skin turgor, dry mucous membranes, tachycardia, and orthostatic hypotension. As dehydration progresses, the patient becomes weak and eyeballs become sunken. Abdominal pain with nausea and vomiting are common. The patient may have Kussmaul respirations, which are rapid and deep as the body attempts to exhale excessive carbon dioxide and reverse metabolic acidosis. Blood glucose level is greater than 250 mg/dL, arterial blood pH is decreased, bicarbonate levels are decreased, and moderate to large ketones are present in the blood or urine. Complications of diabetes include heart disease, stroke, high blood pressure, blindness, kidney disease, peripheral vascular disease.

HANDOFF COMMUNICATION

S Situation	Assess what is currently happening in a short statement.	Patient presents as _____ VS: LOC:	
B Background	Summarize important past assessment data for your patient here. Place lab results and medications on the concept map.	**Age:** **Allergies:** **Isolation:**	**Gender:** **Fall Risk:**
A Assessment	Use the assessment data to complete your concept map.	**Nursing Diagnosis:** Place the Nursing Diagnoses in prioritized order on the concept map and add any needed for your specific patient. **Plan:** Place any further Nursing Interventions Classifications (NIC) needed on the map.	

Implement Your Plan of Care

		EVALUATE YOUR CARE		
R Recommendation	Evaluate your nursing care and make recommendations related to the achievement of your desired outcomes. Were they met, or do new goals need to be established?	**Diag**	**Nursing Outcomes Classification (NOC)**	**Outcome met**
		1	Patient demonstrates stable VS, palpable peripheral pulses, good capillary refill, appropriate urine output, and electrolyte levels within normal range.	☐ Yes ☐ No
		2	Patient verbalizes an increase in energy level and displays an improved ability to participate in desired activities.	☐ Yes ☐ No
		3	Patient maintains glucose in satisfactory range and acknowledges factors that lead to unstable glucose and DKA.	☐ Yes ☐ No
		4	Patient identifies interventions to reduce the risk of infection.	☐ Yes ☐ No
		5	Patient reports limited peripheral discomfort or distorted tactile sensation.	☐ Yes ☐ No

Nursing Diagnosis 1

Deficient fluid volume related to osmotic diuresis from hyperglycemia evidenced by hypotension, tachycardia, poor skin turgor, increased urinary output.

NIC:
1) Monitor BP lying, sitting, standing, and note orthostatic changes, use of accessory muscles, Kussmaul respirations; **2)** Assess peripheral pulses, capillary refill, skin turgor, mucous membranes; **3)** Monitor I&O, note urine specific gravity; **4)** Weigh patient daily and note changes; **5)** Maintain IV access with large-bore catheter; and **6)** Begin fluid resuscitation with 0.9% NaCl solution until BP stabilizes and urine output is over 30 mL/hr.

Nursing Diagnosis 2

Fatigue related to altered body chemistry, insufficient insulin evidenced by listlessness, overwhelming lack of energy.

NIC:
1) Plan schedule with patient and identify activities that lead to fatigue; **2)** Alternate periods of activity with uninterrupted rest or sleep; **3)** Administer oxygen as prescribed; monitor pulse, respiratory rate, and BP before and after activity; and **4)** Perform active or passive ROM exercises and discuss methods of conserving energy during ADL.

Nursing Diagnosis 3

Unstable blood glucose related to lack of adherence to diabetes action plan, inadequate medication management evidenced by increased ketones.

NIC:
1) Perform fingerstick glucose testing and treat hyperglycemia as needed; **2)** Review patient's dietary program; identify deviations from the therapeutic plan; **3)** Administer continuous regular insulin drip IV as prescribed; **4)** Monitor ketones and assess ABGs for metabolic acidosis; **5)** Monitor serum glucose and serum potassium levels; and **6)** Provide liquids containing nutrients and electrolytes and progress diet to solid foods when tolerated.

Nursing Diagnosis 4

Risk for infection related to high glucose levels, decreased leukocyte function.

NIC:
1) Observe for fever, inflammation, flushed appearance, wound drainage, cloudy urine, purulent sputum; **2)** Promote good hand-washing techniques by staff, patient, family; **3)** Maintain aseptic technique for IV insertion, site care, and rotate sites as needed; **4)** Reposition patient and encourage coughing and deep breathing; and **5)** Encourage incentive spirometry.

Condition:
Diabetic Ketoacidosis (DKA) and Diabetes Mellitus

Age:

Link & Explain
• Nursing Interventions Classification (NIC)
• Laboratory and Diagnostic Procedures
• Medications

Nursing Diagnosis 5

Risk for disturbed sensory perception (peripheral neurovascular) related to endogenous chemical alteration: glucose, insulin, electrolyte imbalance.

NIC:
1) Investigate reports of hyperesthesia, pain, sensory loss in feet and legs; **2)** Assess for reddened areas, pressure points, loss of pedal pulses; **3)** Keep hands and feet warm, avoid use of hot water or heating pads; and **4)** Assist with ambulation.

Medications

a. Isotonic (NaCl 0.9%) solution (replaces fluid deficit for the treatment of DKA)

b. Regular insulin (administration by continuous IV infusion to correct hyperglycemia and ketones in the urine or blood; decrease of hyperglycemia should be slow to prevent cerebral edema)

c. Potassium (added to IV as needed to prevent hypokalemia)

d. Bicarbonate (administered IV if pH is less than 7.1 and hypotension is present to correct metabolic acidosis)

Laboratory & Diagnostic Procedures

a. Fasting plasma glucose: used to diagnose elevated blood glucose levels; normal fasting levels are 70–110 mg/dL

b. Hemoglobin A1c (HgbA1C): determines glycemic control over the past 3–4 months; recommended level is 7%; result greater than 8% indicates changes are needed in treatment

c. Ketones: measure the amount of acetone in the urine and blood resulting from incomplete fat metabolism; positive results can indicate diabetic acidosis

d. Potassium: in DKA, hyperkalemia results from metabolic acidosis, but potassium is lost in the urine, and the potassium level in the body is depleted; after insulin is replaced and acidosis is corrected, potassium levels need to be monitored

CONDITION: Diabetes Mellitus: Type 1 and Type 2

PHYSIOLOGY: Diabetes mellitus (DM) is a chronic metabolic disorder in which the body cannot metabolize carbohydrates, fats, and proteins because of lack of insulin.

Type 1 Diabetes

Beta cells in the pancreas are destroyed, and exogenous insulin is required to survive. Without insulin, the patient will develop diabetic ketoacidosis (DKA), a life-threatening emergency caused by a deficiency of insulin. (See concept map for diabetic ketoacidosis.)

Type 2 Diabetes

Decreased ability to use the insulin produced in the pancreas results in inadequate insulin secretion for glucose levels. Risk factors include age over 35, overweight, with a tendency to run in families. The onset is usually gradual. Patients with hyperglycemia usually do not develop DKA because of the endogenous insulin but will develop hyperosmolar hyperglycemic syndrome (HHS) with a blood glucose level above 500 mg/dL. HHS is a life-threatening emergency caused by deficiency of insulin, which results in severe hyperglycemia, osmotic diuresis, extracellular fluid depletion, but not ketosis. Precipitating factors include infections and acute illness.

Complications of diabetes include heart disease, stroke, high blood pressure, blindness, kidney disease, peripheral vascular disease.

HANDOFF COMMUNICATION

S Situation	Assess what is currently happening in a short statement.	Patient presents as _____ VS: LOC:	
B Background	Summarize important past assessment data for your patient here. Place lab results and medications on the concept map.	**Age:** **Allergies:** **Isolation:**	**Gender:** **Fall Risk:**
A Assessment	Use the assessment data to complete your concept map.	**Nursing Diagnosis:** Place the Nursing Diagnoses in prioritized order on the concept map and add any needed for your specific patient. **Plan:** Place any further Nursing Interventions Classifications (NIC) needed on the map.	

Implement Your Plan of Care

R Recommendation	Evaluate your nursing care and make recommendations related to the achievement of your desired outcomes. Were they met, or do new goals need to be established?	**EVALUATE YOUR CARE**	

	Diag	Nursing Outcomes Classification (NOC)	Outcome met
	1	Patient discusses role in management of disease and prevention of complications.	☐ Yes ☐ No
	2	Patient uses a diary to monitor glucose, participates in recommended exercise program, decreases weight to what is appropriate for height and frame.	☐ Yes ☐ No
	3	Patient follows preventative foot-care practices and reports any nonhealing breaks in skin.	☐ Yes ☐ No
	4	Patient identifies healthy ways to deal with feelings.	☐ Yes ☐ No
	5		☐ Yes ☐ No

Nursing Diagnosis 1

Deficient knowledge regarding disease related to misinterpretation of information evidenced by inaccurate statements about diabetes and its management.

NIC:
1) Discuss lifestyle changes required to prevent complications: yearly eye exams, yearly screening for nephropathy, checking feet daily for skin irritation, diligent dental hygiene practices, frequent glucose monitoring; **2)** Encourage patient to demonstrate use of self-monitoring blood glucose equipment and insulin administration; **3)** Discuss the need for identification of hypoglycemia: headache, cold clammy skin, slurred speech, tremors, emotional changes, tachycardia. Discuss treatment with immediate-acting carbohydrates 15–20 g; **4)** Follow sick-day rules during times of illness; **5)** Obtain an A1c blood test every 3–6 months to monitor long-term glucose control; **6)** Discuss the peak and duration of insulin/use of oral agents; and **7)** Instruct the patient to carry medical identification at all times.

Nursing Diagnosis 2

Imbalanced nutrition: more than body requirements related to intake in excess of activity expenditure evidenced by weight gain, hyperglycemia.

NIC:
1) Encourage use of sugar substitutes; **2)** Decrease dietary fats and increase complex carbohydrates, especially those with high fiber; **3)** Assist patient to incorporate food preferences into prescribed diet; **4)** Encourage daily exercise; **5)** Monitor for symptoms of hyperglycemia: polyuria, polydipsia, polyphagia, weakness, blurred vision; **6)** Take medications as prescribed and monitor glucose as scheduled; **7)** Obtain weight daily and record; and **8)** Schedule sessions for dietary counseling.

Nursing Diagnosis 3

Risk for injury related to decreased tactile sensation.

NIC:
1) Avoid wearing open-toe sandals or going barefoot; **2)** Caution against use of heat, cold, strong antiseptics, or chemicals on feet; **3)** Inspect inside of shoes for rough areas that may be irritating to skin; **4)** Recommend that specialist care for ingrown toenails, fungus, corns, or calluses; and **5)** Report breaks in skin to primary physician.

Nursing Diagnosis 4

Powerlessness related to long-term progressive illness evidenced by apathy, withdrawal, anger.

NIC:
1) Encourage patient to express feelings about hospitalization and disease in general; **2)** Assess how the patient has handled problems in the past; **3)** Discuss goals and expectations; **4)** Encourage patient to make decisions regarding care and activities; and **5)** Support participation in self-care and provide positive feedback.

Condition:
Diabetes Mellitus: Type I and Type II

Age:

Link & Explain
• Nursing Interventions Classification (NIC)
• Laboratory and Diagnostic Procedures
• Medications

Nursing Diagnosis 5

NIC:

Medications
a. Insulin
b. Antidiabetic oral agents
c.
d.

Laboratory & Diagnostic Procedures
a. Fasting plasma glucose: used to diagnose elevated blood glucose levels; normal fasting levels are 70–110 mg/dl
b. Hemoglobin A1c (HgbA1c): determines glycemic control over the past 3–4 months; recommended level is 7%; result greater than 8% indicates changes are needed in treatment
c.
d.

CONDITION: Disk Surgery

PHYSIOLOGY: Laminectomy is the surgical excision of a vertebral posterior arch performed in the presence of a herniated disk to relieve pressure on the spinal cord nerve roots and remove the source of pain. Procedures include combinations of disk excision, nerve decompression, and bone fusion. Damaged disks may be replaced with artificial disks. The procedure can be successful with an open laminectomy or a minimally invasive procedure in which a small incision is made in the skin with the use of a surgical microscope for guidance.

HANDOFF COMMUNICATION

S	Situation	Assess what is currently happening in a short statement.	Patient presents as _____
B	Background	Summarize important past assessment data for your patient here. Place lab results and medications on the concept map.	Age: Gender: Allergies: Fall Risk: Isolation:
A	Assessment	Use the assessment data to complete your concept map.	**Nursing Diagnosis:** Place the Nursing Diagnoses in prioritized order on the concept map and add any needed for your specific patient. **Plan:** Place any further Nursing Interventions Classifications (NIC) needed on the map.

Implement Your Plan of Care

		EVALUATE YOUR CARE		
	Evaluate your nursing care and make recommendations related to the achievement of your desired outcomes. Were they met, or do new goals need to be established?	**Diag**	**Nursing Outcomes Classification (NOC)**	**Outcome met**
R Recommendation		1	Patient reports normal sensations and movement as appropriate.	☐ Yes ☐ No
		2	Patient maintains proper alignment of spine.	☐ Yes ☐ No
		3	Patient maintains a normal, effective breathing pattern free of hypoxemia.	☐ Yes ☐ No
		4	Patient reports pain is relieved or controlled.	☐ Yes ☐ No
		5	Patient maintains strength and function of affected body part.	☐ Yes ☐ No

Nursing Diagnosis 1

Ineffective tissue perfusion (spinal) related to diminished or interrupted blood flow: edema of operative site, hematoma formation evidenced by paresthesia or numbness.

NIC:
1) Check neurological signs periodically and compare with baseline. Assess movement and sensation of hands and arms (cervical) and lower extremities (lumbar); 2) Keep patient flat on back for several hours. Monitor VS, note color, warmth, and capillary refill; 3) Monitor I&O and wound drains, such as Jackson-Pratt or Hemovac; 4) Visually check and palpate operative site for swelling. Inspect dressing for cerebrospinal drainage, and 5) Monitor Hgb/Hct and RBCs, monitor for headache.

Nursing Diagnosis 2

Risk for peripheral neurovascular dysfunction related to pressure on the spinal cord nerve roots.

NIC:
1) Limit activities, as prescribed, when patient has had a spinal fusion; 2) Logroll patient from side to side, keeping shoulders and pelvis straight. Use pillow between legs while repositioning; 3) Avoid sudden stretching, twisting, flexing, or jarring of the spine; 4) Monitor BP and note reports of dizziness or weakness. Have patient wear firm, flat walking shoes; and 5) Apply lumbar brace or cervical collar if prescribed.

Nursing Diagnosis 3

Risk for ineffective breathing pattern related to decreased lung expansion.

NIC:
1) Inspect surgical area for edema especially in the first 24–48 hours; 2) Auscultate breath sounds. Note presence of decreased breath sounds, crackles, or rhonchi; 3) Assist with coughing, turning, and deep breathing. Encourage the use of incentive spirometry. Administer supplemental oxygen as needed; and 4) Monitor pulse oximetry and ABGs.

Nursing Diagnosis 4

Acute pain related to physical agent: surgical manipulation, edema, inflammation, or harvesting of bone graft evidenced by guarding, distraction behaviors, or restlessness.

NIC:
1) Observe and document location, severity (0–10 scale), characteristics of pain (steady, intermittent, colicky); 2) Provide comfort measures such as mouth care, back rub (avoiding surgical area), and repositioning; 3) Encourage use of relaxation techniques such as guided imagery and visualization. Provide diversional activities; 4) Investigate patient reports of radicular pain; 5) Administer medication for pain as needed; and 6) Note response to medication; report if pain is not relieved.

Condition:
Disk Surgery
Age:

Link & Explain
• Nursing Interventions Classification (NIC)
• Laboratory and Diagnostic Procedures
• Medications

Nursing Diagnosis 5

Impaired physical mobility related to neuromuscular impairment evidenced by decreased muscle strength and control.

NIC:
1) Schedule activity or procedures with rest periods. Encourage participation in ADL within individual limitations; 2) Provide or assist with passive and active ROM and strengthening exercises, depending on progressive ambulation; and 3) Review proper body mechanics or techniques for participation in activities.

Medications

a. Opioids

b. Cyclobenzaprine (Flexeril), metaxalone (Skelaxin)

c.

d.

Laboratory & Diagnostic Procedures

a. CBC, ABGs

b.

c.

d.

CONDITION: Endocarditis—Infective

PHYSIOLOGY: Infective endocarditis is an infection of the endocardium (innermost layer) of the heart, which affects the heart valves.

There are two forms: *subacute* affects a patient who has a preexisting condition of heart valve problems; *acute* affects a patient who has previously healthy valves, and this illness progresses rapidly. The infection can occur from a bacteria, fungi, or viruses.

Conditions that increase the risk for infective endocarditis include prosthetic valves, congenital heart disease, IV drug use, intravascular devices such as pulmonary artery catheters.

The clinical manifestations of infective endocarditis are:
- Low-grade fever, chills, headache, and muscle pain
- Splinter hemorrhages in nailbeds
- Petechiae of the lips, oral mucosa, feet, and ankles
- Osler's nodes (red pea-size lesions) on the fingertips and toes
- Janeway's lesions (flat, red, circular lesions) on the palms of the hands and soles of the feet

The patient should be assessed for a murmur that is new or changed. A thorough assessment is indicated because embolization to the spleen, kidneys, peripheral blood vessels, or brain can occur.

HANDOFF COMMUNICATION

S Situation	Assess what is currently happening in a short statement.	Patient presents as _____
B Background	Summarize important past assessment data for your patient here. Place lab results and medications on the concept map.	Age: Gender: Allergies: Fall Risk: Isolation:
A Assessment	Use the assessment data to complete your concept map.	**Nursing Diagnosis:** Place the Nursing Diagnoses in prioritized order on the concept map and add any needed for your specific patient. **Plan:** Place any further Nursing Interventions Classifications (NIC) needed on the map.

Implement Your Plan of Care

			EVALUATE YOUR CARE	
R Recommendation	Evaluate your nursing care and make recommendations related to the achievement of your desired outcomes. Were they met, or do new goals need to be established?	**Diag**	**Nursing Outcomes Classification (NOC)**	**Outcome met**
		1	Patient maintains stable VS, cardiac output, adequate urine output, absence of dysrhythmias.	☐ Yes ☐ No
		2	Patient demonstrates a decrease in physiological signs of intolerance: pulse, respirations, BP within normal range for patient.	☐ Yes ☐ No
		3	Patient maintains normal body temperature, no report of chills.	☐ Yes ☐ No
		4	Patient identifies inadequacies of prior coping behaviors, identifies available resources/support systems, and initiates new coping strategies.	☐ Yes ☐ No
		5	Patient follows instructions and explains reason for actions.	☐ Yes ☐ No

Nursing Diagnosis 1

Risk for decreased cardiac output reduced myocardial contractility.

NIC:
1) Auscultate heart for murmurs; **2)** Monitor VS and hemodynamic parameters and report appropriately; **3)** Note skin color, presence and quality of peripheral pulses; **4)** Assess lung sounds for adventitious sounds; monitor pulse oximetry, ABGs; **5)** Monitor I&O and calculate 24-hour deficit or excess; **6)** Observe monitor for cardiac dysrhythmia; and **7)** Administer supplemental oxygen as needed.

Nursing Diagnosis 2

Activity intolerance related to imbalance between oxygen supply and demand evidenced by weakness and fatigue.

NIC:
1) Monitor BP, pulse, and respirations during and after activity; note adverse response: dysrhythmia, dizziness, dyspnea, tachypnea, cyanosis of mucous membranes; **2)** Recommend bedrest and quiet atmosphere. Limit visitors, phone calls, and repeated interruptions; **3)** Suggest changing positions slowly; monitor for dizziness; **4)** Monitor pulse oximetry and administer supplemental oxygen as needed; **5)** Perform passive and active ROM; and **6)** Apply antiembolism stockings, sequential compression device.

Nursing Diagnosis 3

Hyperthermia related to infection evidenced by fever, chills, tachycardia, muscle aches, and headache.

NIC:
1) Administer antipyretic for temperature elevation; **2)** Place cloth with tepid water on patient's head and pulse points; **3)** Assess temperature q4h; **4)** Cover patient with light blanket; **5)** Provide IV fluids as ordered and oral fluids as tolerated such as water, juice, ginger ale; **6)** Monitor I&O and determine fluid deficit; **7)** Collect blood cultures; and **8)** Administer antibiotic as prescribed.

Nursing Diagnosis 4

Risk for ineffective coping mechanisms related to situational crisis evidenced by inappropriate use of defense mechanisms.

NIC:
1) Assess patient/significant other's perception of current situation and signs of inadequate coping mechanisms; **2)** Encourage verbalization of and assist in identifying personal strengths/resources to cope with current situation; **3)** Include patient/family in planning of comfort/supportive care; and **4)** Encourage patient to share what kinds of support would be most beneficial.

Condition:
Endocarditis—Infective
Age:

Link & Explain
• Nursing Interventions Classification (NIC)
• Laboratory and Diagnostic Procedures
• Medications

Nursing Diagnosis 5

Deficient knowledge regarding condition, prognosis, treatment, self-care, and discharge needs related to lack of exposure, recall evidenced by questions, request for information.

NIC:
1) Review disease process, treatment, and recovery expectations; **2)** Discuss medications: actions, administration schedule, side effects; **3)** Review symptoms that need to be reported such as fever, chills, palpitations, chest pain, dyspnea; and **4)** Recommend gradual resumption of activity.

Medications

a. Antibiotic prophylactic treatment for patients at high risk

b. Acetaminophen (Tylenol), ibuprofen (Motrin)

c. Penicillin G (Pfizerpen), ceftriaxone (Rocephin), vancomycin (Vancocin), nafcillin (Nafcil), amphotericin B (Fungizone)

d.

Laboratory & Diagnostic Procedures

a. Blood cultures, CBC, erythrocyte sedimentation rate (ESR), C-reactive protein (CRP) levels

b. Echocardiography, chest x-ray

c. Valve replacement may be necessary for patients with infective endocarditis caused by fungi or viruses

d.

CONDITION: Eye Trauma

PHYSIOLOGY: Approximately 25 million eye injuries occur yearly in the United States, and approximately 10% of these patients will lose the vision in the affected eye. Symptoms may include redness, tenderness, pain, swelling, ecchymosis, diplopia. Eye injuries can be the result of car accidents, sports or leisure activities, or work-related causes. Injuries may be caused by a blunt injury, penetrating injury (glass, knife), chemical injury (acid or alkaline), thermal injury (welding torch, ultraviolet light), foreign body (wood, plastic, metal), trauma, or burns. The use of protective eye wear in some sports can decrease the number of ocular injuries. It is important to provide individual and community education.

HANDOFF COMMUNICATION

S	Situation	Assess what is currently happening in a short statement.	Patient presents as _____
B	Background	Summarize important past assessment data for your patient here. Place lab results and medications on the concept map.	**Age:** **Gender:** **Allergies:** **Fall Risk:** **Isolation:**
A	Assessment	Use the assessment data to complete your concept map.	**Nursing Diagnosis:** Place the Nursing Diagnoses in prioritized order on the concept map and add any needed for your specific patient. **Plan:** Place any further Nursing Interventions Classifications (NIC) needed on the map.

Implement Your Plan of Care

	EVALUATE YOUR CARE		
	Evaluate your nursing care and make recommendations related to the achievement of your desired outcomes. Were they met, or do new goals need to be established?		
R Recommendation	Diag	Nursing Outcomes Classification (NOC)	Outcome met
	1	Patient regains/maintains visual acuity after completing the treatment regimen.	☐ Yes ☐ No
	2	Patient reports pain is controlled and appears relaxed.	☐ Yes ☐ No
	3	Patient has normal temperature and no purulent drainage from eye.	☐ Yes ☐ No
	4	Patient correctly instills eye drops and verbalizes an understanding of necessary procedures.	☐ Yes ☐ No
	5		☐ Yes ☐ No

Nursing Diagnosis 1

Disturbed sensory perception (visual) related to diminished vision evidenced by decreased visual acuity.

NIC:
1) Assess visual acuity with the Snellen (distance vision) and Jaeger (near vision) eye charts; **2)** Assess the peripheral vision with the confrontation test; **3)** Assess the individual pupil response, consensual and accommodation response; **4)** Obtain information related to the type of injury to the eye; **5)** Obtain information regarding diplopia, photophobia and floaters, or spots; and **6)** Provide documentation of findings prior to treatment.

Nursing Diagnosis 2

Acute pain related to tissue, nerve and ocular trauma evidenced by verbalization and facial grimacing.

NIC:
1) Avoid pressure on eye; **2)** Instruct patient to avoid blowing the nose; **3)** Elevate the head of the bed 45 degrees; **4)** Stabilize foreign objects; **5)** Administer systemic analgesics and instill local anesthetic eye drops as prescribed; **6)** Apply cold pack if prescribed; and **7)** Keep environment quiet with limited visitors, decreased noise, and dim lights when not assessing patient.

Nursing Diagnosis 3

Risk for infection related to traumatized tissue and invasive organisms.

NIC:
1) Provide ocular irrigation with sterile saline or an alternative solution if prescribed; **2)** Cover eye with dry 2 sterile patch and a protective shield; **3)** Administer tetanus prophylaxis as prescribed; and **4)** Encourage patient to avoid touching facial area.

Nursing Diagnosis 4

Deficient knowledge regarding condition, prognosis, treatment regimen, self-care, and discharge needs related to information misinterpretation evidenced by request for information.

NIC:
1) Review pathology and prognosis of condition and need for treatment as indicated; **2)** Demonstrate instillation of eye drops; **3)** Discuss importance of reporting increased pain, decreased vision, purulent drainage, fever; **4)** Keep eye patched with protective shield as prescribed; and **5)** Verbalize the need for protective eye wear in the future to prevent eye trauma.

Condition:
Eye Trauma
Age:

- - - - - - - - - - - - - - - -
Link & Explain
• Nursing Interventions Classification (NIC)
• Laboratory and Diagnostic Procedures
• Medications

Nursing Diagnosis 5

NIC:

Medications

a. Eye drops to treat infection, decrease ocular pressure, decrease photophobia, provide anesthesia

b.

c.

d.

Laboratory & Diagnostic Procedures

a.

b.

c.

d.

CONDITION: Fecal Diversions: Postoperative Care of Ileostomy and Colostomy

PHYSIOLOGY: Ileostomy and colostomy are surgical procedures whereby a passage is constructed through the abdominal wall that allows intestinal contents to move from the bowel through an opening in the skin. The opening, called a stoma, is created when the bowel is brought to the opening and sutured to the skin. This procedure is utilized when the patient has a cancerous tumor blocking the passage of feces from the bowel or has inflammatory bowel disease.

Ileostomy is performed as a permanent diversion when the entire colon, rectum, and anus must be removed. It is performed as a temporary diversion to provide bowel rest in chronic colitis.

A colostomy may be permanent or temporary. It may be performed at several areas of the bowel (ascending, transverse, descending/sigmoid) depending on the underlying pathology.

HANDOFF COMMUNICATION

S Situation	Assess what is currently happening in a short statement.	Patient presents as _____	
B Background	Summarize important past assessment data for your patient here. Place lab results and medications on the concept map.	**Age:** **Allergies:** **Isolation:**	**Gender:** **Fall Risk:**
A Assessment	Use the assessment data to complete your concept map.	**Nursing Diagnosis:** Place the Nursing Diagnoses in prioritized order on the concept map and add any needed for your specific patient. **Plan:** Place any further Nursing Interventions Classifications (NIC) needed on the map.	

Implement Your Plan of Care

			EVALUATE YOUR CARE	
R Recommendation	Evaluate your nursing care and make recommendations related to the achievement of your desired outcomes. Were they met, or do new goals need to be established?	**Diag**	**Nursing Outcomes Classification (NOC)**	**Outcome met**
		1	Patient demonstrates behaviors and techniques to promote healing and prevent skin breakdown.	☐ Yes ☐ No
		2	Patient demonstrates beginning acceptance by viewing and touching stoma and participating in self-care.	☐ Yes ☐ No
		3	Patient verbalizes relief or control of pain and appears relaxed, able to sleep appropriately.	☐ Yes ☐ No
		4	Patient maintains adequate hydration with stable VS, good skin turgor, strong peripheral pulses, and appropriate urine output.	☐ Yes ☐ No
		5	Patient correctly performs necessary procedures and explains reasons for the action.	☐ Yes ☐ No

Nursing Diagnosis 1

Risk for impaired skin integrity related to character and flow of drainage.

NIC:
1) Inspect stoma and note irritation, bruises (dark bluish color), and rashes; **2)** Measure stoma with the measurement guide weekly for the first 6 weeks and then monthly for 6 months to alter appliance fit as edema decreases; **3)** Verify that the opening on the back of the adhesive backing to the pouch is only 1/16- to 1/8-inch (2–3 mm) larger than the base of the stoma; **4)** Use a transparent, odor-proof drainable pouch to allow observation of stoma; **5)** Cleanse ostomy pouch on a routine basis, using a vinegar solution or commercial solution; **6)** Apply sealant barrier to protect skin from pouch adhesive; and **7)** Investigate any complaints of burning or itching around the stoma.

Nursing Diagnosis 2

Disturbed body image related to disease process: cancer, colitis, and associated treatment regimen evidenced by actual change in structure and function.

NIC:
1) Review reason for surgery and future expectations; **2)** Encourage patient to verbalize feelings regarding the ostomy. Acknowledge normal feelings of anger, depression, and grief; **3)** Note behaviors such as withdrawal, increased dependency, manipulation, noninvolvement in care; **4)** Provide opportunities for the patient to view and touch stoma while discussing positive signs of healing; and **5)** Maintain positive approach during care activities.

Nursing Diagnosis 3

Acute pain related to physical factors: disruption of skin and tissue (incisions, drains) evidenced by guarding, distraction behaviors, restlessness.

NIC:
1) Assess pain, noting location, characteristics, and intensity (0–10 scale); **2)** Encourage patient to verbalize concerns and provide support; **3)** Provide comfort measures, such as mouth care, back rub, sitz bath if indicated, and repositioning; **4)** Encourage use of relaxation therapy, guided imagery, and visualization; and **5)** Administer medications as indicated, such as opioids, analgesics, and patient-controlled analgesia (PCA).

Nursing Diagnosis 4

Risk for deficient fluid volume related to excessive losses through gastric suction and high-volume ileostomy output.

NIC:
1) Monitor I&O, note enteric losses such as gastric aspirate and stool; **2)** Assess capillary refill, skin turgor, peripheral pulses, and mucous membranes; **3)** Monitor VS and note postural hypotension and tachycardia; **4)** Monitor laboratory values such as Hgb/Hct, sodium, albumin to determine hydration status; and **5)** Administer IV fluids as indicated.

Condition:
Fecal Diversions: Postoperative Care of Ileostomy and Colostomy

Age:

Link & Explain
• Nursing Interventions Classification (NIC)
• Laboratory and Diagnostic Procedures
• Medications

Nursing Diagnosis 5

Deficient knowledge regarding condition, prognosis, treatment, self-care, and discharge needs related to lack of exposure evidenced by statements of misconception.

NIC:
1) Review anatomy and physiology and implications of surgical intervention. Include written and picture resources; **2)** Instruct patient about stomal care and allow time for return demonstration; **3)** Identify symptoms of electrolyte depletion, such a anorexia, abdominal muscle cramps, feelings of faintness, cold extremities, decreased sensation in extremities; **4)** Stress importance of chewing food well and adequate intake of fluids. Avoid foods that increase flatus such as cabbage, beans, beer. Avoid foods that can cause diarrhea such as green beans, broccoli, and spicy foods; **5)** Encourage regular exercise and activity; and **6)** Identify community resources for continued support after discharge.

Medications
a. Antibiotics
b.
c.
d.

Laboratory & Diagnostic Procedures
a. CBC, electrolytes
b. Colonoscopy
c.
d.

CONDITION: Fractures

PHYSIOLOGY: Fractures are a break in the bone that can be associated with serious injury to nerves, blood vessels, muscles, or organs. Common causes are trauma, overuse injury, osteoporosis, and bone tumors. Clinical manifestations include pain, edema, bruising, impaired pulses at the site, bone fragments possibly extending through the muscle and skin, nausea, vomiting. Nonsurgical treatment (closed reduction) may include a simple brace, splint, cast, metal brace, or traction. Surgical intervention (open reduction) may be necessary to stabilize the fracture using pins, screws, and plates.

HANDOFF COMMUNICATION

S	**Situation**	Assess what is currently happening in a short statement.	Patient presents as _____
B	**Background**	Summarize important past assessment data for your patient here. Place lab results and medications on the concept map.	**Age:** **Gender:** **Allergies:** **Fall Risk:** **Isolation:**
A	**Assessment**	Use the assessment data to complete your concept map.	**Nursing Diagnosis:** Place the Nursing Diagnoses in prioritized order on the concept map and add any needed for your specific patient. **Plan:** Place any further Nursing Interventions Classifications (NIC) needed on the map.

Implement Your Plan of Care

R	**Recommendation**	Evaluate your nursing care and make recommendations related to the achievement of your desired outcomes. Were they met, or do new goals need to be established?	**EVALUATE YOUR CARE**	
			Diag / **Nursing Outcomes Classification (NOC)**	**Outcome met**
			1 Patient maintains stabilization and alignment of the fracture.	☐ Yes ☐ No
			2 Patient displays a relaxed manner, participates in activities, sleeps appropriately.	☐ Yes ☐ No
			3 Patient maintains tissue perfusion with palpable pulses, warm dry skin, normal sensation, stable VS, and adequate urinary output.	☐ Yes ☐ No
			4 Patient maintains adequate respiratory function with absence of dyspnea or cyanosis; respiratory rate and ABGs are within normal range for patient.	☐ Yes ☐ No
			5 Patient demonstrates techniques that enable resumption of activities, especially ADL.	☐ Yes ☐ No

Nursing Diagnosis 1

Risk for additional trauma related to loss of skeletal integrity and movement of bone fragments.

NIC:
1) Maintain rest of the affected part as indicated. Provide support of the joints above and below the fracture site, especially during movement; **2)** If a cast is applied, use the palms of the hand, not fingers, when touching the wet cast. Use pillows or sandbags to maintain cast in neutral position; **3)** Evaluate extremity for edema; **4)** Maintain position and integrity of traction; **5)** Review restrictions, weight-bearing activities, symptoms of unrelieved pain, severe swelling, discoloration of skin, coolness of the extremity; and **6)** Assess tissue around cast edges for roughness or pressure points. Investigate burning sensation under cast.

Nursing Diagnosis 2

Acute pain related to movement of bone fragments, edema, and injury to soft tissue evidenced by reports of pain.

NIC:
1) Observe and document location, severity (0–10 scale), characteristics of pain (steady, intermittent); **2)** Encourage patient to report pain early before it becomes severe; **3)** Maintain immobilization of affected area by cast, splint, or traction. Elevate injured extremity; **4)** Provide comfort measures such as mouth care, back rub (avoiding surgical area), and repositioning; **5)** Encourage use of relaxation techniques such as guided imagery and visualization. Provide diversional activities; **6)** Administer medications for pain as needed; and **7)** Note response to medication, report if pain is not relieved.

Nursing Diagnosis 3

Risk for peripheral neurovascular dysfunction related to excessive edema or thrombus formation.

NIC:
1) Evaluate presence and quality of peripheral pulse distal to injury via palpation or Doppler. Compare with uninjured limb; **2)** Assess capillary refill, pulses, skin color, and warmth distal to the fracture; **3)** Apply ice to fracture site intermittently for the initial 24–72 hours; **4)** Note appearance and spread of hematoma; **5)** Report severe unrelieved pain, paresthesia, change in pulse quality distal to injury, decreased skin temperature, pallor; and **6)** Monitor VS; note general pallor, cyanosis, cool skin, or changes in mentation.

Nursing Diagnosis 4

Risk for impaired gas exchange related to altered blood flow, blood, or fat emboli.

NIC:
1) Monitor respiratory rate and effort. Note stridor, use of accessory muscles, retractions, and development of cyanosis; **2)** Auscultate breath sounds, noting development of unequal or decreased breath sounds, crackles; **3)** Instruct patient about incentive spirometry, deep-breathing and coughing exercises; **4)** Inspect skin for petechiae above nipple line, in axilla, spreading to trunk, oral area; and **5)** Monitor pulse oximetry and ABGs.

Condition:
Fractures
Age:

Link & Explain
- Nursing Interventions Classification (NIC)
- Laboratory and Diagnostic Procedures
- Medications

Nursing Diagnosis 5

Impaired physical mobility related to neuromuscular skeletal impairment, pain or discomfort, restrictive therapies: limb immobilization evidenced by inability to move purposefully within the physical environment, imposed restrictions.

NIC:
1) Assess degree of immobility produced by injury and note patient's perception of immobility; **2)** Encourage participation in diversional activities; **3)** Instruct patient while assisting with passive or active ROM exercises; **4)** Encourage self-care activities such as bathing, shaving, and oral hygiene; **5)** Assist with mobility with the use of wheelchair, walker, crutches, cane as needed; **6)** Monitor BP when resuming activity, note reports of dizziness; and **7)** Encourage increased fluid intake of 2,000–3,000 ml/day as tolerated. Increase fiber and roughage in the diet.

Medications
a. Opioids
b. NSAIDs
c. Cyclobenzaprine (Flexeril), metaxalone (Skelaxin)
d. Enoxaparin (Lovenox)

Laboratory & Diagnostic Procedures
a. X-rays, bone scans, CT scans, MRI, arteriograms
b. CBC, coagulation profile
c.
d.

CONDITION: Gastric Partitioning, Gastroplasty, and Gastric Bypass

PHYSIOLOGY: Changing the weight of a severely obese person by surgical intervention demonstrates an improvement in diabetes, hypertension, hyperlipidemia, and sleep apnea. The surgery can be completed by an open approach or by laparoscopy. Open approach is used for those patients who have had previous abdominal surgery or complicated medical problems.

Surgical procedures can be restrictive: the size of the stomach is reduced so that less food is required to make the patient feel full. The food is digested normally, which reduces the risk for anemia or cobalamin deficiency. Malabsorptive surgeries include bypassing various lengths of the small intestine so that less food is absorbed. Weight loss occurs because most of the calories are not absorbed but are routed to the colon.

HANDOFF COMMUNICATION

S	Situation	Assess what is currently happening in a short statement.	Patient presents as _____
B	Background	Summarize important past assessment data for your patient here. Place lab results and medications on the concept map.	Age: Gender: Allergies: Fall Risk: Isolation:
A	Assessment	Use the assessment data to complete your concept map.	**Nursing Diagnosis:** Place the Nursing Diagnoses in prioritized order on the concept map and add any needed for your specific patient. **Plan:** Place any further Nursing Interventions Classifications (NIC) needed on the map.

Implement Your Plan of Care

		EVALUATE YOUR CARE		
	Evaluate your nursing care and make recommendations related to the achievement of your desired outcomes. Were they met, or do new goals need to be established?	Diag	Nursing Outcomes Classification (NOC)	Outcome met
R Recommendation		1	Patient experiences no cyanosis or other signs of hypoxia, with ABGs within acceptable range.	☐ Yes ☐ No
		2	Patient demonstrates behaviors to improve or maintain circulation.	☐ Yes ☐ No
		3	Patient maintains adequate fluid volume with balanced I&O.	☐ Yes ☐ No
		4	Patient demonstrates appropriate weight loss with normalization of laboratory values.	☐ Yes ☐ No
		5	Patient verbalizes necessary lifestyle changes and participates in treatment regimen.	☐ Yes ☐ No

Nursing Diagnosis 1

Ineffective breathing pattern related to decreased lung expansion evidenced by tachypnea, respiratory depth changes, reduced vital capacity.

NIC:
1) Observe respiratory rate and depth; **2)** Elevate head of bed 30–45 degrees; **3)** Auscultate breath sounds. Note presence of wheezes or rhonchi; **4)** Assist with coughing, turning, and deep breathing. Encourage the use of incentive spirometry. Demonstrate splinting of incision; and **5)** Monitor pulse oximetry and ABGs. Administer supplemental oxygen as needed.

Nursing Diagnosis 2

Risk for ineffective tissue perfusion (gastrointestinal) related to diminished blood flow.

NIC:
1) Monitor VS, palpate peripheral pulses, evaluate capillary refill and changes in mentation; **2)** Encourage ambulation and maintain schedule for sequential compression devices (SCD). Assess for redness, edema, and discomfort in calf; **3)** Monitor I&O and wound drains, such as Jackson-Pratt or Hemovac; **4)** Visually check and palpate operative area for swelling. Inspect dressing for excessive drainage; **5)** Monitor Hgb/Hct and RBCs; and **6)** Evaluate for complications such as rigid abdomen, nonincisional abdominal pain, fever, tachycardia, and low blood pressure.

Nursing Diagnosis 3

Risk for deficient fluid volume related to excessive gastric losses: nasogastric suction, diarrhea.

NIC:
1) Assess VS, skin turgor, mucous membranes, peripheral pulses, and capillary refill; **2)** Maintain accurate I&O, noting output less than intake and increased urine specific gravity; **3)** Monitor drainage from NG tube and drains. Assess color and amount of drainage; **4)** Monitor BUN, creatinine, CBC, and electrolytes; and **5)** Administer IV fluids and blood products as prescribed.

Nursing Diagnosis 4

Risk for imbalanced nutrition: less than body requirements related to malabsorption of nutrients and impaired absorption of vitamins.

NIC:
1) Assess abdomen, noting presence and character of bowel sounds, abdominal distention, and reports of nausea; **2)** When oral intake resumes, establish frequent small meals in amounts specified; **3)** Emphasize importance of recognizing satiety and stopping intake; **4)** Avoid taking fluids with meals for 30 minutes before and after meals. Encourage frequent sipping of fluids between meals; and **5)** Maintain IV fluids or total parenteral nutrition as needed.

Condition:
Gastric Partitioning, Gastroplasty, and Gastric Bypass

Age:
- - - - - - - - - - - - - - - - - - - -
Link & Explain
• Nursing Interventions Classification (NIC)
• Laboratory and Diagnostic Procedures
• Medications

Nursing Diagnosis 5

Deficient knowledge regarding condition, prognosis, treatment, self-care, and discharge needs related to lack of exposure evidenced by request for instructions.

NIC:
1) Review disease process, surgical procedure, and prognosis; **2)** Demonstrate care of incisions and dressings and drains; **3)** Emphasize importance of eating small meals slowly, chewing food well, sitting in a calm, relaxed atmosphere; **4)** Identify signs of hypokalemia such as diarrhea, muscle cramps, weakness of lower extremities, irregular pulse, dizziness with position change; **5)** Discuss symptoms of dumping syndrome such as weakness, profuse perspiration, nausea, vomiting, fainting, flushing, and epigastric discomfort during or immediately after meals; and **6)** Review symptoms that need to be reported such as persistent nausea, vomiting, abdominal distention, change in bowel pattern, fever, purulent wound drainage, plateauing of weight or weight gain.

Medications
a. Vitamin and mineral supplements: calcium, vitamin B$_{12}$, folate, thiamine
b.
c.
d.

Laboratory & Diagnostic Procedures
a. CBC, electrolytes, BUN, creatinine
b. Psychological consultation
c.
d.

CONDITION: Glaucoma

PHYSIOLOGY: Irreversible process in which the retinal ganglion cell (nerve cells in front of the eye) die. Atrophy of the optic nerve fibers cause loss of peripheral vision leading to blindness.

Three Major Categories of Glaucoma

1. *Chronic open-angle (primary open-angle) glaucoma:* drainage of aqueous humor from the eye is obstructed; may be associated with diabetes mellitus type II; loss of peripheral vision is gradual.
2. *Primary narrow-angle (closed-angle) glaucoma:* related to trauma, inflammatory process.
3. *Acute angle-closure glaucoma:* sudden, excruciating pain in or around eye, blurred vision, ocular redness.

   Risk factors include age over 45, myopia, long-term steroid use, family history of glaucoma.

HANDOFF COMMUNICATION

S Situation	Assess what is currently happening in a short statement.	Patient presents as _____
B Background	Summarize important past assessment data for your patient here. Place lab results and medications on the concept map.	**Age:** **Gender:** **Allergies:** **Fall Risk:** **Isolation:**
A Assessment	Use the assessment data to complete your concept map.	**Nursing Diagnosis:** Place the Nursing Diagnoses in prioritized order on the concept map and add any needed for your specific patient. **Plan:** Place any further Nursing Interventions Classifications (NIC) needed on the map.

Implement Your Plan of Care

		EVALUATE YOUR CARE	
R Recommendation	Evaluate your nursing care and make recommendations related to the achievement of your desired outcomes. Were they met, or do new goals need to be established?	**Diag**	**Nursing Outcomes Classification (NOC)**	**Outcome met**
		1	Patient maintains current visual field and acuity without further loss.	☐ Yes ☐ No
		2	Patient demonstrates positive problem-solving skills.	☐ Yes ☐ No
		3	Patient verbalizes the understanding of the condition, prognosis, and treatment.	☐ Yes ☐ No
		4		☐ Yes ☐ No
		5		☐ Yes ☐ No

Nursing Diagnosis 1

Disturbed visual sensory perception related to altered sensory reception: altered status of sense organs—increased IOP, ocular trauma, or infection—evidenced by reported changes in sensory acuity: photosensitivity, visual distortions, progressive loss of visual field, measured change in sensory acuity.

NIC:
1) Determine type and degree of visual loss; 2) Encourage expression of feelings about loss of vision; 3) Recommend measures to assist patient to manage visual limitations and provide safety: turn head to view subjects, arrange furniture out of path, reduce clutter, lighting; 4) Keep head of bed elevated; 5) Explain the importance of medication administration; 6) Demonstrate eye drop instillation using correct procedure; and 7) Adhere to medication schedule and avoid missing doses.

Nursing Diagnosis 2

Anxiety (specific level) related to physiological factors, change in health status, presence of pain, possibility or reality of loss of vision evidenced by expressed concern regarding changes in life events.

NIC:
1) Assess anxiety level, degree of pain experienced, sudden onset of symptoms, and current knowledge of condition; 2) Provide accurate, honest information. Discuss probability that careful monitoring and treatment can prevent additional loss of vision; and 3) Encourage patient to acknowledge concerns and express feelings.

Nursing Diagnosis 3

Deficient knowledge regarding condition, prognosis, treatment, and self-care needs related to information misinterpretation evidenced by inaccurate follow-through of instruction.

NIC:
1) Review pathology and prognosis of condition and lifelong treatment needs; 2) Identify potential side effects and adverse reactions to treatment such as change in appetite, nausea, vomiting, diarrhea, fatigue, decreased libido; 3) Encourage patient to make necessary changes in lifestyle; 4) Recommend regular use of sunglasses; 5) Recommend that exercise and activity restrictions be discussed with health-care provider; 6) Avoid constipation by increasing dietary fiber and adequate fluids; 7) Advise patient to report severe eye pain, increased photophobia, existence of veil-like curtain or flashing lights or particles floating; and 8) Identify strategies for socialization and resources such as organizations for the visually impaired and temporary services.

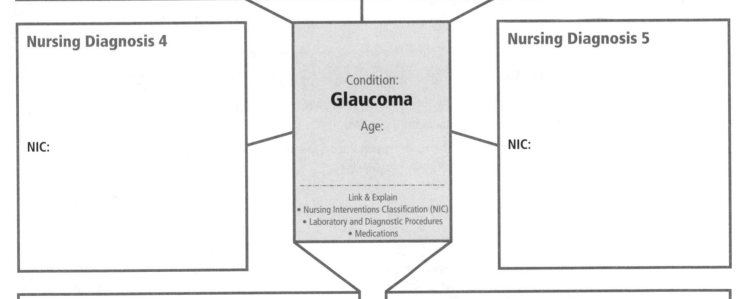

Nursing Diagnosis 4

NIC:

Condition:
Glaucoma
Age:

- - - - - - - - - - - - - - - - - - - -
Link & Explain
• Nursing Interventions Classification (NIC)
• Laboratory and Diagnostic Procedures
• Medications

Nursing Diagnosis 5

NIC:

Medications

a. Chronic open-angle: miotics, anticholinesterase, beta-blockers, carbonic anhydrase inhibitors, prostaglandin agonists

b. Narrow-angle: miotics, alpha agonists, hyperosmotic agents

c.

d.

Laboratory & Diagnostic Procedures

a. Ophthalmoscopy, tonometry, fundus photography

b. Visual acuity tests, visual field test such as confrontation or tangent screen

c. Heidelberg retina tomography (HRT)

d. Surgical intervention: laser therapy, iridotomy, diathermy

CONDITION: Heart Failure (HF)—Chronic

PHYSIOLOGY: Heart failure occurs when the heart is unable to pump sufficient blood to meet the metabolic needs of the body because of progressive worsening of ventricular function and ventricular remodeling. The Heart Failure Society of America developed the acronym FACES (fatigue, limitations of activity, chest congestion/cough, edema, shortness of breath) to assist with education of patients.

Right-sided failure occurs when the right ventricle cannot maintain an adequate cardiac output, and systemic congestion occurs. Signs and symptoms may include murmurs, jugular vein distention, bilateral edema (pedal, sacrum), weight gain, tachycardia, ascites, hepatomegaly, anorexia, and nausea.

Left-sided failure occurs when the left ventricle cannot produce a cardiac output sufficient to prevent pulmonary congestion. Signs and symptoms may include increased heart rate, crackles in lungs, S3 and S4 heart sounds, restlessness, confusion, shallow respirations 30–40/min, paroxysmal nocturnal dyspnea, orthopnea, frothy pink-tinged sputum.

The severity of chronic heart failure is categorized into four classes: I—physical activity not impaired; II—ordinary physical activity results in symptoms (fatigue, shortness of breath, etc.); III—marked limitation in physical activity; IV—symptoms at rest/minimal exertion.

HANDOFF COMMUNICATION

S Situation	Assess what is currently happening in a short statement.	Patient presents as _____ *Classification and etiology of heart failure—presence of comorbidities.*
B Background	Summarize important past assessment data for your patient here. Place lab results and medications on the concept map.	**Age:** **Gender:** **Allergies:** **Fall Risk:** **Isolation:**
A Assessment	Use the assessment data to complete your concept map.	**Nursing Diagnosis:** Place the Nursing Diagnoses in prioritized order on the concept map and add any needed for your specific patient. **Plan:** Place any further Nursing Interventions Classifications (NIC) needed on the map.

Implement Your Plan of Care

			EVALUATE YOUR CARE	
R Recommendation	Evaluate your nursing care and make recommendations related to the achievement of your desired outcomes. Were they met, or do new goals need to be established?	**Diag**	**Nursing Outcomes Classification (NOC)**	**Outcome met**
		1	Patient reports decreased episodes of dyspnea and angina with VS and urinary output within patient baseline.	☐ Yes ☐ No
		2	Patient demonstrates an increase in activity tolerance and ability to meet self-care needs.	☐ Yes ☐ No
		3	Patient maintains electrolytes within normal range and demonstrates minimal signs/symptoms of circulatory overload.	☐ Yes ☐ No
		4	Patient verbalizes improvement in duration and quality of uninterrupted sleep.	☐ Yes ☐ No
		5	Patient identifies a plan for needed alteration in lifestyle/behavioral changes and understanding of ongoing treatment regimen.	☐ Yes ☐ No

Nursing Diagnosis 1

Decreased cardiac output related to altered myocardial contractility evidenced by symptoms of right or left heart failure such as orthopnea, crackles, liver engorgement, and edema.

NIC:
1) Monitor VS, cardiac rhythm, lung sounds, respiratory effort/effectiveness, mental status, urinary output; 2) Monitor EKG, electrolytes, chest x-ray changes; 3) Inspect lower extremities and sacral area for edema; 4) Administer oxygen and monitor pulse oximetry; 5) Administer medications as prescribed and monitor patient response to treatment; 6) Elevate lower extremities to decrease edema; 7) Position patient in semi-Fowler's for dyspnea; and 8) Provide quiet/stress-free environment.

Nursing Diagnosis 2

Activity intolerance related to imbalance between oxygen supply and demand evidenced by changes in VS, presence of dysrhythmia, decreased pulse oximetry.

NIC:
1) Monitor patient cardiopulmonary response to activity (tachycardia, dyspnea, diaphoresis, pallor); 2) Evaluate other possible causes of fatigue (treatments, pain, cachexia, anemia, depression); 3) Implement cardiac rehabilitation program; 4) Provide a bedside commode; instruct patient in avoidance of activities that will illicit vagal response; and 5) Provide assistance with care activities as needed.

Nursing Diagnosis 3

Excess fluid volume related to reduced glomerular filtration rate, increased antidiuretic hormone production, sodium and water retention evidenced by weight gain, respiratory distress.

NIC:
1) Monitor serial weights, VS, lung sounds, presence of edema/ascites, neck vein distention; 2) Monitor urine output, note amount and color as well as time of day diuresis occurs; 3) Maintain chair rest or bed rest with head in semi-Fowler's position during acute phase; 4) Monitor serum electrolytes, BUN, creatinine; 5) Administer diuretics as prescribed; 6) Establish fluid intake schedule if fluids are restricted. Provide frequent mouth care. Maintain strict I&O; and 7) Weigh daily.

Nursing Diagnosis 4

Disturbed sleep pattern related to facility routines evidenced by verbal reports of not feeling well rested.

NIC:
1) Assess current sleep pattern and sleep history; 2) Assess for possible deterrents to sleep (dyspnea, orthopnea, nocturia, fear); 3) Discourage daytime napping and increase activity daily; 4) Instruct patient to decrease fluid intake before bedtime and adjust medication schedule accordingly; 5) Encourage patient to sleep with head elevated, follow bedtime rituals, and avoid caffeine, smoking; 6) Review how to request assistance at night; and 7) Reduce noise and light. Limit interruptions during sleep.

Condition:
Heart Failure (HF)—Chronic
Age:

Link & Explain
• Nursing Interventions Classification (NIC)
• Laboratory and Diagnostic Procedures
• Medications

Nursing Diagnosis 5

Deficient knowledge regarding illness, treatment, self-care, and discharge needs related to lack of understanding about disease evidenced by statements of concern.

NIC:
1) Discuss normal heart function and patient's variation from normal functioning; 2) Explain/reinforce need for lifestyle changes and strict adherence with treatment regimen; 3) Refer for diet counseling; 4) Review medications, instruct patient in skills related to monitoring heart rate/BP; 5) Discuss patient's role in control of risk factors such as smoking, alcohol abuse, high-salt diet; 6) Review signs/symptoms that need immediate intervention; and 7) Address patient/caregiver questions/concerns and refer for support/services as needed.

Medications
a. Oxygen, anti-anxiety agents, sedatives
b. Diuretics, anticoagulants, electrolytes
c. ACE inhibitors, angiotensin II receptor antagonists, vasodilators (nitrates)
d. Beta blockers, inotropic agents, aldosterone antagonists

Laboratory & Diagnostic Procedures
a. EKG, x-ray, pulse oximetry, ABGs, electrolytes, BUN, creatinine, CBC
b. Bleeding/clotting times, drug levels, thyroid studies, liver enzymes, serum proteins, erythrocyte sedimentation rate (ESR)
c. Atrial natriuretic peptide (ANP), beta natriuretic peptide (BNP)
d. Echocardiogram, stress test, cardiac catheterization, pacemaker, defibrillator

CONDITION: Hepatitis

PHYSIOLOGY: Hepatitis is inflammation of the liver. Virus is the most common cause, although it can also be caused by drugs, alcohol, chemicals, autoimmune diseases. Hepatitis involves swelling of hepatocytes, which reduces ability to detoxify blood and produce clotting factors, plasma proteins, bile, glycogen.

Characteristics of Hepatitis

Hepatitis A is more prevalent in crowded conditions with poor sanitation, poor personal hygiene, or infected food handlers. It is transmitted by fecal-oral route. The source is usually contaminated water, milk, food, shellfish. Hepatitis A can be prevented by immunization with the HAV vaccine.

Hepatitis B is transmitted by percutaneous exposure, sexual contact, or perinatal transmission. The source is contaminated needles, syringes, blood products, sexual contact with infected partners, tattoo/body piercing with contaminated needles, bites. Hepatitis B immunoglobulin (HBIG) is recommended for postexposure prophylaxis.

Hepatitis B can be prevented by immunization with the HBV vaccine. *Hepatitis D* may coexist with hepatitis B.

Hepatitis C is transmitted by percutaneous exposure to blood or blood products, high-risk sexual contact, perinatal contact. The source is blood and blood products, needles and syringes, sexual activities with infected partners.

Hepatitis E is transmitted by the fecal-oral route and through contaminated drinking water in developing countries; it is not prevalent in the United States.

HANDOFF COMMUNICATION

S Situation	Assess what is currently happening in a short statement.	Patient presents as _____ VS: LOC:
B Background	Summarize important past assessment data for your patient here. Place lab results and medications on the concept map.	**Age:** **Gender:** **Allergies:** **Fall Risk:** **Isolation:**
A Assessment	Use the assessment data to complete your concept map.	**Nursing Diagnosis:** Place the Nursing Diagnoses in prioritized order on the concept map and add any needed for your specific patient. **Plan:** Place any further Nursing Interventions Classifications (NIC) needed on the map.

Implement Your Plan of Care

R Recommendation	Evaluate your nursing care and make recommendations related to the achievement of your desired outcomes. Were they met, or do new goals need to be established?	*(see table below)*

Diag	**EVALUATE YOUR CARE** Nursing Outcomes Classification (NOC)	Outcome met
1	Patient performs activities of daily living (ADL) and participates in activities at level of ability.	☐ Yes ☐ No
2	Patient is free of signs of liver failure with liver function studies within normal limits, absence of jaundice, hepatic enlargement, or altered mental status.	☐ Yes ☐ No
3	Patient maintains adequate fluid volume evidenced by stable VS, good skin turgor, capillary refill, and appropriate urine output. Patient is free of signs of hemorrhage with clotting times within normal limits.	☐ Yes ☐ No
4	Patient initiates behaviors and lifestyle changes to regain or maintain appropriate weight.	☐ Yes ☐ No
5	Patient initiates necessary lifestyle changes.	☐ Yes ☐ No

Nursing Diagnosis 1

Fatigue related to altered body chemistry such as changes in liver function evidenced by report of lack of energy, inability to maintain usual routines.

NIC:
1) Determine and prioritize role responsibilities as well as alternative providers and community resources; **2)** Recommend rest periods before meals; **3)** Perform ROM exercises and increase activity as tolerated; **4)** Monitor for anorexia, liver tenderness and enlargement; and **5)** Encourage stress management techniques such as relaxation, visualization, guided imagery.

Nursing Diagnosis 2

Impaired liver function related to viral infection evidenced by presence of virus or antibodies, abnormal liver function tests.

NIC:
1) Discuss risk factors related to exposure to contaminated foods, occupation, or lifestyle that may have contributed to the transmission; **2)** Review all prescribed and OTC medications with increased risk for hepatotoxicity; **3)** Review results of laboratory tests such as hepatitis viral titers and liver function studies; **4)** Administer antiviral medications if indicated to reduce viral load; and **5)** Discuss physiology of disease and possible chronic liver disease.

Nursing Diagnosis 3

Risk for deficient fluid volume/bleeding related to excessive losses through vomiting and diarrhea and altered clotting process.

NIC:
1) Monitor I&O, note enteric losses such as vomiting and diarrhea; **2)** Assess BP, peripheral pulses, and mucous membranes; **3)** Check for ascites, measure abdominal girth; **4)** Observe for signs of bleeding such as hematuria, melena, ecchymosis, and oozing from puncture sites; **5)** Monitor laboratory values such as Hgb/Hct, sodium, BUN, albumin; and **6)** Administer IV fluids as prescribed.

Nursing Diagnosis 4

Imbalanced nutrition less than body requirements related to insufficient intake to meet metabolic demands of anorexia, nausea and vomiting evidenced by abdominal pain and cramping.

NIC:
1) Monitor dietary intake and calorie count. Provide meals in several small servings; **2)** Encourage mouth care before meals; **3)** Position patient sitting up in a chair for meals; **4)** Administer vitamin supplements such as B-complex vitamins as prescribed; **5)** Consult with nutritional support to provide diet according to patient's needs, with fat and protein intake as tolerated; and **6)** Monitor electrolytes, prealbumin, albumin, and protein.

Condition:
Hepatitis
Age:

Link & Explain
• Nursing Interventions Classification (NIC)
• Laboratory and Diagnostic Procedures
• Medications

Nursing Diagnosis 5

Deficient knowledge regarding condition, prognosis, treatment, self-care, and discharge needs related to lack of exposure or recall, information misinterpretation evidenced by questions or statements of misconception, request for information.

NIC:
1) Provide specific information regarding prevention and transmission of disease; **2)** Resume activity as tolerated with adequate rest periods. Restrict strenuous exercise, playing sports, heavy lifting; **3)** Assist with identifying diversional activities; **4)** Encourage a continuation of a balanced diet; **5)** Discuss avoidance of alcohol, illicit drugs, and tobacco; and **6)** Refer to community resources for drug/alcohol treatment program if indicated.

Medications

a. Antivirals: amantadine (Symmetrel), famciclovir (Famvir), entecavir (Baraclude) (inhibit viral reproduction)

b. Biologic response modifiers (BMRs): interferon alpha-2a (Roferon A), interferon alpha-2b (Intron-A) (reduce viral load, may induce remission)

c.

d.

Laboratory & Diagnostic Procedures

a. Serum bilirubin: elevation indicates blockage of bile ducts or liver disease; jaundice is evident when levels are high

b. Prothrombin time (PT)/activated partial prothromboplastin time (aPTT): determines bleeding and clotting time

c. Hepatitis A, B, C, D, E viral panels (antibody/antigen test): determine active infection, prior infection, immunity from vaccine

d. Liver enzymes/isoenzymes: detect hepatitis, obstruction

CONDITION: Herniated Nucleus Pulposus (Ruptured Intervertebral Disk)

PHYSIOLOGY: Herniated nucleus pulposus occurs when all or part of the gelatinous center of the intervertebral disk (nucleus pulposus) is forced through a weakened part or tear in the disk. It is also known as a herniated disk or ruptured disk, which often occurs in the lumbosacral vertebral areas of L4–L5 and L5–S1. If it occurs in the cervical region, it usually involves C5–C6 or C6–C7. Herniated disk is partially related to the aging process or the result of someone with a sedentary lifestyle who suddenly does too much activity. At highest risk are those who have occupations that require repetitive lifting or those who suffer from a trauma or accident.

HANDOFF COMMUNICATION

S	Situation	Assess what is currently happening in a short statement.	Patient presents as _____
B	Background	Summarize important past assessment data for your patient here. Place lab results and medications on the concept map.	**Age:** **Gender:** **Allergies:** **Fall Risk:** **Isolation:**
A	Assessment	Use the assessment data to complete your concept map.	**Nursing Diagnosis:** Place the Nursing Diagnoses in prioritized order on the concept map and add any needed for your specific patient. **Plan:** Place any further Nursing Interventions Classifications (NIC) needed on the map.

Implement Your Plan of Care

			EVALUATE YOUR CARE	
R	Recommendation	Evaluate your nursing care and make recommendations related to the achievement of your desired outcomes. Were they met, or do new goals need to be established?	**Diag** / **Nursing Outcomes Classification (NOC)**	**Outcome met**
			1 Patient demonstrates use of therapeutic interventions, such as relaxation skills or behavior modification to relieve pain.	☐ Yes ☐ No
			2 Patient verbalizes understanding of situation, risk factors, and individual treatment regimen.	☐ Yes ☐ No
			3 Patient appears relaxed and reports anxiety is reduced to a manageable level.	☐ Yes ☐ No
			4 Patient verbalizes an understanding of the condition, prognosis, and treatment.	☐ Yes ☐ No
			5	☐ Yes ☐ No

Nursing Diagnosis 1

Acute/chronic pain related to physical injury agents: nerve compression, muscle spasm evidenced by reports of back pain, stiff neck, decreased tolerance for activity evidenced by verbalizing methods that provide relief.

NIC:
1) Observe and document location, severity (0–10 scale), characteristics of pain (steady, intermittent); 2) Note presence of behaviors related to pain: changes in VS, crying, grimacing, sleep disturbance, withdrawal; 3) Assess for paresthesia in the affected extremity, pain aggravated by coughing or sneezing, loss of bowel or bladder control; 4) Provide comfort measures such as warm moist packs, back rub, stretching exercises, ultrasound, diathermy; 5) Teach relaxation techniques such as guided imagery, progressive muscle relaxation, and visualization; 6) Encourage patient to rest in a semi-Fowler's position with pillow under the knees (Williams' position); and 7) Administer medication for pain as needed. Evaluate response to medication.

Nursing Diagnosis 2

Impaired physical mobility related to pain and discomfort, muscle spasms evidenced by impaired coordination, limited ROM, decreased muscle strength.

NIC:
1) Schedule activity or procedures with rest periods. Encourage participation in ADL within individual limitations; 2) Provide or assist with passive and active ROM and strengthening exercises, depending on progressive ambulation; 3) Review proper body mechanics or techniques for participation in activities; 4) Encourage diet high in fiber and adequate fluid intake; 5) Apply antiembolic stockings; and 6) Encourage use of extension and flexion exercises in collaboration with physical therapy.

Nursing Diagnosis 3

Anxiety/ineffective coping related to threat to change in health status, socioeconomic status, role functioning evidenced by expressed concerns regarding changes in life events.

NIC:
1) Assess level of anxiety. Determine previous coping strategies. Identify strategies to address current perceived or actual problems; 2) Provide accurate information and honest answers; 3) Provide opportunity for expression of concerns, such as possible permanent nerve damage, paralysis, effect on sexual ability, changes in employment, finances, altered role responsibilities; 4) Note behaviors of family that promote the "sick role" for patient; and 5) Refer to appropriate support groups, social services, vocational counseling, psychotherapy as needed.

Nursing Diagnosis 4

Deficient knowledge regarding condition, prognosis, treatment, self-care, and discharge needs related to information misinterpretation evidenced by verbalization of problems, statement of misconception.

NIC:
1) Review disease process, interventions, and prognosis; 2) Instruct patient about body mechanics, ergonomics, and home exercises; 3) Discuss medications and side effects such as drowsiness and irritation of gastric mucosa; 4) Recommend firm mattress or backboard under a soft mattress and small pillow under neck; and 5) Instruct patient to report symptoms such as sharp pain, loss of sensation or mobility, changes in bowel habits.

Condition:
Herniated Nucleus Pulposus (Ruptured Intervertebral Disk)

Age:

Link & Explain
• Nursing Interventions Classification (NIC)
• Laboratory and Diagnostic Procedures
• Medications

Nursing Diagnosis 5

NIC:

Medications
a. Opioids, NSAIDs
b. Cyclobenzaprine (Flexeril), metaxalone (Skelaxin)
c.
d.

Laboratory & Diagnostic Procedures
a. Discography, electromyogram (EMG), MRI, CT, myelogram
b. Treatment: physical therapy, epidural injection of corticosteroid and anesthetic agent, minimally invasive surgical procedure, diskectomy, laminectomy
c.
d.

CONDITION: Hiatal Hernia

PHYSIOLOGY: The two major types of hiatal hernias are sliding hernias and paraesophageal (rolling) hernias. Sliding hernias are the most common type. The esophagogastric junction and a portion of the fundus of the stomach slide upward through the esophageal hiatus into the chest, usually as a result of weakening of the diaphragm. The hernia generally moves freely and slides into and out of the chest during changes in position or intra-abdominal pressure. Although volvulus (twisting) and obstruction do occur rarely, the major concern for a sliding hernia is the development of esophageal reflux and its complications. The development of reflux is related to chronic exposure of the lower esophageal sphincter (LES) to the low pressure of the thorax, which significantly reduces the effectiveness of the LES. Symptoms associated with decreased LES pressure are worsened by positions that favor reflux, such as bending or lying supine. Coughing, obesity, and ascites also increase reflux symptoms. Symptoms commonly associated with sliding hiatal hernias include heartburn, regurgitation, chest pain, dysphagia, and belching.

With rolling hernias, also known as paraesophageal hernias, the gastroesophageal junction remains in its normal intra-abdominal location, but the fundus (and possibly portions of the stomach's greater curvature) rolls through the esophageal hiatus and into the chest beside the esophagus. The herniated portion of the stomach may be small or quite large. In rare cases, the stomach completely inverts into the chest. Reflux is not usually present because the LES remains anchored below the diaphragm. However, the risks for volvulus, obstruction (blockage), and strangulation (stricture) are high. The development of iron-deficiency anemia is common because slow bleeding from venous obstruction causes the gastric mucosa to become engorged and ooze. Significant bleeding or hemorrhage is rare. Rolling hernias are thought to develop from an anatomic defect occurring when the stomach is not properly anchored below the diaphragm rather than from muscle weakness. They can also be caused by previous esophageal surgeries, including sliding hernia repair. Rolling (paraesophageal) hernias are characterized by complaints of fullness/breathlessness after eating, feelings of suffocation, chest pain that mimics angina, and worsening of symptoms when reclining.

Patients with hiatal hernias may be managed either medically or surgically based on the severity of symptoms and risk for serious complications. Sliding hiatal hernias are most commonly treated medically. Large rolling hernias present significant risk for strangulation or obstruction and surgical repair is often preferred (Ignatavicius & Walker, 2010, 1249–50).

HANDOFF COMMUNICATION

S Situation	Assess what is currently happening in a short statement.	Patient presents as _____ *Elicit information regarding onset, relief, character of symptoms.*
B Background	Summarize important past assessment data for your patient here. Place lab results and medications on the concept map.	**Age:** **Gender:** **Allergies:** **Fall Risk:** **Isolation:**
A Assessment	Use the assessment data to complete your concept map.	**Nursing Diagnosis:** Place the Nursing Diagnoses in prioritized order on the concept map and add any needed for your specific patient. **Plan:** Place any further Nursing Interventions Classifications (NIC) needed on the map.

Implement Your Plan of Care

		EVALUATE YOUR CARE		
R Recommendation	Evaluate your nursing care and make recommendations related to the achievement of your desired outcomes. Were they met, or do new goals need to be established?	**Diag**	**Nursing Outcomes Classification (NOC)**	**Outcome met**
		1	Patient reports that pain is relieved or controlled.	☐ Yes ☐ No
		2	Patient reports management of nausea and acceptable level of dietary intake.	☐ Yes ☐ No
		3	Patient verbalizes understanding of ways to maintain adequate nutritional status and minimize recurrence of symptoms related to dietary intake.	☐ Yes ☐ No
		4	Patient appears relaxed and reports anxiety reduced to manageable level.	☐ Yes ☐ No
		5	Patient verbalizes understanding of therapeutic regimen and initiates needed lifestyle changes.	☐ Yes ☐ No

Nursing Diagnosis 1

Acute pain related to gastric reflux evidenced by abdominal guarding, facial grimacing.

NIC:
1) Institute position changes to minimize reflux; **2)** Counsel patient to eliminate constrictive clothing and avoid lifting and straining; **3)** Administer medications as indicated; **4)** Encourage use of breathing/relaxation techniques as adjunct to medications; and **5)** Elevate head of the bed.

Nursing Diagnosis 2

Nausea related to irritating effects of gastric content evidenced by inability to eat meals.

NIC:
1) Educate patient regarding causes of nausea and strategies to minimize reflux; **2)** Administer antacids/histamine receptor antagonists as indicated; **3)** Encourage nutritional counseling program if indicated and refer as needed; **4)** Counsel patient to eliminate alcohol and smoking; and **5)** Administer proton pump inhibitors, H2-receptor blockers, and antacids as prescribed.

Nursing Diagnosis 3

Imbalanced nutrition: less than body requirements related to fear that eating may cause exacerbation of symptoms evidenced by weight 10% below ideal for height and body frame.

NIC:
1) Assess weight, body mass, strength, activity levels; monitor accordingly; **2)** Discuss disease process and effects on nutritional status; **3)** Encourage small/frequent meals; **4)** Record intake and related symptoms; **5)** Promote patient participation in dietary planning/management; **6)** Provide nutritional supplements as indicated; and **7)** Refer to dietician as needed.

Nursing Diagnosis 4

Fear anxiety related to change in health status or exacerbation of symptoms evidenced by statements about feeling stressed.

NIC:
1) Perform physical assessment/health history; **2)** Provide reassurance and complete explanations regarding diagnostic procedures and related therapies; **3)** Provide calm environment; **4)** Assist patient with relaxation techniques; and **5)** Administer medication as indicated.

Condition:
Hiatal Hernia
Age:

Link & Explain
• Nursing Interventions Classification (NIC)
• Laboratory and Diagnostic Procedures
• Medications

Nursing Diagnosis 5

Deficient knowledge regarding condition, treatment, self-care, and ongoing care needs related to information misinterpretation evidenced by verbalization of problems and misunderstanding.

NIC:
1) Teach information regarding disease process, symptom management, and health promotion modifications; **2)** Reinforce need for compliance with therapeutic regimen and follow-up with health-care provider; and **3)** Instruct regarding symptoms that require immediate medical follow-up and possible surgical intervention.

Medications

a. Antacids

b. Histamine receptor antagonists

c. Prokinetic drugs

d. Proton pump inhibitors

Laboratory & Diagnostic Procedures

a. Barium swallow study with fluoroscopy

b. Esophagogastroduodenoscopy (EGD)

c. Laboratory/diagnostic procedures to rule out myocardial infarction or cardiac cause of symptoms

d.

CONDITION: Hip Fracture

PHYSIOLOGY: A fracture is a break or disruption in the structure of a bone. Hip fractures refer to disruption of bone continuity involving the upper third of the femur. They are classified as being intracapsular (within the joint capsule) or extracapsular (outside the joint capsule). The most common treatment is surgical repair, typically using the open reduction with internal fixation (ORIF) technique. The surgeon has direct visualization of the fracture site in open reduction, and the internal fixation method uses metal hardware to immobilize the site during healing. The metal hardware used may include the installment of an intramedullary rod, pins, a prosthetic femoral head or neck, or a fixed sliding plate (such as a compression screw). The need for these devices is determined by the patient's age and prior mobility status. Patient falls are the most common cause of hip fractures, and the most common age group affected is the older adult population. The risk for hip fractures is equal among all ethnic and socioeconomic groups, although patients with chronic skeletal conditions such as osteoporosis are at a higher risk due to decreased bone density. During the first stage of healing, a hematoma forms at the site due to the highly vascular bone tissue. The bone then begins to necrose because of decreased blood supply, prompting the migration of bone-forming cells to the site and the formation of fibrocartilage around the break. With the increased vascularity and cellular repair, the fracture site becomes surrounded by a new vascular tissue called a callus (*Taber's*, 2009).

HANDOFF COMMUNICATION

S	Situation	Assess what is currently happening in a short statement.	Patient presents as _____
B	Background	Summarize important past assessment data for your patient here. Place lab results and medications on the concept map.	**Age:** **Gender:** **Allergies:** **Fall Risk:** **Isolation:**
A	Assessment	Use the assessment data to complete your concept map.	**Nursing Diagnosis:** Place the Nursing Diagnoses in prioritized order on the concept map and add any needed for your specific patient. **Plan:** Place any further Nursing Interventions Classifications (NIC) needed on the map.

Implement Your Plan of Care

			EVALUATE YOUR CARE	
R	Recommendation	Evaluate your nursing care and make recommendations related to the achievement of your desired outcomes. Were they met, or do new goals need to be established?	**Diag** / **Nursing Outcomes Classification (NOC)**	**Outcome met**
			1 Patient avoids infection during hospitalization.	☐ Yes ☐ No
			2 Patient demonstrates improved physical mobility by ambulating to a chair postoperative. Patient has a bowel movement within the first 3 postoperative days.	☐ Yes ☐ No
			3 Patient reports a decreased level of pain on a 0–10 numeric scale following implementation of medication or nonpharmacologic treatments.	☐ Yes ☐ No
			4 Patient bathes and dresses self safely with minimal difficulty.	☐ Yes ☐ No
			5	☐ Yes ☐ No

Nursing Diagnosis 1

Risk for infection related to surgical procedure.

NIC:
1) Assess the patient's incision site often and document findings related to redness, drainage, edema; **2)** Use strict aseptic technique for dressing changes and wound irrigations; **3)** Monitor VS every 4–8 hours, watching for increased temperature indicative of systemic infection; **4)** Monitor the patient's daily laboratory values noting any increase in WBC count; and **5)** Administer prophylactic antibiotics to reduce risk for infection.

Nursing Diagnosis 2

Impaired physical mobility related to weakness and decreased weight-bearing ability evidenced by confinement.

NIC:
1) Discuss the patient's mobility status and independence prior to hip fracture; **2)** Reposition the patient every 2 hours to avoid skin breakdown; **3)** Consult physical therapy for assistance with teaching the patient to use assistive devices such as crutches and walkers; **4)** Treat pain prior to increased patient activity; **5)** Encourage early ambulation; **6)** Increase independence with ADL and encourage independence; and **7)** Advise the patient to ambulate only with assistance and implement risk for falls guidelines to avoid further complications.

Nursing Diagnosis 3

Acute pain related to injury and surgical procedure evidenced by verbal reports, narrowed focus, guarding or protective behaviors, and physical and social withdrawal.

NIC:
1) Assess the pain to determine the onset, location, duration, characteristics, and aggravating and alleviating factors; **2)** Determine the patent's current medication use; **3)** Explore the need for opioid and nonopioid analgesics; **4)** Administer pain medications when the patient reports pain and assess pain relief at least 1 hour following administration; **5)** Discuss alternative therapies for pain relief, such as distraction, massage, and meditation; **6)** Describe the adverse effects of untreated pain; **7)** Discuss the patient's fears of undertreated pain, addiction, and overdose; and **8)** Plan nursing care when the patient is most comfortable, administering pain medication at least 30 minutes prior to activities that may increase pain.

Nursing Diagnosis 4

Self-care deficit (bathing/hygiene) related to musculoskeletal impairment

NIC:
1) Discuss the patient's bathing habits and cultural bathing preferences; **2)** Provide pain relief measures at least 45 minutes prior to initiating a bath; **3)** Obtain a shower chair for the patient to decrease the risk for falls; **4)** Consult occupational therapy to provide assistive devices for bathing; and **5)** Initiate bath during the patient's most energetic time of day.

Condition:
Hip Fracture
Age:

- - - - - - - - - -
Link & Explain
• Nursing Interventions Classification (NIC)
• Laboratory and Diagnostic Procedures
• Medications

Nursing Diagnosis 5

NIC:

Medications

a. Analgesics

b. Broad spectrum antibiotics (infection prevention)

c.

d.

Laboratory & Diagnostic Procedures

a. X-ray, CT scan

b. Bone scan, MRI

c. Decreased hemoglobin and hematocrit due to bleeding

d. Increased erythrocyte sedimentation rate due to inflammatory response

CONDITION: Hospice Care/Death & Dying

PHYSIOLOGY: Hospice care is an interdisciplinary program of palliative care and support services that addresses physical, spiritual, social, and economic needs of terminally ill patients and their families. This care can be provided in the home or in a hospice center (*Taber's*, 2009).

HANDOFF COMMUNICATION

S	Situation	Assess what is currently happening in a short statement.	Patient presents as _____
B	Background	Summarize important past assessment data for your patient here. Place lab results and medications on the concept map.	**Age:** **Gender:** **Allergies:** **Fall Risk:** **Isolation:**
A	Assessment	Use the assessment data to complete your concept map.	**Nursing Diagnosis:** Place the Nursing Diagnoses in prioritized order on the concept map and add any needed for your specific patient. **Plan:** Place any further Nursing Interventions Classifications (NIC) needed on the map.

Implement Your Plan of Care

			EVALUATE YOUR CARE	
R	Recommendation	Evaluate your nursing care and make recommendations related to the achievement of your desired outcomes. Were they met, or do new goals need to be established?	**Diag** **Nursing Outcomes Classification (NOC)**	**Outcome met**
			1 Patient verbalizes concerns and discusses feelings.	☐ Yes ☐ No
			2 Patient identifies a support system.	☐ Yes ☐ No
			3 Patient begins to participate in self-care and ADL.	☐ Yes ☐ No
			4 Patient verbalizes awareness of anxiety and healthy ways to deal with it. Patient reports anxiety is reduced to a manageable level.	☐ Yes ☐ No
			5	☐ Yes ☐ No

Nursing Diagnosis 1

Spiritual distress related to intense inner conflict about the outcome, normal grieving for loss, anger directed at God or a greater power, evidenced by verbalization of inner conflict, questioning beliefs and choices.

NIC:
1) Arrange for religious practices if desired; and **2)** Encourage questions and verbalization.

Nursing Diagnosis 2

Anticipatory grieving related to loss evidenced by verbalization, anger, or tearful behavior.

NIC:
1) Provide emotional support; **2)** Provide comfort measures; **3)** Provide family privacy; and **4)** Ask patient if she/he has a faith community.

Nursing Diagnosis 3

Self-care deficit, total, related to cognitive and/or physical impairment evidenced by disheveled appearance.

NIC:
1) Assess ability to carry out ADL and determine deficits; **2)** Encourage acceptance of assistance as necessary; **3)** Encourage independence while providing assistance as needed; **4)** Schedule care to provide adequate time and rest periods; **5)** Provide frequent positive reinforcement and encouragement; **6)** Provide privacy for toileting and bathing; **7)** Place call bell within reach and encourage use; and **8)** Offer frequent toileting.

Nursing Diagnosis 4

Anxiety related to presence of a specific risk factor, situational crisis, threat to self-concept evidenced by increased tension, apprehension, uncertainty, feelings of inadequacy, expressed concern.

NIC:
1) Promote expression of fears and feelings such as guilt, anger, denial, and depression; **2)** Encourage family and friends to verbalize; and **3)** Explain expected process for palliative care.

Condition:
Hospice Care/Death & Dying

Age:

Link & Explain
• Nursing Interventions Classification (NIC)
• Laboratory and Diagnostic Procedures
• Medications

Nursing Diagnosis 5

NIC:

Medications

a. Pain medication as needed (morphine)

b.

c.

d.

Laboratory & Diagnostic Procedures

a.

b.

c.

d.

CONDITION: Human Immunodeficiency Virus (HIV)

PHYSIOLOGY: In a normal immune response, foreign agents interact with B cells and T cells. The normal CD4 T cell count for an adult is 800–1,200 cells/microliter of blood. HIV destroys CD4 T cells, and the decline impairs immune function. Therefore HIV increases the risk of certain infections and cancer. The disease is transmitted by sexual contact, contamination through IV needle sharing, and mother-to-baby perinatal transmission.

Initial incubation lasts 2–4 weeks during which the individual is asymptomatic and HIV test may be negative, although the infection is present.

Stages

Acute infection (acute seroconversion stage): 4–8 weeks after infection, individual has flu-like symptoms; although HIV-positive, the immune function is still normal.

Early chronic: For years, virus remains active and individual is usually unaware of HIV status during this period. The CD4 T cell count remains above 500 cells/microliter. Patient may have lymphadenopathy, persistent headaches, low-grade fevers, and night sweats.

Intermediate chronic: Years after the infection, the immune system is compromised, symptoms of the early phase—weight loss, drenching night sweats, skin rashes, persistent fevers, persistent diarrhea, severe fatigue—are more severe. T cell count drops to 200–500 cells/microliter.

Late chronic or AIDS: As the viral load increases, there is an increased risk of developing opportunistic infections. There is severe damage to the immune system; the CD4 count drops below 200 cells/microliter. Patients may develop cancers, wasting syndrome, a debilitating or life-threatening infection which may be fungal, viral, protozoal, or bacterial.

HANDOFF COMMUNICATION

S Situation	Assess what is currently happening in a short statement.	Patient presents as _____ VS: LOC:
B Background	Summarize important past assessment data for your patient here. Place lab results and medications on the concept map.	Age: Gender: Allergies: Fall Risk: Isolation:
A Assessment	Use the assessment data to complete your concept map.	**Nursing Diagnosis:** Place the Nursing Diagnoses in prioritized order on the concept map and add any needed for your specific patient. **Plan:** Place any further Nursing Interventions Classifications (NIC) needed on the map.

Implement Your Plan of Care

		EVALUATE YOUR CARE	
R Recommendation	Evaluate your nursing care and make recommendations related to the achievement of your desired outcomes. Were they met, or do new goals need to be established?	**Diag** / **Nursing Outcomes Classification (NOC)**	**Outcome met**
		1 Patient demonstrates increased trust and participation in action plan. Patient initiates lifestyle changes to adapt to present life situation.	☐ Yes ☐ No
		2 Patient maintains adequate muscle mass and stable weight.	☐ Yes ☐ No
		3 Patient verbalizes understanding of condition, disease process, and potential complications.	☐ Yes ☐ No
		4 Patient identifies stable support system and uses resources as needed.	☐ Yes ☐ No
		5 Patient participates in desired activities at level of ability.	☐ Yes ☐ No

Nursing Diagnosis 1

Risk-prone health behavior related to life-threatening disease and ongoing grieving evidenced by failure to take action to prevent further health problems.

NIC:
1) Identify barriers to adjustment; **2)** Encourage expression of feelings, denial, shock, fear; **3)** Determine available community resources and services; **4)** Encourage exercise and reinforce structure in daily life; and **5)** Inform patient about treatments and medical advances.

Nursing Diagnosis 2

Risk for imbalanced nutrition: less than body requirements related to wasting syndrome evidenced by body weight 10% below ideal for height and frame.

NIC:
1) Weigh regularly and establish current anthropometric measurements; **2)** Determine the patient's dietary pattern, intake, and knowledge of nutrition; **3)** Assess for nausea and vomiting; **4)** Discuss and document nutritional side effects of medications; **5)** Provide information about foods and supplements that are high in calories, protein, vitamins, and minerals; and **6)** Monitor laboratory tests such as Hgb, prealbumin, albumin, potassium, and sodium.

Nursing Diagnosis 3

Deficient knowledge regarding disease, prognosis, self-care, and discharge needs related to information misinterpretation evidenced by inappropriate behaviors: hostile, agitated, apathetic, hysterical.

NIC:
1) Provide realistic information during each contact with patient; **2)** Review symptoms related to HIV infection: dry cough, fever, anorexia, skin rash; **3)** Instruct patient to seek medical treatment for any signs of infection; **4)** Review drug therapies, dosing, side effects, and adverse reaction; **5)** Assess continued high-risk behaviors such as drug abuse by injection, sharing needles, unsafe sexual practices; and **6)** Utilize resources: support groups, peer counselors, mental health professionals, case managers.

Nursing Diagnosis 4

Risk for social isolation related to altered state of wellness and changes in physical appearance.

NIC:
1) Discuss concerns regarding employment and leisure activity; **2)** Identify availability and stability of support persons; **3)** Encourage honesty in relationships; **4)** Assist patient to problem-solve regarding measures to avoid communicable disease; and **5)** Assess coping mechanism and previous methods of dealing with life problems.

Condition:
Human Immunodeficiency Virus (HIV)
Age:

Link & Explain
• Nursing Interventions Classification (NIC)
• Laboratory and Diagnostic Procedures
• Medications

Nursing Diagnosis 5

Fatigue related to altered body chemistry: side effects of medications evidenced by verbalization of unremitting, overwhelming lack of energy.

NIC:
1) Assess sleep patterns and other factors that may aggravate fatigue; **2)** Note daily energy patterns, times of increased and decreased ability to remain active; **3)** Assist with setting realistic activity goals, determining priorities and responsibilities; and **4)** Instruct in stress management techniques such as breathing exercises, visualization, music, light therapy.

Medications

a. Nucleoside reverse transcriptase inhibitors (NRTIs): zidovudine ZDV (Retrovir, AZT), abacavir (Ziagen), emtricitabine (Emtriva) (prevent production of new virus)

b. Protease inhibitor: tipranavir (Aptivus), indinavir (Crixivan), nelfinavir (Viracept) (indicated to block viral replication process)

c. Nonnucleoside reverse transcriptase inhibitors (NNRTIs): delavirdine (Rescriptor), etravirine (Intelence) (inhibit viral replication)

d. Entry inhibitors: enfuvirtide (Fuzeon), maraviroc (Selzentry) (prevent HIV from entering healthy CD4 cells)

Laboratory & Diagnostic Procedures

a. HIV antibody test: detects antibodies in the blood 2 weeks after exposure

b. Rapid HIV tests: diagnosis at point-of-care sites outside a traditional laboratory

c. CD4 lymphocyte count: counts below 500 benefit from antiretroviral therapy; counts below 200 define progression to AIDS

d. CBC: anemia and iron metabolism abnormalities are common

CONDITION: Hypertension

PHYSIOLOGY: Normal blood pressure is characterized as a systolic blood pressure less than or equal to 120 mm Hg and/or a diastolic blood pressure less than or equal to 80 mm Hg. Hypertension is an extremely common and dangerous disease and has a direct relationship with many other health problems, including coronary, cerebral, renal, and peripheral vascular disease. The body maintains stabilizing mechanisms to attempt to regulate blood pressure within a normal range. These mechanisms are arterial baroreceptors, fluid volume regulation, the renin-angiotensin system, and vascular regulation. Hypertension may be primary or secondary. Primary hypertension has no known cause but may be based on several risk factors, such as age greater than 60, genetic predisposition, excessive calorie or alcohol intake, sedentary lifestyle, hyperlipidemia, African American ethnicity, obesity, smoking, and stress. Secondary hypertension is caused by specific diseases and medications that may make a person more susceptible to hypertension. Any disease that may damage kidney structure or function, adrenal medulla or adrenal cortex dysfunction, coarctation of the aorta (narrowing of the aorta), or neurogenic disturbances such as brain tumors, encephalitis, and psychiatric disturbances commonly cause secondary hypertension. Medications that lead to secondary hypertension include estrogen, glucocorticoids, mineralocorticoids, sympathomimetics, cyclosporine, and erythropoietin. About one in four adults has hypertension, and it is found across all ethnic groups and socioeconomic classes. Treatment for primary hypertension involves removal of the associated risk factors. Sodium restriction, weight reduction, moderation of alcohol intake, increased physical activity, smoking cessation, and stress reduction have been shown to significantly decrease hypertension. Medications that are used for treatment of hypertension include diuretics (increase urine output to decrease excess fluid in the body), calcium channel blockers (cause vasodilation), angiotensin-converting enzyme inhibitors (prevent vasoconstriction), angiotensin II receptor antagonists (prevent vasoconstriction), aldosterone receptor antagonists (decrease sodium reabsorption in the kidneys), beta-adrenergic blockers (reduce the heart rate and cardiac output), central alpha agonists (prevent norepinephrine reuptake to decrease peripheral vascular resistance), and alpha-adrenergic agonists (dilate arteries and veins). These medications may be used alone or in combination to reduce blood pressure. Treatment for secondary hypertension involves treatment of the underlying disease process (*Taber's*, 2009).

HANDOFF COMMUNICATION

S	Situation	Assess what is currently happening in a short statement.	Patient presents as _____ *Identify associated risk factors, length of identified symptoms, and underlying disease processes. Manually measure the patient's blood pressure and discuss past blood pressure trends.*
B	Background	Summarize important past assessment data for your patient here. Place lab results and medications on the concept map.	**Age:** **Gender:** **Allergies:** **Fall Risk:** **Isolation:**
A	Assessment	Use the assessment data to complete your concept map.	**Nursing Diagnosis:** Place the Nursing Diagnoses in prioritized order on the concept map and add any needed for your specific patient. **Plan:** Place any further Nursing Interventions Classifications (NIC) needed on the map.

Implement Your Plan of Care

		EVALUATE YOUR CARE		
R	Recommendation Evaluate your nursing care and make recommendations related to the achievement of your desired outcomes. Were they met, or do new goals need to be established?	**Diag**	**Nursing Outcomes Classification (NOC)**	**Outcome met**
		1	Patient reports compliance to medication regimen and has blood pressure within normal limits.	☐ Yes ☐ No
		2	Patient identifies own risk factors for hypertension and discusses plan to minimize risk factors.	☐ Yes ☐ No
		3	Patient states the possible complications associated with hypertension.	☐ Yes ☐ No
		4	Patient begins diet and weight loss plan as developed by physical therapist and dietitian.	☐ Yes ☐ No
		5		☐ Yes ☐ No

Nursing Diagnosis 1

Risk for ineffective health maintenance related to ineffective individual or family coping.

NIC:
1) Explore with the patient his/her individualized risk factors for hypertension; **2)** Assess influence of cultural beliefs and values on the patient's ability to modify behavior; **3)** Monitor adherence to prescribed medication; **4)** Recognize resistance to changes in lifelong patterns of personal health care; **5)** Develop a realistic plan with the patient to reduce or eliminate individual risk factors; and **6)** Refer the patient to support groups or outside sources to promote adherence to goals.

Nursing Diagnosis 2

Deficient knowledge related to causes and treatments for hypertension evidenced by request for information.

NIC:
1) Assess the patient's current knowledge level of hypertension; **2)** Discuss risk factors for hypertension, including obesity, alcohol intake, smoking, sedentary lifestyle, and stress; **3)** Discuss treatment options for hypertension, including reduction or elimination of risk factors and medication; **4)** Discuss medications prescribed and information related to scheduling; counsel patient to rise slowly from a lying position; and **5)** Encourage patient to have vision screening regularly.

Nursing Diagnosis 3

Risk for injury related to hypertension and effects of therapy, drug interactions.

NIC:
1) Assess the patient for any potential early complications of hypertension, including confusion, dizziness, headache, lightheadedness, and visual disturbances; **2)** Discuss potential complications of prolonged hypertension, including stroke, myocardial infarction, and retinal hemorrhage; **3)** Teach the patient ways to avoid potential complications: eliminating risk factors and implementing a medication regimen; **4)** Encourage patient to stay on medication schedule as prescribed; and **5)** Advise the patient to have blood pressure checked at regular intervals.

Nursing Diagnosis 4

Imbalanced nutrition: more than body requirements related to imbalance between activity level and caloric intake evidenced by weight 10%–20% more than ideal for height and frame.

NIC:
1) Assess the patient's current diet and exercise patterns; **2)** Assess the patient's current BMI; **3)** Discuss influence of cultural beliefs, norms, and values relating to diet and exercise; **4)** Ask the patient to keep a food and exercise diary for 1 week to assess need for changes; **5)** Consult physical therapist and dietitian for assistance with realistic diet and exercise regimen; **6)** Demonstrate the use of food labels to make healthy choices; **7)** Agree on attainable goals for the patient and follow up with progress; and **8)** Discuss the DASH (Dietary Approaches to Stop Hypertension) diet to assist with appropriate selection of foods.

Condition:
Hypertension
Age:

Link & Explain
• Nursing Interventions Classification (NIC)
• Laboratory and Diagnostic Procedures
• Medications

Nursing Diagnosis 5

NIC:

Medications
a. Diuretics (thiazide, loop, and potassium-sparing types)
b. Calcium channel blockers
c. ACE inhibitors, angiotensin II receptor antagonists, aldosterone receptor antagonists
d. Beta-adrenergic blockers, central alpha agonists

Laboratory & Diagnostic Procedures
a. BP measurement
b. 12-lead EKG to determine cardiac involvement
c. Urinalysis to determine kidney and adrenal involvement
d. BUN and creatinine level to determine kidney involvement

CONDITION: Hyperthyroidism (Graves' Disease, Thyrotoxicosis)

PHYSIOLOGY: Metabolic imbalances resulting in excess circulating levels of triiodothyronine (T3) and thyroxine (T4). Thyrotoxic crisis or thyroid storm is untreated severe hyperthyroidism that creates a life-threatening emergency.

Hyperthyroidism may be caused by autoimmune disorders such as Graves' disease, which accounts for 75% of the cases. Antibodies attach to the receptor cells and stimulate the thyroid gland to release T3, T4, or both.

It may also be caused by toxic nodular goiter, which is a thyroid hormone–secreting nodule independent of TSH stimulation.

Clinical manifestations may include systolic hypertension, bounding rapid pulse, angina, dyspnea with mild exertion, warm moist skin, hair loss, diaphoresis, muscle weakness, nervousness, restlessness, lack of ability to concentrate, exophthalmos.

HANDOFF COMMUNICATION

S	Situation	Assess what is currently happening in a short statement.	Patient presents as _____ VS: LOC:
B	Background	Summarize important past assessment data for your patient here. Place lab results and medications on the concept map.	**Age:** **Gender:** **Allergies:** **Fall Risk:** **Isolation:**
A	Assessment	Use the assessment data to complete your concept map.	**Nursing Diagnosis:** Place the Nursing Diagnoses in prioritized order on the concept map and add any needed for your specific patient. **Plan:** Place any further Nursing Interventions Classifications (NIC) needed on the map.

Implement Your Plan of Care

		EVALUATE YOUR CARE	
		Diag	**Nursing Outcomes Classification (NOC)**	**Outcome met**

R — Recommendation Evaluate your nursing care and make recommendations related to the achievement of your desired outcomes. Were they met, or do new goals need to be established?		
1	Patient maintains adequate cardiac output, stable VS, good capillary refill, absence of dysrhythmias.	☐ **Yes** ☐ **No**
2	Patient verbalizes an increase in level of energy and displays an improved ability to participate in desired activities.	☐ **Yes** ☐ **No**
3	Patient demonstrates stable weight and normal laboratory values, without signs of malnutrition.	☐ **Yes** ☐ **No**
4	Patient reports anxiety reduced to a manageable level and identifies healthy ways to deal with feelings.	☐ **Yes** ☐ **No**
5	Patient maintains moist eye membranes, is free from ulcerations, and identifies measures to prevention of complications.	☐ **Yes** ☐ **No**

Nursing Diagnosis 1

Risk for decreased cardiac output related to alteration in heart rate, rhythm, conduction.

NIC:
1) Monitor blood pressure lying, sitting, standing, and note widening pulse pressure; **2)** Investigate reports of chest pain; **3)** Monitor EKG for heart rate and rhythm; **4)** Auscultate heart sounds for gallops, murmurs, or extra sounds; and **5)** Auscultate breath sounds for adventitious sounds such as crackles.

Nursing Diagnosis 2

Fatigue related to hypermetabolic state with increased energy requirements evidenced by emotional lability and irritability, lack of energy to maintain usual routine.

NIC:
1) Note the development of tachypnea, dyspnea, pallor, and cyanosis; **2)** Provide a quiet environment, cool room, decreased sensory stimuli, soothing colors, relaxing music; **3)** Provide calm diversional activities such as listening to the radio, reading; and **4)** Avoid discussing topics that may cause the patient to become upset.

Nursing Diagnosis 3

Risk for imbalanced nutrition: less than body requirements related to increased metabolism evidenced by increased calorie intake and loss of weight.

NIC:
1) Monitor daily food intake; weigh daily and report weight loss; **2)** Encourage the patient to eat small, frequent meals with increased protein, calories, carbohydrates, and vitamins; **3)** Encourage the patient to eat high-calorie snacks that are easy to digest; and **4)** Avoid foods that increase peristalsis such as tea, coffee, and highly seasoned foods.

Nursing Diagnosis 4

Anxiety related to hypermetabolic state and pseudocatecholamine effect of thyroid hormone evidenced by increased feelings of apprehension, shakiness, loss of control, panic.

NIC:
1) Observe behavior that indicates anxiety and note progression to a panic state; **2)** Monitor physical responses of palpitations, hyperventilation, and insomnia; **3)** Stay with patient during severe anxiety, remain calm, acknowledge fear; **4)** Discuss the reason for emotional lability with patient; and **5)** Reinforce that emotional control will return as drug therapy progresses.

Condition:
Hyperthyroidism (Graves' Disease, Thyrotoxicosis)
Age:

Link & Explain
• Nursing Interventions Classification (NIC)
• Laboratory and Diagnostic Procedures
• Medications

Nursing Diagnosis 5

Risk for impaired tissue integrity related to alterations of protective mechanism of closure of the eye.

NIC:
1) Encourage the use of dark glasses when awake; **2)** Tape the eyelids closed when resting or going to sleep; **3)** Elevate the head of the bed, and restrict salt intake to reduce tissue edema; **4)** Administer artificial tears; and **5)** Provide opportunity for the patient to discuss altered appearance and measures to enhance self-image.

Medications

a. Beta blockers: propranolol (Inderal), atenolol (Tenormin), pindolol (Visken) (treat symptoms such as tachycardia, tremors, and nervousness; propranolol inhibits the conversion of T4 to T3)

b. Thyroid hormone antagonist: propylthiouracil (PTU), methimazole (Tapazole) (block thyroid hormone synthesis and inhibit the conversion of T4 to T3; abrupt withdrawal may cause thyroid storm)

c. Oral iodine solution (Lugol's solution), potassium iodide (SSKI) (prevent the release of thyroid hormone from the gland; may exacerbate the disease)

d. Radioactive iodine therapy is the treatment of choice because it destroys the abnormal functioning gland tissue; results peak in 6–12 weeks)

Laboratory & Diagnostic Procedures

a. Thyroid-stimulating hormone (TSH)
b. Free Thyroxine (free T4, Total T3 and T4)
c. Radioactive iodine uptake (RAIU) scanning: measures size and function; hot spots represent areas of increased production, and cold spots indicate areas of decreased-functioning gland tissue
d.

CONDITION: Inflammatory Bowel Disease

PHYSIOLOGY: Inflammatory bowel disease is caused by an abnormal response of the immune system wherein the tissue damage is related to an overactive sustained inflammation.

Ulcerative colitis starts in the rectum and distal areas of the colon and spreads upward in the colon. The inflammation extends down to the mucosa and submucosa of the large intestine. Patients may have continuous symptoms or exacerbations and remissions. Symptoms include diarrhea, abdominal cramps, fever during attacks, and rectal bleeding. Complications include perforation and carcinoma after 10 years of diseased state. Ulcerative colitis can be cured with a total proctocolectomy because the disease affects only the colon.

Crohn's disease is found in any area of the alimentary tract from the mouth to the anus, although it is commonly found in the terminal ileum. Diseased portions between areas of normal bowel are sometimes called skip lesions. Ulcerations extend to all layers of the bowel (transmural), causing a cobblestone appearance. Symptoms include diarrhea, abdominal cramping, weight loss, and malabsorption problems. Complications include fistulas, strictures, anal abscesses, perforation, and risk for carcinoma of the small intestine is increased.

The onset for ulcerative colitis and Crohn's disease is from teenage years to middle 30s.

HANDOFF COMMUNICATION

S Situation	Assess what is currently happening in a short statement.	Patient presents as _____ VS: LOC:
B Background	Summarize important past assessment data for your patient here. Place lab results and medications on the concept map.	Age: Gender: Allergies: Fall Risk: Isolation:
A Assessment	Use the assessment data to complete your concept map.	**Nursing Diagnosis:** Place the Nursing Diagnoses in prioritized order on the concept map and add any needed for your specific patient. **Plan:** Place any further Nursing Interventions Classifications (NIC) needed on the map.

Implement Your Plan of Care

R Recommendation	Evaluate your nursing care and make recommendations related to the achievement of your desired outcomes. Were they met, or do new goals need to be established?	**EVALUATE YOUR CARE**	
		Diag **Nursing Outcomes Classification (NOC)**	**Outcome met**
		1 Patient reports pain is relieved or controlled. Patient appears relaxed and able to sleep and rest appropriately.	☐ Yes ☐ No
		2 Patient reports reduction in frequency of stools that returns to more normal stool consistency.	☐ Yes ☐ No
		3 Patient maintains adequate hydration with stable VS, good skin turgor, normal capillary refill, and appropriate urine output.	☐ Yes ☐ No
		4 Patient demonstrates progressive weight gain toward goal with normalization of laboratory values.	☐ Yes ☐ No
		5 Patient acknowledges own coping abilities and demonstrates necessary lifestyle changes to limit or prevent recurrent episodes.	☐ Yes ☐ No

Nursing Diagnosis 1

Acute pain related to hyperperistalsis, prolonged diarrhea, skin and tissue irritation, fistulas evidenced by reports of colicky, cramping abdominal pain; grimacing; guarding behaviors.

NIC:

1) Assess reports of abdominal cramping or pain, noting location, duration, and intensity (0–10 scale); **2)** Encourage patient to assume a position of comfort such as knees flexed; **3)** Administer 5-aminosalicylates, corticosteroids to relieve spasms and decrease inflammation; **4)** Observe for abdominal distention, increased temperature, and decreased blood pressure; and **5)** Keep rectal area clean and use a moisture barrier ointment. Provide sitz baths when appropriate.

Nursing Diagnosis 2

Diarrhea related to inflammation, irritation, or malabsorption of the bowel evidenced by increased bowel sounds; frequent, severe watery stools; abdominal cramping.

NIC:

1) Observe and record stool frequency, characteristics, and amount; **2)** Administer antidiarrheals to decrease GI motility; **3)** Identify foods and fluids that precipitate diarrhea, such as raw vegetables and fruits, whole-grain cereals, carbonated beverages, and milk products; **4)** Offer clear liquids hourly and avoid cold fluids; **5)** Keep environment quiet and calm; and **6)** Provide room deodorizers.

Nursing Diagnosis 3

Risk for deficient fluid volume related to excessive losses through diarrhea.

NIC:

1) Monitor I&O. Calculate 24-hour fluid balance and report intake less than output; **2)** Assess BP, peripheral pulses, and mucous membranes; **3)** Monitor laboratory values such as Hgb/Hct and electrolytes to determine hydration status; and **4)** Administer IV fluids as prescribed.

Nursing Diagnosis 4

Imbalanced nutrition less than body requirements related to malabsorption of nutrients evidenced by decreased subcutaneous fat and muscle mass, poor muscle tone, hyperactive bowel sounds, steatorrhea.

NIC:

1) Rest the bowel by keeping the patient on NPO status; **2)** Administer total parenteral nutrition (TPN) or enteral feeding as prescribed; **3)** Administer high-calorie, high-vitamin, high-protein, low-residue, lactose-free (if lactase deficient) diet; **4)** Allow meals to be unhurried and calm. Assess abdomen, noting presence and character of bowel sounds, abdominal distention, and reports of nausea; **5)** Provide frequent mouth care to sooth dry mucous membranes; **6)** Monitor laboratory values such as Hgb/Hct, electrolytes, prealbumin and albumin levels; and **7)** Weigh daily.

Condition:
Inflammatory Bowel Disease
Age:

Link & Explain
• Nursing Interventions Classification (NIC)
• Laboratory and Diagnostic Procedures
• Medications

Nursing Diagnosis 5

Ineffective coping related to multiple stressors, unpredictable nature of disease process, lack of support system evidenced by preoccupation with physical self, chronic worry, emotional stress, poor self-esteem.

NIC:

1) Determine outside stressors, such as family, relationships, social and work environment; **2)** Provide patient an opportunity to discuss how illness has affected relationships; **3)** Help patient identify individual effective coping skills; **4)** Provide active listening in a nonjudgmental manner; **5)** Provide uninterrupted rest periods; **6)** Encourage use of stress management skills, relaxation techniques, visualization, guided imagery, and deep breathing exercises; and **7)** Refer for counseling as needed.

Medications
a. Antidiarrheals, hematinics, and vitamins
b. 5-Aminosalicylates
c. Antimicrobials, steroids
d. Immunosuppressants, biological and targeted therapy

Laboratory & Diagnostic Procedures
a. Serum electrolytes, CBC, serum iron, prealbumin/albumin/total proteins.
b. Esophagogastroduodenoscopy or colonoscopy
c. MRI, CT scan
d. Stool specimens, rectal biopsy

CONDITION: Intestinal Obstruction

PHYSIOLOGY: Intestinal obstruction occurs when a blockage obstructs the normal flow of contents through the intestinal tract. Obstruction of the intestine causes the bowel to become vulnerable to ischemia. The intestinal mucosal barrier can be damaged, allowing intestinal bacteria to invade the intestinal wall and causing fluid exudation, which leads to hypovolemia and dehydration. About 7 liters of fluid per day is secreted into the small intestine and stomach and usually reabsorbed. During obstruction, however, fluid accumulates, causing abdominal distention and pressure on the mucosal wall, which can lead to peritonitis and perforation. Obstructions can be partial or complete. The most common type of intestinal obstruction of the small intestine from fibrous adhesions.

The patient's mortality depends on the type of lesion causing the small bowel obstruction (closed-loop or strangulated) and the time until diagnosis and treatment. When an early diagnosis is made, mortality is low, but if more than 75% of the small bowel is necrotic at the time of surgery, the mortality rate is 65%. Complications of intestinal obstruction include bacteremia, secondary infection, and metabolic alkalosis or acidosis. If it is left untreated, a complete intestinal obstruction can cause death within a few hours from hypovolemic or septic shock and vascular collapse.

The two major types of intestinal obstruction are mechanical and neurogenic (or nonmechanical). Neurogenic obstruction occurs primarily after manipulation of the bowel during surgery or with peritoneal irritation, pain of thoracolumbar origin, or intestinal ischemia. It is also caused by the effect of trauma or toxins on the nerves that regulate peristalsis, electrolyte imbalances, and neurogenic abnormalities such as spinal cord lesions. Mechanical obstruction of the bowel is caused by physical blockage of the intestine. Examples of mechanical obstruction include adhesions and strangulated hernias (usually associated with the small intestine), volvulus (twisting of the intestine) of the cecum or sigmoid, intussusception (telescoping of the bowel), strictures, fecal or barium impaction, carcinomas (usually associated with the large intestine), and foreign bodies such as gallstones and fruit pits.

HANDOFF COMMUNICATION

S Situation	Assess what is currently happening in a short statement.	Patient presents as _____ *Note any predisposing factors: surgery, especially abdominal surgery; radiation therapy; gallstones; Crohn's disease; diverticular disease; ulcerative colitis; or a family history of colorectal cancer.*
B Background	Summarize important past assessment data for your patient here. Place lab results and medications on the concept map.	**Age:** **Gender:** **Allergies:** **Fall Risk:** **Isolation:**
A Assessment	Use the assessment data to complete your concept map.	**Nursing Diagnosis:** Place the Nursing Diagnoses in prioritized order on the concept map and add any needed for your specific patient. **Plan:** Place any further Nursing Interventions Classifications (NIC) needed on the map.

Implement Your Plan of Care

		EVALUATE YOUR CARE		
	Evaluate your nursing care and make recommendations related to the achievement of your desired outcomes. Were they met, or do new goals need to be established?	**Diag**	**Nursing Outcomes Classification (NOC)**	**Outcome met**
R Recommendation		1	Patient demonstrates fluid and electrolyte balance with stable VS and balanced I&O.	☐ Yes ☐ No
		2	Patient appears relaxed and reports that pain is relieved or controlled.	☐ Yes ☐ No
		3	Patient experiences relief of nausea and vomiting.	☐ Yes ☐ No
		4	Patient is free from bowel necrosis or perforation.	☐ Yes ☐ No
		5	Patient verbalizes understanding of disease process, self-care, and plan for follow-up with the health-care provider.	☐ Yes ☐ No

Nursing Diagnosis 1

Fluid volume deficit related to third-space fluid shifts into bowel lumen and peritoneal cavity evidenced by nausea and vomiting.

NIC:
1) Maintain accurate I&O; **2)** Assess and report signs/symptoms of fluid/electrolyte imbalance; **3)** Administer potassium replacement after renal function is verified; **4)** Administer IV resuscitation with normal saline or lactated Ringer's solution; **5)** Monitor VS for symptoms of hypovolemic shock; **6)** Maintain patency of NG tube. Irrigate with saline rather than water if prescribed; and **7)** Assess for symptoms of fluid overload especially in the elderly patient.

Nursing Diagnosis 2

Acute pain related to abdominal distention and increased peristalsis evidenced by maintaining a fetal position and grimacing.

NIC:
1) Assess for abdominal guarding, rebound tenderness, and abdominal rigidity; **2)** Auscultate bowel sounds and report hyperactive, diminished, or absent sounds; **3)** Insert NG tube to decompress the abdomen; **4)** Elevate head of bed to semi-Fowler's to decrease pain from distended abdomen; and **5)** Medicate with analgesics as prescribed and evaluate effectiveness.

Nursing Diagnosis 3

Nausea related to irritation of somatic nerves evidenced by gagging sensation.

NIC:
1) Maintain NPO status in preparation for surgical intervention; **2)** Record color, consistency, amount of vomitus or drainage from NG tube; **3)** Monitor patency of NG tube to ensure drainage; and **4)** Provide frequent mouth care.

Nursing Diagnosis 4

Risk for infection related to necrosis/bowel perforation evidenced by increased WBCs and fever.

NIC:
1) Maintain gastric decompression via NG tube; **2)** Monitor VS, bowel sounds, and abdominal distention; **3)** Administer antimicrobials as prescribed; and **4)** Monitor WBCs and temperature. Assess for chills.

Condition:
Intestinal Obstruction

Age:

Link & Explain
• Nursing Interventions Classification (NIC)
• Laboratory and Diagnostic Procedures
• Medications

Nursing Diagnosis 5

Deficient knowledge regarding condition, therapeutic regimen, self-care, and discharge needs related to lack of exposure evidenced by statements regarding misconceptions.

NIC:
1) Discuss postop care/self-care: dressing changes, color and amount of drainage, monitor temperature, activity; **2)** Instruct regarding progressive diet management; **3)** Instruct the patient to report bowel elimination problems; **4)** Counsel patient to seek medical assistance for recurrent abdominal pain, fever, or vomiting; and **5)** Refer to social services, home care, and community support groups.

Medications

a. Broad spectrum antibiotics

b. Analgesics

c. Parenteral nutrition (if indicated)

d.

Laboratory & Diagnostic Procedures

a. Abdominal x-ray

b. CBC, serum electrolytes, BUN

c. Colonoscopy, sigmoidoscopy

d. Abdominal CT scan, abdominal ultrasound

CONDITION: Leukemia

PHYSIOLOGY: Leukemia is a malignant disorder of the blood and bone marrow characterized by the uncontrolled accumulation of white blood cells (WBCs). The production of normal blood cells decreases, which leads to anemia, thrombocytopenia, neutropenia. There is rapid growth of immature and ineffective WBCs, and accumulations occur in the bone marrow, blood, spleen, and liver.

Categories

Acute: WBCs proliferate rapidly and do not develop into mature cells. Types are acute myelogenous leukemia (AML), acute lymphocytic leukemia (ALL). Acute leukemias progress rapidly if untreated.

Chronic: there are few or no blast cells. Types are chronic myelogenous leukemia (CML), chronic lymphocytic leukemia (CLL). Chronic leukemias develop gradually and progress slowly.

HANDOFF COMMUNICATION

S Situation	Assess what is currently happening in a short statement.	Patient presents as _____ VS: LOC:
B Background	Summarize important past assessment data for your patient here. Place lab results and medications on the concept map.	**Age:**　　　　　　　　　　　　**Gender:** **Allergies:**　　　　　　　　　**Fall Risk:** **Isolation:**
A Assessment	Use the assessment data to complete your concept map.	**Nursing Diagnosis:** Place the Nursing Diagnoses in prioritized order on the concept map and add any needed for your specific patient. **Plan:** Place any further Nursing Interventions Classifications (NIC) needed on the map.

Implement Your Plan of Care

			EVALUATE YOUR CARE	
R Recommendation	Evaluate your nursing care and make recommendations related to the achievement of your desired outcomes. Were they met, or do new goals need to be established?	**Diag**	**Nursing Outcomes Classification (NOC)**	**Outcome met**
		1	Patient demonstrates a decrease in physiological signs of intolerance: pulse, respiration, and BP remain within patient's normal range.	☐ Yes ☐ No
		2	Patient reports pain is relieved or controlled.	☐ Yes ☐ No
		3	Patient maintains adequate fluid volume with stable VS and appropriate urine output.	☐ Yes ☐ No
		4	Patient identifies actions to prevent or reduce risk of infection.	☐ Yes ☐ No
		5	Patient verbalizes understanding of condition, disease process, and potential complications.	☐ Yes ☐ No

Nursing Diagnosis 1

Activity intolerance related to generalized weakness; reduced energy stores, increased metabolic rate from massive production of leukocytes evidenced by reports of fatigue.

NIC:
1) Encourage the patient to keep a diary of daily routines and energy levels, noting activities that need more energy; **2)** Recommend rest periods before meals; **3)** Suggest small, nutritious, high-protein meals and snacks throughout the day; and **4)** Administer blood and blood components.

Nursing Diagnosis 2

Acute pain related to chemical agents: antileukemic treatments evidenced by guarding or distracting behaviors, facial grimacing, alteration in muscle tone.

NIC:
1) Monitor VS and note nonverbal cues, such as muscle tension and restlessness; **2)** Provide a quiet environment and reduce stressful stimuli: noise, lighting, and constant interruptions; **3)** Place in a position of comfort, and support joints and extremities with pillows; and **4)** Provide comfort measures such as massage, cool packs, and psychological support.

Nursing Diagnosis 3

Risk for deficient fluid volume related to excessive losses: vomiting, hemorrhage, diarrhea.

NIC:
1) Monitor I&O, note decreased urine output; **2)** Monitor BP and heart rate; **3)** Evaluate skin turgor, capillary refill, and condition of mucous membranes; **4)** Note presence of nausea or fever; **5)** Encourage intake of 3–4 liters of fluid per day; **6)** Administer IV fluids as prescribed; and **7)** Monitor BUN, Hgb/Hct.

Nursing Diagnosis 4

Risk for infection related to inadequate secondary defenses: alterations in mature WBCs with low granulocyte and abnormal lymphocyte count, increased number of immature lymphocytes; immunosuppression, bone marrow suppression.

NIC:
1) Place in a private room using protective isolation precautions if needed. Screen and limit visitors. Prohibit use of live plants and flowers; **2)** Require good hand-washing techniques for all personnel and visitors; **3)** Monitor temperature and observe for tachycardia, hypotension, and subtle mental changes; **4)** Prevent chilling, force fluids, and administer tepid sponge baths; **5)** Auscultate breath sounds, noting crackles and rhonchi. Observe for changes in sputum; and **6)** Observe for cloudy, foul-smelling urine or presence of urgency and burning.

Condition:
Leukemia
Age:

- -
Link & Explain
• Nursing Interventions Classification (NIC)
• Laboratory and Diagnostic Procedures
• Medications

Nursing Diagnosis 5

Deficient knowledge regarding disease, prognosis, treatment, self-care, prevention of crisis, and discharge needs related to information misinterpretation, lack of recall evidenced by statement of misconception.

NIC:
1) Review type of leukemia and treatment options; **2)** Discuss side effects of treatment and solutions for weakness, nausea, vomiting, hair loss, bruising, mouth sores; **3)** Discuss sperm banking and pregnancy issues before treatment if in childbearing age; and **4)** Refer to community resources, support groups.

Medications
a. Colony-stimulating factors (CSFs): sargramostim (Leukine), filgrastim (Neupogen), and pegfilgrastim (Neulasta) (restore WBCs destroyed by chemotherapy and reduce the risk of infection)
b. Anti-infectives: ofloxacin (Ocuflox), rifampin (Rifadin) (treat infections, especially if the patient has a deficit in mature neutrophils)
c. Antiemetics 5-HT3 receptor antagonist drugs: ondansetron (Zofran), granisetron (Kytril) (relieve nausea and vomiting associated with chemotherapy agents)
d. Antigout medication: allopurinol (Zyloprim) (improves renal excretion of toxic by-products from the breakdown of leukemia cells)

Laboratory & Diagnostic Procedures
a. CBC: evaluates Hgb/Hct, RBC count, WBC count, platelets
b. Prothrombin time (PT)/activated partial prothromboplastin time (aPTT): determines bleeding and clotting time
c. Uric acid: waste product resulting from the breakdown of nitrogen-containing compounds; commonly elevated as a result of chemotherapy
d. Bone marrow aspiration/biopsy: determine the changes of number, size, and shape of blood cells to diagnose the type of anemia

CONDITION: Lung Cancer

PHYSIOLOGY: Lung cancer is a leading cause of cancer-related deaths among both men and women. Prognosis is generally poor with only 16% of lung cancers found at an early, localized stage when the 5-year survival rate is 49%. Approximately 80% of lung cancers are related to cigarette smoking or secondhand smoke. Other risk factors include exposure to carcinogenic materials (chemical or other occupational exposure, pollution, etc.). Specific treatment protocols and individual prognosis depend on the type, stage, and location of the cancer cells and the patient's general state of health.

There are two major types of lung cancer: *small cell lung cancer (SCLC)* and *non–small cell lung cancer (NSCLC)*.

SCLC (sometimes called small cell undifferentiated carcinoma or oat cell carcinoma) accounts for 13% of all lung cancers and is almost always caused by smoking. SCLC is characterized by small, round to oval cells, generally beginning in the neuroendocrine cells of the bronchoepithelium of the lungs. They multiply quickly and form large tumors that can spread to lymph nodes and other organs. At the time of diagnosis, approximately 70% have already metastasized, often to the brain.

NSCLC accounts for almost 87% of all lung cancers and includes three subtypes: squamous cell carcinoma, adenocarcinoma, and large cell undifferentiated carcinoma. Squamous cell carcinoma, also associated with smoking, tends to be located centrally near a bronchus. Adenocarcinoma is usually found in the outer region of the lung. One type of adenocarcinoma tends to produce a better prognosis than other types of lung cancer and is sometimes associated with areas of scarring. Large cell undifferentiated carcinoma starts in any part of the lung and grows and metastasizes quickly, resulting in poor prognosis.

The hilus of the lung, close to the large divisions of the bronchi, is the most frequent site of lung cancer. Abnormal cells divide and proliferate over time. As the cells grow into a carcinoma, the bronchial lining becomes irregular and uneven. The tumor may penetrate the lung wall and surrounding tissue or grow into the opening (lumen) of the bronchus. In more than 50% of patients, the tumor spreads into the lymph nodes and then into other organs.

Systemic effects of the lung tumor that are unrelated to metastasis may affect the endocrine, hematologic, neuromuscular, and dermatologic systems. These changes may cause connective tissue and vascular abnormalities referred to as paraneoplastic syndromes. Complications of lung cancer include emphysema, bronchial obstruction, atelectasis, pulmonary abscesses, pleuritis, bronchitis, and compression of the vena cava.

HANDOFF COMMUNICATION

S — Situation — Assess what is currently happening in a short statement.
Patient presents as _____
Include: type/stage/treatments and related side effects.

B — Background — Summarize important past assessment data for your patient here. Place lab results and medications on the concept map.
Age: | Gender:
Allergies: | Fall Risk:
Isolation:

A — Assessment — Use the assessment data to complete your concept map.
Nursing Diagnosis: Place the Nursing Diagnoses in prioritized order on the concept map and add any needed for your specific patient.
Plan: Place any further Nursing Interventions Classifications (NIC) needed on the map.

Implement Your Plan of Care

R — Recommendation — Evaluate your nursing care and make recommendations related to the achievement of your desired outcomes. Were they met, or do new goals need to be established?

EVALUATE YOUR CARE

Diag	Nursing Outcomes Classification (NOC)	Outcome met
1	Patient verbalizes an understanding of the disease process, diagnostic/treatment plan, and available resources for additional information and support.	☐ Yes ☐ No
2	Patient implements positive coping mechanisms and verbalizes reduction of fear/anxiety.	☐ Yes ☐ No
3	Patient experiences adequate respiratory function free of dyspnea, improved breath sounds, and pulse oximetry within normal range.	☐ Yes ☐ No
4	Patient prevents complications by early reporting and compliance with treatment.	☐ Yes ☐ No
5	Patient verbalizes relief of/or ability to tolerate pain; appears relaxed and comfortable.	☐ Yes ☐ No

Nursing Diagnosis 1

Deficient knowledge related to unfamiliarity with disease process, diagnostic evaluation, treatment regimen evidenced by request for information.

NIC:
1) Assess understanding of disease process and treatment options;
2) Identify and communicate community resources, additional sources of information and support; **3)** Discuss diagnostic evaluation procedures and staging classifications as indicated; **4)** Explain treatment regimen, treatment options, and provide related information; and **5)** Include family/support systems in informational sessions.

Nursing Diagnosis 2

Anxiety related to threat of death, pain, treatments, invasive procedures, unfamiliar environment, separation from support systems evidenced by sleeplessness and fatigue.

NIC:
1) Encourage verbalization of fears and concerns; **2)** Provide thorough explanation of care routines, diagnostic tests, and treatments; **3)** Encourage patient to use yoga, meditation, relaxation exercises, biofeedback; **4)** Assess patient's past experience of coping mechanisms/relaxation techniques; **5)** Offer to consult clergy or support services; and **6)** Include family members or support person in all aspects of care.

Nursing Diagnosis 3

Impaired respiratory function related to lung pathology associated with replacement of lung tissue by neoplastic cells evidenced by dyspnea and coughing.

NIC:
1) Monitor VS, breath sounds, pulse oximetry; **2)** Assess for signs/symptoms of impaired respiratory function (dyspnea, orthopnea, cough, confusion); **3)** Implement measures to improve respiratory status (positioning, pain control, breathing techniques, incentive spirometer); **4)** Maintain adequate hydration/implement measures to reduce thickening of secretions; and **5)** Administer mucolytics, bronchodilators, and corticosteroids as prescribed to help control shortness of breath; **6)** Assess for improved respiratory status after treatments such as stereotactic radiotherapy, bronchoscopic laser therapy, or airway stenting.

Nursing Diagnosis 4

Risk for ineffective protection related to cancer and/or side effects of medication and treatments.

NIC:
1) Obtain baseline physical and neurological assessment and monitor for changes from baseline; **2)** Provide bleeding precautions, assessment, screening, and related education; **3)** Institute infection control/protective isolation as needed; **4)** Monitor nutritional status: prealbumin, albumin, weight; **5)** Monitor for side effects/toxicity of treatments such as chemotherapy or targeted therapy; and **6)** Assess for decreased neutrophils, Hgb/Hct, hypercalcemia, symptoms of syndrome of inappropriate antidiuretic hormone hypersecretion (SAIDH) or Cushing's syndrome.

Condition:
Lung Cancer
Age:
_____
Link & Explain
• Nursing Interventions Classification (NIC)
• Laboratory and Diagnostic Procedures
• Medications

Nursing Diagnosis 5

Acute pain related to tumor and/or metastatic disease and/or treatment regimen evidenced by reports of discomfort, facial grimacing.

NIC:
1) Assess for severity and defining characteristics of pain; use pain scale; administer analgesics; **2)** Monitor effectiveness/side effects of pain relief therapies; **3)** Assess fears and concerns related to pain medication; **4)** Teach nonpharmacologic interventions for pain relief; and **5)** Provide ongoing assessment and early intervention for pain/side effects of treatment.

Medications

a. Chemotherapy
b. Radiation therapy
c. Molecular-targeted therapy
d. NSAIDs; opioid analgesics (short- and long-acting, transdermal); morphine, oxygen

Laboratory & Diagnostic Procedures

a. Diagnostics: chest x-ray, bronchoscopy, percutaneous needle biopsy, bone scan, aspiration/biopsy, CT/PET scans
b. Pulmonary function tests
c. CBC, platelet counts, liver function test and related lab studies indicative of metastasis
d. Medications as indicated for superimposed infection

CONDITION: Lymphoma

PHYSIOLOGY: Lymphoma is malignant growth involving the reticuloendothelial and lymphoid systems, resulting in accumulation of abnormal lymphocytes in lymph tissue–forming masses. It may travel to the lungs, GI tract, meninges, skin, and bones. The major site of lymphoid tissue are lymph nodes, spleen, thymus gland, adenoids, tonsils, digestive tract.

Categories of Lymphoma

1. *Hodgkin's lymphoma (HL):* slow, insidious onset; superficial lymphadenopathy in cervical, supraclavicular, or mediastinal nodes. It spreads in a predictable manner to lymph nodes via the lymphatic channels.
2. *Non-Hodgkin's lymphoma (NHL):* may be low-grade or aggressive lymphomas. Low-grade disease is more difficult to treat, whereas more aggressive disease is more responsive to therapy.

Treatment involves combinations of chemotherapy and sometimes radiation.

HANDOFF COMMUNICATION

S	**Situation**	Assess what is currently happening in a short statement.	Patient presents as _____ VS: LOC:
B	**Background**	Summarize important past assessment data for your patient here. Place lab results and medications on the concept map.	**Age:**　　　　　　　　　　　　　**Gender:** **Allergies:**　　　　　　　　　　 **Fall Risk:** **Isolation:**
A	**Assessment**	Use the assessment data to complete your concept map.	**Nursing Diagnosis:** Place the Nursing Diagnoses in prioritized order on the concept map and add any needed for your specific patient. **Plan:** Place any further Nursing Interventions Classifications (NIC) needed on the map.

Implement Your Plan of Care

			EVALUATE YOUR CARE	
R	**Recommendation**	Evaluate your nursing care and make recommendations related to the achievement of your desired outcomes. Were they met, or do new goals need to be established?	**Diag** / **Nursing Outcomes Classification (NOC)**	**Outcome met**
			1 Patient maintains a normal, effective respiratory pattern.	☐ Yes ☐ No
			2 Patient maintains an acceptable level of dietary intake to maintain weight.	☐ Yes ☐ No
			3 Patient identifies stressors in lifestyle that may contribute to the dysfunction.	☐ Yes ☐ No
			4 Patient identifies signs and symptoms of the disease process and treatment.	☐ Yes ☐ No
			5	☐ Yes ☐ No

Nursing Diagnosis 1

Risk for impaired gas exchange related to altered oxygen-carrying capacity of blood.

NIC:
1) Monitor respiratory rate, depth, rhythm, use of accessory muscles, nasal flaring, altered chest excursion, and pulse oximetry; **2)** Elevate head of bed to 45 degrees; **3)** Encourage the use of energy-saving techniques, rest periods before and after meals; **4)** Observe for neck vein distention, headache, dizziness, periorbital or facial edema, or stridor; and **5)** Administer supplemental oxygen and respiratory treatments as prescribed.

Nursing Diagnosis 2

Nausea related to chemotherapy agents; radiation therapy evidenced by report of nausea and gagging sensation.

NIC:
1) Monitor and record patient's food intake, have patient keep daily food diary; **2)** Weigh weekly and note decreases from previous weight; **3)** Recommend high-calorie, nutrient-rich meals that are small and spaced out throughout the day. Avoid high-fat or spicy foods. Encourage supplements between meals; **4)** Control environmental factors such as strong or noxious odors; and **5)** Adjust diet before and after treatments to provide foods such as crackers, toast, carbonated drinks.

Nursing Diagnosis 3

Sexual dysfunction related to altered body structure, disease process, radiation therapy evidenced by alteration in relationship with significant other.

NIC:
1) Identify preexisting and current stress factors that may be affecting the relationship; **2)** Discuss sperm banking and pregnancy issues if appropriate before beginning chemotherapy or radiation; **3)** Provide factual information about treatments and side effects; **4)** Encourage and accept expressions of concern, anger, grief, and fear; and **5)** Refer to appropriate community resources and support groups for sexual dysfunction.

Nursing Diagnosis 4

Deficient knowledge regarding condition, prognosis, treatment, self-care, prevention of crisis, and discharge needs related to unfamiliarity with information resources evidenced by inaccurate follow-through of instructions, development of preventable complications.

NIC:
1) Review with patient his/her understanding of diagnosis and prognosis; **2)** Provide information about potential treatment and side effects such as radiation, chemotherapy, stem cell transplant; **3)** Emphasize the need for ongoing medical follow-up; **4)** Stress importance of reporting symptoms such as cough, fever, chills, decreased energy level, dizziness, chest pain, syncope; and **5)** Recommend regular exercise in moderation with periods of rest.

Condition:
Lymphoma
Age:

Link & Explain
• Nursing Interventions Classification (NIC)
• Laboratory and Diagnostic Procedures
• Medications

Nursing Diagnosis 5

NIC:

Medications
a. Chemotherapy: ABVD regimen for Hodgkin's lymphoma—Adriamycin (doxorubicin), bleomycin, vinblastine, dacarbazine; (R-CHOP regimen for non-Hodgkin's lymphoma—rituximab, cyclophosphamide, doxorubicin hydrochloride, Oncovin, prednisone)
b. Interferons: interferon-alpha (INFa) (helps the body's natural defenses to attack the tumor)
c. Monoclonal antibodies: rituximab (Rituxan), alemtuzumab (Campath) (laboratory-made antibodies that can destroy lymphoma cells)
d. Histone deacetylase (HDAC) inhibitors: valproic acid (VPA), depsipeptide (romidepsin) (effective therapeutic anticancer agents)

Laboratory & Diagnostic Procedures
a. CBC: evaluates Hgb/Hct, RBC count, WBC count, platelets
b. Serum cytokines: interleukin receptors (IL6, IL10, IL2)—messenger chemicals released by T cells that mobilize other components of the immune system; correlates with prognosis
c. Serum lactate dehydrogenase (LDH): substance released by tumors, prognosis in NHL
d. CT scan, MRI, PET scan

CONDITION: Multiple Sclerosis

PHYSIOLOGY: Multiple sclerosis is demyelination of the brain and spinal cord, a chronic, progressive degenerative disorder of the CNS. It is characterized by disseminated demyelination of the nerve fibers of the brain and spinal cord. Underlying nerve fibers may also be damaged, which leads to permanent neurological damage. It is related to viral infections, immunological and genetic factors. Possible precipitating factors include infection, physical injury, emotional stress, excessive fatigue, pregnancy, and poor state of health. The disease results in various degrees of cognitive, motor, and sensory dysfunction. There are periods of remissions and exacerbations.

HANDOFF COMMUNICATION

S Situation	Assess what is currently happening in a short statement.	Patient presents as _____ VS: LOC:
B Background	Summarize important past assessment data for your patient here. Place lab results and medications on the concept map.	**Age:** **Gender:** **Allergies:** **Fall Risk:** **Isolation:**
A Assessment	Use the assessment data to complete your concept map.	**Nursing Diagnosis:** Place the Nursing Diagnoses in prioritized order on the concept map and add any needed for your specific patient. **Plan:** Place any further Nursing Interventions Classifications (NIC) needed on the map.

Implement Your Plan of Care

			EVALUATE YOUR CARE	
R Recommendation	Evaluate your nursing care and make recommendations related to the achievement of your desired outcomes. Were they met, or do new goals need to be established?	**Diag**	**Nursing Outcomes Classification (NOC)**	**Outcome met**
		1	Patient performs self-care activities within level of own ability.	☐ Yes ☐ No
		2	Patient identifies individual actions affecting fatigue and participates in recommended treatment plan.	☐ Yes ☐ No
		3	Patient verbalizes realistic view and acceptance of body and develops realistic plans for adapting to role changes.	☐ Yes ☐ No
		4	Patient demonstrates techniques to prevent urinary tract infection.	☐ Yes ☐ No
		5	Family verbalizes resources within themselves to deal with the situation. Family identifies resources available in the community. Family interacts appropriately with the patient and health-care providers to maintain support and assistance.	☐ Yes ☐ No

Nursing Diagnosis 1

Self-care deficit related to neuromuscular impairment evidenced by inability to perform tasks of self-care.

NIC:
1) Assess degree of functional impairment using a 0–4 scale; **2)** Provide assistive devices as needed, such as shower chair, elevated toilet seat with arm supports, specialized feeding utensils and drinking cups; **3)** Provide strategies to promote independent feeding; **4)** Allow sufficient time to perform tasks; **5)** Provide active or passive ROM exercises and massage; **6)** Encourage the use of medications, cold packs, splints, and footboards as indicated; and **7)** Administer medications to reduce spasticity and promote muscle relaxation.

Nursing Diagnosis 2

Fatigue related to physiological and emotional demands evidenced by inability to maintain usual routines, decreased performance.

NIC:
1) Identify factors influencing activity levels such as warm temperature, inadequate food intake, insomnia; **2)** Determine need for mobility aids such as walker, cane, wheelchair, scooter; **3)** Plan activities in the morning or with scheduled rest periods during the day; **4)** Stress need for stopping activity before fatigue develops; **5)** Administer CNS stimulants to reduce fatigue; and **6)** Administer antidepressants, tricyclic antidepressants, anticonvulsant medications as prescribed to reduce fatigue.

Nursing Diagnosis 3

Low self-esteem related to dependence and disruption in how patient perceives own body evidenced by denial, withdrawal, anger.

NIC:
1) Note behaviors indicating denial or excessive concern with disease process; **2)** Allow time for the patient to accept information; **3)** Provide an open environment for the patient and significant other to discuss concerns; **4)** Acknowledge the grieving process related to actual or perceived changes; **5)** Explain that labile emotions are common with the disease; and **6)** Note presence of depression, impaired thought process, expression of suicidal ideation.

Nursing Diagnosis 4

Impaired urinary elimination related to neurogenic bladder evidenced by incontinence, nocturia, and frequency.

NIC:
1) Note reports of urinary frequency, urgency, burning, incontinence, nocturia. Check bladder for residual urine; **2)** Utilize a bladder-training program; **3)** Encourage the patient to report foul odor, sediment in urine, fever, increased MS symptoms such as spasticity; **4)** Teach self-catheterization or use of indwelling catheter as needed; **5)** Obtain periodic urinalysis, culture, and sensitivity; and **6)** Administer anticholinergic drugs to decrease urinary frequency and urgency and anti-infective agents to treat bacterial infection.

Condition:
Multiple Sclerosis

Age:

Link & Explain
• Nursing Interventions Classification (NIC)
• Laboratory and Diagnostic Procedures
• Medications

Nursing Diagnosis 5

Compromised/disabled family coping related to prolonged disease and disability progression that exhausts the support system evidenced by neglectful care of patient.

NIC:
1) Note weight loss in a patient who is unable to prepare meals or feed self; **2)** Determine underlying cause if medical appointments are missed or prescriptions are not filled; **3)** Assess patient's skin to determine skin breakdown; **4)** Assess for dehydration; **5)** Provide referral to social services and home care.

Medications

a. Antiviral/antiparkinsonian: Symmetrel (amantadine) (manages fatigue)
b. CNS stimulants: methylphenidate (Ritalin) (manages fatigue)
c. Muscle relaxants: tizanidine (Zanaflex)/baclofen (Lioresal) (relieve spasticity)

d. Anticholinergics: propantheline (Pro-Banthine)/oxybutynin (Ditropan) (relieve urinary frequency and urgency)

Laboratory & Diagnostic Procedures

a. MRI: detects characteristic plaques in the brain related to nerve sheath demyelination
b. Magnetic resonance spectroscopy (MRS): decreased brain chemical N-acetyl aspartate can indicate nerve damage
c. Magnetization transfer imaging (MTI): detects white matter abnormalities before lesions can be seen on MRI
d. Lumbar puncture: detects oligoclonal bands (OCBs) found in 85% of patients with MS

CONDITION: Myasthenia Gravis

PHYSIOLOGY: Myasthenia gravis is an autoimmune disease in which antibodies attack acetycholine (ACh) receptors, which decreases the ACh receptor sites at the neuromuscular junction. Fluctuations of musculoskeletal weakness can cause the following: difficulty in movement of the eyes, ptosis (drooping of the eyelids), diplopia (double vision), dysphagia (difficulty chewing or swallowing), and weakened voice. In advanced cases, all muscles become weak, including those associated with respiratory function and bowel as well as bladder control. The symptoms are known to exacerbate with emotional stress, extremes in temperature, pregnancy, or other illnesses. This illness is three times more common in women than in men.

Myasthenia crisis is an exacerbation of muscle weakness, which may require mechanical ventilation resulting from respiratory insufficiency.

Tumors of the thymus gland may also occur in these patients. Eaton-Lambert syndrome is a form of myasthenia gravis in which the patient also has small cell carcinoma of the lung.

HANDOFF COMMUNICATION

S	Situation	Assess what is currently happening in a short statement.	Patient presents as _____
B	Background	Summarize important past assessment data for your patient here. Place lab results and medications on the concept map.	**Age:** **Gender:** **Allergies:** **Fall Risk:** **Isolation:**
A	Assessment	Use the assessment data to complete your concept map.	**Nursing Diagnosis:** Place the Nursing Diagnoses in prioritized order on the concept map and add any needed for your specific patient. **Plan:** Place any further Nursing Interventions Classifications (NIC) needed on the map.

Implement Your Plan of Care

		EVALUATE YOUR CARE	
R	Recommendation Evaluate your nursing care and make recommendations related to the achievement of your desired outcomes. Were they met, or do new goals need to be established?	**Diag** / **Nursing Outcomes Classification (NOC)**	**Outcome met**
		1 Patient maintains stable weight with laboratory results within normal limits.	☐ Yes ☐ No
		2 Patient maintains adequate ventilation as evidenced by absence of respiratory distress, ABGs within acceptable limits, and pulse oximetry maintained at 90% or greater.	☐ Yes ☐ No
		3 Patient establishes method of communication in which needs can be expressed.	☐ Yes ☐ No
		4 Patient demonstrates behaviors to compensate for, or overcome, deficits.	☐ Yes ☐ No
		5 Patient verbalizes understanding of changes and acceptance of self in the situation.	☐ Yes ☐ No

Nursing Diagnosis 1

Imbalanced nutrition: less than body requirements related to impaired swallowing evidenced by 10% weight loss.

NIC:
1) Assess ability to chew and swallow during meals; **2)** Schedule drug administration so effects peak at meals; **3)** Encourage patient to sit up straight in the chair for meals and concentrate when swallowing with chin slightly down to prevent aspiration; **4)** Assist patient with food choices that are nutritious and easy to chew and swallow; **5)** Maintain suction equipment at bedside; **6)** Assess abdomen, noting presence and character of bowel sounds, abdominal distention, and reports of nausea; **7)** Provide small, more frequent meals during the day; **8)** Provide enough time for patient to eat meals; and **9)** Weigh daily.

Nursing Diagnosis 2

Risk for ineffective breathing pattern related to weakness of muscles associated with respiratory function.

NIC:
1) Auscultate breath sounds. Note areas of absent or diminished breath sounds; **2)** Note strength and effectiveness of cough; **3)** Assess skin color, respiratory rate, depth and use of accessory muscles; **4)** Monitor pulse oximetry and ABGs; **5)** Provide supplemental oxygen depending on ABG results: nasal cannula, Venturi mask, nonrebreather mask, or mechanical ventilation if indicated; and **6)** Assist with coughing, turning, and deep breathing. Encourage the use of incentive spirometry.

Nursing Diagnosis 3

Impaired verbal communication related to muscular weakness of the jaw and pharynx evidenced by impaired articulation: soft speech or cannot speak.

NIC:
1) Keep communication simple. Provide questions that can be answered with a short response; **2)** Provide alternative methods of communication as appropriate: slate board, letter-and-picture board, especially if mechanical ventilation is necessary; **3)** Anticipate needs as much as possible; **4)** Place call bell within reach, respond to call promptly; and **5)** Recognize frustration with inability to communicate needs. Allow time for patient to provide information.

Nursing Diagnosis 4

Disturbed sensory perception (visual) related to impairment in extraocular muscles and ptosis evidenced by reported change in sensory acuity.

NIC:
1) Observe behavioral response such as hostility, crying, inappropriate affect, agitation; **2)** Eliminate extraneous noise and stimuli; speak in a calm, quiet voice; **3)** Evaluate visual deficit and presence of diplopia. Patch one eye for diplopia; and **4)** Validate patient's perception and reorient frequently.

Condition:
Myasthenia Gravis

Age:

Link & Explain
• Nursing Interventions Classification (NIC)
• Laboratory and Diagnostic Procedures
• Medications

Nursing Diagnosis 5

Disturbed body image/chronic low self-esteem related to uncertainty of prognosis, change in role function evidenced by feelings of hopelessness, helplessness, or powerlessness.

NIC:
1) Discuss situation and verbalization of fears; **2)** Explain relationship between nature of disease and symptoms; **3)** Encourage family to verbalize feelings and participate in care; **4)** Support and encourage patient, maintain a positive attitude; and **5)** Refer to support services such as counselors, psychiatric resources, social services.

Medications

a. Anticholinesterase agents

b. Corticosteroids

c. Immunosuppressive agents

d.

Laboratory & Diagnostic Procedures

a. EMG, Tensilon test, acetylcholine receptor antibodies

b. Plasmapheresis

c. Thymectomy

d.

CONDITION: Obstructive Sleep Apnea

PHYSIOLOGY: Sleep apnea is a pause in the breathing pattern that lasts at least 10 seconds and occurs a minimum of five times an hour. The most frequently occurring type is obstructive sleep apnea, in which upper airway is blocked, preventing airflow to the lungs. The blockage may be related to relaxation of the soft tissues of the palate, tongue, and neck, as well as large tonsils and adenoids or abnormal anatomy of the bony structures surrounding the airway. Contributing factors are central obesity, male gender, age over 40, use of alcohol or other sedatives before sleep, supine sleeping position, and African American or Hispanic ethnicity. Signs and symptoms of sleep apnea include daytime sleepiness despite full nights of sleep, irritability, fatigue, confusion, depression, headache, poor judgment, personality changes, snoring, tossing and turning while sleeping, and falling asleep during the day at inappropriate times. Problems arise from sleep apnea due to the disturbed sleep cycle and lack of REM (deep) sleep, which prevent adequate rest. Chronic complications that may be related to obstructive sleep apnea include chronic hypoxia and hypercapnia, pulmonary hypertension and cor pulmonale, systemic hypertension, and atherosclerotic vascular disease. In addition, many chronic conditions, such as diabetes, chronic obstructive pulmonary disease, heart failure, hypothyroidism, atrial fibrillation, and cerebrovascular disease are related to sleep apnea (*Taber's*, 2009).

HANDOFF COMMUNICATION

S	Situation	Assess what is currently happening in a short statement.	Patient presents as _____ *Perform a health history, focusing on patient's sleep patterns and daytime symptoms. Include family member who may witness sleep pattern disturbances and apnea. Question patient and family about snoring at night and periods of apnea.*
B	Background	Summarize important past assessment data for your patient here. Place lab results and medications on the concept map.	**Age:** **Gender:** **Allergies:** **Fall Risk:** **Isolation:**
A	Assessment	Use the assessment data to complete your concept map.	**Nursing Diagnosis:** Place the Nursing Diagnoses in prioritized order on the concept map and add any needed for your specific patient. **Plan:** Place any further Nursing Interventions Classifications (NIC) needed on the map.

Implement Your Plan of Care

		EVALUATE YOUR CARE		
R	Recommendation	Evaluate your nursing care and make recommendations related to the achievement of your desired outcomes. Were they met, or do new goals need to be established?	**Diag**	**Nursing Outcomes Classification (NOC)**	**Outcome met**
			1	Patient experiences fewer periods of apnea and awakes more rested.	☐ Yes ☐ No
			2	Patient demonstrates new knowledge and incorporates it into a health regimen.	☐ Yes ☐ No
			3	Patient verbalizes understanding of weight loss strategies and incorporates them into health regimen.	☐ Yes ☐ No
			4	Patient verbalizes and demonstrates energy conservation activities and reports less fatigue.	☐ Yes ☐ No
			5	Patient demonstrates effective breathing pattern that supports adequate gas exchange and rest.	☐ Yes ☐ No

Nursing Diagnosis 1

Disturbed sleep pattern related to obstructed airway while asleep evidenced by excessive daytime sleepiness, inability to concentrate.

NIC:
1) Assess sleep patterns as they occur in normal environment; 2) Assess patient's perception of sleep difficulties and possible relief measures; 3) Encourage patient to follow consistent daily schedule, including sleep preparation activities; 4) Discourage daytime naps and encourage increased daytime activity; 5) Assist patient in identifying nonpharmacologic sleep enhancement techniques; 6) Discourage use of soporific sleep aids, which may increase the obstruction; and 7) Encourage use of prescribed CPAP/BiPAP.

Nursing Diagnosis 2

Deficient knowledge related to inaccurate information evidenced by statements of concern.

NIC:
1) Include patient and family as part of the collaborative health-care team when determining learning needs and goals; 2) Assess patient's ability to learn, learning styles, and preferences; 3) Utilize strategies that support patient's needs and preferences; 4) Provide information to promote self-management; 5) Use a combination of methods to present materials; and 6) Reinforce learning through follow-up and reassess learning needs routinely.

Nursing Diagnosis 3

Impaired nutrition: more than body requirements related to excessive intake, metabolic needs evidenced by 10%–20% above ideal weight for height and frame.

NIC:
1) Assess weight daily using same scale at the same time of day; 2) Perform nutritional assessment; 3) Assess patient's and family's knowledge regarding nutritional needs; 4) Provide education based on patient's needs and knowledge level, including information on nutritional needs, reading nutritional labels, portion-size control; 5) Assist patient in establishing short- and long-term goals; 6) Encourage increased activity and exercise; and 7) Provide positive reinforcement and encouragement.

Nursing Diagnosis 4

Fatigue related to sleep deprivation evidenced by lack of energy, inability to maintain usual routine.

NIC:
1) Assess patient's level of fatigue and impact on daily life; 2) Assess patient's perception of causes of fatigue and willingness to participate in interventions to help decrease fatigue; 3) Educate patient and family regarding possible causes of fatigue and interventions to prevent exacerbation; 4) Assist patient in scheduling daily activities to decrease fatigue; and 5) Help patient determine priorities for activities and determine activities that can be delegated.

Condition:
Obstructive Sleep Apnea
Age:

Link & Explain
• Nursing Interventions Classification (NIC)
• Laboratory and Diagnostic Procedures
• Medications

Nursing Diagnosis 5

Ineffective breathing pattern related to upper airway obstruction evidenced by hypoxemia and hypercapnia.

NIC:
1) Assess duration and frequency of apneic episodes through questioning of patient and family and through ordered diagnostic testing; 2) Assist the patient in identifying factors that may exacerbate sleep apnea, such as sleep positions, poor sleep hygiene, use of alcohol, obesity; 3) Assess patient's compliance with plan of treatment; 4) Explain the function of CPAP or BiPAP to minimize airway obstruction; and 5) Encourage self-management, including use of CPAP or BiPAP.

Medications
a.
b.
c.
d.

Laboratory & Diagnostic Procedures
a. Sleep studies
b. CBC, chemistries, ABGs
c. Chest x-ay
d.

CONDITION: Osteoarthritis (Degenerative Joint Disease)

PHYSIOLOGY: Osteoarthritis is characterized by chronic pain with deterioration of one or more joints. Loss of cartilage usually occurs in weight-bearing joints such as the hips and knees and may also involve the hands. As the cartilage and bone erode, the joint space becomes narrower. Complications such as bone cysts, inflammation of synovial fluid, subluxation, and deformities occur. The patient may also have crepitus (grating sound during ROM); Heberden nodes, which are located at the distal interphalangeal joint; and Bouchard's nodes, which are located at the proximal interphalangeal joint.

Risk factors for osteoarthritis are smoking, obesity, occupations that require repetitive stress to the joints, and trauma to the joint. It is more common in women 60 years of age or older than in men and younger women.

The patient has symptoms of immobility, pain, muscle spasms, and inflammation of the joint, which diminishes with rest and becomes more intense after activity.

HANDOFF COMMUNICATION

S	Situation	Assess what is currently happening in a short statement.	Patient presents as _____
B	Background	Summarize important past assessment data for your patient here. Place lab results and medications on the concept map.	**Age:** **Gender:** **Allergies:** **Fall Risk:** **Isolation:**
A	Assessment	Use the assessment data to complete your concept map.	**Nursing Diagnosis:** Place the Nursing Diagnoses in prioritized order on the concept map and add any needed for your specific patient. **Plan:** Place any further Nursing Interventions Classifications (NIC) needed on the map.

Implement Your Plan of Care

		EVALUATE YOUR CARE	
	Evaluate your nursing care and make recommendations related to the achievement of your desired outcomes. Were they met, or do new goals need to be established?	**Diag** / **Nursing Outcomes Classification (NOC)**	**Outcome met**
R Recommendation		**1** Patient reports pain is controlled. Patient sleeps without interruption and participates in daily activities.	☐ Yes ☐ No
		2 Patient demonstrates techniques that enable resumption and continuation of therapy.	☐ Yes ☐ No
		3 Patient verbalizes increased confidence in ability to deal with illness and change in lifestyle.	☐ Yes ☐ No
		4 Patient demonstrates behaviors that enable self-care activities.	☐ Yes ☐ No
		5 Patient progresses toward weight goal with normalization of laboratory values.	☐ Yes ☐ No

Nursing Diagnosis 1

Chronic pain related to inflammation of the joint evidenced by guarding, distraction behaviors, or restlessness.

NIC:
1) Observe and document location, severity (0–10 scale), characteristics of pain (steady, intermittent); **2)** Provide heat therapy, which decreases muscle tension around the joint, or provide cold therapy, which numbs nerve endings and decreases joint inflammation; **3)** Encourage use of relaxation techniques such as guided imagery, massage, and visualization. Provide diversional activities; **4)** Immobilize by applying a splint or brace if indicated; **5)** Administer medication for pain as needed; and **6)** Note response to medication, report if pain is not relieved.

Nursing Diagnosis 2

Impaired physical mobility related to weakness, stiffness, and pain with ambulation evidenced by reluctance to attempt movement.

NIC:
1) Maintain bedrest, chair rest as indicated; **2)** Schedule activity or procedures between rest periods. Provide analgesics prior to participation in ADL; **3)** Provide or assist with passive and active ROM exercises; **4)** Discuss use of mobility aids such as cane, walker, wheelchair; **5)** Reposition frequently while in bed; and **6)** Collaborate with physical therapist regarding exercise program.

Nursing Diagnosis 3

Disturbed body image related to changes in ability to perform usual tasks evidenced by change in social involvement, sense of isolation.

NIC:
1) Encourage verbalization about disease process; **2)** Ascertain how patient views self in usual lifestyle functioning; **3)** Accept feelings of grief, hostility, and dependency; and **4)** Set limits on maladaptive behavior, assist patient to identify positive behaviors to aid in coping.

Nursing Diagnosis 4

Self-care deficit related to decreased strength and endurance, pain on movement evidenced by inability to manage ADL.

NIC:
1) Use the Functional Level Classification 0 to 4 to assess exacerbation of illness; **2)** Use shower chair, grab bars, and spray attachment as needed; **3)** Utilize supportive slip-on shoes and remove scatter rugs; **4)** Assess the need for an elevated toilet seat; and **5)** Arrange for other agencies such as Meals on Wheels and home-care services.

Condition:
Osteoarthritis (Degenerative Joint Disease)

Age:

Link & Explain
• Nursing Interventions Classification (NIC)
• Laboratory and Diagnostic Procedures
• Medications

Nursing Diagnosis 5

Imbalanced nutrition: more than body requirements related to sedentary activity level evidenced by weight 10% above ideal for body height and frame.

NIC:
1) Perform initial nutritional assessment: height, weight, BMI, ability to feed self, eating preferences; **2)** Evaluate activity pattern; **3)** Monitor caloric intake; **4)** Provide balanced diet with appropriate protein, complex carbohydrates, and calories; **5)** Encourage an increase in fruits and vegetables; **6)** Discuss the need to eat baked or broiled instead of fried foods; and **7)** Encourage the use of spices instead of adding sodium to the meal.

Medications

a. Ibuprofen (Motrin), acetaminophen (Tylenol), lidocaine 5% patches

b. Hyaluronate (Hyalgan), hylan G-F 20 (Synvisc)

c.

d.

Laboratory & Diagnostic Procedures

a. Erythrocyte sedimentation rate (ESR), high-sensitivity C-reactive protein, x-rays, MRI

b. Treatments: paraffin dip, diathermy (electric current), ultrasonography (sound waves), acupuncture, acupressure

c.

d.

CONDITION: Osteoporosis

PHYSIOLOGY: Osteoporosis is a disease in which the bones become less dense due to demineralization. The result of this decrease in density is increased risk for fractures. Bones are constantly undergoing a process called "remodeling," in which bone building (osteoblastic activity) and bone reabsorption (osteoclastic activity) are taking place at a similar rate. With osteoporosis, the rate of bone resorption exceeds the rate of bone building, which decreases the bone density. This problem could be caused either by decreased osteoblastic activity due to decreased efficiency or life span of osteoblasts (bone-forming cells) or by an increase in osteoblastic activity while osteoclastic activity remains static.

Osteoporosis may occur in many structures of the skeleton (generalized osteoporosis) or in a limb that has been immobilized for a period of time greater than 8–12 weeks (regional osteoporosis). Generalized osteoporosis is further divided into primary and secondary osteoporosis. Primary osteoporosis occurs in men and postmenopausal women, usually around age 60 to 70. It is most common in women and is thought to be caused by the decreased estrogen level that occurs after menopause, as estrogen prevents or decreases the rate of bone resorption. In men, it is caused by decreased testosterone levels and ability to absorb calcium, resulting in a slow loss of bone mass. Secondary osteoporosis is caused by an associated medical condition, such as hyperparathyroidism, long-term corticosteroid use, or prolonged immobilization. The treatment for secondary osteoporosis differs in that it is based on treatment of the primary condition. The exact cause of primary osteoporosis is unknown.

The best defense against this disease is building strong bones as a young person. In addition, other factors such as body build, exercise, protein deficiency, alcohol consumption, cigarette smoking, eating disorders, and diet may contribute to the incidence of this disease. About 80% of women are affected by osteoporosis, whereas only 20% of men are affected. Persons of all ethnic backgrounds are at risk. Osteoporosis is diagnosed based on a standard T-score obtained using dual-energy x-ray absorptiometry. This score compares the patient's bone density to that of the average bone mineral density (BMD) of young, healthy white women. A T-score between 1 and 2.5 standard deviations below the average indicates osteopenia, and a T-score of more than 2.5 standard deviations below the average indicates osteoporosis.

Treatment includes medication such as hormone replacement therapy, calcium and vitamin D supplements, parathyroid hormone (stimulates new bone formation), bisphosphonates (inhibit bone resorption), and calcitonin (inhibits osteoclastic activity). Other lifestyle changes include posture strengthening and weight-bearing exercises, diet modifications, pain management, and the use of orthotic devices (*Taber's*, 2009).

HANDOFF COMMUNICATION

S	Situation	Assess what is currently happening in a short statement.	Patient presents as _____
B	Background	Summarize important past assessment data for your patient here. Place lab results and medications on the concept map.	**Age:** **Gender:** **Allergies:** **Fall Risk:** **Isolation:**
A	Assessment	Use the assessment data to complete your concept map.	**Nursing Diagnosis:** Place the Nursing Diagnoses in prioritized order on the concept map and add any needed for your specific patient. **Plan:** Place any further Nursing Interventions Classifications (NIC) needed on the map.

Implement Your Plan of Care

		EVALUATE YOUR CARE	
		Diag / **Nursing Outcomes Classification (NOC)**	**Outcome met**
R	Recommendation Evaluate your nursing care and make recommendations related to the achievement of your desired outcomes. Were they met, or do new goals need to be established?	**1** Patient increases physical activity by taking a 30-minute walk three times per week.	☐ Yes ☐ No
		2 Patient expresses a decrease in level of pain on the 0–10 numeric pain rating scale.	☐ Yes ☐ No
		3 Patient explains methods to prevent injury and remains free of falls in the future.	☐ Yes ☐ No
		4 Patient describes integration of therapeutic regimen into daily living prior to discharge.	☐ Yes ☐ No
		5	☐ Yes ☐ No

Nursing Diagnosis 1

Impaired physical mobility related to skeletal weakness evidenced by immobility or decreased mobility.

NIC:
1) Assess the patient's current level of activity, including types of activities and duration; **2)** Consult with physical therapist for further evaluation, strength training, gait training, and development of a mobility plan; **3)** Obtain any necessary assistive devices for activity, such as gait belt, walker, cane, or wheelchair; **4)** For an immobile patient, perform passive ROM exercises; and **5)** Increase independence in ADL.

Nursing Diagnosis 2

Acute pain related to fracture evidenced by verbal and nonverbal communication of distress.

NIC:
1) Assess and document characteristics of the pain, such as onset, location, duration, aggravating and relieving factors, and severity; **2)** Assess pain intensity using 0–10 numeric pain rating scale; **3)** Establish an acceptable comfort goal with the patient; **4)** Determine the patient's current medication use; **5)** Explore the need for opioid and nonopioid analgesics; and **6)** Discuss nonpharmacologic pain treatments with the patient, such as massage therapy, reading, watching television, and guided imagery.

Nursing Diagnosis 3

Risk for falls related to decreased activity, skeletal weakness.

NIC:
1) Determine the risk for falls using an evaluation tool such as the Fall Risk Assessment; **2)** Evaluate the patient's medications to determine if they increase the risk of falling; **3)** Orient the patient to the environment, place call light within reach, and advise to ask for assistance; **4)** Teach the patient what to do if he/she falls and is unable to get up. Recommend an emergency response system; and **5)** Ensure that the patient has properly fitted shoes for ambulation.

Nursing Diagnosis 4

Readiness for enhanced knowledge related to disease management and lifestyle changes evidenced by questions.

NIC:
1) Provide knowledge as needed related to the pathophysiology of the disease or illness, recommended activities, medication regimen, and nutrition; **2)** Stress the importance of decreased alcohol consumption and smoking cessation (or continued abstinence), as these behaviors promote acidosis, leading to increased bone loss; and **3)** Stress the importance of exercise, and collaborate on a realistic exercise regimen for the patient.

Condition:
Osteoporosis
Age:

- - - - - - - - - - - -
Link & Explain
• Nursing Interventions Classification (NIC)
• Laboratory and Diagnostic Procedures
• Medications

Nursing Diagnosis 5

NIC:

Medications

a. Hormone replacement therapy and estrogen receptor modulators

b. Parathyroid hormone

c. Calcium and vitamin D supplements

d. Bisphosphonates and calcitonin

Laboratory & Diagnostic Procedures

a. Dual-energy x-ray absorptiometry (DEXA) and T-score

b. Serum calcium, vitamin D, phosphorus, and alkaline phosphate levels

c. Qualitative ultrasound (QUS) of the heel or calcaneus

d.

CONDITION: Paget's Disease of the Bone (Osteitis Deformans)

PHYSIOLOGY: Paget's disease results in the disorganization of bone structure because the bone is broken down and reformed, resulting in weak, deformed bones. The patient usually has a history of pathological fractures and bone pain. Assessment findings may include bowing of long bones, arthritis at the joints, enlargement of vertebrae, kyphosis or scoliosis of the spine, unsteady waddling gait, and enlarged skull.

The increased size and thickness of the skull places pressure on the cranial nerves and can result in deafness, vertigo, diminished vision, impaired swallowing, and changes in speech. Bones may also develop malignancy such as osteosarcoma; therefore, severe pain needs to be investigated thoroughly. Although it is uncommon, an increase in serum and urinary calcium may result in some cases from hyperparathyroidism and gout. Increased calcium levels may also be attributed to immobility. Calcium deposits occur in joint spaces and/or as stones in the urinary tract.

Treatment may include braces or surgical intervention to stabilize spine or replace joints.

HANDOFF COMMUNICATION

S	Situation	Assess what is currently happening in a short statement.	Patient presents as _____
B	Background	Summarize important past assessment data for your patient here. Place lab results and medications on the concept map.	**Age:** **Gender:** **Allergies:** **Fall Risk:** **Isolation:**
A	Assessment	Use the assessment data to complete your concept map.	**Nursing Diagnosis:** Place the Nursing Diagnoses in prioritized order on the concept map and add any needed for your specific patient. **Plan:** Place any further Nursing Interventions Classifications (NIC) needed on the map.

Implement Your Plan of Care

		EVALUATE YOUR CARE	
	Evaluate your nursing care and make recommendations related to the achievement of your desired outcomes. Were they met, or do new goals need to be established?	**Diag** / **Nursing Outcomes Classification (NOC)**	**Outcome met**
R Recommendation		**1** Patient displays relaxed manner, participates in activities, and sleeps and rests appropriately.	☐ Yes ☐ No
		2 Patient demonstrates techniques that enable resumption of activities, especially activities of daily living.	☐ Yes ☐ No
		3 Patient verbalizes understanding of changes and acceptance of self in the situation.	☐ Yes ☐ No
		4 Patient demonstrates behaviors that enable continuation of activities.	☐ Yes ☐ No
		5 Patient verbalizes understanding of condition, prognosis, and treatment.	☐ Yes ☐ No

Nursing Diagnosis 1

Acute/chronic pain related to weakened bones evidenced by self-focus, facial mask of pain.

NIC:
1) Observe and document location, severity (0–10 scale), characteristics of pain (continuous, intermittent); 2) Determine activities that increase the severity of pain; 3) Provide comfort measures such as back rub and repositioning; 4) Encourage use of relaxation techniques such as guided imagery and visualization. Provide diversional activities; 5) Discuss necessity of a firm mattress and small pillow under neck; 6) Teach body mechanics; 7) Administer medication for pain as needed; and 8) Note response to medication, report if pain is not relieved.

Nursing Diagnosis 2

Impaired physical mobility related to musculoskeletal impairment, pain or discomfort evidenced by inability to move purposefully within the physical environment, imposed restrictions.

NIC:
1) Determine degree of functional ability using a 0–4 scale. Note patient's perception of immobility; 2) Encourage participation in diversional activities; 3) Instruct patient while assisting with passive or active ROM exercises; 4) Encourage self-care activities such as bathing, shaving, and oral hygiene; 5) Assist with mobility with the use of wheelchair, walker, crutches, cane as needed; 6) Assist with application of corset or brace prior to ambulation; and 7) Increase fiber and roughage in the diet.

Nursing Diagnosis 3

Disturbed body image/chronic low self-esteem related to uncertainty of prognosis, change in role function evidenced by feelings of hopelessness, helplessness, or powerlessness.

NIC:
1) Discuss situation and verbalization of fears; 2) Explain relationship between nature of disease and symptoms; 3) Allow family to verbalize feelings and participate in care; 4) Encourage patient to maintain a positive attitude; and 5) Refer to support services such as counselors, psychiatric resources, social services.

Nursing Diagnosis 4

Risk for falls related to excessive bone resorption.

NIC:
1) Perform initial and ongoing falls risk assessment, including gait and balance, history, cognition, use of mobility aids; 2) Provide supportive, well-fitting shoes; 3) Encourage use of handrails in bathrooms and hallway. Use shower chair and spray attachment as needed; 4) Keep areas well lighted; 5) Encourage patient to use glasses and hearing aids if necessary; and 6) Discuss the need for alterations to the home environment such as removing throw rugs and clutter, allowing open space for ambulation, using night lights, keeping pets from area when patient is walking.

Condition:
Paget's Disease of the Bone (Osteitis Deformans)

Age:

Link & Explain
• Nursing Interventions Classification (NIC)
• Laboratory and Diagnostic Procedures
• Medications

Nursing Diagnosis 5

Deficient knowledge regarding condition, prognosis, treatment, self-care, and discharge needs related to information misinterpretation evidenced by verbalization of problems, statement of misconception.

NIC:
1) Review disease process, surgical procedures if indicated, and prognosis; 2) Instruct patient about safety, use of assistive devices for ambulation, need for environmental changes to ensure safety, home exercises; and 3) Discuss medications' action, schedule, and side effects.

Medications

a. Ibuprofen (Motrin), alendronate (Fosamax), risedronate (Actonel)

b. Pamidronate (Aredia), zoledronic acid (Reclast)

c. Calcitonin, plicamycin (Mithracin)

d. Salmon cacitonin (Calcimar)

Laboratory & Diagnostic Procedures

a. Serum alkaline phosphatase (ALP), 24-hour urinary hydroxyproline, calcium, x-rays, radionuclide bone scan, CT scan, MRI

b.

c.

d.

CONDITION: Pancreatitis

PHYSIOLOGY: Pancreatitis is an inflammation of the pancreas with activation of pancreatic enzymes, which results in localized damage to the pancreas, autodigestion, and fibrosis of the pancreas. Two local complications of acute pancreatitis are pseudocyst and abscess. Pancreatitis can lead to life-threatening complications such as hypovolemia, shock, acute renal failure, diabetes, acute respiratory distress syndrome (ARDS), and multiorgan failure.

Acute pancreatitis is a sudden inflammation over a short period of time ranging from mild abdominal discomfort to damage of vital organs as a result of the release of enzymes and toxins into the blood.

Chronic pancreatitis follows acute disease, and development may be delayed.

The causes of pancreatitis are biliary tract disease, alcohol abuse, abdominal trauma, viral or bacterial infections, and drugs such as sulfonamides, glucocorticoids, thiazide diuretics, and NSAIDs.

HANDOFF COMMUNICATION

S	Situation	Assess what is currently happening in a short statement.	Patient presents as _____ VS: LOC:
B	Background	Summarize important past assessment data for your patient here. Place lab results and medications on the concept map.	Age: Gender: Allergies: Fall Risk: Isolation:
A	Assessment	Use the assessment data to complete your concept map.	**Nursing Diagnosis:** Place the Nursing Diagnoses in prioritized order on the concept map and add any needed for your specific patient. **Plan:** Place any further Nursing Interventions Classifications (NIC) needed on the map.

Implement Your Plan of Care

			EVALUATE YOUR CARE	
R	Recommendation	Evaluate your nursing care and make recommendations related to the achievement of your desired outcomes. Were they met, or do new goals need to be established?	**Diag** / **Nursing Outcomes Classification (NOC)**	**Outcome met**
			1 Patient reports pain is relieved or controlled and follows prescribed therapeutic regimen.	☐ Yes ☐ No
			2 Patient maintains adequate ventilation with respiratory rate and rhythm within normal for patient, has clear breath sounds, is free of dyspnea and shortness of breath.	☐ Yes ☐ No
			3 Patient maintains adequate hydration and normal blood chemistry results with stable VS, appropriate urine output, and is free of bruising and bleeding.	☐ Yes ☐ No
			4 Patient demonstrates progressive weight gain toward goal with normalization of laboratory values.	☐ Yes ☐ No
			5 Patient initiates necessary lifestyle changes and participates in treatment regimen.	☐ Yes ☐ No

Nursing Diagnosis 1

Acute pain related to chemical contamination of peritoneal surfaces by pancreatic exudate, autodigestion of pancreas evidenced by reports of pain, grimacing, guarding behaviors.

NIC:
1) Maintain bedrest during acute attack and provide quiet, restful environment; **2)** Promote position of comfort, side lying with knees flexed, or sitting up and leaning forward; **3)** Administer analgesics intravenously in a timely manner; consider use of patient-controlled analgesia (PCA); **4)** Keep environment free of food odors, which can activate pancreatic enzymes; and **5)** Note location and intensity (0–10 scale) of pain and factors that aggravate and relieve pain.

Nursing Diagnosis 2

Risk for ineffective breathing pattern/impaired gas exchange related to pain, splinting of respirations, and upper abdominal distention.

NIC:
1) Assess for fluid overload. Evaluate respiratory rate and depth. Note respiratory effort; dyspnea, use of accessory muscles; **2)** Auscultate breath sounds. Note areas of diminished or absent breath sounds and presence of adventitious sounds; **3)** Encourage patient to deep breath, cough, and use incentive spirometer; **4)** Note increased restlessness, confusion, and lethargy; **5)** Monitor pulse oximetry, ABGs, and chest x-ray reports; and **6)** Administer oxygen as needed.

Nursing Diagnosis 3

Risk for deficient fluid volume/bleeding related to excessive losses through vomiting and gastric suction and altered clotting process.

NIC:
1) Monitor I&O, note enteric losses such as vomiting, gastric aspirate, and diarrhea; **2)** Assess BP, peripheral pulses, and mucous membranes; **3)** Observe and record peripheral and dependent edema; **4)** Observe for signs of petechia, hematomas, and bleeding from venipuncture sites; **5)** Observe for signs of ecchymosis on the flank area (Grey-Turner's sign) or periumbilical area (Cullen's sign) from bloody exudate of pancreas; **6)** Observe and report coarse muscle tremors, twitching, and positive Chvostek's or Trousseau's sign from hypocalcemia; **7)** Monitor laboratory values such as Hgb/Hct, electrolytes, BUN; and **8)** Administer IV fluids, blood, blood volume expanders as prescribed.

Nursing Diagnosis 4

Imbalanced nutrition: less than body requirements related to vomiting, decreased oral intake, loss of digestive enzymes evidenced by aversion to eating, altered taste sensation, weight loss, poor muscle tone.

NIC:
1) Assess abdomen, noting presence and character of bowel sounds, abdominal distention, and reports of nausea; **2)** Provide frequent mouth care to sooth dry mucous membranes; **3)** Maintain NPO status and gastric suction during acute phase. Maintain IV fluids or total parenteral nutrition as needed; **4)** Resume oral intake slowly with small, frequent feedings. Maintain high-carbohydrate diet. Assess for exacerbation of symptoms such as pain, increasing abdominal girth, and elevations of serum amylase and lipase; **5)** Assist patient in selection of foods and fluids that meet nutritional needs; and **6)** Assess electrolyte, prealbumin, and albumin levels.

Condition:
Pancreatitis
Age:

Link & Explain
• Nursing Interventions Classification (NIC)
• Laboratory and Diagnostic Procedures
• Medications

Nursing Diagnosis 5

Deficient knowledge regarding condition, prognosis, treatment, self-care, and discharge needs related to lack of exposure or recall, information misinterpretation evidenced by questions or statements of misconception, request for information.

NIC:
1) Provide specific information regarding current episode and prognosis. Discuss factors such as alcohol intake, gallbladder disease, duodenal ulcer, drugs; **2)** Discuss avoidance of alcohol, illicit drugs, and tobacco. Explore available treatment programs for chemical dependency; **3)** Emphasize the importance of follow-up care and reporting symptoms of vomiting, abdominal distention, frothy or foul-smelling stools, intolerance of food; and **4)** Encourage a continuation of bland, high-carbohydrate diet with small, frequent meals and gradual resumption to general diet as tolerated.

Medications
a. Opioid analgesics: meperidine (Demerol), morphine sulfate, tramadol (Ultram)
b. Antispasmodics; carbonic anhydrase inhibitor
c. Histamine (H2-receptor antagonists: lansoprazole (Prevacid), ranitidine (Zantac), famotidine (Pepcid); antacids
d. Pancreatic enzyme products

Laboratory & Diagnostic Procedures
a. Serum amylase, serum lipase, serum bilirubin, alkaline phosphatase
b. Serum electrolytes, CBC, serum glucose, serum triglycerides
c. Partial thromboplastin time (PTT)
d. Abdominal ultrasound, endoscopic retrograde cholangiopancreatography (ERCP)

CONDITION: Parkinson's Disease

PHYSIOLOGY: Parkinson's disease is a progressive neurological disorder caused by the degeneration of the dopamine-producing neurons located in the midbrain. It affects the extrapyramidal motor system, which controls posture and voluntary movement.

Clinical manifestations, known as the triad of Parkinson's disease, include tremor (pill-rolling movement), rigidity (jerky intermittent movement, cogwheel), and bradykinesia (masklike face, drooling of saliva, shuffling gait). As the disease progresses, depression, apathy, difficulty swallowing, akinesia, dementia, and complete dependency for ADL occur.

Diagnosis is made through the patient's medical history and an assessment that confirms two of the three symptoms of the triad are present.

HANDOFF COMMUNICATION

S Situation	Assess what is currently happening in a short statement.	Patient presents as _____
B Background	Summarize important past assessment data for your patient here. Place lab results and medications on the concept map.	Age: Gender: Allergies: Fall Risk: Isolation:
A Assessment	Use the assessment data to complete your concept map.	**Nursing Diagnosis:** Place the Nursing Diagnoses in prioritized order on the concept map and add any needed for your specific patient. **Plan:** Place any further Nursing Interventions Classifications (NIC) needed on the map.

Implement Your Plan of Care

		EVALUATE YOUR CARE	
R Recommendation	Evaluate your nursing care and make recommendations related to the achievement of your desired outcomes. Were they met, or do new goals need to be established?	**Diag** / **Nursing Outcomes Classification (NOC)**	**Outcome met**
		1 Patient demonstrates ability to complete ADL with minimal assistance.	☐ Yes ☐ No
		2 Patient maintains weight with normalization of laboratory values.	☐ Yes ☐ No
		3 Patient verbalizes responses that are easy to understand.	☐ Yes ☐ No
		4 Patient demonstrates behaviors that enable continuation of activities.	☐ Yes ☐ No
		5 Patient demonstrates lifestyle changes to meet own needs.	☐ Yes ☐ No

Nursing Diagnosis 1

Impaired physical mobility related to rigidity and bradykinesia evidenced by difficulty of purposeful movement.

NIC:
1) Determine functional ability using a 0–4 scale and reasons for impairment; 2) Schedule activity or procedures with intermittent rest periods; 3) Encourage participation in ADL within individual limitations; 4) Provide or assist with passive and active stretching exercises, increasing the hold phase and number of repetitions; 5) Encourage patient to rock body from side to side to stimulate balance, decrease akinesia; and 6) Encourage patient to use a wide base of support when ambulating.

Nursing Diagnosis 2

Imbalanced nutrition: less than body requirements related to dysphagia evidenced by difficulty chewing and decreased mobility of mouth and tongue.

NIC:
1) Assess chewing and tongue movements during meals; 2) Encourage patient to sit up straight in the chair for meals and concentrate when swallowing with chin slightly down to prevent aspiration; 3) Maintain suction equipment at bedside; assess abdomen, noting presence and character of bowel sounds, abdominal distention, and reports of nausea; 4) Assist patient with food choices that are nutritious, high in fiber, and easy to chew and swallow; 5) Provide six small meals per day. Cut food into small, bite-size pieces before serving; 6) Provide enough time for patient to eat meals. Assess patient intermittently for food pocketed in mouth; and 7) Weigh daily.

Nursing Diagnosis 3

Impaired verbal communication related to dysarthria and tremor evidenced by slurred speech.

NIC:
1) Keep communication simple. Give one direction at a time. Provide questions that can be answered with a short response; 2) Provide alternative methods of communication as appropriate: slate board, letter-and-picture board; 3) Anticipate needs as much as possible. Assess patient frequently; and 4) Encourage patient to continue speech therapy and exercise muscles used to verbalize by repeating words.

Nursing Diagnosis 4

Risk for falls related to gait disturbance.

NIC:
1) Perform initial and ongoing falls risk assessment, including gait and balance, history, cognition, use of mobility aids; 2) Provide supportive, well-fitting shoes; 3) Encourage use of handrails in bathrooms and hallway; 4) Keep areas well lighted; 5) Encourage patient to use glasses and hearing aids if necessary; and 6) Discuss the need for alterations to the home environment such as removing throw rugs and clutter, allowing open space for ambulation, using night lights, keeping pets from area when patient is walking.

Condition:
Parkinson's Disease
Age:

Link & Explain
• Nursing Interventions Classification (NIC)
• Laboratory and Diagnostic Procedures
• Medications

Nursing Diagnosis 5

Self-care deficit related to loss of mobility, neuromuscular or muscular impairment evidenced by inability to manage ADL, unkempt appearance.

NIC:
1) Use shower chair and spray attachment as needed; 2) Utilize supportive slip-on shoes; 3) Encourage family to provide Velcro closures for clothing; and 4) Assess the need for an elevated toilet seat.

Medications

a. Carbidopa (Sinemet), bromocriptine (Parlodel), pergolide (Permax)

b. Ropinirole (Requip), pramipexole (Mirapex)

c.

d.

Laboratory & Diagnostic Procedures

a. CBC, chemistry

b.

c.

d.

CONDITION: Peptic Ulcer

PHYSIOLOGY: Peptic ulcer disease is an ulcerative disorder in the lower esophagus, upper duodenum, or stomach (usually along the lesser curvature). Peptic ulcers are sharply circumscribed breaks of the mucosa that may extend through the tissue layers of the muscle and serosa into the abdominal cavity.

Factors that contribute to the development of peptic ulcers include a genetic predisposition to ulcer formation; poor cell restitution; excessive acid secretion; stress; excessive alcohol or caffeine intake; smoking; ingestion of aspirin and NSAIDs; and chronic use of drugs such as steroidal, potassium, or iodine compounds. The *Helicobacter pylori* bacterium, the principal causative agent of type B chronic gastritis, is also thought to be a major cause of peptic ulcers. Associated diseases include hyperparathyroidism, chronic lung disease, and alcoholic cirrhosis.

Patients with peptic ulcers may be asymptomatic or have gnawing epigastric pain, especially in the middle of the night or when no food has been eaten for several hours. Heartburn, nausea, vomiting, hematemesis, melena, or unexplained weight loss may also be associated with peptic ulcer disease. Food intake often relieves the discomfort.

Peptic ulcers that perforate the upper gastrointestinal tract may penetrate the pancreas, causing symptoms of pancreatitis (severe back pain), and may cause chemical peritonitis followed by bacterial peritonitis or an acute abdomen as irritating GI contents and bacteria enter the abdominal cavity. Bacterial peritonitis can lead to sepsis shock and death. Other complications include abdominal or intestinal infarction or erosion of the ulcer into the liver or biliary tract.

HANDOFF COMMUNICATION

S	Situation	Assess what is currently happening in a short statement.	Patient presents as _____ *Obtain information regarding precipitating symptoms if possible.*
B	Background	Summarize important past assessment data for your patient here. Place lab results and medications on the concept map.	**Age:** **Gender:** **Allergies:** **Fall Risk:** **Isolation:**
A	Assessment	Use the assessment data to complete your concept map.	**Nursing Diagnosis:** Place the Nursing Diagnoses in prioritized order on the concept map and add any needed for your specific patient. **Plan:** Place any further Nursing Interventions Classifications (NIC) needed on the map.

Implement Your Plan of Care

			EVALUATE YOUR CARE	
R	Recommendation	Evaluate your nursing care and make recommendations related to the achievement of your desired outcomes. Were they met, or do new goals need to be established?	**Diag** / **Nursing Outcomes Classification (NOC)**	**Outcome met**
			1 Patient appears relaxed and reports that pain is relieved or controlled.	☐ Yes ☐ No
			2 Patient reports decreased fatigue and improved well-being.	☐ Yes ☐ No
			3 Patient identifies effective coping strategies and enhanced support mechanisms.	☐ Yes ☐ No
			4 Patient maintains adequate fluid volume evidenced by stable VS, good skin turgor, balanced I&O, and absence of postural hypotension.	☐ Yes ☐ No
			5 Patient verbalizes understanding of disease process, possible complications, treatment regimen, needed lifestyle changes, discharge instructions, and importance of follow-up care.	☐ Yes ☐ No

Nursing Diagnosis 1

Acute pain related to inflammation and irritation of mucosa from gastric secretions evidenced by reports of pain, self-focus.

NIC:
1) Perform comprehensive pain assessment using 0–10 pain scale; **2)** Administer analgesic and prescribed medications and evaluate effectiveness; **3)** Assess past experiences with pain and effectiveness of pain management methods; **4)** Note nonverbal cues of pain; **5)** Review factors that aggravate or alleviate pain; and **6)** Implement prescribed dietary modifications.

Nursing Diagnosis 2

Fatigue related to blood loss/chronic illness evidenced by lethargy, overwhelming lack of energy.

NIC:
1) Assess severity of fatigue and associated factors; **2)** Monitor for signs and symptoms of anemia/bleeding: tachycardia, hypotension, decreased Hgb/Hct; **3)** Evaluate adequacy of nutrition and sleep patterns; **4)** Structure care and activities to accommodate frequent rest periods; **5)** Encourage patient to keep journal of activities and symptoms of fatigue; and **6)** Refer to physical therapy/occupational therapy as indicated.

Nursing Diagnosis 3

Ineffective coping related to pain and disease processes evidenced by depression and dependency.

NIC:
1) Assess patient's level of stress and coping skills; **2)** Provide opportunity for patient to discuss how illness has impacted life and relationships; **3)** Assist patient in identifying personally effective coping skills; **4)** Provide emotional support; **5)** Encourage use of relaxation techniques, yoga, biofeedback; and **6)** Refer to social services/support groups.

Nursing Diagnosis 4

Risk for deficient fluid volume related to decreased intake, gastric irritation. Hemorrhage.

NIC:
1) Assess VS, mucous membranes, skin turgor capillary refill, and urinary output; **2)** Monitor I&O; observe for early signs of hypovolemia; **3)** Monitor BUN, Hgb/Hct, electrolytes; **4)** Monitor factors predisposing to deficient fluid volume; and **5)** Provide supplemental IV fluids, PRBC as prescribed.

Condition:
Peptic Ulcer
Age:

Link & Explain
• Nursing Interventions Classification (NIC)
• Laboratory and Diagnostic Procedures
• Medications

Nursing Diagnosis 5

Deficient knowledge regarding condition, prognosis, treatment, self-care, and discharge needs related to unfamiliarity with resources evidenced by request for information.

NIC:
1) Determine patient's understanding/perception of disease process, treatment, self-care needs, and discharge instructions; **2)** Reinforce the need to avoid the following: aspirin products and NSAIDs, alcohol intake, caffeine products, and smoking; **3)** Review signs and symptoms that should be reported—those that may indicate recurrence or complications, including pain, nausea, vomiting, black tarry stools, fatigue, and frank bleeding; **4)** Instruct patient regarding adherence to treatment regimen and follow-up care: recurrence is greater than 50% with noncompliance; and **5)** Refer to social services, home care, community support groups as indicated.

Medications
a. Antibiotics (clarithromycin, amoxicillin)
b. Antisecretory proton pump inhibitors (lansoprazole, omeprazole)
c. Coating agents (Bismuth)
d. H2 blockers (Ranitidine)

Laboratory & Diagnostic Procedures
a. Esophagogastroduodenoscopy (EGD); gastroscopy
b. Barium swallow; upper GI x-ray series
c. Serum gastrin levels, Hgb/Hct, CBC
d. Tests for *H. pylori*: **1)** antibody detection (immunoglobulin G [IgG]) to *H. pylori* is measured in serum, plasma, or whole blood; **2)** urea breath tests detect active *H. pylori* infection by identifying enzymatic activity of bacterial urease; and **3)** fecal antigen testing detects presence of *H. pylori* antigens in stools

CONDITION: Peritonitis

PHYSIOLOGY: Peritonitis is inflammation of the serous membrane that lines the abdominal cavity and its viscera. Intra-abdominal infection may be localized or generalized, with or without abscess formation. Most common pathogens include *Escherichia coli, Klebsiella pneumoniae*, and *Streptococcus*. Resistant and unusual pathogens include *Enterococcus, Candida*, and *Enterobacter*, which occur when the initial therapy for the infection is inadequate.

Causes

Primary peritonitis: chronic liver disease with ascites formation is the most common cause.
Secondary peritonitis: rupture or perforation of an internal organ or instillation of irritating substance causing irritation, which can occur in the GI tract, ovaries, and uterus. It can also be the result of a blunt or penetrating trauma, or it may be a complication from a medical procedure.

HANDOFF COMMUNICATION

S Situation	Assess what is currently happening in a short statement.	Patient presents as _____
B Background	Summarize important past assessment data for your patient here. Place lab results and medications on the concept map.	Age: Gender: Allergies: Fall Risk: Isolation:
A Assessment	Use the assessment data to complete your concept map.	**Nursing Diagnosis:** Place the Nursing Diagnoses in prioritized order on the concept map and add any needed for your specific patient. **Plan:** Place any further Nursing Interventions Classifications (NIC) needed on the map.

Implement Your Plan of Care

			EVALUATE YOUR CARE	
R Recommendation	Evaluate your nursing care and make recommendations related to the achievement of your desired outcomes. Were they met, or do new goals need to be established?	**Diag**	**Nursing Outcomes Classification (NOC)**	**Outcome met**
		1	Patient achieves healing in a timely manner. Patient is free of purulent drainage, erythema, and fever.	☐ Yes ☐ No
		2	Patient demonstrates improved fluid balance with adequate urinary output, stable VS, moist mucous membranes, good skin turgor, normal capillary refill.	☐ Yes ☐ No
		3	Patient reports pain is relieved or controlled.	☐ Yes ☐ No
		4	Patient maintains usual weight and positive nitrogen balance.	☐ Yes ☐ No
		5	Patient correctly performs necessary procedures and explains reason for actions.	☐ Yes ☐ No

Nursing Diagnosis 1

Risk for infection (septicemia) related to inflammatory process of the peritoneum.

NIC:
1) Assess VS, note unresolved or progressing hypotension, decreased pulse pressure, tachycardia, fever, tachypnea; **2)** Note changes in mental status such as new-onset confusion and stupor; **3)** Note skin color, temperature, and moisture; **4)** Maintain strict aseptic technique in care of abdominal wounds and drains. Monitor compliance with hand washing; and **5)** Obtain specimens for culture and monitor results.

Nursing Diagnosis 2

Deficient fluid volume related to fluid shifts from extracellular, intravascular, and interstitial compartments into intestines and/or peritoneal space evidenced by hypotension; tachycardia.

NIC:
1) Maintain accurate I&O, noting output less than intake and increased urine-specific gravity. Assess skin, mucous membranes, peripheral pulses, and capillary refill. Weigh patient periodically; **2)** Take BP in standing, sitting, and lying positions. Note presence of hypotension, tachycardia, tachypnea, fever; **3)** Maintain NPO status with patent NG tube; **4)** Monitor laboratory studies, such as protein, electrolytes, albumin, Hgb/Hct, BUN, and creatinine; and **5)** Administer IV fluids, plasma, blood products as indicated.

Nursing Diagnosis 3

Acute pain related to accumulation of fluid in the abdomen and peritoneal cavity evidenced by muscle guarding, rebound tenderness.

NIC:
1) Observe and document location, severity (0–10 scale); have patient clarify if pain is typical; **2)** Observe for nonverbal cues, such as body positioning, facial expression, inability to find a position of comfort. Assess for shallow respiration, which may indicate pain; **3)** Discuss which pain relief measures were effective in the past; **4)** Encourage use of relaxation techniques such as guided imagery and visualization. Provide comfort measures such as massage and deep breathing; **5)** Maintain semi-Fowler's position. Teach patient to splint incision; and **6)** Administer pain medication as prescribed.

Nursing Diagnosis 4

Risk for imbalanced nutrition: less than body requirements related to anorexia, nausea and vomiting.

NIC:
1) Auscultate bowel sounds, noting hyperactive or absence of bowel sounds; **2)** Monitor NG tube output, note presence of vomiting and diarrhea. Weigh daily; **3)** Measure abdominal girth; **4)** Access abdomen for return to softness, reappearance of normal bowel sounds, and passage of flatus; **5)** Monitor labs such as BUN, protein, prealbumin, albumin, glucose, nitrogen balance; **6)** Maintain IV fluids or total parenteral nutrition as needed; and **7)** Advance diet as tolerated from clear liquids to soft food.

Condition:
Peritonitis
Age:

Link & Explain
• Nursing Interventions Classification (NIC)
• Laboratory and Diagnostic Procedures
• Medications

Nursing Diagnosis 5

Deficient knowledge regarding condition, prognosis, treatment, self-care, and discharge needs related to lack of exposure, recall evidenced by questions, request for information.

NIC:
1) Review disease process, surgical procedure, and recovery expectations; **2)** Demonstrate care of incisions, dressings, and drains; **3)** Review symptoms that need to be reported such as recurrent abdominal pain or abdominal distention, fever, chills, or presence of purulent wound drainage; and **4)** Recommend gradual resumption of activity, no heavy lifting.

Medications

a. Antipyretics

b. Opioids

c. Antiemetics

d.

Laboratory & Diagnostic Procedures

a. CBC, serum protein/albumin, ABG, cultures

b. CT scan, abdominal x-ray, ultrasound scan (abdominal/pelvic)

c. Chest x-ray, peritoneal tap (paracentesis)

d.

CONDITION: Pneumonia

PHYSIOLOGY: Pneumonia is inflammation of the lung parenchyma associated with alveolar edema and congestion that impairs gas exchange. Common pathogens include viruses, bacteria, or fungi. Pneumonia is characterized according to the causative agent and site of inflammation (lobar, bronchial, interstitial). Primary pneumonia is caused by inhalation of a pathogen. Secondary pneumonia is caused by lung damage from an infectious agent (bacterial, viral, or fungal) from another site of the body or from chemical irritants (including gastric aspiration or smoke inhalation), or radiation therapy. Pneumonia is categorized according to the infectious cause of the disease: gram-positive pneumonia, gram-negative pneumonia, anaerobic bacterial pneumonia, mycoplasma pneumonia, and parasitic pneumonia.

Common risk factors include debilitating illness and comorbidities, diabetes, smoking/COPD, malnutrition, immobility, previous antibiotic therapy, abdominal or thoracic procedures, endotracheal intubation/mechanical ventilation. Patients most at risk are the elderly, the very young, and individuals who are immunocompromised.

HANDOFF COMMUNICATION

S	Situation	Assess what is currently happening in a short statement.	Patient presents as _____ *Type of pneumonia/infecting organism; comorbidities/debilitating illnesses.*
B	Background	Summarize important past assessment data for your patient here. Place lab results and medications on the concept map.	**Age:** **Gender:** **Allergies:** **Fall Risk:** **Isolation:**
A	Assessment	Use the assessment data to complete your concept map.	**Nursing Diagnosis:** Place the Nursing Diagnoses in prioritized order on the concept map and add any needed for your specific patient. **Plan:** Place any further Nursing Interventions Classifications (NIC) needed on the map.

Implement Your Plan of Care

		EVALUATE YOUR CARE		
R	Recommendation	Evaluate your nursing care and make recommendations related to the achievement of your desired outcomes. Were they met, or do new goals need to be established?	**Diag**	**Nursing Outcomes Classification (NOC)**	**Outcome met**

Diag	Nursing Outcomes Classification (NOC)	Outcome met
1	Patient maintains airway with clear breath sounds, minimal coughing or suctioning, and absence of dyspnea or cyanosis.	☐ Yes ☐ No
2	Patient demonstrates optimal gas exchange with no symptoms of respiratory distress. ABGs are within patient's normal baseline.	☐ Yes ☐ No
3	Patient experiences timely resolution of current infection without complications.	☐ Yes ☐ No
4	Patient demonstrates adequate nutritional status/hydration with normal skin turgor, moist mucous membranes, and balanced I&O.	☐ Yes ☐ No
5	Patient verbalizes relief/control of pain, demonstrates relaxed demeanor, and engages in activities.	☐ Yes ☐ No

Nursing Diagnosis 1

Ineffective airway clearance related to edema formation and increased sputum formation evidenced by abnormal breath sounds.

NIC:
1) Assess respiratory effort and lung sounds; **2)** Teach cough/deep-breathing techniques; **3)** Provide suctioning/chest PT and nebulizer treatments as needed; **4)** Encourage fluids/monitor hydration; and **5)** Administer medications in a timely manner and auscultate lungs before and after nebulizer treatment.

Nursing Diagnosis 2

Impaired gas exchange related to alveolar capillary membrane changes evidenced by dyspnea and cyanosis.

NIC:
1) Assess respiratory status/mental status such as restlessness or anxiety; **2)** Monitor pulse oximetry/ABGs; **3)** Monitor temperature; encourage rest to decrease metabolic demands; **4)** Elevate head to high Fowler's and encourage frequent position changes; and **5)** Monitor for deterioration in condition. **6)** Administer humidified oxygen as prescribed.

Nursing Diagnosis 3

Risk for infection related to inadequate primary and secondary defenses.

NIC:
1) Monitor VS, quantity/quality of secretions; **2)** Teach/model good hand washing and standard precautions; institute isolation as needed; **3)** Monitor effectiveness of antimicrobial therapy; and **4)** Monitor for deteriorating condition (fever, altered sensorium, changes in sputum).

Nursing Diagnosis 4

Risk for deficient nutrition/fluid volume related to increased metabolic needs due to disease process and decreased intake.

NIC:
1) Evaluate nutritional status and baseline weight; **2)** Monitor intake and ability to tolerate oral intake; **3)** Provide small, frequent meals; **4)** Schedule respiratory treatments not to interfere with meal schedule; and **5)** Assess VS, skin turgor; monitor I&O; and force fluids to individual tolerance, maintain IV fluids.

Condition:
Pneumonia
Age:

- - - - - - - - - - - - -
Link & Explain
• Nursing Interventions Classification (NIC)
• Laboratory and Diagnostic Procedures
• Medications

Nursing Diagnosis 5

Acute pain related to inflammation of the lung parenchyma evidenced by reports of pleuritic pain.

NIC:
1) Perform comprehensive pain assessment; **2)** Provide comfort measures; **3)** Encourage relaxation exercises; **4)** Administer antitussive, analgesics as prescribed; and **5)** Instruct patient in splinting techniques to minimize pain with cough/deep breathing.

Medications

a. Antimicrobials

b. Antipyretics

c. Fluid management/IV therapy

d. Antitussives

Laboratory & Diagnostic Procedures

a. Chest x-ray, pulmonary function studies, bronchoscopy

b. Lab tests: CBC with differential, electrolytes, Hgb/Hct, BUN, serum albumin, prealbumin, urinalysis

c. Oximetry and ABGs

d. Gram stain and cultures (sputum, empyema, pleural, transtracheal or transthoracic fluid), lung biopsies, blood cultures

CONDITION: Radical Neck Surgery—Laryngectomy

PHYSIOLOGY: Radical neck surgery is the result of malignancy that may be in the mouth, nasal cavity, larynx, pharynx, vocal cords, or epiglottis. Disability is the result of potential loss of voice, disfigurement, and social consequences. Approximately 85% of head and neck cancers result from tobacco products or excessive consumption of alcohol. Additional risk factors include chronic candidiasis, poor oral hygiene, ill-fitting dentures, human papillomavirus, and acid reflux disease.

   Symptoms, depending on the location of the cancer, may include weakness, loss of voice, difficulty swallowing, choking easily, chronic sore throat, changes in taste.

HANDOFF COMMUNICATION

S	Situation	Assess what is currently happening in a short statement.	Patient presents as _____ VS: LOC:
B	Background	Summarize important past assessment data for your patient here. Place lab results and medications on the concept map.	**Age:** **Gender:** **Allergies:** **Fall Risk:** **Isolation:**
A	Assessment	Use the assessment data to complete your concept map.	**Nursing Diagnosis:** Place the Nursing Diagnoses in prioritized order on the concept map and add any needed for your specific patient. **Plan:** Place any further Nursing Interventions Classifications (NIC) needed on the map.

Implement Your Plan of Care

			EVALUATE YOUR CARE	
R	Recommendation	Evaluate your nursing care and make recommendations related to the achievement of your desired outcomes. Were they met, or do new goals need to be established?	**Diag** — **Nursing Outcomes Classification (NOC)**	**Outcome met**
			1 Patient maintains patent airway with clear breath sounds.	☐ Yes ☐ No
			2 Patient displays timely wound healing without complications.	☐ Yes ☐ No
			3 Patient demonstrates appropriate feeding methods and maintains desired body weight.	☐ Yes ☐ No
			4 Patient indicates understanding of the communication problem and establishes a method to express needs.	☐ Yes ☐ No
			5 Patient acknowledges presence of impairment.	☐ Yes ☐ No

Nursing Diagnosis 1

Ineffective airway clearance may be related to temporary or permanent change to neck breathing dependent on stoma, edema formation, copious thick secretions evidenced by changes in rate and depth of respirations, use of accessory muscles.

NIC:
1) Monitor respiratory rate and depth; auscultate breath sounds; pulse oximetry; assess for restlessness, dyspnea, and development of cyanosis; **2)** Elevate head 30–45 degrees; **3)** Encourage effective coughing and deep breathing; **4)** Suction tracheostomy tube and oral cavity. Note color and consistency of secretions; **5)** Demonstrate and encourage patient to self-suction using clean technique before discharge; **6)** Observe tissue around tube for bleeding or infection. Check for pooling of secretions or blood behind neck; **7)** Change inner cannula as indicated; instruct patient about importance of procedure to avoid mucous plugs; and **8)** Provide humidification of oxygen to tracheostomy tube and increase fluids as tolerated.

Nursing Diagnosis 2

Impaired skin/tissue integrity related to surgical removal of tissues and grafting evidenced by disruption of skin and tissue surface.

NIC:
1) Assess skin color, temperature, capillary refill in operative areas; **2)** Keep head of bed elevated 30–45 degrees and monitor facial edema; **3)** Monitor bloody drainage from surgical sites, suture lines, and drains. Measure and record each shift; **4)** Cleanse incisions with sterile saline or per protocol. Teach stoma care; **5)** Monitor donor site if graft was performed; and **6)** Report signs of unusual redness, increasing edema, exudate, and temperature elevation.

Nursing Diagnosis 3

Imbalanced nutrition: less than body requirements related to temporary or permanent alteration in mode of food intake evidenced by aversion to eating, lack of interest in food, reported altered taste sensation.

NIC:
1) Auscultate bowel sounds; **2)** Maintain feeding tube: check for placement and flush as indicated to keep patent; **3)** Monitor I&O and weight; **4)** Instruct patient or family in self-feeding techniques; **5)** Note signs of gastric fullness, regurgitation, and diarrhea; **6)** Provide supplemental water by feeding tube or orally to maintain hydration; **7)** Encourage a pleasant environment for meals; and **8)** Consult with dietitian as indicated.

Nursing Diagnosis 4

Impaired verbal communication related to anatomical deficit (removal of vocal cords) or physical barrier (tracheostomy tube) evidenced by inability to speak.

NIC:
1) Discuss why speech and breathing are altered and use anatomical drawing for explanation; **2)** Determine if patient has any other communication deficit such as hearing or vision; **3)** Provide call bell and instructions for contacting nurse. Check on patient periodically; **4)** Provide alternative methods of communication such as pad and pencil, magic slate, picture board, gestures; **5)** Allow sufficient time for communication; **6)** Encourage patient to maintain awareness of outside events with newspaper, television, radio, calendar, clock; and **7)** Discuss voice prosthesis and tracheostomy valve.

Condition:
Radical Neck Surgery— Laryngectomy

Age:

Link & Explain
• Nursing Interventions Classification (NIC)
• Laboratory and Diagnostic Procedures
• Medications

Nursing Diagnosis 5

Disturbed body image/ineffective role performance related to loss of voice, presence of chronic illness evidenced by negative feelings about body change, failure of family members to adapt to change.

NIC:
1) Identify perception of situation and future expectations; **2)** Note nonverbal body language and negative attitudes. Assess for self-destructive or suicidal behavior; **3)** Note emotional reactions such as grieving, depression, and anger; **4)** Maintain a calm, reassuring manner. Acknowledge and accept feelings of grief and hostility; **5)** Set limits on maladaptive behaviors, assisting the patient to identify positive behaviors that will aid in recovery; **6)** Provide positive reinforcement for efforts and progress achieved; and **7)** Refer to psychiatric counseling, support group.

Medications
a. Opioids (pain relief)
b.
c.
d.

Laboratory & Diagnostic Procedures
a. CBC
b. Chest x-ray
c. Direct/indirect laryngoscopy, laryngeal CT scan
d. Pulmonary function studies

CONDITION: Renal Dialysis—General Considerations

PHYSIOLOGY: Renal dialysis is a process that substitutes for kidney function in patients with acute renal failure or chronic end-stage renal disease by removing excess fluid and accumulated toxins.

The two primary types of dialysis are:
1. *Hemodialysis (HD)*, which requires the placement of a venous access and a machine that removes the blood from the body, runs it through a dialyzer, and then returns it to the body.
2. *Peritoneal dialysis (PD)*, which requires the placement of an abdominal catheter for infusing dialysate fluid into the peritoneal cavity for a determined dwell time and then draining it out.

S Situation	Assess what is currently happening in a short statement.	Patient presents as _____ VS: LOC:
B Background	Summarize important past assessment data for your patient here. Place lab results and medications on the concept map.	**Age:** **Gender:** **Allergies:** **Fall Risk:** **Isolation:**
A Assessment	Use the assessment data to complete your concept map.	**Nursing Diagnosis:** Place the Nursing Diagnoses in prioritized order on the concept map and add any needed for your specific patient. **Plan:** Place any further Nursing Interventions Classifications (NIC) needed on the map.

Implement Your Plan of Care

			EVALUATE YOUR CARE	
R Recommendation	Evaluate your nursing care and make recommendations related to the achievement of your desired outcomes. Were they met, or do new goals need to be established?	**Diag**	**Nursing Outcomes Classification (NOC)**	**Outcome met**
		1	Patient demonstrates stable weight with normal laboratory values and no signs of malnutrition.	☐ Yes ☐ No
		2	Patient maintains optimal mobility and function. Patient displays increased strength and is free of associated complications such as contractures and decubitus ulcers.	☐ Yes ☐ No
		3	Patient participates in ADL within level of own ability and constraints of illness.	☐ Yes ☐ No
		4	Patient demonstrates adaptation to changes by setting realistic goals and actively participating in care.	☐ Yes ☐ No
		5	Patient verbalizes understanding of condition and relationship of signs and symptoms of the disease process.	☐ Yes ☐ No

Nursing Diagnosis 1

Imbalanced nutrition: less than body requirements related to dietary restrictions and loss of peptides and amino acids during dialysis evidenced by inadequate food intake, altered taste sensation.

NIC:
1) Monitor food and fluid ingested and calculate daily caloric intake; **2)** Note presence of nausea and anorexia; **3)** Encourage patient to participate in menu planning; **4)** Recommend small, frequent meals. Schedule meals according to dialysis; **5)** Encourage frequent mouth care; and **6)** Suggest socialization during meals.

Nursing Diagnosis 2

Impaired physical mobility related to restrictive therapy: lengthy dialysis procedure, decreased strength and endurance evidenced by decreased muscle mass, tone, and strength.

NIC:
1) Assess activity limitations, noting presence and degree of restriction; **2)** Encourage frequent change of position when on bed rest and support body parts and joints with pillows; **3)** Provide gentle massage; **4)** Encourage deep breathing and coughing, elevate head of bed; and **5)** Instruct patient in active and passive ROM exercises.

Nursing Diagnosis 3

Self-care deficit related to intolerance to activity, decreased strength and endurance evidenced by disheveled and unkempt appearance, strong body odor.

NIC:
1) Determine patient's ability to participate in self-care activities on a 1–4 scale; **2)** Provide assistance with activities as necessary; **3)** Encourage use of energy-saving techniques: using shower chair, completing tasks in small increments, sitting instead of standing; and **4)** Allow sufficient time to accomplish tasks to the fullest extent of ability.

Nursing Diagnosis 4

Disturbed body image/situational low self-esteem related to chronic illness with changes in usual roles and body image evidenced by continuous physical deterioration.

NIC:
1) Note withdrawal behavior, ineffective use of denial, or behaviors indicative of concern with body and its functions; **2)** Assess for use of addictive substances, self-destructive behaviors, suicidal behavior; **3)** Determine stage of grieving; and **4)** Identify strengths, past successes, and previous methods the patient has used to deal with life stressors.

Condition:
Renal Dialysis— General Considerations
Age:

Link & Explain
• Nursing Interventions Classification (NIC)
• Laboratory and Diagnostic Procedures
• Medications

Nursing Diagnosis 5

Deficient knowledge regarding condition, prognosis, treatment, self-care, and discharge needs related to unfamiliarity with information resources evidenced by questions, request for information, statement of misconception.

NIC:
1) Provide education regarding disease progression, prognosis, and potential complications in clear terms; **2)** Provide opportunity for patient to ask questions; **3)** Review medications and encourage patient to discuss any OTC and herbal medications with health-care provider; **4)** Stress importance of adhering to dialysis schedule; and **5)** Emphasize the need to read all product labels for foods, beverages, and OTC drugs.

Medications

a. Erythropoietin exogenous: darbepoetin alfa (Aranesp) (for treatment of anemia resulting from renal failure)
b. Antihypertensives: clonidine (Catapres), prazosin (Minipress) (for treatment of hypertension; counteracts effects of decreased renal blood flow and volume overload)
c. ACE inhibitors: dopamine (Intropin) (protects kidneys from further damage)
d.

Laboratory & Diagnostic Procedures

a. BUN/creatinine ratio: normal ratio is 10:1; in late stages of failure, the ratio decreases because of impaired filtration
b. CBC: hemoglobin may be as low as 7–8 g/dl; bone marrow stimulation for RBC production is depressed because of decreased synthesis of erythropoietin
c. Proteins (especially albumin): decreased serum level indicates protein loss from urine, fluid shifts, or malnutrition; predicts mortality in patients receiving dialysis
d.

CONDITION: Rheumatoid Arthritis (RA)

PHYSIOLOGY: RA is a general term for acute and chronic conditions marked by inflammation, muscle soreness and stiffness, and pain in the joints and associated structures. The rheumatoid factor or antibodies are present in 80% of patients with rheumatoid arthritis and in many patients with other rheumatologic and infectious illnesses (*Taber's*, 2009).

HANDOFF COMMUNICATION

S	Situation	Assess what is currently happening in a short statement.	Patient presents as _____
B	Background	Summarize important past assessment data for your patient here. Place lab results and medications on the concept map.	Age: Gender: Allergies: Fall Risk: Isolation:
A	Assessment	Use the assessment data to complete your concept map.	**Nursing Diagnosis:** Place the Nursing Diagnoses in prioritized order on the concept map and add any needed for your specific patient. **Plan:** Place any further Nursing Interventions Classifications (NIC) needed on the map.

Implement Your Plan of Care

		EVALUATE YOUR CARE	
R Recommendation	Evaluate your nursing care and make recommendations related to the achievement of your desired outcomes. Were they met, or do new goals need to be established?	**Diag** | **Nursing Outcomes Classification (NOC)**	**Outcome met**
		1 Patient reports a decreased level of pain on a 0–10 numeric scale following implementation of medication or nonpharmacologic treatments.	☐ Yes ☐ No
		2 Patient demonstrates improved physical mobility.	☐ Yes ☐ No
		3 Patient uses methods to bathe, dress, and feed self safely with minimal difficulty.	☐ Yes ☐ No
		4 Patient establishes a more realistic body image and acknowledges self as individual.	☐ Yes ☐ No
		5	☐ Yes ☐ No

Nursing Diagnosis 1

Chronic pain related to accumulation of fluid, inflammatory process, degeneration of joint, and deformity evidenced by verbal reports, narrowed focus, guarding or protective behaviors, and physical and social withdrawal.

NIC:
1) Monitor patient's pain characteristics, including onset, location, duration, quality, severity, alleviating and precipitating factors; **2)** Assess patient's expectations for pain control; **3)** Assess patient's knowledge of pain control measures and educate accordingly; **4)** Administer analgesics and anti-inflammatories as ordered, monitoring for effects and side effects; **5)** Teach nonpharmacologic pain relief measures; and **6)** Encourage adequate rest and decrease environmental stressors.

Nursing Diagnosis 2

Impaired physical mobility related to musculoskeletal deformity, pain or discomfort, decreased muscle strength, evidenced by limited ROM, impaired coordination, reluctance to attempt movement, and decreased muscle strength, control, and mass.

NIC:
1) Discuss the patient's mobility status and independence; **2)** Reposition the patient every 2 hours to avoid skin breakdown; **3)** Consult physical therapy for assistance with teaching the patient to use assistive devices such as cane and walkers; **4)** Treat pain prior to increased patient activity; **5)** Encourage early ambulation; **6)** Increase independence with ADL and encourage patient to do things for him/herself; and **7)** Advise patient to ambulate only with assistance and implement risk for falls guidelines to avoid further complications.

Nursing Diagnosis 3

Self-care deficit (bathing, dressing, eating related to musculoskeletal impairment, decreased muscle strength and endurance, limited ROM, pain on movement) evidenced by inability to manage activities of daily living (ADL).

NIC:
1) Discuss the patient's bathing and eating habits and cultural preferences; **2)** Provide pain relief measures at least 45 minutes before initiating task; **3)** Obtain a shower chair for the patient to decrease the risk for falls; **4)** Consult occupational therapy to provide assistive devices for bathing, dressing, and eating; and **5)** Initiate bath and dressing during the patient's most energetic time of day.

Nursing Diagnosis 4

Disturbed body image/ineffective role performance related to change in body structure or function; impaired mobility or ability to perform usual tasks; focus on past strength, function, or appearance evidenced by negative self-talk, feelings of helplessness, change in lifestyle or physical abilities, dependence on others for assistance, or decreased social involvement.

NIC:
1) Involve in a personal development program; **2)** Establish a therapeutic nurse-patient relationship; **3)** Assist patient to assume control; and **4)** Assist patient to formulate goals for self.

Condition:
Rheumatoid Arthritis (RA)
Age:

Link & Explain
• Nursing Interventions Classification (NIC)
• Laboratory and Diagnostic Procedures
• Medications

Nursing Diagnosis 5

NIC:

Medications

a. Methotrexate (Rheumatrex) or leflunomide (Arava)

b. Anti-inflammatory medications: aspirin, NSAIDs, ibuprofen.

c. Celecoxib (Celebrex)

d.

Laboratory & Diagnostic Procedures

a. CBC, synovial fluid analysis

b. C-reactive protein, rheumatoid factor test

c. Erythrocyte sedimentation rate

d. Joint ultrasound or MRI, x-rays

CONDITION: Risk for Falls

PHYSIOLOGY: A fall is any unexplained event that results in the patient's inadvertently coming to rest on the floor or ground. Falls are the leading cause of nonfatal injury in older adults. Injuries from these falls are a leading cause of death in the elderly. Lacerations; head injuries; and fractures of the extremities, ribs, hip, and spine occur as a result of falls. It is important to assess for risk factors that may lead to a patient fall. These include 1) history of a previous fall, 2) female gender, 3) age greater than 65, 4) decreased vision, 5) decreased hearing, 6) peripheral neuropathy, 7) musculoskeletal disorders, 8) decreased cognitive status, and 9) medications (e.g., antihypertensives, sedatives, antidepressants, and/or daily use of four or more medications) (*Taber's*, 2009).

HANDOFF COMMUNICATION

S	Situation	Assess what is currently happening in a short statement.	Patient presents as _____
B	Background	Summarize important past assessment data for your patient here. Place lab results and medications on the concept map.	Age: Gender: Allergies: Fall Risk: Isolation:
A	Assessment	Use the assessment data to complete your concept map.	**Nursing Diagnosis:** Place the Nursing Diagnoses in prioritized order on the concept map and add any needed for your specific patient. **Plan:** Place any further Nursing Interventions Classifications (NIC) needed on the map.

Implement Your Plan of Care

R	Recommendation	Evaluate your nursing care and make recommendations related to the achievement of your desired outcomes. Were they met, or do new goals need to be established?	**EVALUATE YOUR CARE**	
			Diag / **Nursing Outcomes Classification (NOC)**	**Outcome met**
			1 Patient identifies individual risk factors contributing to a risk for falls and modifies environment to maintain safety.	☐ Yes ☐ No
			2 Patient demonstrates measures to reduce the risk for falls.	☐ Yes ☐ No
			3 Patient describes integration of therapeutic regimen into daily living.	☐ Yes ☐ No
			4 Patient is free from complications associated with self-care deficit, and ADL are completed with assistance, as necessary.	☐ Yes ☐ No
			5	☐ Yes ☐ No

Nursing Diagnosis 1

Risk for falls related to patient's age, medical status, and medications.

NIC:
1) Conduct a falls risk assessment; **2)** Assist with isometric and isotonic exercises as appropriate to increase muscle strength; **3)** Place bed in lowest position, with half side rail for patient to use to position self; **4)** Lock beds, wheel chairs when not in motion; **5)** Provide nonskid slippers or shoes; **6)** Orient patient to environment; **7)** Provide assistive devices as needed (e.g., cane, walker, wheel chair); and **8)** Use bed/chair alarm to alert staff when patient has moved from bed/chair.

Nursing Diagnosis 2

Risk for injury related to unsafe environmental conditions

NIC:
1) Conduct a in-home falls risk assessment; **2)** Provide adequate room lighting; **3)** Provide vision and hearing devices as needed; **4)** Clear environment of hazards (throw rugs, obstructing furniture, small objects); **5)** Advise to use safety rails in the bathroom; and **6)** Provide supervision as needed during ambulation.

Nursing Diagnosis 3

Insufficient knowledge related to community resources evidenced by inability to state available resources to assist the disabled evidenced by patient being alone most of the time.

NIC:
1) Provide patient/family education about available community resources (e.g., structural maintenance of home, clearing of snow and ice from walks and steps); **2)** Assess patient/family for needed resources and make referrals (e.g., financial assistance, home modifications, home care, installation of safety equipment, placement in extended care); and **3)** Promote community awareness about problems with design of buildings, pavements, transportation, and relationship to potential for falls.

Nursing Diagnosis 4

Self-care deficit, total, related to cognitive and/or physical impairment.

NIC:
1) Assess patient's ability to carry out ADL and determine deficits; **2)** Assist patient to accept assistance as necessary; **3)** Encourage patient to be as independent as possible while providing assistance as needed; **4)** Schedule care to provide adequate time and rest periods; **5)** Provide frequent positive reinforcement and encouragement; **6)** Provide privacy for toileting and bathing; **7)** Place call bell within reach and encourage use; and **8)** Offer frequent toileting.

Condition:
Risk for Falls
Age:

Link & Explain
• Nursing Interventions Classification (NIC)
• Laboratory and Diagnostic Procedures
• Medications

Nursing Diagnosis 5

NIC:

Medications

a.

b.

c.

d.

Laboratory & Diagnostic Procedures

a.

b.

c.

d.

CONDITION: Seizure Disorders

PHYSIOLOGY: Seizure disorders are characterized by convulsions or other clinically detectable events caused by a sudden discharge of electrical activity that temporarily interrupts brain activity. In idiopathic seizures, which encompass 75% of all seizures, no cause is identified. In acquired seizure disorder, the causes include acidosis, electrolyte imbalances, hypoglycemia, hypoxia, hyperthermia, alcohol and drug withdrawal, septicemia, brain tumors, head trauma.

Classification

The source of the seizure within the brain can be localized, called partial, or distributed, called generalized.
1. *Partial seizures* can be simple (consciousness is unaffected) or complex (consciousness is affected).
2. *Generalized seizure* involves loss of consciousness and is further classified by the effect on the body: absence (brief periods of impaired consciousness without convulsions), myoclonic (brief jerky motor movements), clonic (rhythmic jerky movements involving upper and lower extremities), tonic (sudden tonic extension or flexion of neck, head, trunk, extremities), tonic-clonic or grand mal (rhythmic clonic movements with prolonged postictal phase), atonic (brief loss of postural tone resulting in falls and injury).

HANDOFF COMMUNICATION

S	Situation	Assess what is currently happening in a short statement.	Patient presents as _____
B	Background	Summarize important past assessment data for your patient here. Place lab results and medications on the concept map.	**Age:** **Gender:** **Allergies:** **Fall Risk:** **Isolation:**
A	Assessment	Use the assessment data to complete your concept map.	**Nursing Diagnosis:** Place the Nursing Diagnoses in prioritized order on the concept map and add any needed for your specific patient. **Plan:** Place any further Nursing Interventions Classifications (NIC) needed on the map.

Implement Your Plan of Care

R	Recommendation	Evaluate your nursing care and make recommendations related to the achievement of your desired outcomes. Were they met, or do new goals need to be established?	**EVALUATE YOUR CARE**	
			Diag / **Nursing Outcomes Classification (NOC)**	**Outcome met**
			1 Patient demonstrates behaviors and lifestyle changes to reduce risk factors and protects self from future seizure events and injury.	☐ Yes ☐ No
			2 Patient maintains effective respiratory pattern with patent airway and prevention of aspiration.	☐ Yes ☐ No
			3 Patient verbalizes increased sense of self-esteem in relation to diagnosis.	☐ Yes ☐ No
			4 Patient verbalizes a positive attitude toward life changes.	☐ Yes ☐ No
			5 Patient verbalizes identification of options and use of resources.	☐ Yes ☐ No

Nursing Diagnosis 1

Risk for injury related to loss of muscle coordination, emotional difficulties.

NIC:
1) Explore with patient the various stimuli such as alcohol, drugs, flashing lights that may precipitate seizure activity; 2) Maintain bedrest when prodromal signs or aura is present; 3) Stay with patient before and after seizure; 4) Keep padded side rails up or in accordance with facility protocol. Keep bed in lowest position. Utilize a floor mat if side rails are not available; 5) If patient is out of bed when a seizure begins, assist patient to the floor and place head on a soft surface; 6) Discuss safety measures regarding activities such as climbing ladders, swimming, use of mechanical equipment, driving; 7) Perform neurological and VS checks after seizure. Reorient patient; and 8) Document preseizure activity, presence of aura, type of seizure, type and duration of motor activity, incontinence, eye activity, vocalizations, respiratory impairment.

Nursing Diagnosis 2

Risk for ineffective airway clearance/breathing pattern related to neuromuscular impairment.

NIC:
1) Encourage patient to empty mouth of dentures or food if aura occurs. Avoid chewing gum or sucking lozenges if seizure can occur without warning; 2) Place patient in a lying position on a flat surface during seizure. Turn head to the side; 3) Loosen clothing around the neck, chest, and abdominal area; 4) Turn head to side and suction airway as needed; 5) Administer supplemental oxygen as needed postictally; and 6) Use bag-valve mask and prepare for intubation if needed.

Nursing Diagnosis 3

Self-esteem (situational or chronic low) related to stigma associated with condition evidenced by fear of rejection; negative feelings about body.

NIC:
1) Discuss feelings about diagnosis and perception of threat to self. Encourage expression of feelings; 2) Identify possible public reaction to condition. Encourage patient to refrain from concealing problem; 3) Avoid overprotecting patient, encourage participation in activities; 4) Stress importance of family remaining calm during seizure activity; and 5) Refer patient to a support group such as Epilepsy Foundation to gain information and ideas for dealing with problems.

Nursing Diagnosis 4

Deficient knowledge regarding condition, prognosis, treatment regimen, self-care, and discharge needs related to information misinterpretation evidenced by increased frequency and lack of control of seizure activity.

NIC:
1) Review pathology and prognosis of condition and lifelong need for treatment as indicated; 2) Discuss trigger factors such as loud noises, video games, blinking lights, TV viewing; 3) Discuss importance of maintaining general health such as adequate rest, moderate exercise, avoidance of alcohol, caffeine, and stimulant drugs; 4) Evaluate the need for head gear if frequent severe seizures are common; 5) Discuss local laws pertaining to persons with a seizure disorder; 6) Recommend taking medications with meals when possible; 7) Review prescribed drugs and discuss the need to continue therapy; and 8) Discuss the adverse effects of drugs such as drowsiness, hyperactivity, visual disturbances, rashes, syncope.

Condition:
Seizure Disorders
Age:

Link & Explain
• Nursing Interventions Classification (NIC)
• Laboratory and Diagnostic Procedures
• Medications

Nursing Diagnosis 5

Ineffective coping related to threat of physical and social well-being evidenced by lack of correct information about frequency of seizures.

NIC:
1) Encourage the patient to express feelings, including hostility and anger, denial, depression, and sense of disconnectedness; 2) Identify previous methods of dealing with life problems; 3) Determine presence and quality of support systems; 4) Support behaviors such as increased interest and participation in care; and 5) Monitor for sleep disturbance, increased difficulty concentrating, statements of lethargy, withdrawal.

Medications
a. Carbamazepine (Tegretol), divalproex (Depakote), gabapentin (Neurontin), topiramate (Topamax)
b. Valproic acid (Depakene), clonazepam (Klonopin), phenobarbital, phenytoin (Dilantin)
c.
d.

Laboratory & Diagnostic Procedures
a. Electrolytes, glucose, BUN, liver function tests, CBC
b. Serum drug levels, toxicology screen
c. Electroencephalogram (EEG), CT scan, MRI
d.

CONDITION: Sickle Cell Crisis (Vaso-Occlusive Crisis)

PHYSIOLOGY: Formation of abnormal hemoglobin chains containing hemoglobin S. When red blood cells are exposed to low levels of oxygen saturation, hemoglobin S causes the beta cells to contract and clump together, causing a distortion of the cell and an obstruction of blood flow, resulting in painful crisis.

Patients have painful occlusions of blood vessels in bones, the chest, the lungs, kidney, or liver, which can result in infarction and tissue death. This is often triggered by infection, dehydration, fever, or local trauma. Pain episodes are accompanied by swelling, tenderness, tachypnea, hypertension, nausea and vomiting

Sickle cell disease is an inherited, autosomal recessive disorder.

HANDOFF COMMUNICATION

S	Situation	Assess what is currently happening in a short statement.	Patient presents as _____
B	Background	Summarize important past assessment data for your patient here. Place lab results and medications on the concept map.	Age: Gender: Allergies: Fall Risk: Isolation:
A	Assessment	Use the assessment data to complete your concept map.	**Nursing Diagnosis:** Place the Nursing Diagnoses in prioritized order on the concept map and add any needed for your specific patient. **Plan:** Place any further Nursing Interventions Classifications (NIC) needed on the map.

Implement Your Plan of Care

			EVALUATE YOUR CARE	
R	Recommendation	Evaluate your nursing care and make recommendations related to the achievement of your desired outcomes. Were they met, or do new goals need to be established?	**Diag** / **Nursing Outcomes Classification (NOC)**	**Outcome met**
			1 Patient demonstrates improved ventilation and oxygenation evidenced by respiratory rate within normal limits, absence of cyanosis, use of accessory muscles, and clear breath sounds.	☐ Yes ☐ No
			2 Patient verbalizes relief or control of pain.	☐ Yes ☐ No
			3 Patient demonstrates improved tissue perfusion evidenced by stabilized VS, palpable pulses, adequate urine output, usual mentation, absence of paresthesias.	☐ Yes ☐ No
			4 Patient maintains adequate fluid balance evidenced by appropriate urine output, stable VS, good skin turgor, and prompt capillary refill.	☐ Yes ☐ No
			5 Patient maintains or increases function and strength and function of affected body parts.	☐ Yes ☐ No

Nursing Diagnosis 1

Impaired gas exchange related to increased blood viscosity: occlusions created by sickle cells packing together within the capillaries evidenced by tachypnea, tachycardia, and cyanosis.

NIC:
1) Monitor respiratory rate and depth, use of accessory muscles, and areas of cyanosis; **2)** Auscultate breath sounds, noting diminished or adventitious breath sounds. Observe for fever and cough; **3)** Monitor VS and note changes in cardiac rhythm; **4)** Assist in turning, coughing and deep-breathing exercises, and incentive spirometry; **5)** Promote adequate fluid intake, such as 2–3 L/day as tolerated; **6)** Monitor CBC, pulse oximetry, and ABGs. Administer oxygen as needed; and **7)** Administer exchange packed RBCs as ordered.

Nursing Diagnosis 2

Acute/chronic pain related to sickling with localized stasis, occlusion, infarction, and necrosis evidenced by pain described as throbbing, gnawing, or incapacitating.

NIC:
1) Observe and document location, severity (0–10 scale); have patient clarify if pain is typical; **2)** Observe for nonverbal cues, such as gait disturbances, body positioning, facial expression, elevated BP, tachycardia, increased respiratory rate; **3)** Discuss which pain relief measures were effective in the past; **4)** Encourage use of relaxation techniques such as guided imagery and visualization. Provide diversional activities; **5)** Apply warm, moist compresses to affected joints; and **6)** Administer opioids as indicated.

Nursing Diagnosis 3

Ineffective tissue perfusion (venous) related to vaso-occlusive nature of sickling, inflammatory response evidenced by changes in VS, diminished peripheral pulses, and capillary refill.

NIC:
1) Monitor VS, note color and warmth of skin and capillary refill. Report hypotension, rapid weak pulse, and tachypnea; **2)** Note changes in LOC, report headaches, dizziness, development of sensory or motor deficits. Observe for paralysis or seizure activity; **3)** Investigate reports of change in character of pain, development of bone pain, angina, tingling of extremities, vision changes; **4)** Monitor liver and kidney function tests; **5)** Administer IV fluids and electrolytes as needed; and **6)** Administer anticoagulants as prescribed to decrease risk of deep vein thrombosis.

Nursing Diagnosis 4

Risk for deficient fluid volume related to regulatory failure causing increased blood viscosity.

NIC:
1) Maintain accurate I&O, noting output less than intake and increased urine-specific gravity. Assess skin, mucous membranes, peripheral pulses, and capillary refill. Weigh patient periodically; **2)** Take BP in standing, sitting, and lying positions; **3)** Monitor laboratory studies, such as Hgb/Hct, electrolytes; and **4)** Administer IV fluids and blood products as prescribed.

Condition:
Sickle Cell Crisis (Vaso-Occlusive Crisis)

Age:

Link & Explain
• Nursing Interventions Classification (NIC)
• Laboratory and Diagnostic Procedures
• Medications

Nursing Diagnosis 5

Impaired physical mobility related to multiple recurrent bone infarctions: weight-bearing bones evidenced by reports of severe pain.

NIC:
1) Determine functional ability using a 0–4 scale. Note emotional response to altered ability; **2)** Schedule activity or procedures with rest periods. Encourage participation in ADL within individual limitations; **3)** Provide or assist with passive and active ROM exercises; **4)** Assist with transfers and ambulation if indicated. Provide well-fitting nonskid slippers; **5)** Perform initial and ongoing fall risk assessment; and **6)** Collaborate with physical therapy and occupational therapy.

Medications
a. Hydroxyurea (Droxia), deferoxamine (Desferal), vitamin C
b. Morphine (Astramorph, Duramorph)
c. Hydromorphone (Dilaudid)
d. Nalbuphine (Nubain)

Laboratory & Diagnostic Procedures
a. CBC, stained RBC, hemoglobin electrophoresis
b. Sickle-turbidity tube test (Sickledex), erythrocyte sedimentation rate (ESR), erythrocyte fragility
c. Acid phosphatase (ACP), alkaline phosphatase (ALP), lactate dehydrogenase (LDH), serum iron
d. Abdominal/pelvic ultrasound

CONDITION: Systemic Lupus Erythematosus (SLE)

PHYSIOLOGY: SLE is a chronic multisystem inflammatory autoimmune disease of connective tissue involving multiple organ systems and marked by periodic acute episodes. Its name is derived from the characteristic erythematous "butterfly" rash over the nose and cheeks, although this rash is present in less than 50% of patients. This disease is most prevalent in women of childbearing age. It typically affects the skin, joints, and serous membranes (pleura and pericardium) as well as the renal, hematologic, and neurologic systems.

HANDOFF COMMUNICATION

S	Situation	Assess what is currently happening in a short statement.	Patient presents as _____
B	Background	Summarize important past assessment data for your patient here. Place lab results and medications on the concept map.	**Age:** **Gender:** **Allergies:** **Fall Risk:** **Isolation:**
A	Assessment	Use the assessment data to complete your concept map.	**Nursing Diagnosis:** Place the Nursing Diagnoses in prioritized order on the concept map and add any needed for your specific patient. **Plan:** Place any further Nursing Interventions Classifications (NIC) needed on the map.

Implement Your Plan of Care

			EVALUATE YOUR CARE	
R	Recommendation	Evaluate your nursing care and make recommendations related to the achievement of your desired outcomes. Were they met, or do new goals need to be established?	**Diag** / **Nursing Outcomes Classification (NOC)**	**Outcome met**
			1 Patient reports pain is relieved or controlled and demonstrates use of relaxation skills and diversional activities.	☐ Yes ☐ No
			2 Patient demonstrates behaviors and techniques to promote healing and prevent skin breakdown.	☐ Yes ☐ No
			3 Patient participates in desired activities; meets own self-care needs.	☐ Yes ☐ No
			4 Patient demonstrates stable weight or progressive gain toward goal with normal laboratory results and absence of signs of malnutrition.	☐ Yes ☐ No
			5 Patient identifies causative factors and verbalizes understanding of therapeutic needs.	☐ Yes ☐ No

Nursing Diagnosis 1

Acute pain related to inflammatory process evidenced by verbalization of joint pain.

NIC:
1) Observe and document location, severity (0–10 scale), characteristics of pain and precipitating factors; **2)** Administer analgesic and note response to medication; **3)** Utilize massage and hot/cold therapy to relieve discomfort; and **4)** Encourage relaxation exercises, guided imagery, visualization, deep breathing, distraction.

Nursing Diagnosis 2

Risk for impaired skin integrity related to photosensitivity.

NIC:
1) Inspect skin daily and note irritation, rashes, and breakdown; **2)** Document the size, location, and stage of skin breakdown; implement appropriate treatment; **3)** Discuss use of sunscreens and lifestyle changes to prevent future complications; **4)** Note areas of alopecia, discoid erythema, petechiae, and purpura; and **5)** Encourage the use of mild soap and protein shampoos. Apply moisturizing lotion to dry skin areas.

Nursing Diagnosis 3

Activity intolerance related to chronic inflammation evidenced by weakness and fatigue.

NIC:
1) Assess patient's ability to perform ADL, noting reports of weakness and fatigue; **2)** Assist patient to prioritize activities; **3)** Encourage patient to schedule periods of rest to recuperate between activities; and **4)** Identify energy-saving techniques such as shower chair and sitting to perform tasks.

Nursing Diagnosis 4

Imbalanced nutrition related to failure to ingest food evidenced by weight loss.

NIC:
1) Observe and record patient's food intake; **2)** Weigh weekly and note decreases from previous weight; **3)** Recommend small, frequent meals with between-meal nourishment; **4)** Encourage patient to report nausea, vomiting, or abdominal pain; and **5)** Instruct patient to use good oral hygiene with a soft-bristle toothbrush and alcohol-free mouthwash.

Condition:
Systemic Lupus Erythematosus (SLE)

Age:

Link & Explain
• Nursing Interventions Classification (NIC)
• Laboratory and Diagnostic Procedures
• Medications

Nursing Diagnosis 5

Deficient knowledge regarding condition, prognosis, treatment, self-care, prevention of crisis, and discharge needs related to unfamiliarity with information resources evidenced by inaccurate follow-through of instructions, development of preventable complications.

NIC:
1) Provide information about treatment and therapy options to increase the probability of successful management; **2)** Stress importance of reporting symptoms such as fever, edema, decreased urine output, chest pain, dyspnea; **3)** Discuss cessation of smoking if indicated; **4)** Encourage family to provide support during exacerbation of illness; and **5)** Refer patient to the local community Lupus Foundation or the Arthritis Foundation.

Medications

a. Hydroxychloroquine (Plaquenil)

b. NSAIDs

c. Methotrexate (Rheumatrex) or azathioprine (Imuran), glucocorticoids

d. Plasmapheresis

Laboratory & Diagnostic Procedures

a. Rheumatoid factor, antinuclear antibody, erythrocyte sedimentation rate, immunoglobulins

b. Anti-Smith (anti-Sm)

c. CBC, electrolytes, BUN, creatinine

d.

CONDITION: Thrombophlebitis and Pulmonary Emboli

PHYSIOLOGY: Thrombophlebitis is related to three factors comprising the Virchow triad: stasis of blood flow, vessel wall injury, and alterations in the clotting mechanism. Complications of thrombophlebitis are pulmonary embolism, chronic venous insufficiency, and vein valve destruction.

Pulmonary embolism is the blockage of the pulmonary arteries by a thrombus, fat or air embolism, or tumor. Emboli are small clots that continue to be mobile until they become lodged and obstruct perfusion of the alveoli. Most pulmonary emboli are the product of a thrombosis in the deep veins of the legs (deep vein thrombosis [DVT]).

Smoking, immobility, paralysis, surgery, hypertension, history of atrial fibrillation, stroke, and DVT increase the risk of pulmonary emboli.

Less common are fat emboli, which may occur after a fracture of a long bone, or air emboli, which may occur when air enters the vascular system through improper IV medication administration. Tumor emboli are the product of primary or metastatic tumors.

HANDOFF COMMUNICATION

S Situation	Assess what is currently happening in a short statement.	Patient presents as _____ VS: LOC:
B Background	Summarize important past assessment data for your patient here. Place lab results and medications on the concept map.	**Age:** **Gender:** **Allergies:** **Fall Risk:** **Isolation:**
A Assessment	Use the assessment data to complete your concept map.	**Nursing Diagnosis:** Place the Nursing Diagnoses in prioritized order on the concept map and add any needed for your specific patient. **Plan:** Place any further Nursing Interventions Classifications (NIC) needed on the map.

Implement Your Plan of Care

			EVALUATE YOUR CARE	
R Recommendation	Evaluate your nursing care and make recommendations related to the achievement of your desired outcomes. Were they met, or do new goals need to be established?	**Diag**	**Nursing Outcomes Classification (NOC)**	**Outcome met**
		1	Patient demonstrates improved perfusion by equal skin color, positive peripheral pulses, absence of edema, and increased activity tolerance.	☐ Yes ☐ No
		2	Patient reports that pain is alleviated or controlled.	☐ Yes ☐ No
		3	Patient demonstrates adequate ventilation and oxygenation by ABG results within patient's normal range and is free of symptoms of respiratory distress.	☐ Yes ☐ No
		4	Patient verbalizes the understanding of the disease process and treatment regimen.	☐ Yes ☐ No
		5		☐ Yes ☐ No

Nursing Diagnosis 1

Ineffective peripheral tissue perfusion related to decreased blood flow and venous stasis (partial or complete venous obstruction) evidenced by tissue edema, pain, diminished peripheral pulses and capillary refill.

NIC:
1) Complete a circulation, sensory, and motor evaluation of the involved extremity. Note capillary refill, pulses, skin color, temperature change, edema, calf circumference; 2) Initiate active or passive ROM exercises as indicated; 3) Elevate affected extremity; 4) Encourage deep-breathing exercises; 5) Instruct patient to avoid rubbing legs, crossing legs, and flexing knees, which will impair blood flow; 6) Increase fluids to 1,500 or 2,000 mL/day within cardiac tolerance; 7) Apply warm, moist compresses to affected extremity; and 8) Administer anticoagulant therapy and assess for signs of bleeding such as bloody stool or urine, coffee-ground emesis.

Nursing Diagnosis 2

Acute pain related to diminished arterial circulation and oxygenation of tissues with production of lactic acid in tissues evidenced by reports of pain, tenderness, aching, burning, and guarding of affected limb.

NIC:
1) Assess degree and characteristics of pain; 2) Maintain bedrest during acute phase and increase ambulation slowly and cautiously; 3) Measure for antiemboli stockings when edema is resolved; 4) Provide foot cradle; 5) Encourage patients to change positions frequently; and 6) Investigate new pain or reports of sudden chest pain accompanied by dyspnea, tachycardia, apprehension.

Nursing Diagnosis 3

Impaired gas exchange (pulmonary embolism) related to altered blood flow to alveoli or major portions of the lung evidenced by severe dyspnea, restlessness, apprehension, cyanosis.

NIC:
1) Note respiratory rate and depth of respirations, use of accessory muscles, nasal flaring; 2) Observe for cyanosis of lips, tongue, buccal membranes, ears; 3) Auscultate lungs for decreased or absent breath sounds or crackles; 4) Monitor VS, pulse oximetry, and note changes in cardiac rhythm; 5) Assess level of consciousness and changes in behavior; 6) Initiate measure to maintain the patient's airway, administer supplemental oxygen by appropriate method; and 7) Administer IV fluids and keep IV access patent.

Nursing Diagnosis 4

Deficient knowledge regarding condition, treatment program, self-care, and discharge needs related to misinterpretation of information evidenced by inaccurate follow-through of instructions, development of preventable complications.

NIC:
1) Review pathophysiology of disease process and signs and symptoms of complications; 2) Establish appropriate balance between activity and rest; 3) Problem-solve issues that involve prolonged sitting, standing, wearing restrictive clothing, use of oral contraceptives, prolonged immobility; 4) Identify safety issues with anticoagulant medications such as soft toothbrush, gloves for gardening, forceful blowing of nose; 5) Avoid use of OTC medications and herbal supplements while taking anticoagulants; 6) Wear a medication identification alert tag or bracelet; 7) Instruct to report severe bleeding after minimal trauma or development of petechiae; and 8) Stress importance of medical follow-up and laboratory testing.

Condition:
Thrombophlebitis and Pulmonary Emboli

Age:

Link & Explain
- Nursing Interventions Classification (NIC)
- Laboratory and Diagnostic Procedures
- Medications

Nursing Diagnosis 5

NIC:

Medications
a. Intravenous thrombolytics: tissue plasminogen activator (tPA), alteplase (Activase), recombinant prourokinase (Prourokinase) (minimize infarcted area with early treatment of ischemic stroke)
b. Anticoagulants: warfarin sodium (Coumadin), enoxaparin (Lovenox) (prevent further clotting)
c. Anti-anxiety medications
d.

Laboratory & Diagnostic Procedures
a. Prothrombin time (PT), partial thromboplastin time (PTT), international normalized ratio (INR) baseline information for anticoagulant therapy
b. Spiral (helical) CT scan or ventilation/perfusion (V/Q) scan
c. ABGs
d.

CONDITION: Thyroidectomy

PHYSIOLOGY: Thyroidectomy is a procedure to remove thyroid tissue by an open approach; a minimally invasive, video-assisted approach; or an endoscopic procedure done through a puncture site under the arm. The procedure may be indicated for patients with thyroid cancer, hyperthyroidism, or large goiters that constrict tissue or structures in the neck.

Procedures Include:

Total thyroidectomy: removal of the entire gland and surrounding lymph nodes to treat malignancy.

Lobectomy: removal of the lobe with or without the isthmus between the lobes to treat nodules in a single lobe.

Subtotal thyroidectomy: removal of up to five-sixths of the gland to treat hyperthyroidism when antithyroid drugs do not correct and radioactive iodine (RAI) therapy is contraindicated.

HANDOFF COMMUNICATION

S	Situation	Assess what is currently happening in a short statement.	Patient presents as _____
B	Background	Summarize important past assessment data for your patient here. Place lab results and medications on the concept map.	Age: Allergies: Isolation: Gender: Fall Risk:
A	Assessment	Use the assessment data to complete your concept map.	**Nursing Diagnosis:** Place the Nursing Diagnoses in prioritized order on the concept map and add any needed for your specific patient. **Plan:** Place any further Nursing Interventions Classifications (NIC) needed on the map.

Implement Your Plan of Care

		EVALUATE YOUR CARE		
R	Recommendation	Evaluate your nursing care and make recommendations related to the achievement of your desired outcomes. Were they met, or do new goals need to be established?	**Diag** / **Nursing Outcomes Classification (NOC)**	**Outcome met**
			1 Patient maintains patent airway with aspiration prevented.	☐ Yes ☐ No
			2 Patient establishes method of communication in which needs can be understood.	☐ Yes ☐ No
			3 Patient demonstrates absence of injury with complications minimized or controlled.	☐ Yes ☐ No
			4 Patient reports pain is relieved and controlled.	☐ Yes ☐ No
			5 Patient verbalizes understanding of surgical procedure, prognosis, and potential complications.	☐ Yes ☐ No

Nursing Diagnosis 1

Risk for ineffective airway clearance related to swelling, bleeding, laryngeal spasms.

NIC:
1) Observe respiratory rate, depth, use of accessory muscles; 2) Auscultate breath sounds, noting presence of rhonchi; 3) Assess for dyspnea, stridor, "crowing," and cyanosis. Note quality of voice. Investigate reports of difficulty swallowing or drooling; 4) Elevate head of bed to semi-Fowler's position at 30–45 degrees. Caution patient to avoid bending neck; support head with pillows; 5) Check dressings frequently, especially posterior area; 6) Assist patient with repositioning, deep-breathing exercises, and coughing; and 7) Have suction and emergency tracheostomy equipment at bedside. Suction mouth if indicated; note color and consistency of secretions.

Nursing Diagnosis 2

Impaired verbal communication related to vocal cord injury, laryngeal nerve damage evidenced by impaired articulation, inability to speak, use of nonverbal cues such as gestures.

NIC:
1) Assess speech periodically and encourage voice rest; 2) Keep communication simple. Ask questions requiring a yes or no response; 3) Provide alternative methods of communication as appropriate: slate board, letter-and-picture board; and 4) Anticipate needs as much as possible. Assess patient frequently and answer call light promptly.

Nursing Diagnosis 3

Risk for injury (tetany, thyroid storm) related to hypocalcemia, increased release of thyroid hormones, central nervous system stimulation.

NIC:
1) Monitor VS, noting elevated temperature, tachycardia, dysrhythmia, respiratory distress, and cyanosis: developing pulmonary edema or heart failure; 2) Evaluate reflexes periodically. Observe for neuromuscular irritability: twitching, numbness, paresthesia, positive Chvostek's and Trousseau's signs, and seizure activity; 3) Monitor serum calcium levels; and 4) Administer calcium gluconate as indicated.

Nursing Diagnosis 4

Acute pain related to surgical interruption and manipulation of tissue and muscles evidenced by reports of pain.

NIC:
1) Observe and document location, severity (0–10 scale), characteristics of pain (steady, intermittent); 2) Support head and neck in neutral position with sandbags or small pillows. Teach patient to use hands to support neck during movement; 3) Keep call light and frequently used items within easy reach; 4) Provide cool liquids or soft foods such as juice, ice cream, popsicles; 5) Encourage use of relaxation techniques such as guided imagery and visualization. Provide diversional activities; 6) Assist with ambulation; and 7) Note response to medication, report if pain is not relieved.

Condition:
Thyroidectomy
Age:

Link & Explain
• Nursing Interventions Classification (NIC)
• Laboratory and Diagnostic Procedures
• Medications

Nursing Diagnosis 5

Deficient knowledge regarding condition, prognosis, treatment, self-care, and discharge needs related to lack of exposure and recall, misinterpretation evidenced by questions, request for information, statement of misconception.

NIC:
1) Review disease process, surgical procedure, and future expectations; 2) Discuss need for well-balanced, nutritious meals and the use of iodized salt if needed; 3) Identify foods high in calcium and vitamin D such as dairy products and liver; 4) Recommend avoidance of goitrogenic foods (excessive seafood, soybeans); 5) Review postoperative exercises after incision heals: flexion, extension, lateral movement of the head and neck; 6) Recommend the use of loose-fitting clothes or scarves to cover scar; 7) Report fever, chills, purulent drainage, erythema, gaps in wound edges, sudden weight loss, intolerance to heat or cold, nausea, vomiting, diarrhea; and 8) Review drug therapy and the need to continue as prescribed.

Medications
a. Analgesics, throat spray, lozenges
b. Phosphate-binding agents, thyroid replacement
c. Sedatives, anticonvulsants
d. Calcium (gluconate or chloride)

Laboratory & Diagnostic Procedures
a. CBC, electrolytes, triiodothyronine (T3), thyroxine (T4), thyroid-stimulating hormone (TSH)
b.
c.
d.

CONDITION: Total Nutritional Support: Parenteral/Enteral

PHYSIOLOGY: Malnutrition is a disorder in which the intake is less than required, and it results in reduced organ function, abnormalities in blood chemistry, reduced body mass, and worsened clinical outcomes. Nutritional status is affected by multiple factors, such as eating behaviors, disease states, economics, and environment. In an acutely ill patient, the impact of malnutrition includes muscle mass loss, progressive weakness, potential for infection, poor healing, and an increased rate of systemic complications.

When oral intake is inadequate or not possible, specifically designed nutritional therapy can be administered via enteral or parenteral route to prevent or correct protein-calorie malnutrition. Inadequate nutrition can be the result of an unbalanced diet, digestive difficulties, absorption problems, or other medical conditions. Malnutrition may result in patients with surgery, burns, trauma, infection, celiac disease, cystic fibrosis, cancer, or those having difficulty swallowing.

HANDOFF COMMUNICATION

S	Situation	Assess what is currently happening in a short statement.	Patient presents as _____
B	Background	Summarize important past assessment data for your patient here. Place lab results and medications on the concept map.	**Age:** **Gender:** **Allergies:** **Fall Risk:** **Isolation:**
A	Assessment	Use the assessment data to complete your concept map.	**Nursing Diagnosis:** Place the Nursing Diagnoses in prioritized order on the concept map and add any needed for your specific patient. **Plan:** Place any further Nursing Interventions Classifications (NIC) needed on the map.

Implement Your Plan of Care

		EVALUATE YOUR CARE	
R	Recommendation — Evaluate your nursing care and make recommendations related to the achievement of your desired outcomes. Were they met, or do new goals need to be established?	**Diag**	**Nursing Outcomes Classification (NOC)**	**Outcome met**

Diag	Nursing Outcomes Classification (NOC)	Outcome met
1	Patient demonstrates stable weight or progressive weight gain toward goal, with normalization of laboratory values and no signs of malnutrition.	☐ Yes ☐ No
2	Patient experiences no fever or chills.	☐ Yes ☐ No
3	Patient is free of complications associated with nutritional support.	☐ Yes ☐ No
4	Patient maintains clear airway, free of signs of aspiration.	☐ Yes ☐ No
5	Patient displays moist skin, moist mucous membranes, stable VS, and adequate urinary output.	☐ Yes ☐ No

Nursing Diagnosis 1

Imbalanced nutrition: less than body requirements related to conditions that interfere with nutrient intake or increase nutrient need of metabolic demand evidenced by body weight 10% or more under ideal.

NIC:
1) Assess nutritional status; note energy level, condition of skin, hair, nails, oral cavity, and desire to eat; **2)** Weigh daily and compare with admission weight; **3)** Administer nutritional solutions at prescribed rate, note electrolyte content; **4)** Observe appropriate hang time for total parenteral nutrition (TPN), monitor blood glucose; **5)** Assess tolerance of enteral feedings, auscultate bowel sounds, investigate symptoms of nausea or abdominal discomfort. Check gastric residual, and hold feeding if necessary; **6)** During transition to oral feedings, assess gag reflex, ability to chew or swallow, and motor skills; **7)** Provide self-help utensils as needed. Allow adequate time for chewing, swallowing, and socializing; and **8)** Monitor labs such as electrolytes, BUN, creatinine, total protein, prealbumin, albumin, glucose.

Nursing Diagnosis 2

Risk for infection related to insertion of venous catheter, placement of gastrostomy or jejunostomy tube.

NIC:
1) Stress importance of correct hand washing; **2)** Ensure aseptic environment during insertion of a central line catheter; **3)** Perform central line dressing change per protocol. Inspect insertion site for erythema, induration, drainage, tenderness; **4)** Observe 24-hour hang time for TPN and 12-hour hang time for fat emulsions; **5)** Provide daily and as-needed site care to abdominally placed enteral tubes; **6)** Observe hang time for enteral feeding recommended by manufacturer; and **7)** Assess VS, and report hypotension, decreased pulse pressure, tachycardia, fever, tachypnea, chills.

Nursing Diagnosis 3

Risk for injury related to catheter-related complications such as air emboli and septic thrombophlebitis.

NIC:
1) Maintain closed central IV system using Luer-Lok connections; **2)** Assess catheter for signs of displacement such as extended length of tubing from insertion, leakage, neck or arm pain, swelling at site; **3)** Investigate reports indicating air embolism such as severe chest pain and coughing. Turn patient to left side in Trendelenburg position; **4)** Assess gastrostomy tube or jejunostomy tube for evidence of malposition; and **5)** Monitor for fever or increased serum WBC.

Nursing Diagnosis 4

Risk for aspiration related to presence of GI tube, bolus tube feeding, medication administration.

NIC:
1) Confirm placement of nasoenteral feeding tube with gastric fluid pH of 0–5; **2)** Keep head of bed elevated at 30–45 degrees during and for 1 hour after feeding; **3)** Inflate tracheostomy tube cuff during and for 1 hour after feeding; **4)** Monitor gastric residuals before bolus feeding. Hold feeding according to policy; and **5)** Investigate development of dyspnea, cough, tachypnea, cyanosis.

Condition:
Total Nutritional Support: Parenteral/ Enteral

Age:

Link & Explain
• Nursing Interventions Classification (NIC)
• Laboratory and Diagnostic Procedures
• Medications

Nursing Diagnosis 5

Risk for imbalanced fluid volume related to active loss or failure of regulatory mechanisms specific to underlying disease process.

NIC:
1) Assess for signs of dehydration such as thirst, dry skin and mucous membranes, hypotension; **2)** Assess for signs of fluid excess such as peripheral edema, tachycardia, crackles when auscultating breath sounds; **3)** Provide additional water when flushing tubing if indicated; **4)** Maintain accurate I&O, calculating fluid balance and urine-specific gravity; **5)** Monitor laboratory studies, such as electrolytes, Hgb/Hct, serum albumin, prealbumin, serum transferrin.

Medications
a.
b.
c.
d.

Laboratory & Diagnostic Procedures
a. Body mass index, serum albumin, serum transferrin, prealbumin (PAB), retinol-binding protein, C-reactive protein, CBC, electrolytes, nitrogen balance studies, 24-hour creatinine excretion study
b. Chest x-ray, EKG
c.
d.

CONDITION: Transplantation Considerations—Postoperative and Lifelong

PHYSIOLOGY: Transplant is the transfer of whole or partial organs such as heart, lung, kidney, liver, pancreas, or intestines from one location to another. Heart and lung transplants are more successful than hand and limb transplants, which are still at the experimental stage. Major concerns are immunological response of the patient to donor tissue and the ability of the immune system to distinguish self from non-self leading to rejection of the transplant. Special considerations necessitate meticulous measures to prevent infection and identify early signs of rejection.

Bone, bone marrow, heart valves, cartilage, vein, pancreatic islet, cornea, and stem cell transplants are performed on a daily basis.

HANDOFF COMMUNICATION

S	Situation	Assess what is currently happening in a short statement.	Patient presents as _____
B	Background	Summarize important past assessment data for your patient here. Place lab results and medications on the concept map.	**Age:** **Gender:** **Allergies:** **Fall Risk:** **Isolation:**
A	Assessment	Use the assessment data to complete your concept map.	**Nursing Diagnosis:** Place the Nursing Diagnoses in prioritized order on the concept map and add any needed for your specific patient. **Plan:** Place any further Nursing Interventions Classifications (NIC) needed on the map.

Implement Your Plan of Care

			EVALUATE YOUR CARE	
R	Recommendation	Evaluate your nursing care and make recommendations related to the achievement of your desired outcomes. Were they met, or do new goals need to be established?	**Diag** / **Nursing Outcomes Classification (NOC)**	**Outcome met**
			1 Patient achieves timely wound healing.	☐ Yes ☐ No
			2 Patient verbalizes awareness of feelings.	☐ Yes ☐ No
			3 Patient meets psychological needs evidenced by appropriate expression of feelings and identifies options and resources.	☐ Yes ☐ No
			4 Patient verbalizes understanding of surgical procedure, prognosis, and potential complications.	☐ Yes ☐ No
			5	☐ Yes ☐ No

Nursing Diagnosis 1

Risk for infection related to medically induced immunosuppression.

NIC:
1) Screen visitors and staff for signs of infection. Assign a nurse to care for a transplant patient who is not caring for another patient with an infection; 2) Maintain neutropenic precautions; 3) Monitor compliance with hand washing of staff and visitors; 4) Provide meticulous care of invasive lines, incisions, and wounds. Remove invasive devices as soon as possible; 5) Encourage deep breathing and coughing; 6) Monitor results of serum WBC and blood glucose levels; and 7) Administer antimicrobials as ordered.

Nursing Diagnosis 2

Anxiety/fear related to perceived or actual threat to self-concept, organ rejection, threat of death evidenced by increased tension, apprehension, uncertainty.

NIC:
1) Discuss patient's transplant expectations and fears, including physical appearance, lifestyle changes, and concern about recurrence of disease process; 2) Assess level of anxiety. Determine previous coping strategies. Identify strategies to address current perceived or actual problems; 3) Provide opportunity for patient and family to meet other patients with transplants; 4) Discuss beliefs and concerns commonly held regarding the source of the organ; 5) Identify possible actions to limit physical effects or manifestations of long-term steroid or cyclosporine use; and 6) Refer to appropriate support groups, social services, vocational counseling, psychotherapy as needed.

Nursing Diagnosis 3

Risk for ineffective coping or disabled family coping related to prolonged disease exhausting supportive family.

NIC:
1) Encourage and support patient and family in evaluating lifestyle. Discuss implications for the future; 2) Assess patient and family's current functional status; 3) Determine additional outside stressors: family, social, work environment, or health-care management; 4) Discuss normalcy and monitor progression of recuperation and potential course of recovery; 5) Have patient list previous methods of dealing with problems and outcomes of actions; and 6) Refer to spiritual resource, psychiatric specialist, or social worker as indicated.

Nursing Diagnosis 4

Deficient knowledge regarding condition, prognosis, treatment, self-care, and discharge needs related to lack of exposure, recall evidenced by questions, request for information.

NIC:
1) Review general signs of transplant rejection and infection such as malaise, fever, chills, delayed wound healing, nausea, vomiting, syncope; 2) Emphasize necessity of periodic laboratory tests and routine examinations; 3) Counsel patient to avoid use of OTC medications and adjustment of prescribed medication doses as indicated; 4) Counsel patient to wear ID tag at all times; 5) Discuss self-monitoring routine to chart temperature, weight, BP, pulse, medication dosage, functional ability; 6) Counsel patient to avoid changing cat litter and receiving live vaccines, use gloves when gardening, take proper care of wounds; 7) Instruct patient to avoid any activity that places pressure on incision.

Condition:
Transplantation Considerations— Postoperative and Lifelong
Age:

Link & Explain
• Nursing Interventions Classification (NIC)
• Laboratory and Diagnostic Procedures
• Medications

Nursing Diagnosis 5

NIC:

Medications
a. Levofloxacin (Levaquin), cefazolin (Ancef), cefepime (Maxipime), vancomycin (Lyphocin), ciprofloxacin (Cipro)
b. Methylprednisolone (Solu-Medrol), cyclosporine (Sandimmune), mycophenolate mofetil (CellCept, Myfortic), azathioprine (Imuran), muromonab-CD3 (Orthoclone OKT3), lymphocyte immune globulin (Atgam)
c.
d.

Laboratory & Diagnostic Procedures
a. CBC, serology screening tests, donor-recipient matching, blood typing, tissue matching, cross-matching, CT scan, MRI, total body scan, EKG, pulmonary function studies, renal function studies, dental evaluation
b.
c.
d.

CONDITION: Tuberculosis (TB)

PHYSIOLOGY: TB is an infectious disease caused by *Mycobacterium tuberculosis*, an aerobic acid-fast bacillus. Although it is most frequently a pulmonary disease, more than 15% of patients experience extrapulmonary TB that can infect the meninges, kidneys, bones, or other tissues. Pulmonary TB can range from a small infection of bronchopneumonia to diffuse, intense inflammation, necrosis, pleural effusion, and extensive fibrosis. TB is transmitted by respiratory droplets through sneezing or coughing by an infected person.

Mycobacteria lie dormant until there is a decrease in the host's resistance. TB can affect both genders at any age but is most common in the elderly population and in those who are immunosuppressed. Other high-risk groups are hospital employees, recent immigrants, urban dwellers, drug and alcohol abusers, nursing home residents, and people who are incarcerated. Patients with HIV should be tested for TB, and all patients with TB should be tested for HIV, because the incidence of comorbidities is 25% in these groups.

Clinical manifestations include fatigue, malaise, anorexia, unexplained weight loss, low-grade fevers, night sweats, and a cough that becomes frequent and produces purulent sputum.

HANDOFF COMMUNICATION

S	Situation	Assess what is currently happening in a short statement.	Patient presents as _____ *Note if patient may be immunocompromised, malnourished, in high-risk group, or has had possible recent exposure to newly diagnosed TB patient.*
B	Background	Summarize important past assessment data for your patient here. Place lab results and medications on the concept map.	**Age:** **Gender:** **Allergies:** **Social Alerts:** Living arrangements, recent travel **Mental Status:** **Safety Risk:**
A	Assessment	Use the assessment data to complete your concept map.	**Nursing Diagnosis:** Place the Nursing Diagnoses in prioritized order on the concept map and add any needed for your specific patient. **Plan:** Place any further Nursing Interventions Classifications (NIC) needed on the map.

Implement Your Plan of Care

		EVALUATE YOUR CARE		
R	Recommendation	Evaluate your nursing care and make recommendations related to the achievement of your desired outcomes. Were they met, or do new goals need to be established?	**Diag**	**Nursing Outcomes Classification (NOC)**	**Outcome met**
			1	Patient identifies interventions to prevent or reduce risk of spread of infection.	☐ Yes ☐ No
			2	Patient maintains patent airway and reports absence of (or decreased) dyspnea.	☐ Yes ☐ No
			3	Patient demonstrates progressive weight gain toward goal and is free of signs of malnutrition.	☐ Yes ☐ No
			4	Patient reports feeling less fatigued and demonstrates increased tolerance for activity without distress.	☐ Yes ☐ No
			5	Patient verbalizes understanding of disease process, prognosis, prevention, therapeutic regimen, and plan for follow-up care.	☐ Yes ☐ No

Nursing Diagnosis 1

Risk for infection related to lowered resistance, suppressed inflammatory process.

NIC:
1) Assess for signs/symptoms of active infection; **2)** Review infection control measures such as airborne isolation, proper disposal of tissues with expectorate, wearing mask outside room during transport; **3)** Teach proper hand-washing techniques; **4)** Identify patient risk factors for reactivation/spread of disease (hemoptysis, bone or back pain, bloody urine); **5)** Administer anti-infective agents as indicate; and **6)** Notify local health department.

Nursing Diagnosis 2

Ineffective airway clearance related to thick, purulent secretions evidenced by abnormal breath sounds: rhonchi, wheezes, stridor.

NIC:
1) Assess respiratory function (breath sounds, dyspnea, presence of pallor/cyanosis, pulse oximetry, mentation); **2)** Evaluate effectiveness of patient cough and document amount/character of sputum; **3)** Administer humidified oxygen/respiratory treatments, mucolytic agents, bronchodilators, corticosteroids as indicated; **4)** Teach coughing/deep-breathing exercises; **5)** Position in semi-Fowler's or high-Fowler's if indicated; and **6)** Prepare for intubation and mechanical ventilation as needed.

Nursing Diagnosis 3

Imbalanced nutrition: less than body requirements related to frequent cough and sputum production evidenced by reported lack of interest in food, altered taste sensation.

NIC:
1) Assess nutritional status including physical assessment, recent weight loss, skin integrity; **2)** Obtain diet history; **3)** Monitor I&O/daily weights; encourage small, frequent meals high in protein and carbohydrates; **4)** Provide oral care before/after respiratory treatments; monitor lab studies associated with nutritional status; and **5)** Consult dietician as needed.

Nursing Diagnosis 4

Activity intolerance related to increased metabolic demands of disease process evidenced by frequent coughing, fatigue, shortness of breath.

NIC:
1) Evaluate patient's ability for activity tolerance; **2)** Assess for dyspnea and fatigue; **3)** Schedule frequent rest periods in between ADL and treatment activities; **4)** Assist with self-care as needed to avoid excess energy expenditure; and **5)** Implement measures to promote sleep.

Condition:
Tuberculosis (TB)
Age:

- - - - - - - - - - - -

Link & Explain
• Nursing Interventions Classification (NIC)
• Laboratory and Diagnostic Procedures
• Medications

Nursing Diagnosis 5

Risk for ineffective health management related to lack of knowledge, complexity of therapeutic regimen, discharge needs, and follow-up care evidenced by expressed misconceptions about health status.

NIC:
1) Evaluate patient understanding of disease process and treatment plan; **2)** Evaluate patient's ability to self-manage therapeutic regimen effectively; **3)** Provide teaching and written instructions regarding disease process and ongoing treatment regimen; **4)** Evaluate social/economic support systems; **5)** Explain medications, common side effects, and reason for long treatment period; **6)** Discuss concerns such as treatment failure, drug-resistant TB, and relapse; and **7)** Refer to public health agency and home health care as appropriate.

Medications
a. Isoniazid (INH)
b. Rifampin (RIF)
c. Pyrazinamide (PZAP)
d. Ethambutol (EMB), streptomycin

Laboratory & Diagnostic Procedures
a. Sputum smear for acid-fast bacillus/sputum culture
b. Immunoassay blood analysis: QuantiFERON-TB Gold (QFT-G)
c. Mantoux test (PPD)
d. Chest x-ray, ABGs

CONDITION: Upper Gastrointestinal Bleeding/Esophageal Bleeding

PHYSIOLOGY: Upper gastrointestinal bleeding may be from an arterial, venous, or capillary source. Bleeding that is arterial is usually profuse and bright red, arising from the branches of the celiac artery and superior mesenteric artery. Vomitus that is coffee ground in color is blood that has been in the stomach. Black tarry stools called melena are the result of slow bleeding from an upper gastrointestinal site.

Bleeding from the esophagus is a result of chronic esophagitis, Mallory-Weiss tear, or esophageal varices. Bleeding from the stomach or duodenum may be a side effect of medications such as aspirin, NSAIDs, or corticosteroids. Bleeding from stress-related mucosal disease (SRMD) can occur as a result of a severe physiological event such as burns, trauma, or surgery.

HANDOFF COMMUNICATION

S	Situation	Assess what is currently happening in a short statement.	Patient presents as _____ VS: LOC:
B	Background	Summarize important past assessment data for your patient here. Place lab results and medications on the concept map.	Age: Gender: Allergies: Fall Risk: Isolation:
A	Assessment	Use the assessment data to complete your concept map.	**Nursing Diagnosis:** Place the Nursing Diagnoses in prioritized order on the concept map and add any needed for your specific patient. **Plan:** Place any further Nursing Interventions Classifications (NIC) needed on the map.

Implement Your Plan of Care

			EVALUATE YOUR CARE	
R	Recommendation	Evaluate your nursing care and make recommendations related to the achievement of your desired outcomes. Were they met, or do new goals need to be established?	**Diag** / **Nursing Outcomes Classification (NOC)**	**Outcome met**
			1 Patient reports pain is relieved or controlled, demonstrates relaxed body posture, and sleeps appropriately.	☐ Yes ☐ No
			2 Patient demonstrates problem-solving and effective use of resources.	☐ Yes ☐ No
			3 Patient has stable VS, warm skin, good skin turgor, adequate urine output.	☐ Yes ☐ No
			4 Patient verbalizes understanding of cause of health problem and treatment of modalities used. Patient discusses own role in preventing recurrence.	☐ Yes ☐ No
			5	☐ Yes ☐ No

Nursing Diagnosis 1

Acute pain related to physical response, such as reflex muscle spasm in the stomach wall evidenced by reports of pain, grimacing, rigid body posture, guarding behaviors.

NIC:
1) Maintain bedrest and provide quiet, restful environment; **2)** Provide and implement prescribed dietary modifications; **3)** Administer analgesics intravenously in a timely manner; consider use of morphine sulfate, ketorolac (Toradol); **4)** Discuss factors that aggravate or alleviate pain; and **5)** Note location and intensity (0–10 scale) of pain and factors that aggravate and relieve pain.

Nursing Diagnosis 2

Anxiety related to change in health status, threat of death evidenced by increased tension, restlessness, irritability, fearfulness, tachycardia, diaphoresis.

NIC:
1) Monitor physiological responses such as tachypnea, palpitations, dizziness, headache, restlessness, irritability, lack of eye contact; **2)** Encourage verbalization of concerns. Assist patient in expressing feelings by use of active listening; **3)** Provide accurate, concrete information about procedures; **4)** Provide a calm and restful environment; **5)** Demonstrate and encourage relaxation techniques such as visualization, deep-breathing exercises, and guided imagery; and **6)** Administer medications such as diazepam (Valium), clorazepate (Tranxene), alprazolam (Xanax) as indicated.

Nursing Diagnosis 3

Deficient fluid volume related to acute loss of blood and gastric secretions evidenced by decreased systolic BP and increased heart rate.

NIC:
1) Note patient's physiological response to bleeding such as changes in mentation, weakness, restlessness, anxiety, pallor, diaphoresis, tachypnea; **2)** Note color and characteristics of vomitus, NG tube drainage, and stools; **3)** Assess VS and compare with baseline and previous readings. Take BP in lying, sitting, and standing positions when possible; **4)** Observe for renewed bleeding after cessation of initial bleed; **5)** Administer blood volume expanders, normal saline 0.9% or lactated Ringer's IV; **6)** Insert and maintain NG tube in acute bleeding. Perform gastric lavage as prescribed; and **7)** Monitor laboratory values such as Hgb/Hct, RBCs, BUN, creatinine.

Nursing Diagnosis 4

Deficient knowledge regarding disease process, prognosis, treatment, self-care, and discharge needs related to lack of information or recall, information misinterpretation evidenced by verbalization of the problem, request for information, statement of misconceptions.

NIC:
1) Provide and review information regarding etiology of bleeding, relationship of lifestyle behaviors, and ways to reduce risk and contributing factors; **2)** Assist patient to identify the relationship between food intake and epigastric pain. Encourage avoidance of gastric irritants such as pepper, caffeine, alcohol, fruit juices, fatty and spicy foods; **3)** Emphasize the importance of reading labels on OTC drugs and avoiding products containing aspirin; **4)** Review the significance of coffee-ground emesis, tarry stools, abdominal distention, severe epigastric or abdominal pain radiating to the shoulder; **5)** Discuss importance of smoking cessation; and **6)** Refer to support groups or counseling for lifestyle and behavior changes.

Condition:
Upper Gastrointestinal Bleeding/ Esophageal Bleeding

Age:

Link & Explain
• Nursing Interventions Classification (NIC)
• Laboratory and Diagnostic Procedures
• Medications

Nursing Diagnosis 5

NIC:

Medications
a. Sodium chloride 0.9% IV, lactated Ringer's solution IV, volume expanders, fresh frozen plasma, packed red blood cells
b. Proton pump inhibitors (PPIs), antacids: aluminum based, antiemetics, vitamin B$_{12}$
c. Vasopressin (Pitressin), vitamin K (AquaMephyton)
d. Anti-infectives

Laboratory & Diagnostic Procedures
a. ABGs
b. Serum electrolytes, CBC, coagulation profile, BUN
c. Esophagogastroduodenoscopy (EGD) with control of bleeding such as injection therapy, variceal ligation, sclerotherapy, balloon tamponade, surgical intervention, radiological intervention, transjugular intrahepatic portosystemic shunt (TIPS)
d. Gastrin analysis, parietal cell antibodies, gastric biopsies

CONDITION: Urinary Diversion/Urostomy/Nephrostomy

PHYSIOLOGY: Urinary diversion is the surgical redirection of urine flow. With an incontinent diversion, the urine is diverted out of the body through an opening in the abdominal wall, which requires a tube to drain or a pouch to be worn outside the body. A continent diversion involves the creation of a pouch or bladder inside the body, which is constructed with the use of bowel from the digestive tract.

Urinary Diversions

Nephrostomy: catheter is inserted into the pelvis of the kidney.
Ileal conduit: ureters are attached to a segment of the ileum to form an abdominal stoma.
Cutaneous ureterostomy: ureters are removed from the bladder and brought through the abdominal wall to create a stoma.
Kock pouch: section of the intestine is used to form a pouch inside the abdomen and create a reservoir that is emptied with a catheter.
Orthotopic continent urinary diversion (neobladder): section of the intestine is used to form a pouch inside the abdomen; may use spontaneous method to void.

HANDOFF COMMUNICATION

S *Situation* — Assess what is currently happening in a short statement.

Patient presents as _____

B *Background* — Summarize important past assessment data for your patient here. Place lab results and medications on the concept map.

Age:　　Gender:
Allergies:　　Fall Risk:
Isolation:

A *Assessment* — Use the assessment data to complete your concept map.

Nursing Diagnosis: Place the Nursing Diagnoses in prioritized order on the concept map and add any needed for your specific patient.
Plan: Place any further Nursing Interventions Classifications (NIC) needed on the map.

Implement Your Plan of Care

R *Recommendation* — Evaluate your nursing care and make recommendations related to the achievement of your desired outcomes. Were they met, or do new goals need to be established?

EVALUATE YOUR CARE

Diag	Nursing Outcomes Classification (NOC)	Outcome met
1	Patient demonstrates behaviors and techniques to promote healing and prevent skin breakdown.	☐ Yes ☐ No
2	Patient demonstrates acceptance by viewing and touching stoma and participating in self-care.	☐ Yes ☐ No
3	Patient verbalizes relief or control of pain and appears relaxed.	☐ Yes ☐ No
4	Patient displays continuous flow of urine with output adequate for individual situation.	☐ Yes ☐ No
5	Patient correctly performs necessary procedures and explains reasons for the action.	☐ Yes ☐ No

Nursing Diagnosis 1

Risk for impaired skin integrity related to absence of sphincter at stoma and continuous flow of urine.

NIC:
1) Inspect stoma and note irritation, bruises, rash, status of sutures; **2)** Measure stoma periodically with measurement guide to alter appliance fit as edema decreases; **3)** Use a transparent, odor-proof drainage pouch to allow observation of stoma; **4)** Cleanse ostomy pouch on a routine basis, using a vinegar solution or commercial solution; **5)** Apply sealant barrier to protect skin from pouch adhesive; **6)** Change appliance every 3–5 days. Use adhesive removers to prevent skin irritation; and **7)** Investigate any complaints of burning or itching of the skin.

Nursing Diagnosis 2

Disturbed body image related to disease process and associated treatment regimen evidenced by actual change in structure and function.

NIC:
1) Review reason for surgery and future expectations; **2)** Answer all questions regarding urostomy and its function; **3)** Note behaviors such as withdrawal, increased dependency, manipulation, excuses to avoid involvement in care; **4)** Maintain positive approach during care activities; and **5)** Discuss sexual function, physical changes, medications that may affect sexual function.

Nursing Diagnosis 3

Acute pain related to physical factors: disruption of skin and tissue evidenced by guarding, distraction behaviors, restlessness.

NIC:
1) Assess pain, noting location, characteristics, and intensity (0–10 scale); **2)** Auscultate bowel sounds; note passage of flatus; **3)** Assist with ROM exercises and encourage early ambulation; **4)** Administer medications as indicated, such as opioids, analgesics; use patient-controlled analgesia (PCA); and **5)** Provide sitz baths if needed.

Condition:
Urinary Diversion/ Urostomy/ Nephrostomy
Age:

Link & Explain
• Nursing Interventions Classification (NIC)
• Laboratory and Diagnostic Procedures
• Medications

Nursing Diagnosis 4

Impaired urinary elimination related to surgical diversion, tissue trauma, postoperative edema evidenced by loss of continence and changes in amount, character of urine, and urinary retention.

NIC:
1) Evaluate and maintain urinary catheters and drains, discuss use of stents in the immediate postoperative period; **2)** Note presence of drains and label, observe urine flow through each; **3)** Observe and record color of urine, note hematuria or bleeding from stoma; **4)** Position tubing and drainage pouch so the flow of urine is not obstructed; and **5)** Encourage increased fluids and maintain accurate I&O.

Nursing Diagnosis 5

Deficient knowledge regarding condition, prognosis, treatment, self-care, and discharge needs related to lack of exposure evidenced by statements of misinformation.

NIC:
1) Review anatomy and physiology and implications of surgical intervention. Include written and picture resources; **2)** Review signs of reservoir overdistention and need for intervention; **3)** Discuss use of acid-ash diet: cranberries, prunes, plums, cereals, rice, poultry to decrease risk of crystals and stone formation; **4)** Stress importance of increased fluid intake of at least 2–3 L/day so urine is pale yellow; and **5)** Encourage regular exercise and activity.

Medications
a. Antibiotics
b.
c.
d.

Laboratory & Diagnostic Procedures
a. Urine cytology
b. Intravenous pyelogram (IVP), cystoscope with biopsy, pelvic MRI, CT scan
c.
d.

CONDITION: Urinary Incontinence

PHYSIOLOGY: Urinary incontinence is the involuntary loss of urine, which can cause problems with socialization and hygiene. It is not a normal age-related change. Continence occurs when the pressure in the urethra is greater than the pressure in the bladder.

Types of Incontinence

Stress incontinence: weak pelvic muscles and support structure; urine loss with coughing or sneezing.
Urge incontinence: overactivity of detrusor muscle; noted in central nervous system disorders such as Parkinson's disease, brain tumor.
Reflex incontinence: involuntary urination in day and night; noted with neurologic impairment such as stroke, multiple sclerosis, or spinal cord lesion.
Functional incontinence: related to cognitive, functional, or environmental factors; noted in elderly with balance and mobility problems.
Overflow incontinence: overfull bladder that overcomes sphincter control; noted with urethral stricture, pelvic organ prolapse.

HANDOFF COMMUNICATION

S	Situation	Assess what is currently happening in a short statement.	Patient presents as _____
B	Background	Summarize important past assessment data for your patient here. Place lab results and medications on the concept map.	**Age:** **Gender:** **Allergies:** **Fall Risk:** **Isolation:**
A	Assessment	Use the assessment data to complete your concept map.	**Nursing Diagnosis:** Place the Nursing Diagnoses in prioritized order on the concept map and add any needed for your specific patient. **Plan:** Place any further Nursing Interventions Classifications (NIC) needed on the map.

Implement Your Plan of Care

		EVALUATE YOUR CARE		
R	Recommendation Evaluate your nursing care and make recommendations related to the achievement of your desired outcomes. Were they met, or do new goals need to be established?	**Diag**	**Nursing Outcomes Classification (NOC)**	**Outcome met**
		1	Patient expresses increased sense of self-esteem and uses resources for assistance.	☐ Yes ☐ No
		2	Patient maintains skin integrity and demonstrates behaviors to promote healing and prevent skin breakdown.	☐ Yes ☐ No
		3	Patient demonstrates acceptance of health problem by participating in self-care.	☐ Yes ☐ No
		4	Patient demonstrates techniques or lifestyle changes to reduce risk of infection.	☐ Yes ☐ No
		5	Patient verbalizes understanding of therapeutic needs and initiates necessary lifestyle changes.	☐ Yes ☐ No

Nursing Diagnosis 1

Risk for social isolation related to altered state of wellness.

NIC:
1) Determine patient's response to condition, feelings about self, concerns, and fears; **2)** Assess coping mechanisms and previous methods for dealing with life problems; **3)** Discuss concerns about employment and leisure; and **4)** Assist patient to differentiate between isolation and loneliness.

Nursing Diagnosis 2

Risk for impaired skin integrity related to irritation from urine.

NIC:
1) Clean skin area gently and pat dry, or use hair dryer on cool setting; **2)** Change pad and protective briefs as soon as they become wet; **3)** Instruct patient to wear cotton undergarments; and **4)** Check skinfolds in groin and perineum daily for breakdown with the use of a mirror.

Nursing Diagnosis 3

Disturbed body image related to disease process and associated treatment regimen evidenced by refusal to participate in self-care.

NIC:
1) Note behaviors of withdrawal, increased dependency, manipulation, or decreased involvement in care; **2)** Acknowledge feelings of anger, depression, grief; and **3)** Provide information to assist patient with toileting schedule and odor problems.

Nursing Diagnosis 4

Risk for infection related to depression or immunological defenses.

NIC:
1) Document urine characteristics and note changes indicating urinary tract infection; **2)** Obtain urine specimen as indicated; **3)** Monitor VS and report any elevation in temperature; and **4)** Note decrease in urine output.

Condition:
Urinary Incontinence
Age:

Link & Explain
• Nursing Interventions Classification (NIC)
• Laboratory and Diagnostic Procedures
• Medications

Nursing Diagnosis 5

Deficient knowledge regarding condition, prognosis, treatment, self-care, and discharge needs related to lack of exposure, recall evidenced by inaccurate follow-through of instructions.

NIC:
1) Instruct patient to perform Kegel exercises that stop and start urinary stream; **2)** Encourage patient to keep a diary to determine urinary incontinence related to diet, medications, behavioral interventions; **3)** Avoid foods that have a direct bladder-stimulating or diuretic effect such as caffeine, alcohol, citrus, artificial sweeteners; **4)** Space fluids at regular intervals throughout the day, limit fluids after dinner hour; **5)** Encourage weight reduction and regular exercise; and **6)** Administer drug therapy to improve urethral resistance.

Medications

a. Muscarinic receptor antagonists

b. α-Adrenergic antagonists, α-adrenergic agonists, 5α-reductase inhibitors, tricyclic antidepressants

c. Calcium channel blockers

d. Hormone replacement

Laboratory & Diagnostic Procedures

a. Urine, urine culture and sensitivity

b. Urography, voiding cystourethrogram (VCUG), ultrasonographic bladder scanner

c. Cystourethroscopy

d. Cystometrogram (CMG)

CONDITION: Urolithiasis/Renal Calculi

PHYSIOLOGY: Urolithiasis is the presence of stones anywhere in the urinary tract. Stones formed in the kidneys are called *nephrolithiasis*, and stones formed in the ureters are called *ureterolithiasis*. The calculi are formed from mineral deposits, which are usually calcium oxalate or calcium phosphate. Calculi may also develop from uric acid, struvite, or cystine. The calculi may cause damage to the lining of the urinary tract. Severe pain and obstruction of urine flow occurs when the stone is in the ureter. Dehydration; excessive intake of vitamin C and D, grapefruit juice, purines; congenital renal abnormalities; and heredity place patients at increased risk for urolithiasis.

HANDOFF COMMUNICATION

S Situation	Assess what is currently happening in a short statement.	Patient presents as _____ VS: LOC:
B Background	Summarize important past assessment data for your patient here. Place lab results and medications on the concept map.	Age: Gender: Allergies: Fall Risk: Isolation:
A Assessment	Use the assessment data to complete your concept map.	**Nursing Diagnosis:** Place the Nursing Diagnoses in prioritized order on the concept map and add any needed for your specific patient. **Plan:** Place any further Nursing Interventions Classifications (NIC) needed on the map.

Implement Your Plan of Care

R Recommendation	Evaluate your nursing care and make recommendations related to the achievement of your desired outcomes. Were they met, or do new goals need to be established?	**EVALUATE YOUR CARE**		
		Diag	**Nursing Outcomes Classification (NOC)**	**Outcome met**
		1	Patient is relaxed and able to sleep and rest appropriately.	☐ Yes ☐ No
		2	Patient voids every 3–4 hours in normal amounts greater than or equal to 30 ml/hr.	☐ Yes ☐ No
		3	Patient maintains adequate fluid balance with VS and weight within normal range for patient.	☐ Yes ☐ No
		4	Patient verbalizes understanding of disease process and potential complications.	☐ Yes ☐ No
		5		☐ Yes ☐ No

Nursing Diagnosis 1

Acute pain related to tissue trauma, edema formation, cellular ischemia evidenced by reports of colicky pain.

NIC:
1) Document location, duration, intensity of pain (1–10 scale), and radiation. Note elevated BP and pulse, restlessness, moaning, medicate with analgesic as ordered; **2)** Explain cause of pain and importance to notify the caregiver of change in the characteristics of the pain; **3)** Provide comfort measures, guided imagery, focused breathing, diversional activities, quiet environment; **4)** Apply warm compresses to the back area.

Nursing Diagnosis 2

Impaired urinary elimination related to mechanical obstruction, inflammation evidenced by urgency, frequency, oliguria.

NIC:
1) Monitor I&O and characteristics of urine; **2)** Strain all urine. Document if stones are expelled and send them to the laboratory for analysis; **3)** Encourage increased oral fluid intake if nausea is not present; **4)** Assess reports of bladder fullness, palpate for suprapubic distention; and **5)** Observe for the presence of periorbital edema and dependent edema.

Nursing Diagnosis 3

Risk for deficient fluid volume related to nausea, vomiting, generalized abdominal and pelvic nerve irritation from renal or ureteral colic.

NIC:
1) Increase fluid intake to 3–4 liters/ 24 hours within cardiac tolerance; **2)** Monitor I&O; **3)** Note frequency and characteristics of vomiting and diarrhea; **4)** Administer IV fluids; and **5)** Monitor Hgb/Hct and electrolytes, BUN, and creatinine.

Nursing Diagnosis 4

Deficient knowledge regarding condition, prognosis, treatment, self-care, and discharge needs related to unfamiliarity with information resources evidenced by questions, request for information, statement of misconception.

NIC:
1) Review disease process, prognosis, precipitating factors; **2)** Encourage regular activity and an exercise program; **3)** Review dietary plan and restrictions related to type of stone; **4)** Identify symptoms requiring medical evaluation such as recurrent pain, hematuria, oliguria; and **5)** Review medications and encourage the patient to discuss any OTC and herbal medications with health-care provider.

Condition:
Urolithiasis/ Renal Calculi

Age:

Link & Explain
- Nursing Interventions Classification (NIC)
- Laboratory and Diagnostic Procedures
- Medications

Nursing Diagnosis 5

NIC:

Medications
a. Opioids: morphine sulfate (Duramorph) (decrease ureteral colic and promote muscle relaxation)
b. Antispasmodics: flavoxate (Urispas), oxybutynin (Ditropan) (decrease reflex spasm and relax ureteral smooth muscle to facilitate stone passage)
c. Corticosteroids: prednisone (Deltasone) (reduce tissue edema to facilitate movement of stone)
d. Diuretic: hydrochlorothiazide (Esidrix, HydroDIURIL) (prevent urinary stasis and decrease calcium stone formation if not caused by an underlying disease process)

Laboratory & Diagnostic Procedures
a. BUN/creatinine ratio: normal ratio is 10:1; blockage below the kidney will cause postrenal azotemia (ratio greater than 15:1 without renal disease
b. CBC: Hgb/Hct abnormal if dehydration or anemia is present
c. Urinalysis: color may be yellow, dark brown, or bloody; commonly shows RBCs, WBCs, crystals, casts, bacteria, pus; pH may help identify type of stones
d. Kidney ultrasound and intrarenal Doppler ultrasound: determine the obstructive changes and location of the stone without the risk of kidney failure caused by contrast medium

CONDITION: Venous Stasis Ulcer

PHYSIOLOGY: Venous stasis ulcers are the result of poor, sluggish circulation in the lower extremities. They account for up to 70% of all lower extremity ulcers, more than diabetic and arterial ulcers combined. Venous stasis ulcers are most frequently caused by chronic venous insufficiency, which is usually related to nonfunctioning or incompetent valves and venous hypertension. Venous ulcers are difficult to treat and may persist and recur frequently.

Risk factors for development of chronic venous insufficiency and venous stasis ulcers include family history, varicose veins, deep vein thrombosis, heart failure, atherosclerotic vascular disease, hypertension, obesity, immobility, hypothyroidism, and advanced age. The development of venous stasis ulcers results from increased venous pressure, which increases capillary leakage and edema, leading to buildup of toxic waste materials and hypoxia. This, in turn, leads to tissue ischemia and breakdown. Signs and symptoms of venous stasis ulcers include edema; brownish skin discoloration; superficial wound depth with pink, moist base; irregular wound edges; aching, throbbing pain; and exudate. Most venous stasis ulcers form on the medial aspect of the ankle and lower third of the legs (*Taber's*, 2009).

HANDOFF COMMUNICATION

S	*Situation*	Assess what is currently happening in a short statement.	Patient presents as _____ *Assess patient's history and risk factors. Assess lower extremities, checking for edema, pain, impaired tissue integrity, old scars, fibrotic changes, skin discoloration, and varicose veins. Assess wounds for signs and symptoms of infection. Determine previous treatment.*
B	*Background*	Summarize important past assessment data for your patient here. Place lab results and medications on the concept map.	**Age:** **Gender:** **Allergies:** **Fall Risk:** **Isolation:**
A	*Assessment*	Use the assessment data to complete your concept map.	**Nursing Diagnosis:** Place the Nursing Diagnoses in prioritized order on the concept map and add any needed for your specific patient. **Plan:** Place any further Nursing Interventions Classifications (NIC) needed on the map.

Implement Your Plan of Care

			EVALUATE YOUR CARE	
R	*Recommendation*	Evaluate your nursing care and make recommendations related to the achievement of your desired outcomes. Were they met, or do new goals need to be established?	**Diag** / **Nursing Outcomes Classification (NOC)**	**Outcome met**
			1 Patient identifies strategies to increase venous return and decrease venous congestion.	☐ Yes ☐ No
			2 Patient's wounds decrease in size and have increased granulation tissue.	☐ Yes ☐ No
			3 Patient maintains or attains appropriate weight for height, serum albumin and electrolyte levels.	☐ Yes ☐ No
			4 Patient describes or demonstrates strategies to meet health-care goals.	☐ Yes ☐ No
			5 Patient has decreased edema and verbalizes strategies to prevent and/or decrease edema.	☐ Yes ☐ No

Nursing Diagnosis 1

Ineffective peripheral tissue perfusion related to poor venous return and venous congestion evidenced by tissue edema and pain.

NIC:
1) Routinely assess peripheral vascular system to include distal circulation, sensation, and motion; pedal pulses; pain; pallor and paresthesias; and presence of impaired tissue integrity; 2) Encourage patient to elevate legs when sitting; 3) Apply compression stockings or alternating compression devices as ordered; 4) Teach patient active ROM exercises and encourage frequent performance; 5) Encourage ambulation several times per day; 6) Discourage sitting for prolonged periods, especially with legs or ankles crossed; 7) Discourage standing for long periods of time; 8) Educate and assist patient with smoking cessation; and 9) Provide patient with knowledge and tools for self-management.

Nursing Diagnosis 2

Impaired tissue integrity related to altered tissue perfusion evidenced by skin breakdown and draining wound.

NIC:
1) Inspect wound for signs of healing or wound deterioration; 2) Assess for signs and symptoms of infection: fever, malaise, purulent wound drainage, increased heat and redness surrounding wound, necrotic tissue, increased pain, and loss of function; 3) Apply dressings as ordered, maintaining aseptic technique; 4) Promote compression therapy with tubular support bandages, Velcro wrap (CircAid), Unna's boots; 5) Teach patient and family strategies to improve wound healing and to prevent future skin breakdown; and 6) Improve nutritional status with adequate protein, vitamin A, vitamin C, and zinc.

Nursing Diagnosis 3

Impaired nutrition: less than body requirements related to increased metabolic demand evidenced by weight 10% less than normal weight for frame.

NIC:
1) Obtain nutritional history; 2) Monitor laboratory data that indicates nutritional status: albumin, RBC count, WBC count, and electrolytes; 3) Monitor nutritional intake; 4) Consult dietician for assessment and recommendations; 5) Encourage nutritional supplements as needed; 6) Provide information and strategies to the patient and family to assist them in meeting nutritional needs; and 7) Refer to community resources for meal assistance.

Nursing Diagnosis 4

Ineffective health maintenance related to deficient knowledge regarding disease process and self-management evidenced by lack of knowledge of basic health practices.

NIC:
1) Assess patient's and family's knowledge and possible misconceptions regarding disease process and treatment; 2) Provide patient and family teaching regarding disease process, treatment options, and self-management; 3) Include patient and family as members of the health-care team and in determining goals and plan of care; 4) Refer to home health care or community resources as needed; 5) Provide positive reinforcement and encouragement; and 6) Follow patient progression via phone calls or follow-up office visits.

Condition:
Venous Stasis Ulcer
Age:

Link & Explain
• Nursing Interventions Classification (NIC)
• Laboratory and Diagnostic Procedures
• Medications

Nursing Diagnosis 5

Excess fluid volume related to venous congestion and capillary leakage evidenced by edema.

NIC:
1) Routinely monitor extent and location of edema; 2) Monitor I&O and daily weights; 3) Encourage active ROM exercises and ambulation to increase venous return; 4) Elevate lower extremities when patient is sitting; and 5) Teach patient and family about disease process and strategies to decrease/prevent edema.

Medications
a. Antibiotics
b. Pain medications
c. Topical wound treatments
d.

Laboratory & Diagnostic Procedures
a. CBC, chemistries
b. Ultrasound
c. x-ray
d.

CONDITION: Ventilation Assistance (Mechanical)

PHYSIOLOGY: Impairment of respiratory function affecting oxygenation and carbon dioxide elimination requires mechanical assistance to support spontaneous breathing.

Mechanical ventilation is utilized in the following situations:
1. Inability to maintain adequate oxygenation (hypoxia).
2. Inability to maintain adequate ventilation due to apnea causing a rise in carbon dioxide and fall in pH (respiratory acidosis).
3. Inability to continue the work of breathing (respiratory muscle weakness or failure).

HANDOFF COMMUNICATION

S Situation	Assess what is currently happening in a short statement.	Patient presents as _____ VS: LOC:
B Background	Summarize important past assessment data for your patient here. Place lab results and medications on the concept map.	**Age:** **Gender:** **Allergies:** **Fall Risk:** **Isolation:**
A Assessment	Use the assessment data to complete your concept map.	**Nursing Diagnosis:** Place the Nursing Diagnoses in prioritized order on the concept map and add any needed for your specific patient. **Plan:** Place any further Nursing Interventions Classifications (NIC) needed on the map.

Implement Your Plan of Care

		Diag	EVALUATE YOUR CARE
			Nursing Outcomes Classification (NOC) · Outcome met

	Diag	Nursing Outcomes Classification (NOC)	Outcome met
R Recommendation — Evaluate your nursing care and make recommendations related to the achievement of your desired outcomes. Were they met, or do new goals need to be established?	1	Patient maintains an effective respiratory pattern via ventilator with absence of cyanosis, hypoxemia.	☐ Yes ☐ No
	2	Patient reports that anxiety or fear is reduced to manageable level.	☐ Yes ☐ No
	3	Patient maintains patent airway with clear breath sounds and remains free of aspiration.	☐ Yes ☐ No
	4	Patient reestablishes independent respiration with ABGs within acceptable range and is free of signs of respiratory failure.	☐ Yes ☐ No
	5	Patient demonstrates behaviors or skills to meet individual needs and prevent complications.	☐ Yes ☐ No

Nursing Diagnosis 1

Ineffective breathing pattern/impaired spontaneous ventilation related to alteration of patient's usual oxygen/carbon dioxide ratio evidenced by dyspnea, increased work of breathing, use of accessory muscles.

NIC:
1) Observe overall breathing pattern. Note respiratory rate, auscultate periodically, note adventitious breath sounds and symmetry of chest movement; **2)** Count patient's respirations for 1 full minute and compare with desired ventilator set rate; **3)** Inflate tracheal/endotracheal cuff. Check cuff inflation every 4–8 hours; **4)** Respond to high-pressure alarms (need for suction, patient biting on tube placed orally, patient is anxious and fighting the ventilator, water in tubing); **5)** Respond to low-pressure alarms (disconnection in system, leak in the cuff). Ventilate manually for high or low alarms if source of ventilator alarm cannot be identified and rectified; **6)** Keep resuscitation bag at bedside to ventilate manually as needed; and **7)** Monitor pulse oximetry and ABG.

Nursing Diagnosis 2

Fear/severe anxiety related to threat of death, dependency of mechanical support evidenced by hypervigilance.

NIC:
1) Identify patient's perception of threat presented by the situation; **2)** Observe and monitor physical responses such as restlessness, changes in VS, repetitive movements; **3)** Encourage patient to acknowledge and express fears; **4)** Identify previous coping strengths of the patient; and **5)** Demonstrate and encourage the use of relaxation techniques, guided imagery, progressive relaxation.

Nursing Diagnosis 3

Ineffective airway clearance related to foreign body (artificial airway) in the trachea evidenced by changes in rate and depth of respirations, cyanosis, abnormal breath sounds.

NIC:
1) Monitor endotracheal (ET) tube placement. Note line marking and compare with desired placement. Secure tube carefully with tube holder; **2)** Note excessive coughing, increased dyspnea, high-pressure alarm sounding on ventilator, visible secretions in tracheal/ET tube; **3)** Suction as needed for coughing or if experiencing respiratory distress. Limit duration of suctioning to 15 seconds. Hyperventilate before and after catheter passes; and **4)** Note color and consistency of sputum.

Nursing Diagnosis 4

Risk for dysfunctional ventilatory weaning response related to depression, limited energy stores.

NIC:
1) Assess physical factors involved in weaning as follows: stable heart rate, stable BP, and improved breath sounds; **2)** Explain weaning techniques such as spontaneous breathing trial, equipment, and individual expectations; **3)** Evaluate patient's progress. Note restlessness and changes in respiratory rate, use of accessory muscles; and **4)** Avoid stressful procedures and nonessential activities. Provide undisturbed rest periods.

Condition:
Ventilation Assistance (Mechanical)
Age:

Link & Explain
• Nursing Interventions Classification (NIC)
• Laboratory and Diagnostic Procedures
• Medications

Nursing Diagnosis 5

Deficient knowledge regarding condition, prognosis and therapy, self-care, and discharge needs related to stress of situational crisis evidenced by inaccurate follow-through of instructions.

NIC:
1) Discuss specific condition requiring ventilatory support, what measures are being tried for weaning, and short- and long-term goals; **2)** Encourage patient to evaluate impact of ventilator dependence on lifestyle and changes patient would like to make; **3)** Instruct patient or caregiver about hand-washing techniques, suctioning, stoma care, chest physiotherapy; **4)** Emphasize need for smoking cessation if indicated; and **5)** Review nutrition, assistance with feeding and meal preparation, and graded exercise.

Medications
a. Corticosteroids
b. Bronchodilators
c.
d.

Laboratory & Diagnostic Procedures
a. ABGs, CBC, electrolytes
b. Chest x-ray
c. Pulmonary function studies
d.

Concept Maps for Patients With Psychiatric/Mental Health Disorders

6

Understanding psychiatric concepts is becoming more and more important in nursing care today. This chapter provides care maps that describe psychiatric or mental health conditions that a nurse may come across in a specific unit (inpatient or outpatient) for mental health or as comorbidities for patients in other specialties. We have included the major conditions that are likely to be diagnosed.

The conditions included in this chapter are:

1. Alcohol Withdrawal Syndrome (AWS)
2. Anorexia (Anorexia Nervosa)/Bulimia
3. Antisocial Personality Disorder
4. Attention Deficit-Hyperactivity Disorder (ADHD)
5. Bipolar I Disorder (Axis I)
6. Borderline Personality Disorder
7. Domestic Violence/Intimate Partner Abuse
8. Generalized Anxiety Disorder (Axis I)
9. Major Depressive Disorder (Axis I)
10. Obsessive-Compulsive Disorder (OCD)
11. Posttraumatic Stress Disorder (Axis I)
12. Rape-Trauma Syndrome
13. Risk for Suicide
14. Schizophrenia (Axis I)
15. Sleep Disorders (Insomnia)
16. Substance Abuse

CONDITION: Alcohol Withdrawal Syndrome (AWS)

PHYSIOLOGY: AWS is the neurological, psychiatric, and cardiovascular signs and symptoms that result when a person accustomed to consuming large quantities of alcohol suddenly becomes abstinent. Alcohol withdrawal usually follows a predictable pattern. In the first hours of abstinence, patients are often irritable, anxious, tremulous, and easily startled. Their blood pressure and pulse rise, but they remain alert and oriented. If they do not consume alcohol (or receive drug treatment) in the first 12 to 48 hours, they may suffer an alcohol withdrawal seizure. Abstinence for 72 to 96 hours may result in severe agitation, hallucinations, and marked fluctuations in blood pressure and pulse. This stage of withdrawal is known as delirium tremens, or alcoholic delirium; it may prove fatal in as many as 15% of patients (*Taber's*, 2009).

HANDOFF COMMUNICATION

S Situation	Assess what is currently happening in a short statement.	Patient presents with _____
B Background	Summarize important past assessment data for your patient here. Place lab results and medications on the concept map.	**Age:** **Gender:** **Allergies:** **Fall Risk:** **Isolation:**
A Assessment	Use the assessment data to complete your concept map.	**Nursing Diagnosis:** Place the Nursing Diagnoses in prioritized order on the concept map and add any needed for your specific patient. **Plan:** Place any further Nursing Interventions Classifications (NIC) needed on the map.

Implement Your Plan of Care

			EVALUATE YOUR CARE	
R Recommendation	Evaluate your nursing care and make recommendations related to the achievement of your desired outcomes. Were they met, or do new goals need to be established?	**Diag**	**Nursing Outcomes Classification (NOC)**	**Outcome met**
		1	Maintain effective breathing pattern with respiratory rate within normal range, lungs clear, and free of cyanosis or other signs and symptoms of hypoxia.	☐ Yes ☐ No
		2	Display vital signs (VS) within patient's normal range and absence or reduced frequency of dysrhythmias. Demonstrate an increase in activity tolerance.	☐ Yes ☐ No
		3	Demonstrate absence of untoward effects of withdrawal. Experience no physical injury.	☐ Yes ☐ No
		4	Regain or maintain level of consciousness (LOC). Report absence of or reduced hallucinations. Identify external factors that effect sensory-perceptual abilities.	☐ Yes ☐ No
		5		☐ Yes ☐ No

Nursing Diagnosis 1

Risk for ineffective breathing pattern related to alcohol toxicity, sedative drugs used to decrease effects of withdrawal, tracheobronchial obstruction, or fatigue.

NIC:
1) Monitor respiratory rate, depth, and pattern; **2)** Auscultate breath sounds; **3)** Elevate head of bed (HOB); **4)** Encourage coughing and deep breathing; **5)** Have suction equipment available; and **6)** Administer supplemental O_2 as needed.

Nursing Diagnosis 2

Risk for decreased cardiac output related to direct effect of alcohol on the cardiac muscle, altered systemic vascular resistance, or electronic alteration in rate, rhythm, or conduction.

NIC:
1) Monitor VS frequently in acute withdrawal; **2)** Monitor cardiac rhythm and rate; **3)** Monitor I&O; **4)** Monitor laboratory values; **5)** Monitor K+ levels closely; **6)** Be prepared to assist in CPR; **7)** Administer fluids and electrolytes; and **8)** Administer medications as indicated.

Nursing Diagnosis 3

Risk for injury related to cessation of alcohol intake with varied autonomic nervous system responses to the system's suddenly altered state: seizures, equilibrium and balance difficulties, and reduced hand-eye coordination.

NIC:
1) Identify stages of AWS: *Stage 1*— hyperactivity, tremors, sleeplessness, nausea and vomiting (N&V), diaphoresis, tachycardia, and hypertension. *Stage 2*—increased hyperactivity, seizures, and hallucinations. *Stage 3*— DTs (delirium tremens), extreme autonomic hyperactivity, confusion, anxiety, insomnia, and fever; **2)** Monitor and document seizure activity; **3)** Check DTRs (deep tendon reflexes); **4)** Assist with ambulation and self-care activities; and **5)** Administer medications as indicated.

Nursing Diagnosis 4

Disturbed sensory perception related to chemical alteration due to alcohol consumption or electrolyte imbalance, sleep deprivation, or psychological stress; anxiety or fear evidenced by disorientation to time, place, and person; changes in response to stimuli; bizarre thinking; listlessness; irritability; apprehension, fear, or anxiety.

NIC:
1) Assess LOC and ability to speak and respond to stimuli and commands; **2)** Observe for behavioral responses such as hyperactivity; **3)** Note hallucinations and document; **4)** Provide quiet environment; **5)** Consistent personal care; **6)** Encourage SO (significant other) to stay; **7)** Reorient frequently; **8)** Provide environmental safety; **9)** Limit bedside talking; **10)** Provide seclusion and restraints if needed; **11)** Monitor laboratory studies; and **12)** Administer medications as indicated.

Condition:
Alcohol Withdrawal Syndrome (AWS)

Age:

Link & Explain
• Nursing Interventions Classification (NIC)
• Laboratory and Diagnostic Procedures
• Medications

Nursing Diagnosis 5

NIC:

Medications
a. Benzodiazepines (Librium, Valium, Ativan, Serax, antiseizure medication carbamazepine [Tegretol])
b. Haloperidol (Haldol)
c. Magnesium sulfate
d. Thiamine, vitamins C & B, multivitamins

Laboratory & Diagnostic Procedures
a. Chest x-ray, EKG
b. Blood alcohol level (BAL)
c. CBC, electrolytes, glucose and ketones, blood ammonia, albumin and prealbumin
d. Liver function tests

CONDITION: Anorexia (Anorexia Nervosa)/Bulimia

PHYSIOLOGY: Anorexia nervosa is an eating disorder marked by weight loss, emaciation, a disturbance in body image, and a fear of weight gain that results in self-imposed starvation. Patients with the disorder lose weight either by excessive dieting, compulsive exercising, self-induced vomiting, or laxative or diuretic abuse to purge themselves of calories they have ingested. The illness is typically found in industrialized nations and usually begins in the teenage years. Young women are 10 to 20 times more likely than men to suffer from the disorder. Weight loss of greater than 15% of body mass is typical, often with significant metabolic consequences, which may include severe electrolyte disturbances, hypoproteinemia with associated edema, and endocrine dysfunction. Immune disturbances, anemia, and secondary cardiac arrhythmias may occur. In women, amenorrhea is also characteristically accompanied by infertility and loss of libido. Repeated vomiting can cause esophageal erosion, ulceration, tears, and bleeding, as well as dental caries and tooth and gum erosion. The disease often resists therapy.

Diagnosis is made by the following criteria: intense fear of becoming obese. This fear does not diminish as weight loss progresses. The patient claims to feel fat even when emaciated. A loss of 25% of original weight may occur. No known physical illness accounts for the weight loss. Patients with anorexia refuse to maintain body weight over a minimum normal weight for age and height.

Psychiatric therapy in a hospital is usually required if the patient refuses to eat. The patient may need to be fed parenterally (*Taber's*, 2009).

HANDOFF COMMUNICATION

S Situation	Assess what is currently happening in a short statement.	Patient presents with _____	
B Background	Summarize important past assessment data for your patient here. Place lab results and medications on the concept map.	**Age:** **Allergies:** **Isolation:**	**Gender:** **Fall Risk:**
A Assessment	Use the assessment data to complete your concept map.	**Nursing Diagnosis:** Place the Nursing Diagnoses in prioritized order on the concept map and add any needed for your specific patient. **Plan:** Place any further Nursing Interventions Classifications (NIC) needed on the map.	

Implement Your Plan of Care

R Recommendation — Evaluate your nursing care and make recommendations related to the achievement of your desired outcomes. Were they met, or do new goals need to be established?

EVALUATE YOUR CARE

Diag	Nursing Outcomes Classification (NOC)	Outcome met
1	Establish a dietary pattern with caloric intake adequate to regain or maintain appropriate weight.	☐ Yes ☐ No
2	Verbalize understanding of causative factors and behaviors necessary to correct fluid deficit.	☐ Yes ☐ No
3	Verbalize understanding of causative factors and awareness of impairment. Demonstrate behaviors to change or prevent malnutrition. Display improved ability to make decisions and problem solve.	☐ Yes ☐ No
4	Establish a more realistic body image. Acknowledge self as individual, and accept responsibility for own actions.	☐ Yes ☐ No
5		☐ Yes ☐ No

Nursing Diagnosis 1

Imbalanced nutrition: less than body requirements related to psychological restrictions of food intake and/or excessive activity, laxative abuse, or purging evidenced by weight loss, poor skin turgor, decreased muscle tone, denial of hunger, unusual hoarding or handling of food, amenorrhea, electrolyte imbalance, cardiac irregularities, and hypotension.

NIC:
1) Establish a minimum weight goal and daily requirements; **2)** Contract with patient regarding commitment to therapeutic program; **3)** Provide small, frequent, nutritionally dense meals; **4)** Make selective menu available; **5)** Be alert to choices of low-calorie foods, hoarding food, and disposing of food; **6)** Maintain regular weighting schedule and weigh back to scale; **7)** If bulimic, maintain no bathroom privileges 1–2 hours after meals; **8)** Avoid room checks and other control devices; **9)** Monitor exercise programs; **10)** Observe during mealtime and for 30 minutes after; and **11)** Maintain matter-of-fact, nonjudgmental attitude.

Nursing Diagnosis 2

Risk for fluid volume deficit related to inadequate intake of food or fluids, chronic or excessive laxative or diuretic use.

NIC:
1) Monitor vital signs (VS), capillary refill, mucous membrane status, and skin turgor; **2)** Monitor amount and type of fluid intake; **3)** Review electrolyte and renal function tests; and **4)** Administer IV and electrolytes as indicated.

Nursing Diagnosis 3

Disturbed thought processes related to severe malnutrition, electrolyte imbalance, psychological conflicts evidenced by impaired ability to make decisions and problem-solve, non–reality-based verbalizations, ideas of reference, altered sleep patterns, altered attention span or distractibility, perceptual disturbances with failure to recognize hunger, fatigue, anxiety, and depression.

NIC:
1) Be aware of patient's distorted thinking ability; **2)** Listen to but avoid challenging irrational or illogical thinking; **3)** Present reality concisely and briefly; **4)** Adhere strictly to nutritional regimen; and **5)** Review electrolytes and renal function tests.

Nursing Diagnosis 4

Disturbed body image/chronic low self-esteem related to morbid fear of obesity, negative perception of body or self, perceived loss of control in some aspect of life, unmet dependency needs, personal vulnerability, dysfunctional family system evidenced by distorted view of body as fat even in presence of severe emaciation, use of denial, feeling powerless to prevent or make changes, expressions of guilt, overly conforming, or dependant on others' opinions.

NIC:
1) Have patient draw picture of self; **2)** Involve in a personal development program; **3)** Recommend consultation with an image consultant; **4)** Establish a therapeutic nurse-patient relationship; **5)** State rules clearly; **6)** Confront denial and respond with reality when patient makes unrealistic statements; **7)** Assist patient to assume control; and **8)** Assist patient to formulate goals for self.

Condition:
Anorexia (Anorexia Nervosa)/ Bulimia

Age:

Link & Explain
• Nursing Interventions Classification (NIC)
• Laboratory and Diagnostic Procedures
• Medications

Nursing Diagnosis 5

NIC:

Medications
a. Olanzapine
b.
c.
d.

Laboratory & Diagnostic Procedures
a. CBC; urinalysis; thyroid screen
b. Electrolytes
c. Liver function tests; BUN
d. GI series; EKG

CONDITION: Antisocial Personality Disorder

PHYSIOLOGY: Antisocial personality disorder is characterized by disregard for the rights and feelings of others. It usually begins before age 15. In early childhood, lying, stealing, fighting, truancy, and disregard of authority are common. In adolescence, aggressive sexual behavior, excessive use of alcohol and drug use may be characteristic. In adulthood, these behavioral patterns continue with the addition of poor work performance, inability to function responsibly as a parent, and inability to accept normal restrictions imposed by the law. Affected people may repeatedly perform illegal acts (e.g., destroying property, harassing others, or stealing) or pursue illegal occupations. They disregard the safety, wishes, rights, and feelings of others. This type of personality disorder is not due to mental retardation, schizophrenia, or manic episodes. It is much more common in males than females. This condition has been referred to as psychopathy, sociopathy, or dyssocial personality disorder (*Taber's*, 2009).

HANDOFF COMMUNICATION

S	Situation	Assess what is currently happening in a short statement.	Patient presents with _____
B	Background	Summarize important past assessment data for your patient here. Place lab results and medications on the concept map.	**Age:**　　　　　　　　　　　　　　**Gender:** **Allergies:**　　　　　　　　　　　**Fall Risk:** **Isolation:**
A	Assessment	Use the assessment data to complete your concept map.	**Nursing Diagnosis:** Place the Nursing Diagnoses in prioritized order on the concept map and add any needed for your specific patient. **Plan:** Place any further Nursing Interventions Classifications (NIC) needed on the map.

Implement Your Plan of Care

		EVALUATE YOUR CARE	
R Recommendation	Evaluate your nursing care and make recommendations related to the achievement of your desired outcomes. Were they met, or do new goals need to be established?	**Diag** / **Nursing Outcomes Classification (NOC)**	**Outcome met**
		1 Acknowledge realities of the situation. Verbalize understanding of reason(s) for behavior/precipitating factors. Express increased self-concept. Demonstrate self-control evidenced by relaxed posture and nonviolent behavior.	☐ Yes ☐ No
		2 Identify resources within self to deal with situations. Express more realistic understandings.	☐ Yes ☐ No
		3 Verbalize awareness of feelings that lead to poor social interactions. Become involved in achieving positive changes in social behaviors and interpersonal skills.	☐ Yes ☐ No
		4 Verbalize understanding of dynamics of enabling behavior. Participate in individual family programs. Identify ineffective coping behaviors and consequences. Initiate and plan for necessary lifestyle changes. Take action to change self-destructive behaviors and alter behaviors that contribute to patient's behavior.	☐ Yes ☐ No
		5	☐ Yes ☐ No

Nursing Diagnosis 1

Risk for other-directed violence related to contempt for authority or rights of others, inability to tolerate frustration, need for immediate gratification, easy agitation, vulnerable self-concept, inability to verbalize feelings, use of maladjusted coping mechanisms including substance use.

NIC:
1) Observe for early signs of distress and investigate possible causes; **2)** Maintain straightforward communication; **3)** Assist patient to identify adequate solutions and behaviors such as exercise; **4)** Give as much autonomy as possible; **5)** Monitor for suicidal or homicidal ideation; and **6)** Accept patient's anger without reacting.

Nursing Diagnosis 2

Ineffective coping related to very low tolerance for external stress, lack of experience of internal anxiety (guilt, shame), personal vulnerability, unmet expectations, multiple life changes, evidenced by choice of aggression and manipulation to handle problems or conflicts, inappropriate use of defense mechanisms (denial, projection), chronic worry, anxiety, destructive behavior, or high rate of accidents.

NIC:
1) Determine understanding of current situation; **2)** Set limits and confront efforts to get caregivers to grant special privileges; **3)** Encourage verbalization of feelings; **4)** Explore alternative coping mechanisms; **5)** Assist patient to learn relaxation skills; **6)** Structure diversional activity that relates to recovery, such as social activity with support group; **7)** Identify possible and actual triggers for relapse; and **8)** Encourage involvement in writing and verbalization of plans to live realistically.

Nursing Diagnosis 3

Impaired social interaction related to inadequate personal resources (shallow feelings), immature interests, underdeveloped conscience, unacceptable social values evidenced by difficulty meeting expectations of others; lack of belief that rules pertain to self; sense of emptiness or inadequacy covered by expressions of self-conceit, arrogance, or contempt; or behavior unacceptable by dominant cultural group.

NIC:
1) Encourage patient to express perceptions of the problem; **2)** Assess patient's use of coping skills; **3)** Have patient list behaviors that cause discomfort; **4)** Involve in role playing; **5)** Discuss self-concepts and self-talk; and **6)** Refer to ongoing therapy.

Nursing Diagnosis 4

Dysfunctional family processes related to abuse and history of alcoholism or drug use, inadequate coping skills, lack of problem-solving skills, genetic predisposition or biochemical influences evidenced by feelings of anger, frustration, or responsibility for patient's behavior.

NIC:
1) Review family history and explore roles of family members; **2)** Explore how family members have coped with patient's problem; **3)** Assess current level of functioning of family members; **4)** Provide information about enabling behavior; **5)** Encourage participation in therapeutic writing; **6)** Provide factual information to family and patient about addictive behaviors and the effect on families; **7)** Encourage family members to be aware of own feelings and look at the situation with objectivity; and **8)** Involve family in discharge planning and referrals.

Condition:
Antisocial Personality Disorder
Age:

Link & Explain
• Nursing Interventions Classification (NIC)
• Laboratory and Diagnostic Procedures
• Medications

Nursing Diagnosis 5

NIC:

Medications
a.
b.
c.
d.

Laboratory & Diagnostic Procedures
a. Psychological evaluation
b.
c.
d.

CONDITION: Attention Deficit-Hyperactivity Disorder (ADHD)

PHYSIOLOGY: ADHD is a persistent pattern of inattention, hyperactivity, or both, occurring more frequently and severely than is typical in those at a comparable level of development. ADHD is the most common neurobehavioral disorder of childhood. The illness may begin in early childhood but may not be diagnosed until after the symptoms have been present for many years. The prevalence is estimated to be 3% to 5% in children; 4% in adults (Taber's, 2009).

HANDOFF COMMUNICATION

S Situation	Assess what is currently happening in a short statement.	Patient presents with _____	
B Background	Summarize important past assessment data for your patient here. Place lab results and medications on the concept map.	**Age:** **Allergies:** **Isolation:**	**Gender:** **Fall Risk:**
A Assessment	Use the assessment data to complete your concept map.	**Nursing Diagnosis:** Place the Nursing Diagnoses in prioritized order on the concept map and add any needed for your specific patient. **Plan:** Place any further Nursing Interventions Classifications (NIC) needed on the map.	

Implement Your Plan of Care

R Recommendation

Evaluate your nursing care and make recommendations related to the achievement of your desired outcomes. Were they met, or do new goals need to be established?

EVALUATE YOUR CARE

Diag	Nursing Outcomes Classification (NOC)	Outcome met
1	Patient will not harm self or others. Patient will acknowledge realities of the situation. Verbalize understanding of why behavior occurs. Identify precipitating factors. Demonstrate self-control as evidenced by relaxed posture, nonviolent behavior. Express realistic self-evaluation and increased sense of self-esteem. Participate in care and meet own needs in an assertive manner. Use resources and support systems in an effective manner.	☐ Yes ☐ No
2	Demonstrate some acceptance of self as is rather than in an idealized image.	☐ Yes ☐ No
3	Participate in learning process. Identify interferences to learning and specific actions to deal with them. Verbalize understanding of condition, disease process, and treatment. Perform necessary procedures correctly and explain reasons for the actions.	☐ Yes ☐ No
4	Verbalize understanding of dynamics of enabling behavior. Participate in individual family programs. Identify ineffective coping behaviors and consequences. Initiate and plan for necessary lifestyle changes. Take action to change self-destructive behaviors and alter behaviors that contribute to patient's behavior.	☐ Yes ☐ No
5		☐ Yes ☐ No

Nursing Diagnosis 1

Ineffective coping related to situational or maturational crises, retarded ego development, low self-concept evidenced by easy distraction by extraneous stimuli and shifting between uncompleted activities.

NIC:
1) Determine understanding of current situation; 2) Set limits and confront efforts to get caregivers to grant special privileges; 3) Encourage verbalization of feelings; 4) Explore alternative coping mechanisms; 5) Assist patient to learn relaxation skills; 6) Structure diversional activity that relates to recovery, such as social activity with support group; 7) Identify possible and actual triggers for relapse; and 8) Encourage involvement in writing and verbalization of plans to live realistically.

Nursing Diagnosis 2

Chronic low self-esteem related to retarded ego development, lack of positive or repeated negative feedback, negative role models evidenced by lack of eye contact, derogatory self-comments, hesitation to try new tasks, and inadequate level of confidence.

NIC:
1) Spend time with patient and develop trust; 2) Promote open communication; 3) Encourage simple methods of achievement; 4) Teach effective, socially appropriate communication techniques for getting needs met and in interactions with others; and 5) Encourage verbalizations of fears.

Nursing Diagnosis 3

Knowledge deficit regarding pathophysiology of condition, management, and available community resources related to insufficient information and misconceptions evidenced by statements of concerns and questions.

NIC:
1) Ascertain readiness, level of knowledge, and individual learning needs; 2) Provide positive reinforcement; 3) Provide access information for contact person and identify available community resources and support groups; 4) Remain relaxed with patient; 5) Decrease environmental stimuli; and 6) Encourage fluids and a high-protein diet.

Nursing Diagnosis 4

Dysfunctional family processes related to ADHD behaviors, inadequate coping skills, lack of problem-solving skills, genetic predisposition or biochemical influences evidenced by feelings of anger, frustration, or responsibility for patient's behavior.

NIC:
1) Review family history and explore roles of family members; 2) Explore how family members have coped with patient's problem; 3) Assess current level of functioning of family members; 4) Provide information about enabling behavior; 5) Encourage participation in therapeutic writing; 6) Provide factual information to family and patient about behaviors and the effect on families; 7) Encourage family members to be aware of own feelings and look at the situation with objectivity; and 8) Involve family in discharge planning and referrals.

Condition:
Attention Deficit-Hyperactivity Disorder (ADHD)
Age:

Link & Explain
• Nursing Interventions Classification (NIC)
• Laboratory and Diagnostic Procedures
• Medications

Nursing Diagnosis 5

NIC:

Medications
a. Amphetamine-dextroamphetamine (Adderall)
b. Dextroamphetamine (Dexedrine, Dextrostat)
c. Dexmethylphenidate (Focalin); lisdexamfetamine (Vyvanse)
d. Methylphenidate (Ritalin, Concerta, Metadate, Daytrana)

Laboratory & Diagnostic Procedures
a. Developmental, mental, nutritional, physical, and psychosocial tests
b.
c.
d.

CONDITION: Bipolar I Disorder (Axis I)

PHYSIOLOGY: Bipolar I disorder (axis I) is a psychological disorder marked by manic and depressive episodes. The individual experiences, or has experienced, a full syndrome of manic or mixed symptoms. The patient may also have experienced episodes of depression. This diagnosis is further specified by the current or most recent behavioral episode experienced. For example, the specifier might be a single manic episode (to describe individuals having a first episode of mania) or a current (most recent) episode of mania, hypomania, mixed, or depressed behavior (to describe individuals who have had recurrent mood episodes) (*Taber's*, 2009; Townsend, 2009, p. 525).

HANDOFF COMMUNICATION

S	Situation	Assess what is currently happening in a short statement.	Patient presents with _____
B	Background	Summarize important past assessment data for your patient here. Place lab results and medications on the concept map.	**Age:** **Gender:** **Allergies:** **Social Alerts:** **Mental Status:** **Safety Risk:**
A	Assessment	Use the assessment data to complete your concept map.	**Nursing Diagnosis:** Place the Nursing Diagnoses in prioritized order on the concept map and add any needed for your specific patient. **Plan:** Place any further Nursing Interventions Classifications (NIC) needed on the map.

Implement Your Plan of Care

		EVALUATE YOUR CARE	
R	Recommendation — Evaluate your nursing care and make recommendations related to the achievement of your desired outcomes. Were they met, or do new goals need to be established?	**Diag** / **Nursing Outcomes Classification (NOC)**	**Outcome met**
		1 The patient will eat a well-balanced diet. The patient's nutritional status is restored. The patient's weight has stabilized. The patient's laboratory values will be within normal limits.	☐ Yes ☐ No
		2 The patient will accept responsibility for own behaviors. The patient does not manipulate or become intrusive to others for gratification of own needs. The patient interacts with others in an appropriate manner.	☐ Yes ☐ No
		3 Report improvement in sleep or rest pattern. Verbalize increased sense of well-being and feeling rested.	☐ Yes ☐ No
		4 No evidence of physical injury. No longer experiencing physical agitation. Patient will express having no homicidal or suicidal thoughts.	☐ Yes ☐ No
		5	☐ Yes ☐ No

Nursing Diagnosis 1

Imbalanced nutrition: less than body requirements related to poor self-care evidenced by weight loss.

NIC:
1) Provide high-protein, high-calorie finger foods; **2)** Ensure that fruit juices and healthy snacks are available on the unit; **3)** Monitor I&O, calorie count, and daily weights; **4)** Provide favorite foods if possible; **5)** Supplement with vitamins and minerals; and **6)** Sit with or walk with patient during meals.

Nursing Diagnosis 2

Impaired social interaction related to perceptual difficulties evidenced by lack of interactions.

NIC:
1) Recognize purpose of manipulative behavior; **2)** Set limits on manipulative and intrusive behavior; **3)** Provide positive reinforcement for appropriate behavior; **4)** Provide consequences for inappropriate behavior in a matter-of-fact manner; **5)** Escort patient to a quiet area if inappropriate behavior can not be redirected; and **6)** Assist patient to identify positive aspects of self.

Nursing Diagnosis 3

Disturbed sleep pattern related to inability to self-comfort evidenced by insomnia.

NIC:
1) Ascertain usual sleep patterns and changes that are occurring; **2)** Provide comfortable bedding and some of own possessions such as a pillow or an afghan; **3)** Establish new sleep routine incorporating old pattern and new environment; **4)** Encourage light physical activity during the day; **5)** Promote bedtime comfort regimens and avoid caffeine; and **6)** Provide an area with low external stimuli.

Nursing Diagnosis 4

Risk for injury related to altered perceptions.

NIC:
1) Observe patient every 15 minutes on admission; **2)** Remove sharps, belts, and other dangerous objects from environment; **3)** Reduce external stimuli; **4)** Assign private room; **5)** Provide sufficient staff for show of strength if necessary; **6)** Administer tranquilizers as ordered; **7)** Maintain a calm, matter-of-fact, non-judgmental attitude; **8)** Stay with patient when he/she is agitated; and **9)** Provide physical activities.

Condition:
Bipolar I Disorder (Axis I)
Age:

Link & Explain
• Nursing Interventions Classification (NIC)
• Laboratory and Diagnostic Procedures
• Medications

Nursing Diagnosis 5

NIC:

Medications

a. Antimanic (Lithium)

b. Anxiolytics (e.g., benzodiazepam, BuSpar)

c. Anticonvulsants (e.g., carbamazepine, valproic acid, gabapentin)

d. Antipsychotics (e.g., aripiprazole, risperidone, olanzapine)

e. Antidepressant medications (e.g., SSRIs, MAOIs) *used with caution for depressive episodes, not for manic episodes*

Laboratory & Diagnostic Procedures

a. Blood alcohol level and electrolytes

b. Renal function tests

c.

d.

CONDITION: Borderline Personality Disorder

PHYSIOLOGY: Borderline personality disorder is characterized by difficulty in maintaining stable interpersonal relationships and self-image. It manifests as unpredictable and impulsive behavior, outbursts of anger, irritability, sadness, and fear. Self-mutilation or suicidal behavior may be present. Sometimes there is a chronic feeling of emptiness or boredom (*Taber's*, 2009).

HANDOFF COMMUNICATION

S	**Situation**	Assess what is currently happening in a short statement.	Patient presents with _____
B	**Background**	Summarize important past assessment data for your patient here. Place lab results and medications on the concept map.	**Age:**　　　　　　　　　　**Gender:**　　　　　　**Allergies:**　　　　　　　　**Fall Risk:**　　　　**Isolation:**
A	**Assessment**	Use the assessment data to complete your concept map.	**Nursing Diagnosis:** Place the Nursing Diagnoses in prioritized order on the concept map and add any needed for your specific patient.　**Plan:** Place any further Nursing Interventions Classifications (NIC) needed on the map.

Implement Your Plan of Care

R	**Recommendation**	Evaluate your nursing care and make recommendations related to the achievement of your desired outcomes. Were they met, or do new goals need to be established?	(see table below)

EVALUATE YOUR CARE

Diag	Nursing Outcomes Classification (NOC)	Outcome met
1	Acknowledge realities of the situation. Verbalize understanding of reason(s) for behavior/precipitating factors. Express increased self-concept. Demonstrate self-control evidenced by relaxed posture and nonviolent behavior.	☐ Yes ☐ No
2	Patient will appear relaxed and report anxiety is reduced to a manageable level. Verbalize awareness of feelings of anxiety. Identify healthy ways to deal with and express anxiety. Demonstrate problem-solving skills. Use resources/support systems effectively.	☐ Yes ☐ No
3	Demonstrate some acceptance of self as is rather than in an idealized image.	☐ Yes ☐ No
4	Verbalize awareness of feelings that lead to poor social interactions. Become involved in achieving positive changes in social behaviors and interpersonal skills.	☐ Yes ☐ No
5		☐ Yes ☐ No

Nursing Diagnosis 1

Risk for self- or other-directed violence and self-mutilation related to projection as a major defense mechanism, pervasive problems with negative transference, feelings of guilt or need to punish self, distorted sense of self, and inability to deal with increasing psychological or physiological tension in a healthy manner.

NIC:

1) Observe for early signs of distress and investigate possible causes; **2)** Maintain straightforward communication; **3)** Assist patient to identify adequate solutions and behaviors such as exercise; **4)** Give as much autonomy as possible; **5)** Monitor for suicidal or homicidal ideation; and **6)** Accept patient's anger without reacting.

Nursing Diagnosis 2

Anxiety (severe to panic) related to unconscious conflicts (experience of extreme stress), perceived threat to self-concept, unmet needs evidenced by easy frustration and feelings of hurt, abuse of alcohol or other drugs, transient psychotic symptoms, and performance of self-mutilation.

NIC:

1) Assess degree and reality of threat to patient and level of anxiety; **2)** Evaluate coping and defense mechanisms being used to deal with the perceived or real threat; **3)** Review coping mechanisms used in the past, such as problem-solving skills and asking for help; **4)** Maintain frequent contact and therapeutic communication; and **5)** Administer sedatives and tranquilizers as indicated.

Nursing Diagnosis 3

Chronic low self-esteem/disturbed personal identity related to lack of positive feedback, unmet dependency needs, retarded ego development, or fixation at an earlier level of development evidenced by difficulty identifying self or defining self-boundaries, feelings of depersonalization, extreme mood changes, lack of tolerance for rejection or being alone, unhappiness with self, striking out at others, performance of ritualistic self-damaging acts, and belief that punishing self is necessary.

NIC:

1) Spend time with patient and develop trust; **2)** Promote open communication; **3)** Encourage simple methods of achievement; **4)** Teach effective, socially appropriate communication techniques for getting needs met and in interactions with others; and **5)** Encourage verbalizations of fears.

Nursing Diagnosis 4

Social isolation related to immature interests, unacceptable social behavior, inadequate personal resources, and inability to engage in satisfying personal relationships evidenced by alternating clinging and distancing behaviors, difficulty meeting expectations of others, experiencing feelings of difference from others, expressing interests inappropriate to developmental age, and exhibiting behavior unaccepted by dominant cultural group.

NIC:

1) Encourage patient to express perceptions of the problem; **2)** Assess patient's use of coping skills; **3)** Have patient list behaviors that cause discomfort; **4)** Involve in role playing; **5)** Discuss self-concepts and self-talk; and **6)** Refer to ongoing therapy.

Condition:
Borderline Personality Disorder

Age:

Link & Explain
• Nursing Interventions Classification (NIC)
• Laboratory and Diagnostic Procedures
• Medications

Nursing Diagnosis 5

NIC:

Medications
a.
b.
c.
d.

Laboratory & Diagnostic Procedures
a. Dialectical behavioral therapy (DBT)
b.
c.
d.

CONDITION: Domestic Violence/Intimate Partner Abuse

PHYSIOLOGY: Abuse or neglect occurring within families. Domestic violence includes child abuse, spouse abuse, elder abuse, sexual abuse, marital rape, and lapses in household firearm safety (*Taber's*, 2009).

HANDOFF COMMUNICATION

S	Situation	Assess what is currently happening in a short statement.	Patient presents with _____
B	Background	Summarize important past assessment data for your patient here. Place lab results and medications on the concept map.	**Age:** **Gender:** **Allergies:** **Fall Risk:** **Isolation:**
A	Assessment	Use the assessment data to complete your concept map.	**Nursing Diagnosis:** Place the Nursing Diagnoses in prioritized order on the concept map and add any needed for your specific patient. **Plan:** Place any further Nursing Interventions Classifications (NIC) needed on the map.

Implement Your Plan of Care

			EVALUATE YOUR CARE	
R	Recommendation	Evaluate your nursing care and make recommendations related to the achievement of your desired outcomes. Were they met, or do new goals need to be established?	**Diag** / **Nursing Outcomes Classification (NOC)**	**Outcome met**
			1 Modify environment as indicated to prevent trauma.	☐ Yes ☐ No
			2 Be involved in problem-solving solutions for current situation.	☐ Yes ☐ No
			3 Verbalize or demonstrate acceptance of self and an increased sense of self worth.	☐ Yes ☐ No
			4 Demonstrate ability to deal with emotional reactions in an individually appropriate manner.	☐ Yes ☐ No
			5	☐ Yes ☐ No

Nursing Diagnosis 1

Risk for trauma related to dependent position in relationship and vulnerability.

NIC:
1) Refer to appropriate authorities, social service, or case manager to remove from the situation; and **2)** Promote counseling for patient and family.

Nursing Diagnosis 2

Interrupted family processes related to unrealistic expectations, presence of stressors, and lack of support evidenced by verbalization on negative feelings, inappropriate caretaking behaviors, and evidence of physical or psychological trauma to the patient.

NIC:
1) Determine existing situation and patient perception of problem; **2)** Observe family interactions; and **3)** Refer to social service, case manager for counseling.

Nursing Diagnosis 3

Chronic low self-esteem related to deprivation and negative feedback of family members, personal vulnerability, feelings of abandonment evidenced by lack of eye contact, withdrawal from social contacts, discounting own needs, nonassertiveness or passiveness, indecisive or overly conforming behavior.

NIC:
1) Provide opportunity for and encourage verbalization or acting out of individual situation; **2)** Spend time with patient; **3)** Provide reinforcement for positive actions; **4)** Encourage expressions of feelings of guilt, shame, and anger; and **5)** Involve in therapy or group therapy.

Nursing Diagnosis 4

Posttrauma syndrome related to sustained or reoccurring abuse evidenced by acting-out behavior.

NIC:
1) Assess physical trauma or use sexual assault nurse examiner to collect evidence; **2)** Evaluate behavior; **3)** Assess signs or stages of grieving; **4)** Identify support systems; and **5)** Refer to counselor.

Condition:
Domestic Violence/ Intimate Partner Abuse

Age:

Link & Explain
• Nursing Interventions Classification (NIC)
• Laboratory and Diagnostic Procedures
• Medications

Nursing Diagnosis 5

NIC:

Medications

a.

b.

c.

d.

Laboratory & Diagnostic Procedures

a. X-rays of injuries

b.

c.

d.

CONDITION: Generalized Anxiety Disorder (Axis I)

PHYSIOLOGY: Generalized anxiety disorder (axis I) is excessive anxiety and worry predominating for at least 6 months. Restlessness, easy fatigability, difficulty in concentrating, irritability, muscle tension, and disturbed sleep may be present. Adults with this disorder often worry about everyday, routine circumstances such as job responsibilities, finances, the health of family members, misfortune to their children, or minor matters such as being late or completing household chores. Frequently they experience cold, clammy hands; dry mouth; sweating; nausea or diarrhea; urinary frequency; trouble swallowing or a "lump in the throat"; an exaggerated startle response; or depressive symptoms. The intensity, duration, or frequency of the anxiety and worry is far out of proportion to the actual likelihood or impact of the feared event (*Taber's*, 2009).

HANDOFF COMMUNICATION

S	Situation	Assess what is currently happening in a short statement.	Patient presents with _____
B	Background	Summarize important past assessment data for your patient here. Place lab results and medications on the concept map.	**Age:** **Gender:** **Allergies:** **Social Alerts:** **Mental Status:** **Safety Risk:**
A	Assessment	Use the assessment data to complete your concept map.	**Nursing Diagnosis:** Place the Nursing Diagnoses in prioritized order on the concept map and add any needed for your specific patient. **Plan:** Place any further Nursing Interventions Classifications (NIC) needed on the map.

Implement Your Plan of Care

R Recommendation	Evaluate your nursing care and make recommendations related to the achievement of your desired outcomes. Were they met, or do new goals need to be established?	**EVALUATE YOUR CARE**	

Diag	Nursing Outcomes Classification (NOC)	Outcome met
1	The patient will identify ineffective coping behaviors and consequences. Verbalize awareness of own coping and problem-solving abilities. Meet psychological needs evidenced by appropriate expression of feelings, identification of options, and use of resources. Make decisions and express satisfaction with choices.	☐ Yes ☐ No
2	Patient will appear relaxed and report anxiety is reduced to a manageable level. Verbalize awareness of feelings of anxiety. Identify healthy ways to deal with and express anxiety. Demonstrate problem-solving skills. Use resources/support systems effectively.	☐ Yes ☐ No
3	Report improvement in sleep or rest pattern. Verbalize increased sense of well-being and feeling rested.	☐ Yes ☐ No
4	Verbalize awareness of feelings that lead to poor social interactions. Become involved in achieving positive changes in social behaviors and interpersonal relationships.	☐ Yes ☐ No
5		☐ Yes ☐ No

Nursing Diagnosis 1

Ineffective coping related to anxiety evidenced by inability to maintain activities of daily living (ADLs).

NIC:
1) Assess level of anxiety experienced by the patient; **2)** Assess patient's perceptions and expectations; **3)** Observe early signs of distress; **4)** Evaluate patient's current coping and problem-solving patterns; **5)** Assess for abuse of drugs or alcohol; **6)** Assess and promote presence of positive coping skills and inner strengths, such as use of relation techniques, willingness to express feelings, and use of support systems; and **7)** Establish a therapeutic nurse-patient relationship.

Nursing Diagnosis 2

Anxiety (severe to panic) related to inability to modify feelings evidenced by easy frustration and feelings of hurt, abuse of alcohol or other drugs, transient psychotic symptoms, and performance of self-mutilation.

NIC:
1) Assess degree and reality of threat to patient and level of anxiety; **2)** Evaluate coping and defense mechanisms being used to deal with the perceived or real threat; **3)** Review coping mechanisms used in the past, such as problem-solving skills and asking for help; **4)** Maintain frequent contact and therapeutic communication; and **5)** Administer sedatives and tranquilizers as indicated.

Nursing Diagnosis 3

Disturbed sleep pattern related to anxiety evidenced by insomnia.

NIC:
1) Ascertain usual sleep patterns and changes that are occurring; **2)** Provide comfortable bedding and some of own possessions such as a pillow or an afghan; **3)** Establish new sleep routine incorporating old pattern and new environment; **4)** Encourage light physical activity during the day; and **5)** Promote bedtime comfort regimens and avoid caffeine.

Nursing Diagnosis 4

Social isolation/impaired social interaction related to diagnosis evidenced by avoidance of others.

NIC:
1) Assess causative and contributing factors (review of social history);
2) Encourage patient to verbalize perceptions of problem and causes;
3) Determine patient's use of coping skills and defense mechanisms; and
4) Assist patient to recognize/make positive changes in impaired social and interpersonal interactions.

Condition:
Generalized Anxiety Disorder (Axis I)

Age:

Link & Explain
• Nursing Interventions Classification (NIC)
• Laboratory and Diagnostic Procedures
• Medications

Nursing Diagnosis 5

NIC:

Medications

a. Anxiolytics (e.g., benzodiazepam, BuSpar)

b. Antidepressant medications (e.g., SSRIs, MAOIs)

c. Antihypertensive agents (e.g., beta blockers, alpha-2-receptor agonists)

d.

Laboratory & Diagnostic Procedures

a.

b.

c.

d.

CONDITION: Major Depressive Disorder (Axis I)

PHYSIOLOGY: Major depressive disorder (axis I) is a mood disorder characterized by a period of at least 2 weeks of depressed mood or the loss of interest or pleasure in nearly all activities. Establishing the diagnosis requires the presence of at least four of the following: 1) changes in appetite, weight, sleep, and psychomotor activity; 2) decreased energy; 3) feelings of worthlessness or guilt; 4) difficulty thinking, concentrating, or making decisions; 5) recurrent thoughts of death or plans for or attempts to commit suicide. The symptoms must persist for most of the day, nearly every day, for at least two consecutive weeks. The episode must be accompanied by clinical significant distress or impairment in social, occupational, or other important areas of functioning; also the disorder must not be due to bereavement, drugs, alcohol, or the direct effect of a disease such as hypothyroidism (*Taber's*, 2009).

HANDOFF COMMUNICATION

S	Situation	Assess what is currently happening in a short statement.	Patient presents with _____
B	Background	Summarize important past assessment data for your patient here. Place lab results and medications on the concept map.	**Age:** **Gender:** **Allergies:** **Social Alerts:** **Mental Status:** **Safety Risk:**
A	Assessment	Use the assessment data to complete your concept map.	**Nursing Diagnosis:** Place the Nursing Diagnoses in prioritized order on the concept map and add any needed for your specific patient. **Plan:** Place any further Nursing Interventions Classifications (NIC) needed on the map.

Implement Your Plan of Care

		EVALUATE YOUR CARE		
R	Recommendation — Evaluate your nursing care and make recommendations related to the achievement of your desired outcomes. Were they met, or do new goals need to be established?	**Diag**	**Nursing Outcomes Classification (NOC)**	**Outcome met**
		1	Provide safe environment and prevent injury; patient verbalizes reason(s) for behavior or precipitating factors, demonstrates self control through nonviolent behavior, uses resources and support systems in an effective manner.	☐ Yes ☐ No
		2	Patient will appear relaxed and report anxiety is reduced to a manageable level. Verbalize awareness of feelings of anxiety. Identify healthy ways to deal with and express anxiety. Demonstrate problem-solving skills. Use resources/support systems effectively.	☐ Yes ☐ No
		3	Report improvement in sleep or rest pattern. Verbalize increased self of well-being and feeling rested.	☐ Yes ☐ No
		4	Verbalize awareness of feelings that lead to poor social interactions. Become involved in achieving positive changes in social behaviors and interpersonal relationships.	☐ Yes ☐ No
		5		☐ Yes ☐ No

Nursing Diagnosis 1

Risk for self-directed violence related to diagnosis.

NIC:
1) Assess suicidal intent and contributing factors; **2)** Provide safe environment to avoid self-harm (removal of objects that can harm; constant observation); **3)** Observe early signs of distress; **4)** Maintain straightforward and therapeutic communication; and **5)** Encourage verbalization of feelings in a caring and concerned manner.

Nursing Diagnosis 2

Anxiety/disturbed thought processes related to diagnosis evidenced by easy frustration and feelings of hurt, abuse of alcohol or other drugs, transient psychotic symptoms, and performance of self-mutilation.

NIC:
1) Assess degree and reality of threat to patient and level of anxiety; **2)** Evaluate coping and defense mechanisms being used to deal with the perceived or real threat; **3)** Review coping mechanisms used in the past, such as problem-solving skills and asking for help; and **4)** Maintain frequent contact and therapeutic communication.

Nursing Diagnosis 3

Disturbed sleep pattern related to anxiety evidenced by insomnia.

NIC:
1) Ascertain usual sleep patterns and changes that are occurring; **2)** Provide comfortable bedding and some of own possessions such as a pillow or an afghan; **3)** Establish new sleep routine incorporating old pattern and new environment; **4)** Encourage light physical activity during the day; and **5)** Promote bedtime comfort regimens and avoid caffeine.

Nursing Diagnosis 4

Social isolation/impaired social interaction related to depression evidenced by lack of interactions with others or expression of feelings of aloneness or rejection.

NIC:
1) Assess causative and contributing factors (review of social history); **2)** Encourage patient to verbalize perceptions of problem and causes; **3)** Determine patient's use of coping skills and defense mechanisms; **4)** Assist patient to recognize/make positive changes in impaired social and interpersonal interactions.

Condition:
Major Depressive Disorder (Axis I)
Age:

Link & Explain
• Nursing Interventions Classification (NIC)
• Laboratory and Diagnostic Procedures
• Medications

Nursing Diagnosis 5

NIC:

Medications

a. Antidepressant medications (e.g., SSRIs, MAOIs)

b. Anxiolytics (e.g., benzodiazepam)

c.

d.

Laboratory & Diagnostic Procedures

a.

b.

c.

d.

CONDITION: Obsessive-Compulsive Disorder (OCD)

PHYSIOLOGY: The hallmarks of OCD are recurring thoughts, ideas, feelings, or actions that either cause significant psychological distress or interfere with effective living. Common obsessions include concerns about cleanliness, injury, or aggressive or sexual impulses. Common compulsions include repetitive hand washing, cleaning, praying, counting, or making things orderly. A diagnosis of OCD is established if distress is present, the acts are time consuming (i.e., take more than an hour a day), or the illness significantly interferes with the individual's normal routine, occupation, or social activities. In the general population, the lifetime prevalence of this disorder is approximately 2.5%. It is estimated to be present in 35% to 50% of patients with Tourette's syndrome (*Taber's*, 2009).

HANDOFF COMMUNICATION

S	Situation	Assess what is currently happening in a short statement.	Patient presents with _____
B	Background	Summarize important past assessment data for your patient here. Place lab results and medications on the concept map.	**Age:** **Gender:** **Allergies:** **Fall Risk:** **Isolation:**
A	Assessment	Use the assessment data to complete your concept map.	**Nursing Diagnosis:** Place the Nursing Diagnoses in prioritized order on the concept map and add any needed for your specific patient. **Plan:** Place any further Nursing Interventions Classifications (NIC) needed on the map.

Implement Your Plan of Care

		EVALUATE YOUR CARE		
R	Recommendation Evaluate your nursing care and make recommendations related to the achievement of your desired outcomes. Were they met, or do new goals need to be established?	**Diag**	**Nursing Outcomes Classification (NOC)**	**Outcome met**
		1	Verbalize awareness of feelings and healthy ways to deal with anxiety.	☐ Yes ☐ No
		2	Prevent tissue breakdown and/or demonstrate tissue regeneration.	☐ Yes ☐ No
		3	Develop realistic goals and plans for the future.	☐ Yes ☐ No
		4	Express feelings freely and appropriately. Demonstrate individual involvement in problem-solving processes. Encourage and allow patient to handle situation in own way.	☐ Yes ☐ No
		5		☐ Yes ☐ No

Nursing Diagnosis 1

Anxiety (severe) related to earlier life conflicts evidenced by repetitive actions, recurring thoughts, and decreased social and role functioning.

NIC:
1) Assess degree and reality of threat to patient and level of anxiety; **2)** Evaluate coping and defense mechanisms being used to deal with the perceived or real threat; **3)** Review coping mechanisms used in the past, such as problem-solving skills and asking for help; **4)** Maintain frequent contact and therapeutic communication; and **5)** Administer medications as indicated.

Nursing Diagnosis 2

Risk for impaired skin integrity related to repetitive behavior related to cleaning such as hand washing, teeth brushing, showering, and so on.

NIC:
1) Encourage use of cool bath, baking soda, or starch; **2)** Apply calamine lotion as indicated; **3)** Provide age-appropriate diversional activity; and **4)** Administer medications as indicated.

Nursing Diagnosis 3

Risk for ineffective role performance related to psychological stress.

NIC:
1) Assess meaning of condition to patient and family; **2)** Acknowledge and accept feelings of frustration; **3)** Set limits on maladaptive behavior; **4)** Be realistic and positive during treatment; **5)** Give positive reinforcement of progress; **6)** Role play social situations; and **7)** Mediate as indicated.

Nursing Diagnosis 4

Interrupted family processes related to social behavior evidenced by lack of eye contact, withdrawn behavior, and limited outside-the-home exposure.

NIC:
1) Note components of family and other supports, including friends and neighbors; **2)** Identify patterns of communication and interaction among family members; **3)** Identify and encourage use of previously successful coping behaviors; **4)** Stress importance of continuous open dialogue among family members; and **5)** Refer to support groups, clergy, and family therapy as indicated.

Condition:
Obsessive-Compulsive Disorder (OCD)

Age:

Link & Explain
• Nursing Interventions Classification (NIC)
• Laboratory and Diagnostic Procedures
• Medications

Nursing Diagnosis 5

NIC:

Medications

a. Citalopram (Celexa), paroxetine (Paxil)

b. Fluoxetine (Prozac)

c. Fluvoxamine (Luvox)

d. Sertraline (Zoloft)

Laboratory & Diagnostic Procedures

a. Yale-Brown Obsessive Compulsive Scale (YBOCS)

b.

c.

d.

CONDITION: Posttraumatic Stress Disorder (Axis I)

PHYSIOLOGY: Posttraumatic stress disorder (axis I) is intense psychological distress marked by horrifying memories, recurring fears, and feelings of helplessness that develop after a psychologically traumatic event, such as the experience of combat, criminal assault, life-threatening accidents, natural disasters, or rape. The symptoms of PTSD may include re-experiencing the traumatic event (a phenomenon called "flashback"); avoiding stimuli associated with the trauma; memory disturbances; psychological or social withdrawal; or increased aggressiveness, irritability, insomnia, startle responses, and vigilance. Persistent symptoms of increased arousal (not present before the trauma), are indicated by two (or more) of the following: 1) difficulty falling or staying asleep, 2) irritability or outbursts of anger, 3) difficulty concentrating, 4) hypervigilance, 5) exaggerated startle response. Duration of the disturbance is more than 1 month, and the symptoms may last for years after the event but often can be managed with supportive psychotherapy or medications such as antidepressants (*Taber's*, 2009).

HANDOFF COMMUNICATION

S Situation	Assess what is currently happening in a short statement.	Patient presents with _____
B Background	Summarize important past assessment data for your patient here. Place lab results and medications on the concept map.	**Age:** **Gender:** **Allergies:** **Social Alerts:** **Mental Status:** **Safety Risk:**
A Assessment	Use the assessment data to complete your concept map.	**Nursing Diagnosis:** Place the Nursing Diagnoses in prioritized order on the concept map and add any needed for your specific patient. **Plan:** Place any further Nursing Interventions Classifications (NIC) needed on the map.

Implement Your Plan of Care

		EVALUATE YOUR CARE	
R Recommendation	Evaluate your nursing care and make recommendations related to the achievement of your desired outcomes. Were they met, or do new goals need to be established?	**Diag** / **Nursing Outcomes Classification (NOC)**	**Outcome met**
		1 The patient will identify ineffective coping behaviors and consequences. Verbalize awareness of own coping and problem-solving abilities. Meet psychological needs evidenced by appropriate expression of feelings, identification of options, and use of resources. Make decisions and express satisfaction with choices.	☐ Yes ☐ No
		2 Patient will appear relaxed and report anxiety is reduced to a manageable level. Verbalize awareness of feelings of anxiety. Identify healthy ways to deal with and express anxiety. Demonstrate problem-solving skills. Use resources/support systems effectively.	☐ Yes ☐ No
		3 Report improvement in sleep or rest pattern. Verbalize increased sense of well-being and feeling rested.	☐ Yes ☐ No
		4 Patient discusses trauma without experiencing panic. Patient has fewer flashbacks/nightmares. Patient can sleep without medication. Patient demonstrates use of adaptive coping strategies.	☐ Yes ☐ No
		5	☐ Yes ☐ No

Nursing Diagnosis 1

Ineffective coping related to incapacitating stress evidenced by lack of ability to carry out activities of daily living (ADL).

NIC:
1) Assess level of anxiety experienced by the patient; 2) Assess patient's perceptions and expectations; 3) Observe early signs of distress; 4) Evaluate patient's current coping and problem-solving patterns; 5) Assess for abuse of drugs or alcohol; 6) Assess and promote presence of positive coping skills and inner strengths, such as use of relation techniques, willingness to express feelings, and use of support systems; and 7) Establish a therapeutic nurse-patient relationship.

Nursing Diagnosis 2

Anxiety related to constant stress evidenced by verbalizations, and lack of attention.

NIC:
1) Assess degree and reality of threat to patient and level of anxiety; 2) Stay with the patient and remain calm; 3) Use simple explanations; 4) Maintain low-stimuli environment; 5) Review coping mechanisms used in the past, such as problem-solving skills and asking for help; 6) Encourage verbalization of current situation; 7) Maintain frequent contact and therapeutic communication; and 8) Administer sedatives and tranquilizers as indicated.

Nursing Diagnosis 3

Disturbed sleep pattern related to stress evidenced by insomnia.

NIC:
1) Ascertain usual sleep patterns and changes that are occurring; 2) Provide comfortable bedding and some of own possessions such as a pillow or an afghan; 3) Establish new sleep routine incorporating old pattern and new environment; 4) Encourage light physical activity during the day; and 5) Promote bedtime comfort regimens and avoid caffeine.

Nursing Diagnosis 4

Stress overload related to diagnosis evidenced by flashback symptoms.

NIC:
1) Accept patient; establish trust; 2) Stay with patient during flashbacks; 3) Encourage verbalization about the trauma when patient is ready; 4) Discuss coping strategies; and 5) Assist patient to try to comprehend the trauma and how it will be assimilated into his or her persona.

Condition:
Posttraumatic Stress Disorder (Axis I)

Age:

Link & Explain
• Nursing Interventions Classification (NIC)
• Laboratory and Diagnostic Procedures
• Medications

Nursing Diagnosis 5

NIC:

Medications

a. Anxiolytics (e.g., benzodiazepam, BuSpar)

b. Antidepressant medications (e.g., SSRIs, MAOIs)

c. Antihypertensive agents (e.g., beta blockers, alpha2-receptor agonists, clonidine).

d.

Laboratory & Diagnostic Procedures

a. Blood alcohol level, ABGs, electrolytes

b. Renal function tests

c.

d.

CONDITION: Rape-Trauma Syndrome

PHYSIOLOGY: Rape-trauma syndrome is a sustained maladaptive response to a forced, violent sexual penetration against the victim's will or consent. Acute phase: profound emotional responses marked by shame, fear, humiliation, self-blame, self-degradation, anger, and desire for revenge. Symptoms include crying, trembling, talkativeness, statements of disbelief, and emotional shock. Other signs are hostility and power-lessness. Physical responses include sleeplessness, gastrointestinal and genitourinary discomfort (*Taber's*, 2009).

HANDOFF COMMUNICATION

S	Situation	Assess what is currently happening in a short statement.	Patient presents with _____
B	Background	Summarize important past assessment data for your patient here. Place lab results and medications on the concept map.	**Age:** **Gender:** **Allergies:** **Fall Risk:** **Isolation:**
A	Assessment	Use the assessment data to complete your concept map.	**Nursing Diagnosis:** Place the Nursing Diagnoses in prioritized order on the concept map and add any needed for your specific patient. **Plan:** Place any further Nursing Interventions Classifications (NIC) needed on the map.

Implement Your Plan of Care

			EVALUATE YOUR CARE	
R	Recommendation	Evaluate your nursing care and make recommendations related to the achievement of your desired outcomes. Were they met, or do new goals need to be established?	**Diag** / **Nursing Outcomes Classification (NOC)**	**Outcome met**
			1 Verbalize understanding of therapeutic needs.	☐ Yes ☐ No
			2 Recognize need to seek assistance.	☐ Yes ☐ No
			3 Achieve timely wound healing free of purulent drainage or erythema.	☐ Yes ☐ No
			4 Verbalize awareness of own coping abilities. Verbalize acceptance of self in situation.	☐ Yes ☐ No
			5	☐ Yes ☐ No

Nursing Diagnosis 1

Knowledge deficit regarding required medical and legal procedures, prophylactic treatment for individual concerns (STIs or pregnancy), community resources and supports. Patient may be lacking information evidenced by statements of concern, questions, misconceptions, or exacerbation of symptoms.

NIC:
1) Note level of anxiety and fear, which alter thought process; **2)** Review procedures and possible complications in clear, precise terms; **3)** Encourage and provide opportunity for questions; and **4)** Acknowledge that certain feelings and patterns of response are normal reactions.

Nursing Diagnosis 2

Rape-trauma syndrome related to actual or attempted sexual penetration without consent evidenced by wide range of emotional reactions, including anxiety, fear, anger, embarrassment, or multisystem physical complains.

NIC:
1) Attend to physical and health priorities; **2)** Promote trusting, therapeutic relationship; **3)** Use a calm, consistent approach; **4)** Be supportive of patient's views; and **5)** Explain need for procedures.

Nursing Diagnosis 3

Risk for impaired tissue integrity related to forceful sexual penetration and trauma to fragile tissues.

NIC:
1) Assess for wound(s); **2)** Provide wound care if needed; **3)** Monitor temperature; **4)** Place in semi-Fowler position to promote drainage; and **5)** Encourage patient to wear loose-fitting clothing to promote healing.

Nursing Diagnosis 4

Ineffective coping related to personal vulnerability, unmet expectations, unrealistic perceptions, inadequate support systems, coping methods, multiple stressors repeated over time, overwhelming threat to self evidenced by verbalizations of inability to cope or difficulty asking for help, muscular tension, headaches, emotional tension, or chronic worry.

NIC:
1) Assess extent of altered perception; **2)** Identify meaning of loss to patient; **3)** Determine outside stressors; **4)** Encourage patient to express feelings; and **5)** Monitor sleep disturbance.

Condition:
Rape-Trauma Syndrome
Age:

Link & Explain
• Nursing Interventions Classification (NIC)
• Laboratory and Diagnostic Procedures
• Medications

Nursing Diagnosis 5

NIC:

Medications

a. Emergency contraception

b. Antibiotics

c.

d.

Laboratory & Diagnostic Procedures

a. Culture and sensitivity of cervix

b. RPR (rapid plasma reagent) or VDRL (Venereal Disease Research Laboratories)

c. DNA collection: nails, vagina, and possibly other areas

d.

CONDITION: Risk for Suicide

PHYSIOLOGY: Suicidal behavior is the result of a complication of a psychiatric condition such as mood disorders, schizophrenia, substance use, personality disorders, and anxiety disorders, although suicide may occur in someone with no previous history of psychiatric illness. The history of suicidal attempts is a reliable indicator of future risk of attempt or completion of the act.

HANDOFF COMMUNICATION

S Situation	Assess what is currently happening in a short statement.	Patient presents with _____
B Background	Summarize important past assessment data for your patient here. Place lab results and medications on the concept map.	Age: Gender: Allergies: Fall Risk: Social Alerts: Mental Status: Safety Risk:
A Assessment	Use the assessment data to complete your concept map.	**Nursing Diagnosis:** Place the Nursing Diagnoses in prioritized order on the concept map and add any needed for your specific patient. **Plan:** Place any further Nursing Interventions Classifications (NIC) needed on the map.

Implement Your Plan of Care

			EVALUATE YOUR CARE	
R Recommendation	Evaluate your nursing care and make recommendations related to the achievement of your desired outcomes. Were they met, or do new goals need to be established?	**Diag**	**Nursing Outcomes Classification (NOC)**	**Outcome met**
		1	The patient will remain safe and unharmed with absence of verbalization or behaviors related to harming self.	☐ Yes ☐ No
		2	The patient maintains cleanliness and dresses neatly and appropriately. The patient eats most of meals and takes adequate oral fluids.	☐ Yes ☐ No
		3	The patient is able to discuss learned coping behaviors.	☐ Yes ☐ No
		4	The patient will verbalize goals and resume level of functioning.	☐ Yes ☐ No
		5		☐ Yes ☐ No

Nursing Diagnosis 1

Risk for self-directed violence related to life crisis, feelings of worthlessness.

NIC:
1) Assess for behaviors that may indicate level of risk for suicide, such as giving items away, previous attempts, presence of hallucinations or delusions; **2)** Assess patient for self-mutilation: cutting, burns; **3)** Ask patient information about intent or plan to commit suicide; **4)** Remove any items (mirrors, razors, hangers, belts) that could be harmful to patient; **5)** Instruct visitors about restricted items; **6)** Check to make sure all medications are swallowed; **7)** Provide observation of patient per institution policy; and **8)** Create a contract regarding what the patient and nurse will do to keep the patient safe.

Nursing Diagnosis 2

Self-care deficit (hygiene) related to difficulty concentrating evidenced by inappropriate dress and dysfunctional eating habits.

NIC:
1) Encourage independence in ADLs, but intervene as needed; **2)** Offer assistance in grooming and selection of clothing; **3)** Provide positive reinforcement for in- dependent accomplishments; **4)** Monitor oral intake for food and fluids; and **5)** Offer fluids to prevent dehydration and encourage eating of healthy foods.

Nursing Diagnosis 3

Ineffective individual coping related to emotional lability evidenced by crying, irritation, laughing.

NIC:
1) Spend time talking with patient to encourage verbalization of fears and the development of trust; **2)** Patient will verbalize feelings of hopelessness, loneli- ness, anger; **3)** Encourage patient to practice new coping skills in a safe, therapeutic environment; and **4)** Provide positive feedback for adaptive coping.

Nursing Diagnosis 4

Disturbed self-esteem related to expres- sions of shame and guilt evidenced by negative feedback about self.

NIC:
1) Educate patient about appropriate communication techniques for getting needs met; **2)** Provide opportunities for the patient to be successful; **3)** Ask pa- tient about past experiences, pictures of self, personal possessions; and **4)** Allow time to accomplish tasks at own pace.

Condition:
Risk for Suicide
Age:

Link & Explain
• Nursing Interventions Classification (NIC)
• Laboratory and Diagnostic Procedures
• Medications

Nursing Diagnosis 5

NIC:

Medications

a. Antipsychotics (e.g., aripiprazole, risperidone, olanzapine)

b. Anxiolytics (e.g., benzodiazepam, BuSpar)

c. Anticonvulsants (e.g., carbamazepine, valproic acid, gabapentin)

d. Antidepressant medications (e.g., SSRIs, MAOIs)

Laboratory & Diagnostic Procedures

a. Blood alcohol level, toxicology screening, CBC, electrolytes

b.

c.

d.

CONDITION: Schizophrenia (Axis I)

PHYSIOLOGY: Schizophrenia (axis I) is a thought disorder marked by delusions, hallucinations, and disorganized speech and behavior (the "positive" symptoms) and by flat affect, social withdrawal, and absence of volition (the "negative" symptoms). It involves dysfunction in one or more areas, such as interpersonal relations, work or education, or self-care. Associated features include inappropriate affect, anhedonia, dysphoric mood, abnormal psychomotor activity, cognitive dysfunction, confusion, lack of insight, and depersonalization. It is a diagnosis of exclusion, and organic causes that could explain the symptoms must be ruled out before making a diagnosis of schizophrenia. The onset typically occurs between the late teens and mid-30s. The cause of schizophrenia is unknown. Eighty percent of people diagnosed suffer from frequent relapses that may result in periodic hospitalizations, intense treatment, or crisis management. The DSM-IV-TR identifies five types of schizophrenia based on the overall presenting clinical picture: disorganized, catatonic, paranoid, undifferentiated, and residual (*Taber's*, 2009).

HANDOFF COMMUNICATION

S	Situation	Assess what is currently happening in a short statement.	Patient presents with _____
B	Background	Summarize important past assessment data for your patient here. Place lab results and medications on the concept map.	**Age:** **Gender:** **Allergies:** **Social Alerts:** **Mental Status:** **Safety Risk:**
A	Assessment	Use the assessment data to complete your concept map.	**Nursing Diagnosis:** Place the Nursing Diagnoses in prioritized order on the concept map and add any needed for your specific patient. **Plan:** Place any further Nursing Interventions Classifications (NIC) needed on the map.

Implement Your Plan of Care

R	Recommendation	Evaluate your nursing care and make recommendations related to the achievement of your desired outcomes. Were they met, or do new goals need to be established?	**EVALUATE YOUR CARE**		
			Diag	**Nursing Outcomes Classification (NOC)**	**Outcome met**
			1	The patient discusses content of hallucinations with nurse. The patient reports that the hallucinations are eliminated or at least manageable. The patient can identify and use distractions to limit or eliminate hallucinations.	☐ Yes ☐ No
			2	The patient can perform activities of daily living (ADLs) independently. The patient maintains personal hygiene at an acceptable level.	☐ Yes ☐ No
			3	The patient will attend groups willingly and without being accompanied by the nurse. The patient interacts appropriately with others. The patient can identify at least one positive self-attribute.	☐ Yes ☐ No
			4	The patient demonstrates the ability to trust. The patient differentiates between delusional thinking and reality.	☐ Yes ☐ No
			5		☐ Yes ☐ No

Nursing Diagnosis 1

Disturbed sensory perception (auditory) related to diagnosis evidenced by verbalizations.

NIC:
1) Observe for signs of hallucinations; **2)** Be cautious with touch; **3)** Refer to the hallucinations as "the voices" instead of "they" when asking for content of hallucinations; and **4)** Use, and educate the patient on using, distractions to bring the patient back to reality.

Nursing Diagnosis 2

Self-care deficit (hygiene) related to distorted perceptions about self-care evidenced by lack of hygiene.

NIC:
1) Encourage independence in ADLs, but intervene as needed; and **2)** Offer recognition and positive reinforcement for independent accomplishments.

Nursing Diagnosis 3

Low self-esteem related to perceptions evidenced by lack of eye contact, derogatory self-comments, hesitation to try new tasks, and inadequate level of confidence.

NIC:
1) Spend time with patient and develop trust; **2)** Attend groups with patient at first to offer support; **3)** Encourage simple methods of achievement; **4)** Teach effective, socially appropriate communication techniques for getting needs met and in interactions with others; and **5)** Encourage verbalization of fears.

Nursing Diagnosis 4

Disturbed thought processes related to diagnoses evidenced by disorientation.

NIC:
1) Do not whisper to others in patient's presence; **2)** Complete a mouth check for medications; **3)** Be cautious with touch; **4)** Use same staff as much a possible; and **5)** Meet patient needs and keep promises to promote trust.

Condition:
Schizophrenia
(Axis I)

Age:

Link & Explain
• Nursing Interventions Classification (NIC)
• Laboratory and Diagnostic Procedures
• Medications

Nursing Diagnosis 5

NIC:

Medications

a. Antipsychotics (e.g., aripiprazole, risperidone, olanzapine)

b. Anxiolytics (e.g., benzodiazepam, BuSpar)

c. Anticonvulsants (e.g., carbamazepine, valproic acid, gabapentin)

d. Antidepressant medications (e.g., SSRIs, MAOIs)

e. Benzodiazepines (e.g., alprazolam, lorazepam)

Laboratory & Diagnostic Procedures

a. Blood alcohol level and electrolytes

b. EKG and EEG

c.

d.

CONDITION: Sleep Disorders (Insomnia)

PHYSIOLOGY: Any condition that interferes with sleep, excluding environmental factors such as noise, excess heat or cold, movement (as on a train, bus, or ship), travel through time zones, or change in altitude, constitutes insomnia. The major classes of sleep disorders are dyssomnias, parasomnias, and sleep pattern disruption associated with medical illness. Other factors that may interfere with sleep include poor sleep hygiene, effects of drugs or alcohol, and dietary changes (*Taber's*, 2009).

HANDOFF COMMUNICATION

S	Situation	Assess what is currently happening in a short statement.	Patient presents with _____
B	Background	Summarize important past assessment data for your patient here. Place lab results and medications on the concept map.	Age: Gender: Allergies: Fall Risk: Isolation:
A	Assessment	Use the assessment data to complete your concept map.	**Nursing Diagnosis:** Place the Nursing Diagnoses in prioritized order on the concept map and add any needed for your specific patient. **Plan:** Place any further Nursing Interventions Classifications (NIC) needed on the map.

Implement Your Plan of Care

			EVALUATE YOUR CARE	
	Evaluate your nursing care and make recommendations related to the achievement of your desired outcomes. Were they met, or do new goals need to be established?	**Diag**	**Nursing Outcomes Classification (NOC)**	**Outcome met**
R (Recommendation)		**1**	Report improvement in sleep pattern or rest. Verbalize increased sense of well-being and feeling rested.	☐ Yes ☐ No
		2	Recognize changes in thinking and behavior. Identify interventions to deal effectively with situations and deficits.	☐ Yes ☐ No
		3	Verbalize understanding of factors contributing to current situation. Adopt lifestyle changes to support individual health-care needs. Assume responsibility for own health-care needs.	☐ Yes ☐ No
		4	Demonstrate improved communication and relationship skills.	☐ Yes ☐ No
		5		☐ Yes ☐ No

Nursing Diagnosis 1

Disturbed sleep pattern related to lack of sleep privacy, environmental changes, noise, physical or psychological alterations evidenced by change in normal sleep pattern, interrupted sleep, verbal reports of not feeling rested, dissatisfaction with sleep, and decreased ability to function.

NIC:
1) Ascertain usual sleep habits;
2) Provide comfortable bedding and some of patient's own possessions;
3) Establish new sleep routine;
4) Encourage light physical activity during the day; 5) Promote bedtime comfort regimen; 6) Instruct in relaxation techniques; and 7) Avoid or limit interruptions.

Nursing Diagnosis 2

Impaired memory/disturbed thought process related to lack of sleep evidenced by personality changes and altered attention span.

NIC:
1) Allow patient time to respond;
2) Discuss incidents of difficulty and how to promote safety, such as not driving if patient has not slept; 3) Evaluate stress level; and 4) Review laboratory data.

Nursing Diagnosis 3

Ineffective health maintenance related to fatigue evidenced by weight loss, inability to keep health-care provider appointments, or inability to maintain positive lifestyle.

NIC:
1) Assess level of adaptive behavior;
2) Provide information about individual health-care needs; 3) Maintain adequate hydration and balanced diet; and 4) Establish a health maintenance plan with patient.

Nursing Diagnosis 4

Risk for sexual dysfunction related to sleep deprivation.

NIC:
1) Encourage verbalization; 2) Note patient and partner interactions;
3) Assess development and lifestyle;
4) Provide privacy; and 5) Refer to sex counselor or marriage counselor.

Condition:
Sleep Disorders (Insomnia)

Age:

Link & Explain
• Nursing Interventions Classification (NIC)
• Laboratory and Diagnostic Procedures
• Medications

Nursing Diagnosis 5

NIC:

Medications

a.

b.

c.

d.

Laboratory & Diagnostic Procedures

a. Polysomnography

b.

c.

d.

CONDITION: Substance Abuse (Alcohol or Drugs)

PHYSIOLOGY: Substance abuse is a maladaptive pattern of behavior marked by the use of chemically active agents (e.g., prescription or illicit drugs, alcohol, and tobacco). Of all deaths in the United States each year, half are caused by substance abuse. About 33% of all Americans smoke cigarettes, 6% use illicit drugs regularly, and about 14% of all Americans are alcoholics. The consequences of substance abuse include heart disease, cancer, stroke, chronic obstructive lung disease, cirrhosis, trauma, and familial, social, legal, and economic difficulties (*Taber's*, 2009).

HANDOFF COMMUNICATION

S	Situation	Assess what is currently happening in a short statement.	Patient presents with _____
B	Background	Summarize important past assessment data for your patient here. Place lab results and medications on the concept map.	**Age:** **Gender:** **Allergies:** **Fall Risk:** **Isolation:**
A	Assessment	Use the assessment data to complete your concept map.	**Nursing Diagnosis:** Place the Nursing Diagnoses in prioritized order on the concept map and add any needed for your specific patient. **Plan:** Place any further Nursing Interventions Classifications (NIC) needed on the map.

Implement Your Plan of Care

			EVALUATE YOUR CARE	
R	Recommendation	Evaluate your nursing care and make recommendations related to the achievement of your desired outcomes. Were they met, or do new goals need to be established?	**Diag** / **Nursing Outcomes Classification (NOC)**	**Outcome met**
			1 Verbalize awareness of relationship of substance abuse to current situation. Engage in therapeutic program. Verbalize acceptance of and responsibility for own behavior.	☐ Yes ☐ No
			2 Identify consequences of using substance as a method of coping.	☐ Yes ☐ No
			3 Demonstrate progressive weight gain toward goal with normalization of laboratory values and absence of malnutrition.	☐ Yes ☐ No
			4 Verbalize understanding of dynamics of enabling behavior. Participate in individual and family programs. Identify ineffective coping behaviors and consequences. Initiate and plan for necessary lifestyle changes. Take action to change self-destructive behaviors and alter behaviors that contribute to patient's addiction.	☐ Yes ☐ No
			5	☐ Yes ☐ No

Nursing Diagnosis 1

Ineffective denial related to threat of unpleasant reality, lack of emotional support, overwhelming stress evidenced by lack of acceptance that alcohol or drugs is causing the present situation.

NIC:
1) Convey attitude of acceptance of individual, not behavior; **2)** Ascertain reason for beginning abstinence and involvement in therapy; **3)** Review definition of dependence and abuse with categories of symptoms including patterns of use, impairment caused by use, and tolerance to substance; **4)** Answer questions honestly and provide factual information; **5)** Discuss current life situation and the impact of substance abuse; **6)** Confront and examine denial and rationalization; and **7)** Provide positive feedback for expressing awareness of denial.

Nursing Diagnosis 2

Ineffective coping related to personal vulnerability, negative role modeling, inadequate support systems, previous ineffective or inadequate coping skills evidenced by impaired adaptive behavior and problem-solving skills.

NIC:
1) Determine understanding of current situation; **2)** Set limits and confront efforts to get caregivers to grant special privileges; **3)** Encourage verbalization of feelings; **4)** Explore alternative coping mechanisms; **5)** Assist patient to learn relaxation skills; **6)** Structure diversional activity that relates to recovery, such as social activity with support group; **7)** Identify possible and actual triggers for relapse; and **8)** Encourage involvement in writing and verbalization of plans to live without alcohol.

Nursing Diagnosis 3

Imbalanced nutrition: less than body requirements related to insufficient dietary intake to meet metabolic needs for psychological, physiological, or economic reasons evidenced by weight less than normal for height and body build; decreased subcutaneous fat; lack of interest in food; poor muscle tone; sore, inflamed buccal cavity; or laboratory evidence of protein and vitamin deficiencies.

NIC:
1) Assess height, weight, body build, strength, and activity and rest levels; **2)** Note condition of oral cavity; **3)** Note total daily intake; **4)** Monitor weight weekly; **5)** Consult with dietitian; **6)** Arrange dental consultation; and **7)** Review laboratory reports.

Nursing Diagnosis 4

Dysfunctional family processes related to abuse and history of alcoholism or drug use, inadequate coping skills, lack of problem-solving skills, genetic predisposition, or biochemical influences evidenced by feelings of anger, frustration, or responsibility for patient's alcoholic behavior.

NIC:
1) Review family history and explore roles of family members; **2)** Explore how family members have coped with patient's problem; **3)** Assess current level of functioning of family members; **4)** Provide information about enabling behavior; **5)** Encourage participation in therapeutic writing; **6)** Provide factual information to family and patient about addictive behaviors and the effect on families; **7)** Encourage family members to be aware of own feelings and look at the situation with objectivity; and **8)** Involve family in discharge planning and referrals.

Condition:
Substance Abuse (Alcohol or Drugs)
Age:

Link & Explain
- Nursing Interventions Classification (NIC)
- Laboratory and Diagnostic Procedures
- Medications

Nursing Diagnosis 5

NIC:

Medications
a. Acamprosate
b. Disulfiram (Antabuse)
c. Naltrexone (Vivitrol)
d.

Laboratory & Diagnostic Procedures
a. A toxicology screen or blood alcohol level
b. CBC, total protein
c. Folate level, serum magnesium
d. Liver function tests, uric acid

Concept Maps for Geriatric Patients

As the population in the United States increases in age, we are called more often to care for the older adult. Older adults live not only in residential facilities but also in homes and acute care settings. Many times, the older adult patient has chronic health-care needs as well as some specific ones that are listed in this chapter. Caring for older adults involves many psychosocial aspects as well because of a decline in function and the loss of support systems due to the death of loved ones and friends. Nursing care of the older adult is very rewarding; these patients are a wealth of information and history from which we all can learn much.

The conditions included in this chapter are:

1. Alzheimer's Disease
2. Cataracts (Vision Problems)
3. Elder Abuse
4. Extended Care Placement
5. Herpes Zoster (Shingles)

CONDITION: Alzheimer's Disease

PHYSIOLOGY: Alzheimer's disease (dementia, Alzheimer's type) is a progressive, degenerative neurologic disease resulting in progressive cognitive decline, including loss of memory, judgment, and abstraction, as well as personality and behavioral changes. It occurs most frequently in the elderly, with 60% of cases occurring in those older than 65 years of age. Although the exact cause is not known, female gender, increasing age, and family history increase the risk of a person developing Alzheimer's dementia. In addition, repeated head trauma and exposure to certain herpes viruses and some metals may be related to development of the disease, especially at an earlier age. Pathophysiologic changes include progressive atrophy of the cerebral cortex, vascular degeneration, neurofibrillary tangles, neuritic plaques, and decreased neurotransmitters. The progression of Alzheimer's disease is divided into three broad stages: early, middle, and moderate. Patients experience the progression differently and do not move through the stages at the same rate or with the same symptoms (*Taber's*, 2009).

Early-stage symptoms include loss of short-term memory, mild cognitive impairment and loss of judgment, decrease in socialization, subtle personality changes, impaired emotional response to stress, and decreased sense of smell.

Middle-stage symptoms include impairment of all cognitive functions; loss of independence in dealing with finances and day-to-day responsibilities; possible depression or mood swings; disorientation to person, place, and time; wandering; incontinence; and decreased ability to perform activities of daily living.

Late-stage symptoms include complete incapacitation, loss of motor and verbal skills, total dependence in activities of daily living, and agnosia.

HANDOFF COMMUNICATION

S	Situation	Assess what is currently happening in a short statement.	Patient presents as _____
B	Background	Summarize important past assessment data for your patient here. Place lab results and medications on the concept map.	**Age:** **Gender:** **Allergies:** **Fall Risk:** **Isolation:**
A	Assessment	Use the assessment data to complete your concept map.	**Nursing Diagnosis:** Place the Nursing Diagnoses in prioritized order on the concept map and add any needed for your specific patient. **Plan:** Place any further Nursing Interventions Classifications (NIC) needed on the map.

Implement Your Plan of Care

			EVALUATE YOUR CARE	
R	Recommendation Evaluate your nursing care and make recommendations related to the achievement of your desired outcomes. Were they met, or do new goals need to be established?	**Diag**	**Nursing Outcomes Classification (NOC)**	**Outcome met**
		1	This outcome changes depending on staging. In general, the desired outcome is to maintain as high a level of function as possible.	☐ Yes ☐ No
		2	Patient remains free from physical injury.	☐ Yes ☐ No
		3	Caregiver maintains own physical and psychological well-being and beneficial, caring relationship with patient.	☐ Yes ☐ No
		4	Patient remains asleep through most of the night and awake during most of the day.	☐ Yes ☐ No
		5		☐ Yes ☐ No

Nursing Diagnosis 1

Chronic confusion related to disease process evidenced by lack of short-term memory.

NIC:
1) Assess patient's degree of impairment and level of orientation; **2)** Establish therapeutic, trusting relationship with patient; **3)** Re-orient frequently, using verbal and visual cues; **4)** Determine previously effective interventions and implement as appropriate; **5)** Maintain a consistent, structured environment; **6)** Ensure adequate rest and maintain normal sleep–wake cycle; and **7)** Do not challenge illogical thinking.

Nursing Diagnosis 2

Risk for injury related to chronic confusion, wandering, incontinence, and disease progression.

NIC:
1) Routinely assess patient's level of orientation; **2)** Monitor patient frequently through hourly or more frequent rounding as needed; **3)** Provide a sitter; **4)** Reorient frequently; **5)** Encourage use of call bell; **6)** Use bed alarms; **7)** Offer toileting, water, and other services frequently; and **8)** Place bedside table with frequently used patient belongings within reach.

Nursing Diagnosis 3

Caregiver role strain related to progression of chronic debilitating disease process evidenced by caregiver fatigue.

NIC:
1) Establish therapeutic relationship with patient and caregiver; **2)** Assess caregiver's general health and for signs of stress, including anger, depression, withdrawal, irritability, and fatigue; **3)** Assess the patient for abuse or neglect; **4)** Encourage caregiver to participate in support groups and provide referral as needed; **5)** Refer patient and caregiver to social worker or case management; and **6)** Provide emotional support and time for caregiver to discuss problems, concerns, and feelings.

Nursing Diagnosis 4

Disturbed sleep pattern related to anxiety, depression, or changes in sleep phases evidenced by night wandering.

NIC:
1) Assess past normal sleep patterns; **2)** Establish a daily routine that promotes activity and limits naps during the day; **3)** Establish a bedtime routine that promotes relaxation and decreased stress; **4)** Provide a quiet, soothing environment for sleeping; **5)** Adjust treatment and medication regimen to provide uninterrupted sleep; and **6)** Administer hypnotic or anxiolytics medication as ordered, monitoring for effect and side effects.

Condition:
Alzheimer's Disease
Age:

- - - - - - - - - - - - - - - -
Link & Explain
• Nursing Interventions Classification (NIC)
• Laboratory and Diagnostic Procedures
• Medications

Nursing Diagnosis 5

NIC:

Medications

a. Cholinesterase inhibitors

b. *N*-methyl-D-aspartate inhibitors

c. Antidepressants

d. Psychotropics

Laboratory & Diagnostic Procedures

a. CBC, chemistries, and urinalysis to rule out other causes of confusion

b. CT and PET scans

c. Chest x-ray

d.

CONDITION: Cataracts (Vision Problems)

PHYSIOLOGY: A cataract is an opacity of the lens of the eye. This opacity distorts the image that is projected on the retina, thus causing distorted vision. Cataracts are caused by a gradual increase in the density of the lens due to a loss in the amount of water that the lens stores. As the lens becomes denser, it becomes opaque, meaning that it is no longer transparent. Cataracts may be related to old age or caused by other factors, such as trauma or toxic exposure. After age 70, some degree of cataract formation is expected. The patient presents with slightly blurred vision and decreased perception of color. As the condition worsens, vision may be reduced to such an extent that ADLs (activities of daily living) are affected, and without treatment, blindness may occur. Treatment for cataracts is extraction of the affected lens and replacement with a plastic lens (*Taber's*, 2009).

HANDOFF COMMUNICATION

S Situation	Assess what is currently happening in a short statement.	Patient presents as _____	
B Background	Summarize important past assessment data for your patient here. Place lab results and medications on the concept map.	**Age:** **Allergies:** **Isolation:**	**Gender:** **Fall Risk:**
A Assessment	Use the assessment data to complete your concept map.	**Nursing Diagnosis:** Place the Nursing Diagnoses in prioritized order on the concept map and add any needed for your specific patient. **Plan:** Place any further Nursing Interventions Classifications (NIC) needed on the map.	

Implement Your Plan of Care

			EVALUATE YOUR CARE	
R Recommendation	Evaluate your nursing care and make recommendations related to the achievement of your desired outcomes. Were they met, or do new goals need to be established?	**Diag**	**Nursing Outcomes Classification (NOC)**	**Outcome met**
		1	Patient discusses safety measures to cope with decreased visual acuity.	☐ Yes ☐ No
		2	Patient remains free of falls and modifies environment to minimize the incidence of falls.	☐ Yes ☐ No
		3	Patient discusses ways to safely prepare and eat food.	☐ Yes ☐ No
		4	Patient discusses treatment or the surgical procedure for visual deficit.	☐ Yes ☐ No
		5		☐ Yes ☐ No

Nursing Diagnosis 1

Disturbed visual perception related to altered sensory input evidenced by decreased vision.

NIC:
1) Improve the patient's safety by orienting him/her to surroundings and keeping room free of clutter; **2)** Familiarize the patient with your voice, and always make presence and purpose known when entering the patient's room; **3)** Provide a lighted magnifying device to increase the patient's ability to read text or see details; **4)** Determine any factors that increase the patient's visual acuity, such as lighting; and **5)** Refer the patient to a vision specialist for treatment.

Nursing Diagnosis 2

Risk for falls related to decreased visual acuity.

NIC:
1) Determine the patient's risk for falls using an evaluation tool such as the Fall Risk Assessment; **2)** Thoroughly orient the patient to the environment, and place the call light within reach; **3)** Adjust lighting to improve the patient's ability to see; **4)** Provide ambulatory devices such as a walker to improve stability; **5)** Teach the patient what to do if he or she falls and is unable to get up; **6)** Recommend an emergency response system; and **7)** Ensure that the patient has properly fitted shoes for ambulation.

Nursing Diagnosis 3

Self-care deficit (feeding) related to decreased visual acuity evidenced by need for help with food preparation and eating.

NIC:
1) Assess the patient's ability to prepare food and feed self. Inquire about previous methods of meal preparation; **2)** Request a referral for occupational therapy to work with the patient on methods of meal preparation and tools for eating; **3)** Encourage the use of the microwave for safety rather than the oven for meal preparation; **4)** Collaborate with the patient to develop a meal plan that can be easily prepared, implementing the types of food the patient enjoys; and **5)** If necessary, refer the patient to a social worker to set up a meal delivery service or home health care.

Nursing Diagnosis 4

Knowledge deficit related to eye treatment or surgery evidenced by questions.

NIC:
1) Assess the patient's understanding of surgical treatment for cataracts; **2)** Discuss treatment options for cataracts, including the differences between intracapsular and extracapsular extraction of the lens; **3)** Discuss the risks and benefits of surgery; **4)** Discuss postoperative care, including the risks for complications such as increased intraocular pressure and infection; and **5)** Teach the patient about activities to avoid following surgery, such as blowing the nose, sexual intercourse, bending from the waist, and straining to have a bowel movement, which may increase intraocular pressure.

Condition:
Cataracts (Vision Problems)
Age:

Link & Explain
• Nursing Interventions Classification (NIC)
• Laboratory and Diagnostic Procedures
• Medications

Nursing Diagnosis 5

NIC:

Medications

a. Antibiotics (postoperatively to prevent infection)

b. Analgesics (postoperatively)

c.

d.

Laboratory & Diagnostic Procedures

a. Vision test using the Snellen chart

b. Brightness acuity testing

c. Lens evaluation using direct ophthalmoscope

d.

CONDITION: Elder Abuse

PHYSIOLOGY: Elder abuse is emotional, physical, or sexual injury or financial exploitation of a person over the age of 65 years of age. It includes violence, financial exploitation, intimidation, humiliation, isolation, and neglect (failure to provide adequate food, clothing, health care, or shelter). Elders may be exploited by individuals and organizations (*Taber's*, 2009).

HANDOFF COMMUNICATION

S	Situation	Assess what is currently happening in a short statement.	Patient presents as _____
B	Background	Summarize important past assessment data for your patient here. Place lab results and medications on the concept map.	**Age:** **Gender:** **Allergies:** **Fall Risk:** **Isolation:**
A	Assessment	Use the assessment data to complete your concept map.	**Nursing Diagnosis:** Place the Nursing Diagnoses in prioritized order on the concept map and add any needed for your specific patient. **Plan:** Place any further Nursing Interventions Classifications (NIC) needed on the map.

Implement Your Plan of Care

		EVALUATE YOUR CARE
	Diag	Nursing Outcomes Classification (NOC) — Outcome met
R Recommendation — Evaluate your nursing care and make recommendations related to the achievement of your desired outcomes. Were they met, or do new goals need to be established?	**1**	Patient or caregiver modifies environment as indicated to prevent trauma. ☐ Yes ☐ No
	2	Patient acknowledges feelings and healthy ways to deal with them, verbalizes some control over present situation, makes choices related to care, and is involved in self-care. ☐ Yes ☐ No
	3	Patient verbalizes or demonstrates acceptance of self and an increased sense of self-worth. ☐ Yes ☐ No
	4	Caregiver maintains own physical and psychological well-being and beneficial, caring relationship with patient. ☐ Yes ☐ No
	5	☐ Yes ☐ No

Nursing Diagnosis 1

Risk for trauma related to physical abuse or neglect.

NIC:
1) Refer to appropriate authorities, social service, or case manager to remove patient from the situation; 2) Promote counseling for older adult and family; and 3) Assist with safe placement.

Nursing Diagnosis 2

Powerlessness related to potentially dangerous environment evidenced by anger, apathy, withdrawal, or depression.

NIC:
1) Identify factors that have led to patient's feeling of powerlessness; 2) Encourage activities that assist in formulating realistic goals; and 3) Encourage advanced directives, living will, and durable power of attorney.

Nursing Diagnosis 3

Chronic low self-esteem related to deprivation and negative feedback of family members, personal vulnerability, or feelings of abandonment evidenced by lack of eye contact, withdrawal from social contacts, discounting own needs, nonassertiveness or passiveness, indecisive or overly conforming behavior.

NIC:
1) Provide opportunity for and encourage verbalization or acting out of individual situation; 2) Spend time with patient; 3) Provide reinforcement for positive actions; 4) Encourage expressions of feelings of guilt, shame, and anger; and 5) Involve in occupational therapy or group therapy.

Nursing Diagnosis 4

Caregiver role strain related to progression of chronic debilitating disease process evidenced by caregiver fatigue.

NIC:
1) Establish therapeutic relationship with patient and caregiver; 2) Assess caregiver's general health and for signs of stress, including anger, depression, withdrawal, irritability, and fatigue; 3) Assess the caregiver's knowledge of, or role in, abuse or neglect; 4) Encourage caregiver to participate in support groups and provide referral as needed; 5) Refer patient and caregiver to social worker or case management; and 6) Provide emotional support and time for caregiver to discuss problems, concerns, and feelings.

Condition:
Elder Abuse
Age:

Link & Explain
- Nursing Interventions Classification (NIC)
- Laboratory and Diagnostic Procedures
- Medications

Nursing Diagnosis 5

NIC:

Medications

a.

b.

c.

d.

Laboratory & Diagnostic Procedures

a. X-rays if indicated

b. Nutritional panel

c.

d.

CONDITION: Extended Care Placement

PHYSIOLOGY: Extended care facility placement is for patients who require long-term custodial or medical care for chronic illness or rehabilitation therapy (*Taber's*, 2009).

HANDOFF COMMUNICATION

S	Situation	Assess what is currently happening in a short statement.	Patient presents as _____
B	Background	Summarize important past assessment data for your patient here. Place lab results and medications on the concept map.	**Age:** **Gender:** **Allergies:** **Fall Risk:** **Isolation:**
A	Assessment	Use the assessment data to complete your concept map.	**Nursing Diagnosis:** Place the Nursing Diagnoses in prioritized order on the concept map and add any needed for your specific patient. **Plan:** Place any further Nursing Interventions Classifications (NIC) needed on the map.

Implement Your Plan of Care

R	Recommendation	Evaluate your nursing care and make recommendations related to the achievement of your desired outcomes. Were they met, or do new goals need to be established?	**EVALUATE YOUR CARE**

Diag	Nursing Outcomes Classification (NOC)	Outcome met
1	Patient is free from complications associated with self-care deficit, and activities of daily living are completed with assistance, as necessary.	☐ Yes ☐ No
2	Patient verbalizes or demonstrates acceptance of self and an increased sense of self-worth.	☐ Yes ☐ No
3	Patient verbalizes understanding of the extended care process, correctly performs necessary procedures and explains reasons for the actions, initiates necessary lifestyle changes, and participates in treatment regimens.	☐ Yes ☐ No
4	Patient acknowledges feelings and healthy ways to deal with them, verbalizes some control over present situation, makes choices related to care, and is involved in self-care.	☐ Yes ☐ No
5		☐ Yes ☐ No

Nursing Diagnosis 1

Self-care deficit, total, related to cognitive and/or physical impairment evidenced by inability to perform ADLs (activities of daily living).

NIC:
1) Assess patient's ability to carry out ADLs and determine deficits; **2)** Assist patient to accept assistance as necessary; **3)** Encourage patient to be as independent as possible, while providing assistance as needed; **4)** Schedule care to provide adequate time and rest periods; **5)** Provide frequent positive reinforcement and encouragement; **6)** Provide privacy for toileting and bathing; **7)** Place call bell within reach and encourage use; and **8)** Offer frequent toileting.

Nursing Diagnosis 2

Chronic low self-esteem related to deprivation, placement, personal vulnerability, and feelings of abandonment evidenced by lack of eye contact, withdrawal from social contacts, discounting own needs, nonassertiveness or passiveness, indecisive or overly conforming behavior.

NIC:
1) Provide opportunity for and encourage verbalization or acting out of individual situation; **2)** Spend time with patient; **3)** Provide reinforcement for positive actions; **4)** Encourage expressions of feelings of guilt, shame, and anger; and **5)** Involve patient in occupational therapy or group therapy.

Nursing Diagnosis 3

Deficient knowledge related to extended care placement evidenced by questions.

NIC:
1) Identify patient's learning needs and assess willingness to learn; **2)** Determine patient's ability to learn and prior experience with health teaching; **3)** Provide an environment that is conducive to learning at a time best for the patient; **4)** Start with simple concepts, moving to more complex, in multiple teaching sessions, as appropriate; **5)** Provide audio and visual aids as appropriate; and **6)** Encourage questions.

Nursing Diagnosis 4

Powerlessness related to potentially dangerous environment evidenced by anger, apathy, withdrawal, or depression.

NIC:
1) Identify factors that have led to patient's feeling of powerlessness; **2)** Encourage activities that assist in formulating realistic goals; and **3)** Encourage advanced directives, living will, and durable power of attorney.

Condition:
Extended Care Placement
Age:

Link & Explain
• Nursing Interventions Classification (NIC)
• Laboratory and Diagnostic Procedures
• Medications

Nursing Diagnosis 5

NIC:

Medications

a.

b.

c.

d.

Laboratory & Diagnostic Procedures

a.

b.

c.

d.

CONDITION: Herpes Zoster (Shingles)

PHYSIOLOGY: Herpes zoster, also known as shingles, is a skin eruption most common in older adults and immunosuppressed individuals. It is caused by the varicella zoster virus, which also causes chickenpox, and shingles can occur anytime subsequent to having chickenpox. The virus, which lays dormant in the nerve roots, is reactivated and causes vesicular eruptions that occur unilaterally in a dermatomal, linear distribution. The skin eruption is preceded by 48 to 72 hours of deep, somatic-type pain, paresthesia and pruritus in the same area. Outbreaks are usually limited to the face and truncal area, and sufferers typically experience only one outbreak in a lifetime. The cause of reactivation is not clearly understood but may be related to increased stressors or illness. Approximately 20% of persons who have an outbreak of shingles, mostly in the elderly population, may develop postherpetic neuralgia. This is a severe neuralgic pain in the area of the outbreak and may last from weeks to years, causing significant disability. Other, acute complications, occurring rarely, include encephalitis, blindness, pneumonia, and hearing impairment.

Treatment is usually symptomatic, but antivirals may be useful in shortening the outbreak and preventing neuralgia if initiated within 72 hours of first symptom occurrence. Shingles is not itself contagious; however, the virus that causes shingles may be passed to an individual who has not been exposed to chickenpox, resulting in the development of chickenpox. It is passed through direct contact with the vesicular fluid and cannot be transmitted through airborne droplets. Once the vesicles crust over, the person is no longer contagious (*Taber's*, 2009).

HANDOFF COMMUNICATION

S	Situation	Assess what is currently happening in a short statement.	Patient presents as _____
B	Background	Summarize important past assessment data for your patient here. Place lab results and medications on the concept map.	Age: Gender: Allergies: Fall Risk: Isolation:
A	Assessment	Use the assessment data to complete your concept map.	**Nursing Diagnosis:** Place the Nursing Diagnoses in prioritized order on the concept map and add any needed for your specific patient. **Plan:** Place any further Nursing Interventions Classifications (NIC) needed on the map.

Implement Your Plan of Care

			EVALUATE YOUR CARE	
R	Recommendation Evaluate your nursing care and make recommendations related to the achievement of your desired outcomes. Were they met, or do new goals need to be established?	**Diag**	**Nursing Outcomes Classification (NOC)**	**Outcome met**
		1	Patient reports absence or decrease of pruritus and scratching.	☐ Yes ☐ No
		2	Patient reports pain is controlled.	☐ Yes ☐ No
		3	Patient can identify interventions to prevent and reduce risk of infection.	☐ Yes ☐ No
		4	Patient verbalizes understanding of the disease process and potential complications, identifies relationship of signs and symptoms to the disease process and correlates symptoms with causative agents, correctly performs necessary procedures and explains reasons for the actions, initiates necessary lifestyle changes, and participates in treatment regimens.	☐ Yes ☐ No
		5		☐ Yes ☐ No

Nursing Diagnosis 1

Impaired skin integrity related to disease process evidenced by rash.

NIC:
1) Assess skin routinely, noting stage of vesicles and healing and monitoring for signs of infection; **2)** Apply topical treatments as ordered, and monitor for effect and side effects; **3)** Monitor patient's skin care practices; and **4)** Wash hands frequently, and encourage patient and visitors to do so as well.

Nursing Diagnosis 2

Acute pain related to pathology and nerve involvement evidenced by verbal reports, narrowed focus, guarding or protective behaviors, and physical and social withdrawal.

NIC:
1) Monitor patient's pain characteristics, including onset, location, duration, quality, severity, and alleviating and precipitating factors; **2)** Assess patient's expectations for pain control; **3)** Assess patient's knowledge of pain control measures, and educate accordingly; **4)** Administer analgesics as ordered, monitoring for effect and side effects; **5)** Teach nonpharmacologic pain relief measures; and **6)** Encourage adequate rest, and decrease environmental stressors.

Nursing Diagnosis 3

Risk for infection related to impaired skin integrity.

NIC:
1) Monitor the patient for signs and symptoms of infection, including redness, swelling, pain, purulent drainage, fever, and malaise; **2)** Wash hands before and after each patient care activity; **3)** Instruct the patient and family members on proper hand hygiene and infection prevention activities; **4)** Administer antibiotics per orders, monitoring for effect and side effects; **5)** Assess nutritional status; and **6)** Limit visitors.

Nursing Diagnosis 4

Deficient knowledge related to disease process, treatment, and follow-up care evidenced by questions.

NIC:
1) Identify patient's learning needs, and assess willingness to learn; **2)** Determine patient's ability to learn and prior experience with health teaching; **3)** Provide an environment that is conducive to learning at a time best for the patient; **4)** Start with simple concepts, moving to more complex, in multiple teaching sessions, as appropriate; **5)** Provide audio and visual aids as appropriate; and **6)** Encourage questions.

Condition:
Herpes Zoster (Shingles)

Age:

Link & Explain
- Nursing Interventions Classification (NIC)
- Laboratory and Diagnostic Procedures
- Medications

Nursing Diagnosis 5

NIC:

Medications

a. Antivirals

b. Analgesics

c. Antipruritics

d.

Laboratory & Diagnostic Procedures

a. Viral culture

b. White count

c.

d.

Concept Maps for Community or Population Processes

This chapter provides care maps that describe system conditions experienced by nurses who work in the community, with populations of patients, or in acute care facilities, when a crisis occurs and nursing staff must deal with large-impact population issues. Care mapping for communities is very important and is fostered by a thorough assessment of community or population needs, observational experiences in the community, and demographic statistics.

Communities have characteristics, just as individuals do, and are often in need of nursing care. Community nurses make an impact on the living conditions of the entire group as well as on the individuals within the group. Today's lifestyles, as well as the current world of uncertainty, make nurses' responses to community events that affect health more important than ever.

The situations included in this chapter are:

1. Bioterrorism
2. Botulism
3. Obesity
4. Posttraumatic Stress Response
5. Pressure Sore/Ulcer
6. Trauma

CONDITION: Bioterrorism

PHYSIOLOGY: Bioterrorism is the use of biological warfare agents against civilian rather than military targets (*Taber's*, 2009).

HANDOFF COMMUNICATION

S	Situation	Assess what is currently happening in a short statement.	The community or population health issue presents as _____
B	Background	Summarize important past assessment data for your patient here. Place lab results and medications on the concept map.	
A	Assessment	Use the assessment data to complete your concept map.	**Nursing Diagnosis:** Place the Nursing Diagnoses in prioritized order on the concept map and add any needed for your specific patient. **Plan:** Place any further Nursing Interventions Classifications (NIC) needed on the map.

Implement Your Plan of Care

R	Recommendation	Evaluate your nursing care and make recommendations related to the achievement of your desired outcomes. Were they met, or do new goals need to be established?	**EVALUATE YOUR CARE**

Diag	Nursing Outcomes Classification (NOC)	Outcome met
1	Degree of injury is minimized and further injury is prevented.	☐ Yes ☐ No
2	Patients identify interventions to prevent and reduce risk of infection.	☐ Yes ☐ No
3	Patients use resources and support systems effectively.	☐ Yes ☐ No
4	Patients verbalize increased sense of self-concept and hope for the future.	☐ Yes ☐ No
5		☐ Yes ☐ No

Nursing Diagnosis 1

Risk for injury-trauma, suffocation, or poisoning related to contact with chemical pollutants, poisonous gases, exposure to open flame or flammable material, acceleration or deceleration forces, or contamination of water and food.

NIC:
1) Acquire information about nature of emergency, accident, or disaster; **2)** Prepare area and equipment; **3)** Assist in triaging patients for treatment; **4)** Determine primary needs and specific complaints; **5)** Check medical alert tags; **6)** Work with other responding agencies; **7)** Provide therapeutic interventions; and **8)** Identify community resources.

Nursing Diagnosis 2

Risk for infection related to environmental exposure or trauma and tissue destruction.

NIC:
1) Note risk factors for occurrence of infection; **2)** Observe for manifestations of infective agent and systemic infection; **3)** Demonstrate proper hand washing; **4)** Provide infection precautions such as isolation when indicated; **5)** Group cohort individuals; **6)** Obtain appropriate specimens for testing; **7)** Administer and monitor medications as indicated; and **8)** Alert proper authorities of infectious agent.

Nursing Diagnosis 3

Anxiety (severe/panic) related to situational crises and exposure to toxins evidenced by impaired functioning and sympathetic stimulation or extraneous movements such as restlessness.

NIC:
1) Determine degree of anxiety or fear; **2)** Note degree of disorganization; **3)** Create quiet area if able; **4)** Develop trust; **5)** Determine presence of physical symptoms; **6)** Assist patient to correct distortions; and **7)** Administer medications as indicated.

Nursing Diagnosis 4

Spiritual distress related to physical and psychological stress evidenced by anger directed toward deity or engaging in self-blame.

NIC:
1) Determine patient's beliefs; **2)** Establish an environment that promotes free expression; **3)** Listen to patient; **4)** Ask how you can be most helpful; **5)** Refer to resources; **6)** Encourage participation in support groups; and **7)** Make time for nonjudgmental discussion if possible.

Condition:
Bioterrorism

Link & Explain
• Nursing Interventions Classification (NIC)
• Laboratory and Diagnostic Procedures
• Medications

Nursing Diagnosis 5

NIC:

Medications

a. Antidotes

b. Analgesics

c.

d.

Laboratory & Diagnostic Procedures

a. Cultures of substances

b.

c.

d.

CONDITION: Botulism

PHYSIOLOGY: Botulism is a paralytic and occasionally fatal illness caused by exposure to toxins released by *Clostridium botulinum*, an anaerobic, gram-positive bacillus. In adults, the disease usually occurs after food contaminated by the toxin is eaten, after gastrointestinal surgery, or after the toxin is released into an infected wound. In infants (usually between the ages of 3 and 20 weeks of age), the illness results from the intestinal colonization by clostridial spores (possibly related to honey or corn syrup ingestion), then production of the exotoxin within the intestine. Because the toxin is extraordinarily lethal and easy to manufacture and distribute, concern has been raised regarding its use as an agent of biological warfare. Food-borne botulism may result from consumption of improperly cooked and canned meals in which the spores of the bacillus survive and reproduce. Wound botulism may begin in abscesses, where an anaerobic environment promotes the proliferation of the bacterium. In either case, cranial nerve paralysis and failure of the autonomic and respiratory systems may occur; however, gastrointestinal symptoms are likely only in food-borne outbreaks. The poison responsible for botulism damages the nervous system by blocking the release of acetylcholine at the neuromuscular junction, which causes the paralysis associated with the illness (*Taber's*, 2009).

HANDOFF COMMUNICATION

S	Situation	Assess what is currently happening in a short statement.	The community or population health issue presents as _____
B	Background	Summarize important past assessment data for your patient here. Place lab results and medications on the concept map.	
A	Assessment	Use the assessment data to complete your concept map.	**Nursing Diagnosis:** Place the Nursing Diagnoses in prioritized order on the concept map and add any needed for your specific patient. **Plan:** Place any further Nursing Interventions Classifications (NIC) needed on the map.

Implement Your Plan of Care

		EVALUATE YOUR CARE		
R Recommendation	Evaluate your nursing care and make recommendations related to the achievement of your desired outcomes. Were they met, or do new goals need to be established?	**Diag**	**Nursing Outcomes Classification (NOC)**	**Outcome met**
		1	Affected citizens demonstrate improved fluid balance evidenced by adequate urinary output with normal specific gravity, stable VS, moist mucous membranes, good skin turgor, prompt capillary refill, and weight within acceptable range.	☐ Yes ☐ No
		2	Patients demonstrate improved physical mobility.	☐ Yes ☐ No
		3	Patients appear relaxed and report anxiety reduced to a manageable level.	☐ Yes ☐ No
		4	Patients maintain adequate ventilation and respiratory rate and rhythm normal for each individual, breath sounds are clear, and patients are free of dyspnea or shortness of breath.	☐ Yes ☐ No
		5		☐ Yes ☐ No

Nursing Diagnosis 1

Risk for fluid volume deficit related to active losses (vomiting, diarrhea, decreased intake, nausea, dysphagia) evidenced by reports of thirst, dry skin and mucous membranes, decreased BP and urine output, change in mental status, increased hematocrit.

NIC:
1) Monitor VS, capillary refill, mucous membrane status, and skin turgor;
2) Monitor amount and type of fluid intake; 3) Review electrolyte and renal function tests; and 4) Administer IV and electrolytes as indicated.

Nursing Diagnosis 2

Impaired physical mobility related to neuromuscular impairment evidenced by cranial nerve deficits, limited ability to perform gross or fine motor skills, descending paralysis.

NIC:
1) Discuss the patient's mobility status and independence prior to illness;
2) Reposition the patient every 2 hours to avoid skin breakdown; 3) Treat pain prior to increased patient activity;
4) Encourage early ambulation;
5) Increase independence with ADL (activities of daily living) and encourage the patient to do things for himself or herself; and 6) Advise the patient to ambulate only with assistance, and implement risk for falls guidelines to avoid further complications.

Nursing Diagnosis 3

Anxiety (severe) related to threat of death, interpersonal transmission evidenced by expressed concerns, apprehension, awareness of physiological symptoms, and focus on self.

NIC:
1) Evaluate anxiety level; 2) Provide ongoing information; 3) Provide presence; and 4) Provide comfort care.

Nursing Diagnosis 4

Risk for impaired spontaneous ventilation related to neuromuscular impairment and presence of infectious process.

NIC:
1) Evaluate respiratory depth and rate;
2) Auscultate breath sounds; 3) Encourage deep-breathing exercises; 4) Note any increased restlessness; and
5) Administer O_2 as needed.

Condition:
Botulism

Link & Explain
• Nursing Interventions Classification (NIC)
• Laboratory and Diagnostic Procedures
• Medications

Nursing Diagnosis 5

NIC:

Medications

a. IV hydration

b. Antibiotics

c.

d.

Laboratory & Diagnostic Procedures

a. Stool culture

b. Blood cultures

c.

d.

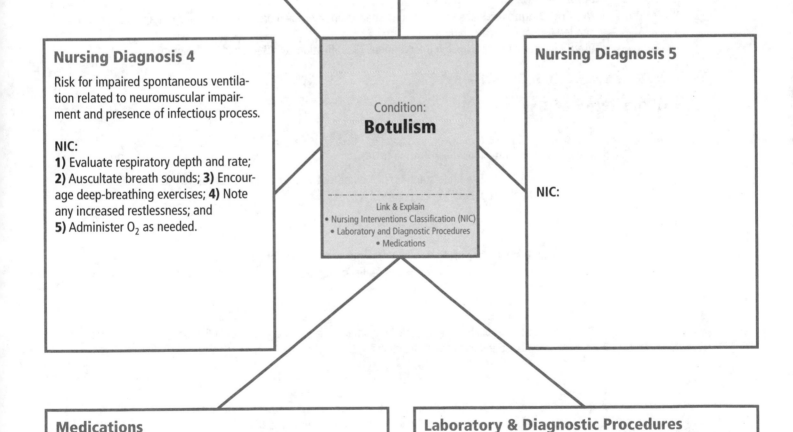

CONDITION: Obesity

PHYSIOLOGY: Obesity is an unhealthy accumulation of body fat. In adults, damaging effects of excess weight are seen when the body mass index exceeds 25kg/m². Obesity is defined as having a body mass index exceeding 30kg/m². Obesity is the most common metabolic/nutritional disease in the United States. More than 65% of the adult population is overweight. Obesity is more common in women, minorities, and the poor. Obese individuals have an increased risk of developing diabetes mellitus, hypertension, heart disease, stroke, fatal cancers, and other illnesses. In addition, obese individuals may suffer psychologically and socially. Obesity is the end result of an imbalance between food eaten and energy expended, but the underlying causes are more complex. Genetic, hormonal, and neurological influences all contribute to weight gain and loss. In addition, some medications may cause patients to gain weight (*Taber's*, 2009).

HANDOFF COMMUNICATION

S	Situation	Assess what is currently happening in a short statement.	The community or population health issue presents as _____
B	Background	Summarize important past assessment data for your patient here. Place lab results and medications on the concept map.	
A	Assessment	Use the assessment data to complete your concept map.	**Nursing Diagnosis:** Place the Nursing Diagnoses in prioritized order on the concept map and add any needed for your specific patient. **Plan:** Place any further Nursing Interventions Classifications (NIC) needed on the map.

Implement Your Plan of Care

			EVALUATE YOUR CARE	
R	Recommendation	Evaluate your nursing care and make recommendations related to the achievement of your desired outcomes. Were they met, or do new goals need to be established?	**Diag** / **Nursing Outcomes Classification (NOC)**	**Outcome met**
			1 Patients verbalize understanding of weight loss strategies and incorporate them into health regimen.	☐ Yes ☐ No
			2 Patients verbalize understanding of importance of regular exercise to weight loss and general well-being; formulate realistic exercise program with gradual increase in activity.	☐ Yes ☐ No
			3 Patients establish more realistic body image; acknowledge self as individual; accept responsibility for own actions.	☐ Yes ☐ No
			4 Patients verbalize understanding of need for lifestyle changes to maintain weight control; establish community goals and plan for attaining goal.	☐ Yes ☐ No
			5	☐ Yes ☐ No

Nursing Diagnosis 1

Imbalanced nutrition: more than body requirements related to food intake that exceeds body's needs, psychological factors, socioeconomic status evidenced by weight of 20% or more over optimum body weight, excess body fat by skinfold or other measurements, reported or observed dysfunctional eating patterns, intake more than body requirements.

NIC:
1) Assess weight using same scale at the same time of day; **2)** Perform nutritional assessment and food availability; **3)** Assess community's knowledge regarding nutritional needs; **4)** Provide education based on needs and knowledge level, including information on nutritional needs, reading nutritional labels, portion size control, etc.; **5)** Assist patients in establishing short- and long-term goals; **6)** Encourage increased activity and exercise; and **7)** Provide positive reinforcement and encouragement.

Nursing Diagnosis 2

Sedentary lifestyle related to lack of interest or motivation, lack of resources, lack of training or knowledge of specific exercise needs, or physical deconditioning evidenced by choice of a daily routine lacking physical exercise.

NIC:
1) Review necessity for and benefits of regular exercise; **2)** Determine current activity level and plan for progressive exercise opportunities; **3)** Identify perceived and actual barriers to exercise; **4)** Discuss appropriate warm-up and cool-down exercises; **5)** Determine optimal heart rates for participants; **6)** Encourage involvement in social activities; and **7)** Involve physical therapy.

Nursing Diagnosis 3

Disturbed body image/chronic low self-esteem related to view of self in contrast to social values, family or subcultural encouragement of overeating, control sex, and love issues evidenced by negative feelings about body.

NIC:
1) Determine patients' view of fat and what it does to individuals; **2)** Promote open communication avoiding criticism and judgment; graph weights on a weekly basis; and **3)** Outline and clearly state expectations.

Nursing Diagnosis 4

Knowledge deficit regarding condition, prognosis, and self-care evidenced by statements of lack of or requests for information about obesity and nutritional requirements.

NIC:
1) Determine level of nutritional knowledge and what patients believe is most urgent; **2)** Identify individual long-term goals for health; **3)** Provide information on how to maintain a satisfactory food intake; **4)** Identify sources of information in the community; and **5)** Discuss alternative ways to reward people for maintaining goals.

Condition:
Obesity

Link & Explain
• Nursing Interventions Classification (NIC)
• Laboratory and Diagnostic Procedures
• Medications

Nursing Diagnosis 5

NIC:

Medications

a. Orlistat (Xenical)

b. Phentermine (Ionamin)

c.

d.

Laboratory & Diagnostic Procedures

a. CBC

b. Nutritional panels

c. Albumin level

d.

CONDITION: Posttraumatic Stress Response

PHYSIOLOGY: Posttraumatic stress response is triggered by events outside the range of usual human experience: serious threat to self/loved ones, serious injury to self/loved ones, serious accidents (e.g., industrial, motor vehicle), abuse (physical and psychosocial), criminal victimization, rape, witnessing mutilation/violent death, tragic occurrence involving multiple deaths, disasters, sudden destruction of home/community, epidemics, wars, being held prisoner of war, torture. Risk factors may include:

- Occupation (e.g., police, fire, rescue, corrections, emergency room staff, mental health worker, [responder family members])
- Perception of event, exaggerated sense of responsibility, diminished ego strength, survivor's role in the event
- Inadequate social support; nonsupportive environment
- Displacement from home; duration of the event
- Nature of incident (catastrophic accident, assault, suicide attempt) and possibly injury/death of other(s) involved; *Taber's*, 2009)

Stages

- Acute subtype: begins within 6 months and does not last longer than 6 months
- Chronic subtype: lasts more than 6 months
- Delayed subtype: period of latency of 6 months or more before onset of symptoms

(Doenges, Moorhouse, & Geissler-Murr, 2004)

HANDOFF COMMUNICATION

S	Situation	Assess what is currently happening in a short statement.	The community or population health issue presents as _____
B	Background	Summarize important past assessment data for your patient here. Place lab results and medications on the concept map.	
A	Assessment	Use the assessment data to complete your concept map.	**Nursing Diagnosis:** Place the Nursing Diagnoses in prioritized order on the concept map and add any needed for your specific patient. **Plan:** Place any further Nursing Interventions Classifications (NIC) needed on the map.

Implement Your Plan of Care

		EVALUATE YOUR CARE		
R	Recommendation	Evaluate your nursing care and make recommendations related to the achievement of your desired outcomes. Were they met, or do new goals need to be established?	**Diag**	**Nursing Outcomes Classification (NOC)**	**Outcome met**
			1	Patients are free of severe anxiety.	☐ Yes ☐ No
			2	Patients demonstrate ability to deal with emotional reactions in an individually appropriate manner.	☐ Yes ☐ No
			3	Patients report absence of physical manifestations (pain, nightmares/flashbacks, insomnia, fatigue) associated with the event.	☐ Yes ☐ No
			4	Patients verbalize increased sense of self-concept and hope for the future.	☐ Yes ☐ No
			5		☐ Yes ☐ No

Nursing Diagnosis 1

Anxiety (severe)/powerlessness related to situational crisis [specify] evidenced by poor eye contact, restlessness, impaired attention, sleep disturbance.

NIC:
1) Assess level of anxiety; 2) Monitor physical responses (palpitations/rapid pulse, diaphoresis); 3) Develop therapeutic relationship with patients; 4) Observe behavior; 5) Consult support services as indicated; and 6) Medicate as indicated.

Nursing Diagnosis 2

Ineffective coping/stress tolerance related to situational crisis evidenced by emotional outbursts (anger, crying) and self-destructive and unhealthy coping strategies (drinking, substance abuse).

NIC:
1) Provide emotional support; 2) Provide opportunity for and encourage verbalization and discussion of individual situation; 3) Assess mental status; 4) Spend time with patients; and 5) Develop a plan for dealing with anxiety.

Nursing Diagnosis 3

Alteration in sleep/rest pattern related to prolonged psychological discomfort, nightmares evidenced by daytime drowsiness, anxiety, restlessness, and irritability.

NIC:
1) Assess causative factors; 2) Use counseling/behavioral modification (relaxation exercises) to help patient; and 3) Assist patient in establishing optimal sleep pattern.

Nursing Diagnosis 4

Spiritual distress related to physical and psychological stress evidenced by anger directed toward deity or engaging in self-blame.

NIC:
1) Determine patient's beliefs; 2) Establish an environment that promotes free expression; 3) Listen to patient; 4) Ask how you can be most helpful; 5) Refer to resources; 6) Encourage participation in support groups; and 7) Make time for nonjudgmental discussion if possible.

Condition:
Posttraumatic Stress Response

Link & Explain
• Nursing Interventions Classification (NIC)
• Laboratory and Diagnostic Procedures
• Medications

Nursing Diagnosis 5

NIC:

Medications

a. Sertraline (Zoloft), 50 mg PO qd

b.

c.

d.

Laboratory & Diagnostic Procedures

a.

b.

c.

d.

CONDITION: Pressure Sore/Ulcer

PHYSIOLOGY: Pressure sore/ulcer is damage to the skin or underlying structures as a result of tissue compression and inadequate perfusion. Pressure sores/ulcers typically occur in patients who are bed or chair bound, such as patients with sensory and mobility deficits (e.g., spinal cord injury, stroke, or coma), malnourished patients, patients with peripheral vascular disease, hospitalized elderly patients, and patients in convalescent homes. Some evidence also suggests that incontinence is a risk factor. The most common sites of skin breakdown are over bony prominences (e.g., sacrum, trochanter, shoulder blade, ischial tuberosity, iliac crest, elbow, lateral malleoli, heel, and occiput). The combination of pressure, shearing forces, friction, and moisture leads to tissue injury and occasionally necrosis. If not treated vigorously, the ulcer will progress from a simple red patch of skin to erosion into the subcutaneous tissues, eventually extending to muscle or bone. Deep ulcers often become infected with bacteria and develop gangrene; *Taber's*, 2009).

HANDOFF COMMUNICATION

S	Situation	Assess what is currently happening in a short statement.	The community or population health issue presents as _____. Patient is at risk for pressure sore/ulcer in the following site(s): _____. Patient has a pressure sore/ulcer in the following sites(s): _____.
B	Background	Summarize important past assessment data for your patient here. Place lab results and medications on the concept map.	**Score on Braden scale predicting pressure ulcer_____** **Serum protein levels (albumin____, prealbumin____)** **Medication(s)_____** **Preexisting conditions: edema____, diabetes___, liver disease___, renal failure___, alcoholism___, heart disease___, peripheral vascular disease___, neurological disease___, decreased mobility___**
A	Assessment	Use the assessment data to complete your concept map.	**Nursing Diagnosis:** Place the Nursing Diagnoses in prioritized order on the concept map and add any needed for your specific patient. **Plan:** Place any further Nursing Interventions Classifications (NIC) needed on the map.

Implement Your Plan of Care

		EVALUATE YOUR CARE		
R	Recommendation — Evaluate your nursing care and make recommendations related to the achievement of your desired outcomes. Were they met, or do new goals need to be established?	Diag	Nursing Outcomes Classification (NOC)	Outcome met
		1	Patient maintains optimum tissue perfusion.	☐ Yes ☐ No
		2	Patient displays timely healing of skin lesions or pressure sores/ulcers without complication.	☐ Yes ☐ No
		3	Patient participates in prevention measures and treatment program.	☐ Yes ☐ No
		4	Patient identifies individual risk factors for development of pressure sore/ulcer.	☐ Yes ☐ No
		5		☐ Yes ☐ No

Nursing Diagnosis 1

Ineffective peripheral tissue perfusion related to reduced or interrupted blood flow evidenced by reddened and/or necrotic tissue.

NIC:
1) Identify underlying condition or pathology involved with ineffective peripheral tissue perfusion; **2)** Assess blood supply (capillary refill, color, warmth, sensation of skin, ability to move extremities); **3)** Review medication list for any drugs with a vasoconstrictive activity; **4)** Use Braden scale to predict pressure ulcer risk; **5)** Encourage mobility, activity, and range of motion to enhance circulation and promote tissue health; **6)** Use proper turning and transfer techniques; **7)** Regularly reposition patient; and **8)** Use appropriate padding or pressure-relieving devices.

Nursing Diagnosis 2

Impaired skin/tissue integrity may be related to altered circulation, edema, inflammation, and/or decreased sensation evidenced by destruction of skin layers, invasion of body structures.

NIC:
1) Describe anatomic location, depth of skin or tissue injury or damage. Stage ulcer using the National Pressure Ulcer Advisory Panel Updated Staging System; **2)** Photograph lesion(s) as appropriate to document status and provide visual baseline for further comparison; **3)** Remeasure wound(s) regularly and observe for complications; **4)** Provide adequate nutrition; **5)** Avoid use of heating pads/ice packs to extremities in cases of decreased tissue perfusion; **6)** Avoid use of plastic material (linen savers), and remove wet or wrinkled linens promptly; **7)** Remove adhesive materials (tape, nonadherent dressings) with care; and **8)** Avoid use of perfumes, dyes, preservatives, alcohol, hydrogen peroxide, and povidone-iodine.

Nursing Diagnosis 3

Deficient knowledge regarding cause, prevention of condition, and potential complications may be related to lack of information or misinterpretation, possibly evidenced by statements of concern and/or questions.

NIC:
1) Review benefits of following medical regimen; **2)** Encourage regular inspection and monitoring of skin for changes or failure to heal; **3)** Identify safety measures for patient with persistent impairments; **4)** Encourage mobility, activity, and range of motion to enhance circulation and promote tissue health; **5)** Avoid use of heating pads/ice packs to extremities in cases of decreased tissue perfusion; **6)** Avoid use of perfumes, dyes, preservatives, alcohol, hydrogen peroxide, and povidone-iodine; **7)** Avoid use of tobacco and tobacco products; and **8)** Review measures to avoid infection of wound.

Nursing Diagnosis 4

Risk for infection at site of pressure sore/ulcer related to nonintact skin.

NIC:
1) Maintain overall skin hygiene; **2)** Consult with physician or wound specialist as indicated to assist with development of plan for care of wound; **3)** Use body-temperature physiologic solutions (e.g., isotonic saline) to clean or irrigate wound; **4)** Cleanse wound with irrigation syringe provided; **5)** Use appropriate barrier dressing or wound coverage; **6)** Assist with débridement or enzymatic therapy as indicated; and **7)** Review measures to avoid infection of wound.

Condition:
Pressure Sore/Ulcer

Link & Explain
• Nursing Interventions Classification (NIC)
• Laboratory and Diagnostic Procedures
• Medications

Nursing Diagnosis 5

NIC:

Medications
a.
b.
c.
d.

Laboratory & Diagnostic Procedures
a.
b.
c.
d.

CONDITION: Trauma

PHYSIOLOGY: Trauma is a physical injury or wound caused by external force or violence. It may be self-inflicted. In the United States, trauma is the principal cause of death between the ages of 1 and 44 years. In addition to each death from trauma, at least two cases of permanent disability are caused by trauma. The principal types of trauma include motor vehicle accidents, military service, falls, burns, gunshot wounds, and drowning. Most deaths occur within the first several hours of the event (*Taber's*, 2009).

HANDOFF COMMUNICATION

S	Situation	Assess what is currently happening in a short statement.	The community or population health issue presents as _____
B	Background	Summarize important past assessment data for your patient here. Place lab results and medications on the concept map.	
A	Assessment	Use the assessment data to complete your concept map.	**Nursing Diagnosis:** Place the Nursing Diagnoses in prioritized order on the concept map and add any needed for your specific patient. **Plan:** Place any further Nursing Interventions Classifications (NIC) needed on the map.

Implement Your Plan of Care

			EVALUATE YOUR CARE	
R	Recommendation	Evaluate your nursing care and make recommendations related to the achievement of your desired outcomes. Were they met, or do new goals need to be established?	**Diag** / **Nursing Outcomes Classification (NOC)**	**Outcome met**
			1 Degree of injury is minimized and further injury is prevented.	☐ Yes ☐ No
			2 Pain level is decreased on a 0–10 numeric scale following implementation of medication or nonpharmacologic treatments.	☐ Yes ☐ No
			3 Patient acknowledges feelings and healthy ways to deal with them, verbalizes some control over present situation, makes choices related to care, and is involved in self-care.	☐ Yes ☐ No
			4 Patient verbalizes increased sense of self-concept and hope for the future.	☐ Yes ☐ No
			5	☐ Yes ☐ No

Nursing Diagnosis 1

Trauma related to loss of skeletal integrity evidenced by fractures, loss of skin integrity, or decreased mobility.

NIC:
1) Acquire information about nature of emergency, accident, or disaster; **2)** Prepare area and equipment; **3)** Assist to triage patients for treatment (Black, Morgue; Red, Immediate; Yellow, Delayed; Green, Minor); **4)** Determine primary needs and specific complaints; **5)** Check medical alert tags; **6)** Work with other responding agencies; **7)** Provide therapeutic interventions; and **8)** Identify community resources.

Nursing Diagnosis 2

Acute pain related to injury and surgical procedure evidenced by verbal reports, narrowed focus, guarding or protective behaviors, and physical and social withdrawal.

NIC:
1) Assess the pain to determine the onset, location, duration, characteristics, and aggravating and alleviating factors; **2)** Determine the patient's current medication use; **3)** Explore the need for opioid and nonopioid analgesics; and **4)** Administer pain medications when the client reports pain, and assess pain relief at least 1 hour following.

Nursing Diagnosis 3

Powerlessness related to potentially dangerous environment evidenced by anger, apathy, withdrawal, or depression.

NIC:
1) Identify factors that led to patient's feeling of powerlessness; **2)** Encourage activities that assist in formulating realistic goals; and **3)** Encourage self-care in situation as much as possible.

Nursing Diagnosis 4

Anxiety (severe/panic). Fear related to situational crises and exposure to toxins evidenced by impaired functioning and sympathetic stimulation or extraneous movements such as restlessness.

NIC:
1) Determine degree of anxiety or fear; **2)** Note degree of disorganization; **3)** Create quiet area if able; **4)** Develop trust; **5)** Determine presence of physical symptoms; **6)** Assist patient to correct distortions; and **7)** Administer medications as indicated.

Condition:
Trauma

Link & Explain
• Nursing Interventions Classification (NIC)
• Laboratory and Diagnostic Procedures
• Medications

Nursing Diagnosis 5

NIC:

Medications

a.

b.

c.

d.

Laboratory & Diagnostic Procedures

a.

b.

c.

d.

Concept Maps for Systems to Promote Leadership Processes

Leadership as a subject in nursing is becoming increasingly important with respect to the nurse's role in safeguarding patient and family outcomes. All nurses are leaders of patient care and are the ones who know best the patients and their physiological and psychological responses to health and illness. Leadership takes practice and, like all other interventions, astute assessment.

This chapter provides care maps that describe system conditions commonly experienced by nurses as leaders in health-care settings. Although it may seem that concept maps best fit specific patient situations, they can also benefit system thinking. For example, if an interprofessional communication breakdown occurs, the communication process concept map can be applied to that situation and can assist you, the student, to "sort it out" and identify areas for improvement.

These concept maps are unique and were made to help you gain professional insight into system issues. The Situation, Background, Assessment, Recommendation (SBAR) model is a mechanism to assist you in framing the problem and therefore make it easier to establish goals and recommend interventions. The SBAR format can also help you organize the issue into a concise description when communicating it to others on your team. The concept maps challenge you to think critically about common system issues using the nursing process.

The conditions included in this chapter are:

1. Delegation to Health-Care Providers (RNs, LPNs, UAP)
2. Ineffective Inter- and/or Intraprofessional Communication Process
3. Ineffective Leadership
4. Infection Rates
5. Medication Errors (Risk for Patient Injury)

CONDITION: Delegation to Health-Care Providers (RNs, LPNs, UAP)

PHYSIOLOGY: Delegation to health-care providers (RNs, LPNs, UAP [Unlicensed Assistive Personnel]) is transferring to a competent individual the authority to perform a selected nursing task in a selected situation. The nurse retains accountability for the delegation. RNs are accountable for supervising those to whom they have delegated tasks. RNs often delegate nursing tasks to other team members, and they are accountable for the decision to delegate and for the adequacy of nursing care to the patient, provided the person to whom the task was delegated performed the task as instructed and delegated by the delegating RN. The RN retains accountability for the outcome of delegation. (ANA, 2005, 2012).

Five Rights of Delegation

1. The right task [based on the scope of practice of the person it is being delegated to].
2. Under the right circumstances [based on patient needs and available resources].
3. To the right person [who has the ability, qualifications, and/or experience required to complete the task].
4. With the right directions and communication [including any unique patient requirements and characteristics; clear expectations regarding what to do, what to report, and when to ask for assistance; and written instructions if required].
5. Under the right supervision and evaluation [by a registered nurse who monitors task and its effectiveness and is available to provide guidance and follow up on problems or need for changes] (ANA & NCSBN, n.d.).

HANDOFF COMMUNICATION

S	Situation	Assess what is currently happening in a short statement.	The system issue presents as _____
B	Background	Summarize important past assessment data for your patient here. Place lab results and medications on the concept map.	
A	Assessment	Use the assessment data to complete your concept map.	**Nursing Diagnosis:** Place the Nursing Diagnoses in prioritized order on the concept map and add any needed for your specific patient. **Plan:** Place any further Nursing Interventions Classifications (NIC) needed on the map.

Implement Your Plan of Care

		EVALUATE YOUR CARE		
R	Recommendation — Evaluate your nursing care and make recommendations related to the achievement of your desired outcomes. Were they met, or do new goals need to be established?	Diag	Nursing Outcomes Classification (NOC)	Outcome met
		1	The delegating nurse should understand possible choices for delegation; identify risks and benefit of delegated decisions.	☐ Yes ☐ No
		2	Express beliefs about the meaning of choices for delegation.	☐ Yes ☐ No
		3	Make decisions that are congruent with the American Nursing Association and National Council of State Boards of Nursing Joint Statement on Delegation as well as the particular State Board of Nursing Nurse Practice Act.	☐ Yes ☐ No
		4	Use reliable evidence in making delegation decisions.	☐ Yes ☐ No
		5		☐ Yes ☐ No

Nursing Diagnosis 1

Readiness for enhanced decision-making related to delegation of appropriate nursing tasks to correct health-care providers evidenced by ability to explain a suitable plan for delegation of patient care.

NIC:
1) Encourage verbalization of ideas, concerns, particular delegation decisions that need to be made; **2)** Develop a plan for safe delegation; and **3)** Use support resources.

Nursing Diagnosis 2

Readiness for enhanced communication related to delegation of nursing tasks evidenced by ability to provide clear expectations for patient care and what to report.

NIC:
1) Encourage verbalization; **2)** Clarify meaning of words associated with delegation; and **3)** Encourage need or desire for pictures, written communications, demonstration, and instructions as part of direction for delegation.

Nursing Diagnosis 3

Decisional conflict during delegation related to lack of experience or interference with decision-making evidenced by feelings of distress while attempting to make a decision regarding delegation.

NIC:
1) Provide opportunity for expressions of indecision and availability and involvement of support persons; **2)** Review information to support the decision to be made; and **3)** Determine effectiveness of current delegation techniques.

Nursing Diagnosis 4

Conflict related to perceived threat, lack of relevant information, multiple or divergent sources of information evidenced by physical signs of distress or self-focusing.

NIC:
1) Encourage verbalization; **2)** Clarify meaning of words associated with delegation; **3)** Encourage need or desire for pictures, written communications, demonstration and instructions as part of direction for delegation; **4)** Use therapeutic communication process; **5)** Review the five rights of delegation and reflect on the appropriateness of each one; and **6)** Follow up on delegated tasks.

Condition:
Delegation to Health-Care Providers (RNs, LPNs, UAP)

Age:

Link & Explain
• Nursing Interventions Classification (NIC)
• Laboratory and Diagnostic Procedures
• Medications

Nursing Diagnosis 5

NIC:

Medications

a.

b.

c.

d.

Laboratory & Diagnostic Procedures

a.

b.

c.

d.

CONDITION: Ineffective Inter- and/or Intraprofessional Communication Process

PHYSIOLOGY: Ineffective inter- and/or intraprofessional communication process is a breakdown in the process of communication, which is the sending of data, messages, or other forms of information from one entity to another. The information communicated must be acknowledged and verified by the receiver in order for the exchange of information to be effective.

Timeliness of giving the information is important especially when communicating with patient care–related issues. When communication between health-care professionals is altered, patient care can become unsafe (Rosenstein & O'Daniel, 2005, 2008; *Taber's* 2009).

HANDOFF COMMUNICATION

S	Situation	Assess what is currently happening in a short statement.	The system issue presents as _____
B	Background	Summarize important past assessment data for your patient here. Place lab results and medications on the concept map.	
A	Assessment	Use the assessment data to complete your concept map.	**Nursing Diagnosis:** Place the Nursing Diagnoses in prioritized order on the concept map and add any needed for your specific patient. **Plan:** Place any further Nursing Interventions Classifications (NIC) needed on the map.

Implement Your Plan of Care

			EVALUATE YOUR CARE		
R	Recommendation	Evaluate your nursing care and make recommendations related to the achievement of your desired outcomes. Were they met, or do new goals need to be established?	**Diag**	**Nursing Outcomes Classification (NOC)**	**Outcome met**
			1	Verbalize or indicate an understanding of the communication difficulty and plan for ways of handling. Establish method of communication that maintains patient safety. Demonstrate congruent verbal and nonverbal communication.	☐ Yes ☐ No
			2	Establish method of communication in which needs can be expressed.	☐ Yes ☐ No
			3	Participate in therapeutic communication.	☐ Yes ☐ No
			4	Verbalize understanding of situation and potential complications.	☐ Yes ☐ No
			5		☐ Yes ☐ No

Nursing Diagnosis 1

Ineffective communication related to difference in individual perceptions evidenced by deficient communication regarding patient situation evidenced by impaired articulation, documentation, or inability to modulate speech professionally.

NIC:
1) Utilize SBAR (Situation, Background, Assessment, and Recommendation) when communicating information on clinical status of patient to health-care providers; **2)** Use at least two patient identifiers when providing care, treatment, and services; **3)** Apply the Transfusion Process Map (available from the Pennsylvania Patient Safety Authority at http://patientsafetyauthority.org/EducationalTools/PatientSafetyTools/blood/Documents/process.pdf) to eliminate patient identification errors when administering a blood transfusion. Two patient identifiers should be used from the time the type and cross specimen is obtained until the blood is transfused; **4)** Report critical results of tests and diagnostic procedures on a timely basis; **5)** Employ the Universal Protocol for Preventing Wrong Site, Wrong Procedure, Wrong Person Surgery by (a) conducting a preprocedure verification process; (b) marking the procedure site; (c) calling a timeout before the procedure is performed to check for signed informed consent form and proper site, patient, and procedure; **6)** Conduct regular safety huddles, which are brief meetings to ascertain what happened to threaten patient or staff safety and what can be done to avoid the same outcome in the future (U.S. Department of Veteran's Affairs, n.d.); **7)** Initiate a hand-off to verbally transfer information, responsibility, and accountability of patient care to another staff. This includes the review of written reports on the pertinent patient information, the latest significant changes in patient status, and the latest recommendation on the plan of care. The receiving staff has to acknowledge the completeness and pertinence of information and accept the responsibilities in providing patient care; **8)** Callout is a technique used when critical information is called out during an emergency situation. The information is said aloud for the benefit of any team members present during an emergency that are hearing and listening to the information; **9)** Check-back is a method to verify information especially when transcribing a doctor's order. Medical orders must be reviewed for completeness and clarity; **10)** Make use of the words "I am concerned, uncomfortable, safety (CUS)" when feeling communication is not effectively conveying the situation. CUS reminds nurses to speak up when they are concerned about the patient's situation, uncomfortable with the patient's current assessment, and/or worried about the patient's safety (AHRQ, 2008); **11)** Exercise the Two-Challenge Rule when there is a patient safety concern. Verbalize this at least twice if concern is not corrected; **12)** "Stop the Line" is a phrase understood by all to indicate a significant safety concern (Pratt et al., 2007); **13)** Use approved medical abbreviations and avoid those that are not approved and may cause confusion; **14)** Create opportunities for various health-care providers to get together to enhance collaboration and communication. Encourage open dialogue, collaborative rounds; implement preop and postop team briefings; and create interdisciplinary committees or task forces that discuss problem areas; and **15)** Develop and implement procedures to handle disruptive behaviors between health-care providers. When a disruptive event does occur, implement a timeout, code white, or red light policy that addresses the issue in real time to prevent any further serious consequences (O'Daniel & Rosenstein, 2008).

Nursing Diagnosis 2

Conflict related to perceived threat, lack of relevant information, multiple or divergent sources of information evidenced by physical signs of distress or self-focusing.

NIC:
1) Identify reason(s) for conflict; **2)** Determine effectiveness of current conflict resolution techniques; **3)** Correct misconceptions individual may have and provide factual information as needed; and **4)** Have individual consider consequences related to not making appropriate decisions to facilitate resolution of conflict.

Condition:
Ineffective Inter- and/or Intraprofessional Communication Process

Age:

Link & Explain
- Nursing Interventions Classification (NIC)
- Laboratory and Diagnostic Procedures
- Medications

Nursing Diagnosis 3

Readiness for enhanced communication related to nursing tasks evidenced by ability to provide clear expectations for patient care and what to report.

NIC:
1) Encourage verbalization; **2)** Clarify meaning of words associated with delegation; and **3)** Encourage need or desire for graphics, written communications, demonstration, instructions, and delegation.

Medications
a.
b.
c.
d.

Nursing Diagnosis 4

Deficient knowledge related to situation evidenced by inability to discuss specifics about situation.

NIC:
1) Ascertain level of knowledge regarding situation and unfolding events; **2)** Determine ability, readiness, and barriers to learning; and **3)** Provide information relevant to situation.

Nursing Diagnosis 5

NIC:

Laboratory & Diagnostic Procedures
a.
b.
c.
d.

CONDITION: Ineffective Leadership

PHYSIOLOGY: Effective leadership is the process of influencing others to accomplish goals. An effective leader is someone who displays the following elements of leadership:

1. Creates a vision for the future.
2. Displays excellent communication skills.
3. Functions as a change agent.
4. Engenders partnerships with others through stewardship.
5. Develops and renews followers as a means of developing the leaders of the future.

Attributes of leaders include emotional intelligence, decision-making skills, being a change agent, delegation ability, demonstrating ethical behavior, understanding relevant laws and being lawful, communicating well, influencing, nurturing a culture of safety, and demonstrating self-management.

HANDOFF COMMUNICATION

S	Situation	Assess what is currently happening in a short statement.	The system issue presents as _____
B	Background	Summarize important past assessment data for your patient here. Place lab results and medications on the concept map.	
A	Assessment	Use the assessment data to complete your concept map.	**Nursing Diagnosis:** Place the Nursing Diagnoses in prioritized order on the concept map and add any needed for your specific patient. **Plan:** Place any further Nursing Interventions Classifications (NIC) needed on the map.

Implement Your Plan of Care

		EVALUATE YOUR CARE	
	Evaluate your nursing care and make recommendations related to the achievement of your desired outcomes. Were they met, or do new goals need to be established?	**Diag**	**Nursing Outcomes Classification (NOC)**	**Outcome met**

		Diag	Nursing Outcomes Classification (NOC)	Outcome met
R	Recommendation	1	Discuss realistic role expectations of team members.	☐ Yes ☐ No
		2	Develop realistic plans for role transition to leadership position.	☐ Yes ☐ No
		3	Express sense of control over the present situation and hopefulness about future team outcomes.	☐ Yes ☐ No
		4	Perform leadership skills correctly and explain rationale for actions. Demonstrate reduced stress reaction.	☐ Yes ☐ No
		5		☐ Yes ☐ No

Nursing Diagnosis 1

Ineffective leadership role performance related to inadequate role preparation evidenced by lack of role competency.

NIC:
1) Determine individual's perceptions of current situation; **2)** Identify available resources (preceptor, education, and role model); **3)** Provide needed resources; and **4)** Use role rehearsal to practice new role.

Nursing Diagnosis 2

Powerlessness related to lack of control over situation evidenced by inadequate coping patterns.

NIC:
1) Determine individual's perception of situation; **2)** Assist individual in noting availability of resources and support system; and **3)** Encourage individual to develop a plan to assist in overcoming powerlessness.

Nursing Diagnosis 3

Deficient knowledge related to leadership skills evidenced by verbalization of the problem.

NIC:
1) Determine barriers to learning; **2)** Assess the level of individual's capabilities and possibilities of the situation; **3)** Differentiate "critical" from "desirable" content; and **4)** Provide needed information.

Nursing Diagnosis 4

Stress overload related to inadequate resources evidenced by psychological and physiological distress.

NIC:
1) Evaluate individual's report of physical/emotional problem; **2)** Assess his/her emotional responses and coping mechanisms being used; **3)** Determine presence or absence of available resources; **4)** Incorporate individual's strengths, assets, and past coping strategies that were successful; **5)** Encourage individual to seek help or assistance in meeting obligations and to delegate tasks as appropriate; **6)** Encourage individual to rest, sleep, and exercise on regular schedule; and **7)** Encourage individual to eat nutritious meals.

Condition:
Ineffective Leadership

Age:

Link & Explain
• Nursing Interventions Classification (NIC)
• Laboratory and Diagnostic Procedures
• Medications

Nursing Diagnosis 5

NIC:

Medications

a.

b.

c.

d.

Laboratory & Diagnostic Procedures

a. Leadership inventory for style and effectiveness

b.

c.

d.

CONDITION: Infection Rates

PHYSIOLOGY: Infection rates are the incidence of disease caused by microorganisms. The most common pathologic organisms are bacteria, viruses, fungi, protozoa, and helminths. Life-threatening infectious disease usually occurs when immunity is weak or suppressed. Many disease-causing agents, however, may afflict those who are young and usually healthy. Transmission of pathogens to their hosts occurs through inhalation, ingestion, injection (via a vector bite), direct or indirect contact. In the health-care environment, infections are often transmitted via the hands of health-care providers (*Taber's*, 2009).

Infection rates for various health-care agencies are monitored by the Joint Commission in an effort to track trends and occurrences and provide suggestions for decreasing hospital-acquired infections (Wright, 2010).

HANDOFF COMMUNICATION

S	Situation	Assess what is currently happening in a short statement.	The system issue presents as _____
B	Background	Summarize important past assessment data for your patient here. Place lab results and medications on the concept map.	
A	Assessment	Use the assessment data to complete your concept map.	**Nursing Diagnosis:** Place the Nursing Diagnoses in prioritized order on the concept map and add any needed for your specific patient. **Plan:** Place any further Nursing Interventions Classifications (NIC) needed on the map.

Implement Your Plan of Care

		EVALUATE YOUR CARE	
R Recommendation	Evaluate your nursing care and make recommendations related to the achievement of your desired outcomes. Were they met, or do new goals need to be established?	**Diag** / **Nursing Outcomes Classification (NOC)**	**Outcome met**
		1 Verbalize risk factors for infection on the nursing care area.	☐ Yes ☐ No
		2 Describe interventions aimed at prevention of infection that can be implemented unitwide.	☐ Yes ☐ No
		3 Demonstrate work-style changes to promote safe environment.	☐ Yes ☐ No
		4 Correct environmental hazards as identified.	☐ Yes ☐ No
		5	☐ Yes ☐ No

Nursing Diagnosis 1

Risk for infection related to surgical site (surgical site infection) or other specific nursing unit.

NIC:
1) Practice strict hand hygiene; **2)** Time preop antibiotics within 1 hour before surgery; **3)** Use recommended antibiotic before surgery; **4)** Ensure duration of postop antibiotics is 24 hours or less; **5)** Maintain blood glucose of patients at or below 150 mg/dL during and after surgery; **6)** Redose antibiotics during longer procedures and increased blood loss; **7)** Maintain body temperature over 36°C for all colon procedures; **8)** Clip rather than shave for hair removal; and **9)** Change dressings using proper technique.

Nursing Diagnosis 2

Risk for infection related to ventilator use (ventilator-associated pneumonia) in critical care units.

NIC:
1) Practice strict hand hygiene; **2)** Raise head of bed to 30–45 degrees; **3)** Wean as soon as possible; **4)** Ensure duration of postop antibiotics is 24 hours or less; **5)** Provide oral care every 6 hours with chlorhexidine oral rinse twice a day; **6)** Avoid gastric overdistention; **7)** Avoid unplanned extubation and reintubation; **8)** Use a cuffed endotracheal tube with in-line or subglottic suctioning; **9)** Maintain an endotracheal cuff pressure of at least 20 cm H_2O; and **10)** Use aseptic techniques when suctioning secretions and handling respiratory therapy equipment.

Nursing Diagnosis 3

Risk for infection related to central intravenous line (central-line-associated bloodstream infection).

NIC:
1) Practice strict hand hygiene; **2)** Use sterile gowns, gloves, masks, drapes, and head covers for insertion of central lines; **3)** Use chlorhexidine antiseptic at time of central line insertion and during site care; and **4)** Use preferred site for central line.

Nursing Diagnosis 4

Risk of infection related to urinary tract infections (UTI) related to catheter use.

NIC:
1) Practice strict hand hygiene; **2)** Evaluate catheter necessity; **3)** Use smallest gauge catheter possible; **4)** Perform antiseptic cleaning of meatus; **5)** Use sterile gowns, gloves, and drapes for insertion of catheter; **6)** Use aseptic technique/sterile technique when handling catheter; **7)** Use closed drainage system; **8)** Properly secure indwelling catheters after insertion to prevent movement and urethral traction; **9)** Do not disconnect the catheter and drainage tube; and **10)** Do not change catheter routinely.

Condition:
Infection Rates
Age:

Link & Explain
• Nursing Interventions Classification (NIC)
• Laboratory and Diagnostic Procedures
• Medications

Nursing Diagnosis 5

Risk for infection related to antibiotic-resistant organisms.

NIC:
1) Practice strict hand hygiene; **2)** Use isolation precautions (masks and contact precautions); **3)** Cohort patients; and **4)** Use dedicated equipment.

Medications

a. Appropriate use of chlorhexidine

b. Appropriate use of antibiotics

c.

d.

Laboratory & Diagnostic Procedures

a. Environmental cultures.

b. Aggregates of patient laboratory data

c.

d.

CONDITION: Medication Errors (Risk for Patient Injury)

PHYSIOLOGY: "A medication error is any preventable event that may cause or lead to inappropriate medication use or patient harm while the medication is in the control of the health care professional, patient, or consumer. Such events may be related to professional practice, health-care products, procedures, and systems, including prescribing; order communication; product labeling, packaging, and nomenclature; compounding; dispensing; distribution; administration; education; monitoring; and use" (NCC MERP, 2010).

HANDOFF COMMUNICATION

S	Situation	Assess what is currently happening in a short statement.	The system issue presents as _____
B	Background	Summarize important past assessment data for your patient here. Place lab results and medications on the concept map.	
A	Assessment	Use the assessment data to complete your concept map.	**Nursing Diagnosis:** Place the Nursing Diagnoses in prioritized order on the concept map and add any needed for your specific patient. **Plan:** Place any further Nursing Interventions Classifications (NIC) needed on the map.

Implement Your Plan of Care

		EVALUATE YOUR CARE	
R Recommendation	Evaluate your nursing care and make recommendations related to the achievement of your desired outcomes. Were they met, or do new goals need to be established?	**Diag** / **Nursing Outcomes Classification (NOC)**	**Outcome met**
		1 Verbalize risk factors for medication error. Describe interventions aimed at prevention of medication error. Modify environment as indicated to enhance medication administration safety. Verbalize correct information regarding patient medications. Administer medications using necessary procedures correctly and provide rationales for actions.	☐ Yes ☐ No
		2 Verbalize understanding of medication administration and potential complications.	☐ Yes ☐ No
		3 Participate in therapeutic communication. Recognize negative and positive factors affecting the situation to meet demands and needs. Identify alternatives to inappropriate activities for adaptation and problem-solving.	☐ Yes ☐ No
		4 Meet psychological needs evidenced by appropriate expression of feelings, identification of options, and use of resources.	☐ Yes ☐ No
		5	☐ Yes ☐ No

Nursing Diagnosis 1

Risk for injury related to medication error(s).

NIC:
1) Assess patient for health status, medication history, age, gender, ethnicity, drug allergies, laboratory values, diet; **2)** Follow regular dosage schedules and adhere to prescribed doses and dosage intervals; **3)** Follow the 10 rights of medication administration: (a) right medication, (b) right dose, (c) right time, (d) right route, (e) right patient, (f) right patient education, (g) right documentation, (h) right to refuse medication, (i) right assessment, (j) right evaluation; **4)** Conduct the safe medication administration check three times; **5)** Clarify any incomplete, illegible, or questionable medication order before administration; **6)** Use computerized order entry, computerized medication administration record, bar coding with appropriate scanning of patient arm band and medication container, and automated medication dispensing system; **7)** Have point-of-care access to patient information during medication administration (diagnosis, medical history, allergies, medication list, laboratory values) and drug information; **8)** Establish a quiet zone for the administration of medications to decrease interruptions; **9)** Use at least two patient identifiers when administering medications; **10)** Calculate all drug doses accurately; **11)** Double check all medication calculations and verify with another nurse; **12)** Verify all high-alert medications with another nurse; **13)** Use only approved medication abbreviations; **14)** Use vigilance in administering medications with a suffix and those with "confused drug names"; **15)** Prevent wrong line administration of medications; **16)** Use only non–free-flow electronic infusion control devices; **17)** Perform medication reconciliation on admission, during transfer between clinical units, in shift reports, in new medication administration records (MARs), and at discharge; **18)** Provide patient education regarding medications; **19)** Use standard order sheets as appropriate; and **20)** Follow organization's medication administration policies (ISMP, 2010; NCC MERP, 2010).

Nursing Diagnosis 2

Deficient knowledge related to medications and medication administration process evidenced by inability to discuss medications and procedure for safe administration evidenced by poor recall, resource retrieval, calculation skills.

NIC:
1) Ascertain level of knowledge regarding medications and medication administration process; **2)** Identify ability to perform psychomotor skills associated with safe medication administration process. Determine ability, readiness, and barriers to learning; and **3)** Provide information relevant to situation.

Nursing Diagnosis 3

Defensive coping related to low level of confidence in others evidenced by projection of blame or responsibility.

NIC:
1) Determine level of anxiety and effectiveness of current coping mechanisms; **2)** Describe all aspects of the problem through the use of therapeutic communication skills; **3)** Encourage control in all situations possible; include individual in decisions and planning; and **4)** Convey attitude of acceptance and respect.

Nursing Diagnosis 4

Readiness for enhanced communication related to situation evidenced by ability to provide clear expectations for patient care and what to report.

NIC:
1) Encourage verbalization; **2)** Clarify meaning of words associated with delegation; and **3)** Encourage need or desire for pictures, written communications, demonstration, instructions, and delegation.

Condition:
Medication Errors (Risk for Patient Injury)

Age:

Link & Explain
• Nursing Interventions Classification (NIC)
• Laboratory and Diagnostic Procedures
• Medications

Nursing Diagnosis 5

NIC:

Medications

a.
b.
c.
d.

Laboratory & Diagnostic Procedures

a.
b.
c.
d.

Concept Maps for Patients in Critical Care

Patients who are hospitalized and require intensive monitoring are admitted to the critical care area. The acute problems are sometimes the result of cardiac disease, infection, or trauma. Hourly VS and assessment, frequent laboratory collection and analysis, as well as EKG and hemodynamic monitoring are common practices in critical care. This close monitoring allows the nurse to determine if the patient is having positive or negative outcomes in response to treatment and to implement changes in care as needed. The key is to act quickly to avoid a failure-to-rescue event because patients in critical care are already compromised.

The conditions included in this chapter are:

1. Acute Renal Failure
2. Acute Respiratory Distress Syndrome (ARDS)
3. Anaphylactic Shock
4. Brain Trauma
5. Cardiac Surgery
6. Cardiogenic Shock
7. Dysrhythmia
8. Guillain-Barré Syndrome
9. Myocardial Infarction (MI)
10. Pneumothorax/Hemothorax
11. Septic Shock
12. Spinal Cord Trauma
13. Stroke/Brain Attack

CONDITION: Acute Renal Failure

PHYSIOLOGY: Acute renal failure is a sudden decrease in kidney function that may not be associated with a decrease in urine output but results in a buildup of toxic wastes such as urea and creatinine in the blood. The stages of renal failure are:

Oliguric: Filtration capability is greatly reduced because of damage to renal tubules, and the output is less than 400 mL/24 hours.

Diuretic: Large quantities of urine occur because of the kidney's inability to concentrate urine. Some patients skip the oliguric stage; others with oliguria progress to the diuretic phase.

Convalescent: Renal blood flow and filtration improve, which is indicated by a decrease in BUN and creatinine levels. Function improves in the first 1 to 2 weeks of this stage, but it may take months to stabilize.

The list of causes of acute kidney damage is extensive; here are a few in each of the three categories:

Prerenal: hypovolemia (burns, hemorrhage), decreased cardiac output (heart failure, cardiogenic shock), decreased peripheral vascular resistance (anaphylaxis, neurologic injury), decreased renovascular blood flow (hepatorenal syndrome, embolism).

Intrarenal: nephrotoxic injury (radiocontrast agents, drugs such as gentamicin), interstitial nephritis (allergies, infection), other (acute glomerulonephritis, systemic lupus erythematosus).

Postrenal: benign prostatic hyperplasia, bladder cancer, calculi formation.

HANDOFF COMMUNICATION

S Situation	Assess what is currently happening in a short statement.	The patient is _____ years of age. VS LOC
B Background	Summarize important past assessment data for your patient here. Place lab results and medications on the concept map.	**Age:** **Gender:** **Allergies:** **Fall Risk:** **Isolation:**
A Assessment	Use the assessment data to complete your concept map.	**Nursing Diagnosis:** Place the Nursing Diagnoses in prioritized order on the concept map and add any needed for your specific patient. **Plan:** Place any further Nursing Interventions Classifications (NIC) needed on the map.

Implement Your Plan of Care

		Diag	EVALUATE YOUR CARE — Nursing Outcomes Classification (NOC)	Outcome met
R Recommendation	Evaluate your nursing care and make recommendations related to the achievement of your desired outcomes. Were they met, or do new goals need to be established?	1	Patient has urinary output with normal specific gravity, laboratory studies near normal, stable VS, and absence of edema.	☐ Yes ☐ No
		2	Patient has BP, heart rate and rhythm within normal range for patient. Patient has strong peripheral pulses and normal capillary refill.	☐ Yes ☐ No
		3	Patient maintains or regains weight as needed; is free of edema.	☐ Yes ☐ No
		4	Patient experiences no signs or symptoms of infection.	☐ Yes ☐ No
		5	Patient verbalizes an understanding of therapeutic needs and initiates necessary lifestyle changes.	☐ Yes ☐ No

Nursing Diagnosis 1

Fluid volume excess related to compromised regulatory mechanism evidenced by intake greater than output, oliguria, changes in urine specific gravity.

NIC:
1) Record accurate I&O, including ice chips, IV medications, GI losses; **2)** Assess skin, face, and dependent areas for edema, and evaluate on a 1–4 scale; **3)** Auscultate heart and lung sounds for evidence of pulmonary edema; **4)** Weigh daily at same time of day and on same scale; **5)** Monitor laboratory studies such as BUN, creatinine, Hgb/Hct, serum sodium, serum potassium.

Nursing Diagnosis 2

Risk for decreased cardiac output related to fluid overload, electrolyte imbalance, and severe acidosis.

NIC:
1) Monitor BP and heart rate; **2)** Observe EKG for changes in rhythm; **3)** Auscultate for development of S3 and S4; **4)** Assess color of skin, mucous membranes, and nailbeds. Note capillary refill; **5)** Assess for development of crackles in lungs and shortness of breath (SOB); **6)** Provide supplemental oxygen as needed; **7)** Monitor electrolytes, pulse oximetry, and ABGs.

Nursing Diagnosis 3

Risk for imbalanced nutrition: less than body requirements related to protein catabolism, dietary restrictions, increased metabolic needs.

NIC:
1) Provide small, frequent feedings to minimize anorexia and nausea; **2)** Offer frequent mouth care and provide hard candy to sooth dry mouth between meals; **3)** Provide high-calorie, low- to moderate-protein diet that includes complex carbohydrates and fat to meet caloric needs; **4)** Restrict potassium, sodium, and phosphorus as needed to prevent hypertension and maintain normal blood levels; **5)** Monitor serum pre-albumin, albumin, transferrin, sodium, and potassium levels; **6)** Administer medications such as iron supplements, B complex, C vitamins, folic acid.

Nursing Diagnosis 4

Risk for infection related to invasive procedures and devices.

NIC:
1) Teach hand-washing technique and discuss the importance to prevent infection; **2)** Provide routine catheter care, remove indwelling catheter as soon as possible; **3)** Assess skin integrity because edema may increase the risk for skin breakdown; **4)** Encourage coughing, deep breathing, and frequent position change; **5)** Use aseptic technique when caring for IV and invasive lines. Change site and dressings per protocol.

Condition:
Acute Renal Failure
Age:

Link & Explain
• Nursing Interventions Classification (NIC)
• Laboratory and Diagnostic Procedures
• Medications

Nursing Diagnosis 5

Deficient knowledge regarding condition, prognosis, treatment, self-care, and discharge needs related to unfamiliarity with information resources evidenced by questions, request for information, and statement of misconception.

NIC:
1) Review disease process, prognosis, precipitating factors; **2)** Discuss renal dialysis or future transplant if needed; **3)** Review dietary plan and restrictions, including fluid restrictions; **4)** Encourage observation of urine amount, frequency, and characteristics; **5)** Review medications and encourage the patient to discuss any OTC and herbal medications with health-care provider.

Medications
a. Diuretics: furosemide (Lasix), bumetanide (Bumex), torsemide (Demadex) (given in the oliguric phase to convert to the diuretic phase)
b. Antihypertensives: clonidine (Catapres), methyldopa (Aldomet), prazosin (Minipress) (treatment of hypertension; counteract effects of decreased renal blood flow and volume overload)
c. Vasodilators: dopamine (Intropin), fenoldopam (Corlopam) (cause dilation of renal vasculature and enhance perfusion)
d. Calcium channel blockers: nifedipine (Adalat) (reduce influx of calcium into kidney cells and improve GFR)

Laboratory & Diagnostic Procedures
a. BUN: measures the by-product of protein metabolism in the liver, filtered by the kidneys, and excreted in urine; elevated in kidney dysfunction, dehydration, and liver disease
b. Creatinine: end product of muscle and protein metabolism, filtered by the kidneys and excreted in urine; increased in kidney disease
c. Electrolytes: sodium, potassium, chloride, magnesium, phosphorus are usually increased but it depends on hydration status; calcium is usually low and needs to be replaced
d. Urine creatinine clearance, glomerular filtration rate (GFR)

CONDITION: Acute Respiratory Distress Syndrome (ARDS)

PHYSIOLOGY: ARDS is an acute, progressive form of pulmonary failure in which the alveoli capillary membrane becomes damaged and permeable to intravascular fluid. The patient has dyspnea and hypoxemia in spite of administration of an increased concentration of oxygen. Radiology results show many pulmonary infiltrates; pulmonary edema is present in the absence of cardiac disease. ARDS may be precipitated by sepsis, trauma, aspiration, drug ingestion, burns, inhalation of toxins, and pneumonia.

The three phases in ARDS are:

Injury phase (1–7 days): insult occurs, alveoli fill with fluid, oxygenation is limited, surfactant dysfunction occurs, patient develops atelectasis
Reparative phase (1–2 weeks): influx of neutrophils, monocytes, lymphocytes, and fibroblasts occurs; pulmonary vasculature is destroyed, decreased lung compliance; hypoxemia progresses
Fibrotic phase (2–3 weeks): remodeling of the lung, scarring, fibrosis, decreased gas exchange, severe hypoxemia

As ARDS progresses, interventions focus on prevention of sepsis and multiple organ dysfunction syndrome (MODS). The goal is to wean the patient from the ventilator if possible and return the patient to optimal health. The survival rate decreases as the patient progresses through the stages. MODS is the major cause of death in ARDS.

HANDOFF COMMUNICATION

S Situation	Assess what is currently happening in a short statement.	Patient presents as _____
B Background	Summarize important past assessment data for your patient here. Place lab results and medications on the concept map.	**Age:** **Gender:** **Allergies:** **Fall Risk:** **Isolation:**
A Assessment	Use the assessment data to complete your concept map.	**Nursing Diagnosis:** Place the Nursing Diagnoses in prioritized order on the concept map and add any needed for your specific patient. **Plan:** Place any further Nursing Interventions Classifications (NIC) needed on the map.

Implement Your Plan of Care

			EVALUATE YOUR CARE	
R Recommendation	Evaluate your nursing care and make recommendations related to the achievement of your desired outcomes. Were they met, or do new goals need to be established?	**Diag**	**Nursing Outcomes Classification (NOC)**	**Outcome met**
		1	Patient demonstrates improved ventilation and adequate oxygenation of tissue with improvement of ABGs.	☐ Yes ☐ No
		2	Patient maintains patent airway with improvement in breath sounds.	☐ Yes ☐ No
		3	Patient reports that anxiety or fear is reduced to a manageable level.	☐ Yes ☐ No
		4	Patient displays appropriate urinary output with specific gravity, BUN, and creatinine near normal.	☐ Yes ☐ No
		5	Patient has dry skin, moist mucous membranes, stable VS, and adequate urinary output.	☐ Yes ☐ No

Nursing Diagnosis 1

Impaired gas exchange related to alveoli destruction evidenced by abnormal ABGs—hypoxia and hypercapnia.

NIC:
1) Assess VS, monitor ABGs. Note if (ARDSNet) protocol is being used; **2)** Assess endotracheal tube for placement and cuff leak. Auscultate lungs for complications from overdistended alveoli; **3)** Monitor tidal volume pressures and positive end-expiratory pressure (PEEP) on mechanical ventilator; **4)** Assess color, capillary refill, peripheral pulses; **5)** Sedate patient as indicated to provide adequate ventilation and reduce tissue oxygen requirements; **6)** Change patient positions frequently to improve perfusion.

Nursing Diagnosis 2

Ineffective airway clearance related to secretions evidenced by changes in rate and depth of respirations, cyanosis, abnormal breath sounds.

NIC:
1) Monitor endotracheal (ET) tube placement. Note line marking and compare with desired placement. Secure tube carefully with tube holder; **2)** Note excessive coughing, increased dyspnea, high-pressure alarm sounding on ventilator, visible secretions in tracheal/ET tube; **3)** Suction as needed. Note color and amount of secretions. Limit duration of suctioning to 15 seconds. Hyperventilate before and after each catheter passes; **4)** Maintain adequate hydration.

Nursing Diagnosis 3

Fear/severe anxiety related to threat of death, dependency on mechanical support evidenced by hypervigilance.

NIC:
1) Identify patient's perception of threat presented by the situation; **2)** Observe and monitor physical responses such as restlessness, changes in VS, repetitive movements; **3)** Encourage patient to acknowledge and express fears; **4)** Identify previous coping strengths of the patient; **5)** Demonstrate and encourage the use of relaxation techniques, guided imagery, progressive relaxation.

Nursing Diagnosis 4

Risk for excess fluid related to decreased renal tissue oxygenation because of hypoxemia.

NIC:
1) Monitor BUN, creatinine, electrolytes, Hgb/Hct; **2)** Assess patient for edema of the face, extremities, sacral area; **3)** Monitor BP, heart rate, lung sounds, LOC, I&O, urine specific gravity, daily weight; **4)** Administer diuretics as prescribed; **5)** Apply antiembolism stockings, sequential compression device.

Condition:
Acute Respiratory Distress Syndrome (ARDS)

Age:
_____
Link & Explain
• Nursing Interventions Classification (NIC)
• Laboratory and Diagnostic Procedures
• Medications

Nursing Diagnosis 5

Imbalanced nutrition: less than body requirements related to conditions that interfere with nutrient intake evidenced by body weight 10% or more under ideal.

NIC:
1) Assess nutritional status; note energy level and condition of skin, hair, nails, oral cavity; **2)** Administer prophylactic medications such as proton pump inhibitors or H2-receptor antagonists to prevent mucosal damage; **3)** Weigh frequently and compare with admission weight; **4)** Administer nutritional solutions at prescribed rate, note electrolyte content; **5)** Assess tolerance of enteral feedings, auscultate bowel sounds, investigate symptoms of nausea or abdominal discomfort. Check gastric residual and hold feeding if necessary; **6)** Monitor labs such as electrolytes, BUN, creatinine, total protein, prealbumin, albumin, glucose.

Medications
a. Corticosteroids, surfactant replacement, antibiotic therapy
b. Proton pump inhibitors, H2-receptor antagonists
c. Diuretics
d.

Laboratory & Diagnostic Procedures
a. ABG, pulse oximetry, chest x-ray, pulmonary artery catheter (Swan-Ganz) measurements
b. CBC, electrolytes, BUN, creatinine
c. Bronchoscopy, sputum culture
d.

CONDITION: Anaphylactic Shock

PHYSIOLOGY: Rapidly developing, systemic anaphylaxis can produce life-threatening acute airway obstruction followed by vascular collapse after exposure to an antigen (*Taber's*, 2009). The patient experiences a sudden onset of symptoms such as flushing, pruritus, urticaria, angioedema (edema of the eyes, lips, tongue), nasal congestion, hoarseness because of edema of the larynx and vocal cords. Stridor may be auscultated as the result of laryngeal edema. Lower airway obstruction is evident with clinical manifestations of wheezing, chest tightness, tachycardia, and hypotension.

Treatment goals include the following: **1)** Remove the antigen such as by discontinuing the IV drug being infused if that is the cause of the reaction, turning off the blood if a reaction is noticed during blood administration, removing a stinger if the reaction occurred after a bee sting. **2)** Reverse effects of the mediators—epinephrine is administered to promote bronchodilation and vasoconstriction. Usually, diphenhydramine (Benadryl) is administered to block histamine release. Corticosteroids are used to reduce inflammation. **3)** Promote adequate tissue perfusion—oxygen is administered related to SpO_2 (saturation of peripheral oxygen). IV fluids are replaced. Positive ionotropic agents and vasopressors may be administered.

HANDOFF COMMUNICATION

S Situation	Assess what is currently happening in a short statement.	Patient presents as _____
B Background	Summarize important past assessment data for your patient here. Place lab results and medications on the concept map.	**Age:** **Gender:** **Allergies:** **Fall Risk:** **Isolation:**
A Assessment	Use the assessment data to complete your concept map.	**Nursing Diagnosis:** Place the Nursing Diagnoses in prioritized order on the concept map and add any needed for your specific patient. **Plan:** Place any further Nursing Interventions Classifications (NIC) needed on the map.

Implement Your Plan of Care

R Recommendation	Evaluate your nursing care and make recommendations related to the achievement of your desired outcomes. Were they met, or do new goals need to be established?	**EVALUATE YOUR CARE**	
		Diag **Nursing Outcomes Classification (NOC)**	**Outcome met**
		1 Patient demonstrates adequate perfusion with stable VS, good peripheral pulses, warm and dry skin, normal mentation, appropriate urine output.	☐ Yes ☐ No
		2 Patient achieves adequate oxygenation evidenced by lack of signs and symptoms of respiratory distress, respiratory rate below 24, heart rate and pulse oximetry within baseline.	☐ Yes ☐ No
		3 Patient verbalizes understanding of condition and initiates necessary lifestyle changes.	☐ Yes ☐ No
		4 Patient identifies inadequacies of prior coping behaviors, identifies available resources/support systems, and initiates new coping strategies.	☐ Yes ☐ No
		5 Patient appears relaxed, verbalizes fears/concerns, and reports decreased anxiety.	☐ Yes ☐ No

Nursing Diagnosis 1

Ineffective perfusion related to decreased oxygenation and third spacing of fluid evidenced by hypoxemia, tachypnea, tachycardia, hypotension.

NIC:
1) Remove stimuli responsible for reaction; **2)** Assess LOC, VS, skin color, and temperature; **3)** Monitor peripheral pulses, lung sounds, pulse oximetry, ABGs; **4)** Administer epinephrine, diphenhydramine (Benadryl) as prescribed and evaluate response. Prepare to repeat epinephrine as prescribed; **5)** Administer fluid replacement; **6)** Administer positive ionotropic agents and vasopressors if required; **7)** Assess urine output.

Nursing Diagnosis 2

Impaired gas exchange related to airway edema evidenced by wheezing, stridor, edema of the larynx and epiglottis.

NIC:
1) Assess VS, presence of retractions, angioedema, dyspnea, cyanosis; **2)** Assess lung sounds and report adventitious sounds; **3)** Assess pulse oximetry and ABGs and report hypoxemia or alteration in acid/base balance; **4)** Administer oxygen or prepare for intubation; **5)** Administer nebulized bronchodilators and intravenous corticosteroids as prescribed.

Nursing Diagnosis 3

Deficient knowledge regarding disease process, treatment, self-care, and discharge needs related to reaction to antigens evidenced by inaccurate follow-through of instructions.

NIC:
1) Avoid triggers such as foods, environmental factors, medications, vectors; **2)** Discuss importance of regular medical follow-up care; **3)** Identify adverse symptoms to medications such as fatigue, daytime drowsiness; **4)** Discuss prophylactic medications and those to be used during an emergency situation.

Nursing Diagnosis 4

Risk for ineffective coping mechanisms related to situational crisis.

NIC:
1) Assess patient/significant other's perception of current situation and signs of inadequate coping mechanisms; **2)** Encourage verbalization and assist in identifying personal strengths/resources to cope with current situation; **3)** Include patient/family in planning of comfort/supportive care; **4)** Encourage patient to share what kinds of support would be most beneficial.

Condition:
Anaphylactic Shock
Age:

Link & Explain
- Nursing Interventions Classification (NIC)
- Laboratory and Diagnostic Procedures
- Medications

Nursing Diagnosis 5

Risk for spiritual distress related to physical and psychological stress.

NIC:
1) Assess patient's spiritual beliefs, cultural practices, and religious affiliations; **2)** Implement measures to promote spiritual well-being and support patient in related activities; **3)** Support grieving process of patient and significant others; **4)** Consult clergy or other spiritual counselor as identified by the patient.

Medications

a. Epinephrine

b. Diphenhydramine (Benadryl)

c. Nebulized bronchodilators, corticosteroids

d. Positive ionotropic agents, vasopressors

Laboratory & Diagnostic Procedures

a. Chest x-ray, pulmonary function tests

b.

c.

d.

CONDITION: Brain Trauma

PHYSIOLOGY: Traumatic brain injury is a physical injury to the cranium and intracranial structures. It may be a minor injury such as a concussion or a major injury such as an intracranial hemorrhage. The injury is defined by the region of the brain that is affected.

Acute subdural hematoma is caused by bleeding between the dura mater and the arachnoid layer of the meninges. It is usually venous but may be arterial in origin. With a venous bleed, the hematoma is slower to develop. Symptoms include headache and decreasing LOC. The size of the hematoma reflects the clinical manifestations and the outcome.

Epidural hematoma is caused by bleeding between the dura and the inner surface of the skull. The hematoma develops rapidly, and emergency treatment is necessary. This bleeding is usually arterial but may be venous in origin. Initial loss of consciousness usually occurs, followed by a brief lucid interval and later a decrease in LOC.

Intracerebral hematoma is caused by bleeding in the parenchyma within the frontal or temporal lobes. The bleeding is from rupture of the intracerebral vessel at the time of injury.

HANDOFF COMMUNICATION

S	Situation	Assess what is currently happening in a short statement.	The patient is _____ years of age. VS LOC	
B	Background	Summarize important past assessment data for your patient here. Place lab results and medications on the concept map.	**Age:** **Allergies:** **Isolation:**	**Gender:** **Fall Risk:**
A	Assessment	Use the assessment data to complete your concept map.	**Nursing Diagnosis:** Place the Nursing Diagnoses in prioritized order on the concept map and add any needed for your specific patient. **Plan:** Place any further Nursing Interventions Classifications (NIC) needed on the map.	

Implement Your Plan of Care

		EVALUATE YOUR CARE		
R	Recommendation	Evaluate your nursing care and make recommendations related to the achievement of your desired outcomes. Were they met, or do new goals need to be established?	**Diag**	**Nursing Outcomes Classification (NOC)**	**Outcome met**

Diag	Nursing Outcomes Classification (NOC)	Outcome met
1	Patient maintains improved LOC, cognition, and motor or sensory function. Patient has normal VS and absence of symptoms of increased intracranial pressure (ICP).	☐ Yes ☐ No
2	Patient maintains a normal or effective respiratory pattern, free of cyanosis, with pulse oximetry and ABGs within acceptable range.	☐ Yes ☐ No
3	Patient demonstrates ability to resume activities.	☐ Yes ☐ No
4	Patient maintains afebrile state and achieves timely wound healing.	☐ Yes ☐ No
5	Patient maintains appropriate weight for height and body frame without evidence of malnutrition.	☐ Yes ☐ No

Nursing Diagnosis 1

Ineffective cerebral tissue perfusion related to interruption of blood flow by cerebral edema evidenced by altered LOC.

NIC:

1) Monitor neurological status and compare with baseline using Glasgow Coma Scale (GCS); 2) Evaluate eye-opening (e.g., spontaneous, opens only to painful stimuli, keeps eyes closed); 3) Assess verbal response: note if alert; oriented to person, place, time or confused; uses inappropriate words and phrases or does not respond; 4) Assess motor response to simple commands, noting purposeful and nonpurposeful movements. Document right and left sides separately; 5) Evaluate pupils, noting size, shape, equality, and reaction to light and accommodation; 6) Monitor VS, BP, noting increased systolic or widening pulse pressure; heart rate, noting bradycardia, tachycardia, or other dysrhythmias; respirations, noting periods of apnea, Cheyne-Stokes respiration; 7) Monitor ICP, vision difficulties, nausea/vomiting, increased headache; 8) Maintain head in midline position to prevent compression of jugular veins and cerebral venous drainage; 9) Avoid activities that increase intrathoracic or intra-abdominal pressure, such as coughing, vomiting, straining at stool; 10) Monitor for hyperthermia from hypothalamic injury, use measures to reduce temperature and prevent shivering; 11) Elevate head of bed 20–30 degrees to promote venous drainage from head.

Nursing Diagnosis 2

Risk for ineffective breathing pattern related injury to respiratory center of brain.

NIC:

1) Monitor rate, rhythm, depth of respirations; 2) Elevate head 30 degrees as prescribed; 3) Auscultate breath sounds; 4) Suction if indicated no longer than 10–15 seconds; 5) Provide supplemental oxygen; 6) Monitor pulse oximetry and ABGs.

Nursing Diagnosis 3

Impaired physical mobility related to perceptual or cognitive impairment evidenced by inability to purposefully move extremities.

NIC:

1) Provide flotation mattress. Position patient to avoid skin and tissue pressure damage. Turn at regular intervals; 2) Massage skin with emollients and keep bedding clean and wrinkle free; 3) Provide eye care with artificial tears and eye patches as indicated; 4) Monitor bowel elimination and provide for regular bowel elimination program; 5) Monitor urine output and inspect for color and odor of urine. Assist with bladder training when indicated; 6) Inspect for localized tenderness, redness, skin warmth, edema in lower extremities; 7) Apply sequential compression devices (SCD) to lower extremities.

Nursing Diagnosis 4

Risk for infection related to traumatized tissue, broken skin, invasive procedures, stasis of body fluids.

NIC:

1) Provide aseptic care. Maintain good handwashing techniques; 2) Observe areas of impaired skin, note drainage characteristics and inflammation; 3) Monitor fever, presence of chills, diaphoresis, change in mentation; 4) Encourage deep breathing, observe sputum for odor and color; 5) Provide adequate hydration and note color and clarity of urine. Maintain integrity of closed urinary drainage system.

Condition:
Brain Trauma
Age:

Link & Explain
• Nursing Interventions Classification (NIC)
• Laboratory and Diagnostic Procedures
• Medications

Nursing Diagnosis 5

Altered ability to ingest nutrients because of decreased LOC, weakness of muscles required for chewing and swallowing.

NIC:

1) Assess ability to chew, swallow, and handle secretions; 2) Weigh and evaluate changes; 3) Auscultate bowel sounds and note decreasing, hyperactive, or absence; 4) Prevent aspiration by elevating head of bed during meals or tube feeding; 5) Observe labs for indications of malnutrition, dehydration, or electrolyte imbalance; 6) Collaborate with speech, occupational, and physical therapist; 7) Assess for impaired swallowing, contractures of hands, paralysis.

Medications
a. Osmotic diuretic: Mannitol (decreases ICP in treatment of cerebral edema)
b. Steroid: dexamethasone (Decadron) (decreases cerebral edema)
c. Anticonvulsant: phenytoin sodium (Dilantin) (prevention of seizures with increased ICP). Sedative: lorazepam (Ativan) (decreases agitation and the negative effects on ICP)
d. Antipyretics: acetaminophen (Tylenol) (reduces fever and its effect on cerebral metabolism)

Laboratory & Diagnostic Procedures
a. MRI scan: detects bleeding and swelling in the brain
b. CT scan: detects bleeding and swelling in the brain
c. Spinal x-ray: rules out cervical fracture from trauma ICP measurement to monitor the increase in pressure

CONDITION: Cardiac Surgery

PHYSIOLOGY: Coronary artery bypass graft (CABG) is a procedure in which one or more blocked coronary arteries are bypassed by a blood vessel graft to restore normal blood flow to the heart.

Valve replacement surgery is a procedure in which the incompetent valve of the heart is replaced by a natural (biological) or an artificial (mechanical) valve.

HANDOFF COMMUNICATION

S	Situation	Assess what is currently happening in a short statement.	Patient presents as _____
B	Background	Summarize important past assessment data for your patient here. Place lab results and medications on the concept map.	**Age:** **Gender:** **Allergies:** **Fall Risk:** **Isolation:**
A	Assessment	Use the assessment data to complete your concept map.	**Nursing Diagnosis:** Place the Nursing Diagnoses in prioritized order on the concept map and add any needed for your specific patient. **Plan:** Place any further Nursing Interventions Classifications (NIC) needed on the map.

Implement Your Plan of Care

Evaluate your nursing care and make recommendations related to the achievement of your desired outcomes. Were they met, or do new goals need to be established?

R Recommendation

EVALUATE YOUR CARE

Diag	Nursing Outcomes Classification (NOC)	Outcome met
1	Patient displays hemodynamic stability, such as stable BP, cardiac output.	☐ Yes ☐ No
2	Patient maintains an effective respiratory pattern free of cyanosis, symptoms of hypoxia, with breath sounds equal bilaterally.	☐ Yes ☐ No
3	Patient verbalizes relief or absence of pain. Patient differentiates surgical discomfort from angina or preoperative heart pain.	☐ Yes ☐ No
4	Patient demonstrates behaviors and techniques to promote healing and prevent complications.	☐ Yes ☐ No
5	Patient participates in learning process; verbalizes understanding of condition, prognosis, and potential complications.	☐ Yes ☐ No

Nursing Diagnosis 1

Risk for decreased cardiac output related to altered myocardial contractility secondary to temporary factors.

NIC:
1) Observe for bleeding from incisions and chest tube; 2) Monitor for decrease in BP, dysrhythmias, chest pain, dyspnea; 3) Assess changes in mental status, orientation, and for onset of confusion, restlessness, reduced response to stimuli; 4) Record skin temperature, color, quality of peripheral pulses; 5) Measure and document I&O and calculate fluid balance; 6) Administer IV fluids or blood products as needed.

Nursing Diagnosis 2

Risk for ineffective breathing pattern related to decreased lung expansion, diminished oxygen-carrying capacity (blood loss).

NIC:
1) Assess respiratory rate and depth. Note respiratory effort, presence of dyspnea, use of accessory muscle and nasal flaring; 2) Auscultate breath sounds. Note areas of diminished or absent sounds and presence of adventitious sounds such as crackles or rhonchi; 3) Observe character of cough and sputum production; 4) Elevate head of bed in semi-Fowler's position. Assist with early ambulation; 5) Reinforce splinting of chest with pillows during deep breathing and coughing.

Nursing Diagnosis 3

Acute pain/impaired comfort related to sternotomy (mediastinal incision), tissue inflammation, edema formation evidenced by increased heart rate and reports of incisional discomfort.

NIC:
1) Note type and location of incision; 2) Encourage patient to report type, location, and intensity of pain on a rating scale; 3) Observe for anxiety, irritability, crying, restlessness, and sleep disturbances; 4) Identify and encourage use of behaviors such as guided imagery, distractions, visualizations, and deep breathing; 5) Medicate before procedures and activity as indicated.

Nursing Diagnosis 4

Impaired skin integrity related to surgical incisions and puncture wounds evidenced by disruption of skin surface.

NIC:
1) Inspect all incisions. Evaluate healing progress. Review expectations for healing; 2) Suggest wearing soft cotton shirts, loose-fitting clothing; leave incisions open to air as much as possible; 3) Encourage showering in warm water, washing incisions gently; 4) Review normal signs of healing such as itching along wound line, bruising, slight redness, and scabbing. (5) Instruct to watch for incision that does not heal, bloody or purulent drainage, localized area that is swollen and red, and to report temperature elevation.

Condition:
Cardiac Surgery
Age:

Link & Explain
- Nursing Interventions Classification (NIC)
- Laboratory and Diagnostic Procedures
- Medications

Nursing Diagnosis 5

Deficient knowledge regarding condition, postoperative care, self-care, and discharge needs related to lack of exposure or recall evidenced by request for information.

NIC:
1) Reinforce breathing exercises with incentive spirometer; 2) Discuss routine and prophylactic medications. Stress importance of checking with physician before taking any nonprescribed medications; 3) Reinforce schedule for routine laboratory tests and follow-up visits; 4) Review prescribed cardiac rehabilitation exercise program and realistic goals; 5) Reinforce limitations regarding lifting, driving, return to work, sexual activity, exercising.

Medications

a. Antithrombotic/antiplatelet

b. Vasodilators

c. Diuretics

d. Vasopressors

Laboratory & Diagnostic Procedures

a. CBC, electrolyte panel, coagulation studies, cardiac enzymes

b. ABG

c. EKG

d. Chest x-ray

CONDITION: Cardiogenic Shock

PHYSIOLOGY: Cardiogenic shock occurs when the heart is an ineffective pump, resulting in a decreased cardiac output and impaired tissue perfusion. The most common cause of cardiogenic shock is an extensive left ventricular myocardial infarction. Other causes include dysrhythmias, cardiomyopathy, myocardial contusion, valvular dysfunction, ventricular septal rupture, and severe heart failure.

The pathophysiology of cardiogenic shock is directly related to cardiac dynamics. When damage to the myocardium occurs, contractility is reduced, leading to a decreased stroke volume. Cardiac output and ejection fraction decrease, causing hypotension. The hypotension causes peripheral vasoconstriction and increased afterload (the amount of resistance the ventricles need to overcome to empty the ventricles effectively). The backup of blood into the pulmonary circulation causes decreased oxygen perfusion across the alveoli, which reduces oxygen in the blood ultimately being delivered to the tissues. An increased demand is placed on the myocardium to perfuse the cells, which may increase the infarction.

Clinical manifestations include left ventricular failure (S3, crackles, dyspnea, hypoxemia); right ventricular failure (jugular vein distention, peripheral edema, hepatomegaly); tachycardia; hypotension; tachypnea; oliguria; cool, pale skin; and decreased mentation.

Monitoring: cardiac output (CO), cardiac index (CI), right arterial pressure (RAP), pulmonary artery occlusion (wedge) pressure (PAOP or PAWP), systemic vascular resistance (SVR).

HANDOFF COMMUNICATION

S Situation	Assess what is currently happening in a short statement.	Patient presents as _____
B Background	Summarize important past assessment data for your patient here. Place lab results and medications on the concept map.	**Age:** **Gender:** **Allergies:** **Fall Risk:** **Isolation:**
A Assessment	Use the assessment data to complete your concept map.	**Nursing Diagnosis:** Place the Nursing Diagnoses in prioritized order on the concept map and add any needed for your specific patient. **Plan:** Place any further Nursing Interventions Classifications (NIC) needed on the map.

Implement Your Plan of Care

			EVALUATE YOUR CARE	
R Recommendation	Evaluate your nursing care and make recommendations related to the achievement of your desired outcomes. Were they met, or do new goals need to be established?	**Diag**	**Nursing Outcomes Classification (NOC)**	**Outcome met**
		1	Patient achieves adequate cardiac output with normal VS, strong peripheral pulses, warm/dry skin, and urine output <30 mL/hr.	☐ Yes ☐ No
		2	Patient achieves adequate oxygenation with respirations less than 24 and pulse oximetry within normal limits.	☐ Yes ☐ No
		3	Patient verbalizes reduction of anxiety or fear.	☐ Yes ☐ No
		4	Patient expresses a sense of spiritual well-being, maintains connectedness with significant others, and participates in usual spiritual practices.	☐ Yes ☐ No
		5	Patient identifies inadequacies of prior coping behaviors and accesses available resources/support systems.	☐ Yes ☐ No

Nursing Diagnosis 1

Altered tissue perfusion (cardiac) related to decreased myocardial contractility evidenced by increased heart rate, dysrhythmias, EKG changes.

NIC:
1) Medicate for pain with morphine and evaluate effectiveness of medication; 2) Auscultate heart, note rhythm, rate, presence of dysrhythmias, S3; 3) Monitor VS and report decrease in BP, tachycardia, weak thready pulse, narrowing pulse pressure, angina; 4) Assess peripheral pulses, capillary refill, and skin; report delayed capillary refill and cool, pale, clammy skin; 5) Monitor urine output, report hourly output less than 30 mL; 6) Assess for changes in hemodynamic monitoring; 7) Administer medications as prescribed, assess for hypotension from nitroglycerin and nitroprusside; 8) Prepare for intraaortic balloon pump or ventricular assist device (VAD) if needed.

Nursing Diagnosis 2

Risk for impaired gas exchange related to alveolar-capillary membrane changes such as fluid collection and shifts into interstitial space or alveoli.

NIC:
1) Assess respiratory rate, lung sounds, and monitor for dyspnea, tachypnea, crackles, wheezes, and rhonchi; 2) Assess pulse oximetry, sensorium, ABGs, and report hypoxia, decreased LOC, or alteration in acid/base balance; 3) Assess skin, nailbeds, and mucous membranes for cyanosis or pallor; 4) Administer oxygen as prescribed; 5) Maintain head of bed elevated at 20 to 30 degrees if tolerated.

Nursing Diagnosis 3

Anxiety related to threat of death evidenced by fearful attitude.

NIC:
1) Use a calm, confident approach without false reassurance; 2) Acknowledge patient's perception of stressful situation; 3) Stay with patient to promote safety and reduce fear; 4) Answer all questions factually with consistent information; 5) Administer medications for anxiety as prescribed. Provide rest periods and quiet surroundings.

Nursing Diagnosis 4

Risk for spiritual distress related to physical and psychological stress.

NIC:
1) Assess patient's spiritual beliefs, cultural practices, and religious affiliations; 2) Implement measures to promote spiritual well-being and support patient in related activities; 3) Support grieving process of patient and significant others; 4) Consult clergy or other spiritual counselor as identified by the patient.

Condition:
Cardiogenic Shock
Age:

Link & Explain
• Nursing Interventions Classification (NIC)
• Laboratory and Diagnostic Procedures
• Medications

Nursing Diagnosis 5

Risk for ineffective coping related to situational crisis evidenced by inappropriate use of defense mechanisms.

NIC:
1) Assess patient/significant other's perception of current situation and signs of inadequate coping mechanisms; 2) Encourage verbalization and assist in identifying personal strengths/resources to cope with current situation; 3) Include patient/family in planning of comfort/supportive care; 4) Encourage patient to share what kinds of support would be most beneficial.

Medications
a. Nitroglycerine (Tridil)—venodilation, dilates coronary arteries
b. Diuretics
c. Norepinephrine (Levophed)—cardiac stimulation, peripheral vasoconstriction
d. nitroprusside (Nipride)—arterial and venous vasodilation

Laboratory & Diagnostic Procedures
a. Cardiac markers, B-type natriuretic peptide (BNP), CBC, electrolyte panel
b. Glucose
c. Echocardiogram, chest x-ray, EKG
d.

CONDITION: Dysrhythmia

PHYSIOLOGY: Dysrhythmia is abnormal formation of conduction of the electrical impulses within the heart. Decreased intrinsic pacemaker may result from a block in conduction in the atrioventricular (AV) junction or His-Purkinje system. These dysrhythmias may be classified as second-degree AV block Type I, second-degree AV block Type II, or third-degree AV block.

Tachydysrhythmias are caused by reentry, often due to enhanced or abnormal automaticity. These dysrhythmias may be classified as sinus tachycardia, atrial flutter, atrial fibrillation, paroxysmal atrial tachycardia, ventricular tachycardia, or ventricular fibrillation.

Other dysrhythmias include:

Premature atrial contractions: electrical impulse starts in the atrium before the next normal impulse of the sinus node.
Premature ventricular contractions: electrical signal originates in the ventricles, causing them to contract before receiving the electrical signal from the atrium.

HANDOFF COMMUNICATION

S Situation	Assess what is currently happening in a short statement.	Patient presents as _____
B Background	Summarize important past assessment data for your patient here. Place lab results and medications on the concept map.	**Age:** **Gender:** **Allergies:** **Fall Risk:** **Isolation:**
A Assessment	Use the assessment data to complete your concept map.	**Nursing Diagnosis:** Place the Nursing Diagnoses in prioritized order on the concept map and add any needed for your specific patient. **Plan:** Place any further Nursing Interventions Classifications (NIC) needed on the map.

Implement Your Plan of Care

R Recommendation	Evaluate your nursing care and make recommendations related to the achievement of your desired outcomes. Were they met, or do new goals need to be established?	**EVALUATE YOUR CARE**	
		Diag / **Nursing Outcomes Classification (NOC)**	**Outcome met**
		1 Patient maintains or achieves adequate cardiac output with BP and pulse within normal range.	☐ **Yes** ☐ **No**
		2 Patient verbalizes understanding of prescribed medications and how they interact with other drugs.	☐ **Yes** ☐ **No**
		3 Patient verbalizes diet and activity restrictions, medications, and symptoms requiring immediate medical attention.	☐ **Yes** ☐ **No**
		4 Patient displays reduced frequency or absence of dysrhythmia.	☐ **Yes** ☐ **No**
		5	☐ **Yes** ☐ **No**

Nursing Diagnosis 1

Risk for decreased cardiac output related to altered electrical conduction.

NIC:
1) Palpate radial, carotid, femoral, and dorsalis pulses, noting rate, regularity, amplitude (full or thready), and symmetry; **2)** Auscultate heart sounds, noting rhythm, rate, presence of extra heart beats, or dropped beats; **3)** Determine type of dysrhythmia and document with rhythm strip if cardiac monitoring is available; **4)** Monitor VS, assess adequacy of cardiac output and tissue perfusion, noting significant variations in BP, pulse rate equality, respirations, changes in skin color and temperature, LOC, and urine output during episodes of dysrhythmia; **5)** Investigate reports of chest pain, documenting location, duration, intensity (0–10 scale); **6)** Prepare for CPR if emergency occurs; **7)** Monitor electrolytes, cardiac enzymes, drug levels; **8)** Monitor I&O, BUN, creatinine.

Nursing Diagnosis 2

Risk for poisoning (digoxin toxicity) related to limited range of therapeutic effectiveness, lack of education, reduced vision, cognitive limitations.

NIC:
1) Explain patient's type of digoxin (Lanoxin) preparation and its specific therapeutic use; **2)** Instruct patient to maintain the prescribed dose and not to omit or take extra doses; **3)** Advise patient that digoxin may interact with many other drugs, such as barbiturates, neomycin, and antacids; **4)** Advise patient not to take OTC drugs, such as laxatives, antidiarrheals, antacids, cold remedies, diuretics, and herbals without discussing with the health-care provider; **5)** Discuss the necessity of periodic laboratory evaluations to check therapeutic range of digoxin; **6)** Discuss symptoms of digoxin toxicity such as anorexia, nausea, vomiting, blurred vision, halos, fatigue; **7)** Monitor electrolytes, BUN, creatinine, and liver function studies.

Nursing Diagnosis 3

Deficient knowledge regarding cause, treatment, self-care, and discharge needs related to lack of information, misunderstanding of medical condition or therapy needs evidenced by questions, statements of misconception.

NIC:
1) Assess the patient's level of knowledge, ability and desire to learn; **2)** Be alert to signs of avoidance such as changing the subject from the information being presented; **3)** Present information with pictures, reading material, videos, question-and-answer sessions in group sessions; **4)** Reinforce explanations of diet and activity restrictions, medications, and symptoms requiring immediate medical attention; **5)** Identify complications such as fatigue, dependent edema, progressive changes in mentation, vertigo, and psychological manifestations; **6)** Demonstrate accurate pulse-taking technique; **7)** Discuss monitoring and environmental safety concerns if the patient has a pacemaker or implantable cardioverter defibrillator (ICD); **8)** Recommend wearing medical alert bracelet or necklace and carrying pacemaker card identification.

Nursing Diagnosis 4

Risk for decreased cardiac tissue perfusion related to altered electrical imbalance.

NIC:
1) Recognize the electrical conduction problem and prepare for interventions as prescribed; **2)** Administer oxygen; **3)** Avoid activities that increase vagal tone such as gagging, suctioning, or vomiting since this may cause bradydysrhythmias; **4)** Administer atropine or prepare for cardiac pacemaker for bradydysrhythmias; **5)** Provide electrical cardioversion or defibrillation for unstable tachycardias; **6)** Administer appropriate drugs for supraventricular tachycardia such as adenosine (Adenocard); **7)** Monitor the patient's cardiac rhythm, VS, and LOC during drug administration and procedure.

Condition:

Dysrhythmia

Age:

Link & Explain
• Nursing Interventions Classification (NIC)
• Laboratory and Diagnostic Procedures
• Medications

Nursing Diagnosis 5

NIC:

Medications
a. Antidysrhythmics
b. Beta-adrenergic blockers, calcium channel blockers, adenosine (Adenocard)
c. Atropine
d.

Laboratory & Diagnostic Procedures
a. Electrolytes, drug screen, thyroid studies, C reactive protein (CRP)
b. Arterial blood gases, EKG
c. Holter monitor
d. Electrophysiology (EP) studies, radiofrequency ablation (RFA), cryoablation (CA)

CONDITION: Guillain-Barré Syndrome

PHYSIOLOGY: Guillain-Barré syndrome is the result of destruction of the myelin sheath of the peripheral nerves, which results in the rapid progression of paralysis. Symptoms begin symmetrically in the lower extremities and spread in an ascending manner to the abdomen and chest as well as the upper extremities. The patient has decreased or absent deep tendon reflexes, loss of bowel and bladder control, respiratory compromise, difficulty speaking, and diplopia. The blood pressure may become labile with cardiac dysrhythmia and tachycardia present.

The patient's history usually identifies that the patient had a respiratory infection, gastrointestinal infection, or virus within the past few weeks.

The three stages of the disease are:
Acute initial phase: begins with the onset of symptoms and ends when no further deterioration occurs (1–4 weeks)
Plateau phase: no changes occur (days–2 weeks)
Recovery phase: remyelination and axonal regeneration (4 months–2 years)

HANDOFF COMMUNICATION

S	Situation	Assess what is currently happening in a short statement.	Patient presents as _____	
B	Background	Summarize important past assessment data for your patient here. Place lab results and medications on the concept map.	**Age:** **Allergies:** **Isolation:**	**Gender:** **Fall Risk:**
A	Assessment	Use the assessment data to complete your concept map.	**Nursing Diagnosis:** Place the Nursing Diagnoses in prioritized order on the concept map and add any needed for your specific patient. **Plan:** Place any further Nursing Interventions Classifications (NIC) needed on the map.	

Implement Your Plan of Care

		EVALUATE YOUR CARE		
Recommendation	Evaluate your nursing care and make recommendations related to the achievement of your desired outcomes. Were they met, or do new goals need to be established?	**Diag**	**Nursing Outcomes Classification (NOC)**	**Outcome met**
		1	Patient maintains pulse oximetry within normal range without mechanical ventilation.	☐ Yes ☐ No
		2	Patient maintains optimal position of function evidenced by absence of contractures and footdrop.	☐ Yes ☐ No
R		3	Patient displays decreased frequency or absence of dysrhythmia.	☐ Yes ☐ No
		4	Patient demonstrates a calm facial appearance, appears relaxed.	☐ Yes ☐ No
		5	Patient maintains weight for height and frame, laboratory values within normal limits.	☐ Yes ☐ No

Nursing Diagnosis 1

Ineffective breathing pattern/impaired spontaneous ventilation related to musculoskeletal impairment evidenced by dyspnea and changes in depth and quality of respirations.

NIC:
1) Discuss the pathology of the disease and the possible need for intubation; **2)** Monitor VS, pulse oximetry, and ABGs; **3)** Observe breathing pattern and symptoms of air hunger. Note respiratory rate, auscultate every 2 hours, note decreased breath sounds and decreased depth of chest movement; **4)** Collaborate with respiratory therapist to monitor vital capacity every 2 hours; **5)** Prepare for intubation and mechanical ventilation; **6)** Check mechanical ventilator settings; **7)** Check tubing for obstruction, such as kinking, secretions, or accumulation of water. Drain tubing as needed; **8)** Ventilate manually for high or low alarms if source of ventilator alarm cannot be identified and rectified; **9)** Keep resuscitation bag at bedside to ventilate manually as needed.

Nursing Diagnosis 2

Impaired physical mobility related to neuromuscular impairment evidenced by impaired coordination, decreasing muscle strength.

NIC:
1) Schedule activity or procedures with rest periods; **2)** Provide or assist with passive and active ROM, report the need for increased assistance with movement; **3)** Provide means for communication such as communication board if speech is weak and moving finger or blinking once or twice for yes and no as paralysis progresses. Electronic devices may also be available for use; **4)** Consult with physical therapy, occupational therapy, speech therapy; **5)** Encourage family/significant other to participate in care.

Nursing Diagnosis 3

Risk for decreased cardiac output related to affected sympathetic and parasympathetic systems.

NIC:
1) Monitor for changes in BP, dysrhythmias, chest pain; **2)** Auscultate heart sounds; note rate, rhythm, presence of extra beats, and dropped beats; **3)** Determine type of dysrhythmia and document with a rhythm strip; **4)** Keep IV line patent. Report dysrhythmia, bradycardia, hypertension, or hypotension; **5)** Administer beta blocker or nitroprusside (Nitropress) for hypertension; **6)** Increase IV fluids for hypotension and place patient in a supine position; **7)** Provide calm and quiet environment.

Nursing Diagnosis 4

Fear/severe anxiety related to threat of death, dependency on mechanical support evidenced by hypervigilance.

NIC:
1) Identify patient's perception of threat presented by the situation; **2)** Observe and monitor physical responses such as facial expression, changes in VS; **3)** Decrease environmental stimuli. Encourage family to sit with patient; **4)** Discuss previous coping strengths with the family or significant other; **5)** Demonstrate and encourage the use of relaxation techniques, guided imagery, massage; **6)** Offer services from chaplain or spiritual resources; **7)** Discuss recovery period, which can be 6 months to 2 years while remyelination and axonal regeneration occur.

Condition:
Guillain-Barré Syndrome
Age:

Link & Explain
• Nursing Interventions Classification (NIC)
• Laboratory and Diagnostic Procedures
• Medications

Nursing Diagnosis 5

Imbalanced nutrition: less than body requirements related to impaired swallowing evidenced by ascending paralysis.

NIC:
1) Assess ability to chew and swallow during meals, and assist patient with nutritious food choices; **2)** Weigh daily and compare with admission weight; **3)** Determine need for enteral feedings as paralysis progresses to trunk; **4)** Administer nutritional solutions at prescribed rate via infusion control device. Assess abdomen, noting bowel sounds, abdominal distention, and reports of nausea; **5)** Monitor gastric residuals, placement of tube with measurement of pH (0–5); **6)** Monitor CBC, serum glucose, electrolytes, prealbumin, albumin; **7)** Maintain suction equipment at bedside.

Medications
a. Immunoglobulin (Sandoglobulin)
b. Treatment of BP changes and dysrhythmia
c.
d.

Laboratory & Diagnostic Procedures
a. CBC, cerebrospinal fluid analysis
b. Electromyographic (EMG), nerve conduction studies
c. MRI, CT, ABG
d. Plasmapheresis

CONDITION: Myocardial Infarction (MI)

PHYSIOLOGY: Myocardial infarction is irreversible myocardial cell death as a result of coronary artery occlusion. MI usually occurs when plaque in a coronary artery breaks away and the resulting clot obstructs the injured blood vessel. Perfusion of the muscular tissue downstream from the blocked artery is lost, resulting in myocardial ischemia and necrosis if blood flow is not restored. Cellular ischemia and necrosis can affect the heart's rhythm, pumping action, and general circulation, resulting in heart failure, life-threatening dysrhythmias, and death. Patients with ST-segment-elevation myocardial infarction (STEMI) usually have a more extensive MI associated with prolonged and complete coronary occlusion. Patients with unstable angina (UA) or non-ST-segment-elevation myocardial infarction (NSTEMI) usually have transient thrombosis or incomplete coronary occlusion.

Classic symptoms of MI include gradual onset of dull pain or pressure felt mostly in the substernal region of the chest, radiating to the neck, shoulders, arms, or jaw. Pain is often associated with difficulty breathing, nausea, vomiting, and diaphoresis. Clinical presentations vary considerably, however, especially in women and the elderly in whom unexplained breathlessness is the primary symptom. Patients often mistake symptoms for indigestion, gas pain, or muscle aches.

HANDOFF COMMUNICATION

S	Situation	Assess what is currently happening in a short statement.	Patient presents as _____ Type of MI and areas of ventricle affected by occlusion:
B	Background	Summarize important past assessment data for your patient here. Place lab results and medications on the concept map.	**Age:** **Gender:** **Allergies:** **Fall Risk:** **Isolation:**
A	Assessment	Use the assessment data to complete your concept map.	**Nursing Diagnosis:** Place the Nursing Diagnoses in prioritized order on the concept map and add any needed for your specific patient. **Plan:** Place any further Nursing Interventions Classifications (NIC) needed on the map.

Implement Your Plan of Care

			EVALUATE YOUR CARE		
R	Recommendation	Evaluate your nursing care and make recommendations related to the achievement of your desired outcomes. Were they met, or do new goals need to be established?	**Diag**	**Nursing Outcomes Classification (NOC)**	**Outcome met**
			1	Patient verbalizes relief or control of chest pain within appropriate period after administration of medications.	☐ Yes ☐ No
			2	Patient demonstrates measurable, progressive increase in tolerance of activity with heart rate, rhythm, and BP within normal limits.	☐ Yes ☐ No
			3	Patient verbalizes reduction in anxiety and fear through recognition of feelings, concerns, and use of effective coping mechanisms.	☐ Yes ☐ No
			4	Patient maintains hemodynamic stability (BP/cardiac output) within normal range, adequate urinary output, decreased frequency or absence of dysrhythmias	☐ Yes ☐ No
			5	Patient demonstrates adequate tissue perfusion with skin warm and dry, normal peripheral pulses and capillary refill.	☐ Yes ☐ No

Nursing Diagnosis 1

Acute pain related to tissue ischemia (coronary artery occlusion) evidenced by reports of chest pain.

NIC:
1) Assess pain by using the PQRST assessment of chest pain; 2) Administer medication for pain as prescribed and evaluate patient response; 3) Assess VS before and after administration of opioid medication; 4) Administer supplemental oxygen by nasal cannula or face mask, monitor pulse oximetry; 5) Administer aspirin (ASA) and nitrates as prescribed; 6) Provide quiet environment, calm activities, and comfort measures.

Nursing Diagnosis 2

Activity intolerance related to imbalance between myocardial oxygen supply and demand evidenced by alterations in heart rate and BP with activity.

NIC:
1) Assess for changes in VS, pain, or shortness of breath before, during, and after activity; 2) Explain gradual schedule for resumption of activities of daily living; 3) Provide frequent rest periods; 4) Instruct patient to avoid increasing abdominal pressure (Valsalva maneuver); 5) Refer to cardiac rehabilitation program.

Nursing Diagnosis 3

Anxiety/fear related to change in health, threat of loss/death, or internal conflicts about values, beliefs, and goals in life evidenced by focus on self.

NIC:
1) Encourage patient to share concerns and ask questions as needed; 2) Explain all procedures and medications to patient and provide time for questions; 3) Maintain confident, caring manner; 4) Provide reassurance that feelings are normal response to situation; 5) Encourage participation in treatment and post-discharge planning.

Nursing Diagnosis 4

Risk for decreased cardiac output related to changes in rate, rhythm, electrical conduction, reduced preload, increased systemic vascular resistance.

NIC:
1) Auscultate heart sounds for S3 and S4; 2) Auscultate breath sounds for rales; assess for dyspnea, tachypnea; 3) Monitor heart rate and observe for dysrhythmias; 4) Measure cardiac output; monitor ABGs, electrolytes, and cardiac enzymes; 5) Observe for pallor, cyanosis, cool and clammy skin.

Condition:
Myocardial Infarction (MI)

Age:

Link & Explain
• Nursing Interventions Classification (NIC)
• Laboratory and Diagnostic Procedures
• Medications

Nursing Diagnosis 5

Risk for ineffective tissue perfusion (myocardial) related to interruption of blood flow, plaque formation in coronary arteries.

NIC:
1) Obtain 12-lead EKG; 2) Measure cardiac enzymes; 3) Prepare for percutaneous coronary intervention/or thrombolytic therapy; 4) Monitor VS and observe for changes in neurological status such as anxiety, lethargy, stupor; 5) Monitor I&O, assess for urine output below 30 mL/hr; 6) Apply anti-emboli stockings or intermittent pneumatic compression device.

Medications

a. Aspirin, antianginals, antidysrhythmics, ACE inhibitors, angiotension receptor blockers, beta blockers

b. Anticoagulants/antiplatelets

c. Thrombolytic agents

d. Antiemetics/stool softeners

Laboratory & Diagnostic Procedures

a. Cardiac enzymes

b. ABGs

c. Percutaneous coronary intervention (PCI)

d.

CONDITION: Pneumothorax/Hemothorax

PHYSIOLOGY: Complete or partial collapse of the lung from an accumulation of air (pneumothorax), blood (hemothorax), or fluid (pleural effusion) occurs in the pleural space. Intrathoracic pressure changes occur from increased volumes in the pleural space and a reduction in lung capacity. It causes respiratory distress, problems with gas exchange, and tension on mediastinal structures that can impede cardiac and systemic circulation. Complications include hypoxemia, respiratory failure, and cardiac arrest.

Closed pneumothorax: rupture of blebs of the visceral pleura, which is more common with airway inflammation, heavy smokers, broken ribs, positive pressure during mechanical ventilation, insertion of central line catheter.
Open pneumothorax: air enters the pleural space when there is a penetrating injury to the chest wall from chest trauma. Air enters the pleural space during inspiration and is therefore called a *sucking chest wound.*
Tension pneumothorax: high intrapleural pressures resulting from an open or closed chest wound. The pressure results in a mediastinal shift toward the unaffected lung. Clinical manifestations include chest pain radiating to the shoulder, neck vein distention, and tracheal deviation.

HANDOFF COMMUNICATION

S Situation — Assess what is currently happening in a short statement.
Patient presents as _____
VS
LOC

B Background — Summarize important past assessment data for your patient here. Place lab results and medications on the concept map.
Age:　　Gender:
Allergies:　　Fall Risk:
Isolation:

A Assessment — Use the assessment data to complete your concept map.
Nursing Diagnosis: Place the Nursing Diagnoses in prioritized order on the concept map and add any needed for your specific patient.
Plan: Place any further Nursing Interventions Classifications (NIC) needed on the map.

Implement Your Plan of Care

R Recommendation — Evaluate your nursing care and make recommendations related to the achievement of your desired outcomes. Were they met, or do new goals need to be established?

EVALUATE YOUR CARE

Diag	Nursing Outcomes Classification (NOC)	Outcome met
1	Patient establishes a normal and effective respiratory pattern with ABGs within patient's normal range.	☐ Yes ☐ No
2	Patient demonstrates adequate coping methods, has relaxed facial expression, sleeps 8 hours at night.	☐ Yes ☐ No
3	Patient is careful to maintain safety of equipment when turning and getting out of bed.	☐ Yes ☐ No
4	Patient verbalizes understanding of cause of problem and identifies symptoms requiring medical follow-up.	☐ Yes ☐ No
5		☐ Yes ☐ No

Nursing Diagnosis 1

Ineffective breathing pattern related to decreased lung expansion due to air or fluid accumulation evidenced by dyspnea, tachycardia, change in depth and quality of respirations, abnormal ABGs.

NIC:
1) Identify precipitating factors such as trauma, malignancy, infection, or complication of mechanical ventilation; 2) Evaluate respiratory function, noting rapid or shallow respirations, dyspnea, reports of air hunger, development of cyanosis, changes in VS; 3) Assess for flail chest if patient has fractured ribs. During inspiration, the affected portion is sucked in, and during expiration it bulges out. Respirations are rapid and shallow; 4) Auscultate breath sounds, note chest excursion and position of trachea; 5) Maintain position of comfort, elevate head of bed, turn to affected side; 6) Assist with insertion of Heimlich (flutter) valve or chest tube, which is connected to suction with water-seal chamber or dry suction control chamber; 7) Assist client with splinting painful area when coughing or deep breathing.

Nursing Diagnosis 2

Fear/severe anxiety related to threat of death and threat to self-concept evidenced by increased muscle and facial tension.

NIC:
1) Identify patient's feelings and concerns about the situation; 2) Observe and monitor physical responses such as restlessness, changes in VS, repetitive movements; 3) Encourage patient to acknowledge and express fears; 4) Identify previous coping strengths of the patient; 5) Demonstrate and encourage the use of relaxation techniques, guided imagery, progressive relaxation.

Nursing Diagnosis 3

Risk for trauma/suffocation related to dependence on external device (chest drainage system).

NIC:
1) Monitor for change in respiratory pattern, tachypnea, dyspnea, air hunger, chest pain; (2) Secure all connection sites, monitor equipment; 3) Monitor thoracic insertion site for drainage around catheter; 4) Check water-seal chamber for correct fluid level; check presence of bubbling, presence of tidaling; 5) Check chest tube drainage for blood, assess Hgb/Hct, prepare for autotransfusion if necessary; 6) Do not disconnect or clamp unless prescribed.

Nursing Diagnosis 4

Deficient knowledge regarding condition, treatment regimen, self-care, and discharge needs related to lack of exposure to information evidenced by expressions of concern, request for information.

NIC:
1) Identify chance of recurrence or long-term complications; 2) Review symptoms requiring immediate evaluation, such as sudden chest pain, dyspnea, air hunger, respiratory distress; 3) Review significance of good health practices, adequate nutrition, rest, exercise; 4) Emphasize need for smoking cessation if indicated.

Condition:
Pneumothorax/ Hemothorax
Age:

Link & Explain
• Nursing Interventions Classification (NIC)
• Laboratory and Diagnostic Procedures
• Medications

Nursing Diagnosis 5

NIC:

Medications
a. NSAIDs: pain relief
b. Opioids: pain relief
c.
d.

Laboratory & Diagnostic Procedures
a. ABGs, Hgb/Hct
b. Chest x-ray
c. Thoracic CT
d. Thoracic ultrasound

CONDITION: Septic Shock

PHYSIOLOGY: Septic shock is a clinical syndrome associated with severe systemic infection that stimulates the inflammatory/immune system. Septic shock can be caused by gram-negative and gram-positive bacteria, viruses, fungi, or parasites. Diagnostic criteria include perfusion abnormalities, which typically result in lactic acidosis, oliguria, and an acute alteration in mental status. Clinical manifestations include infection with fever or hypothermia, hypotension unresponsive to fluid resuscitation, tachycardia, tachypnea, and hypoxemia. Laboratory findings may include leukocytosis (increased WBC count) or leukopenia (decreased WBC count), increased serum creatinine, coagulation abnormalities. Septic shock is a major cause of death in intensive care units. The incidence has increased because of the number of patients who are immunocompromised, the use of invasive devices, and a longer life span for the elderly.

Common factors or conditions associated with septic shock include diabetes mellitus, malnutrition, alcohol abuse, cirrhosis, respiratory infections, chronic kidney disease, hemorrhage, cancer, and surgery. People with traumatic injuries with either peritoneal contamination, burns, abscesses, or multiple blood transfusions are at particular risk as well.

HANDOFF COMMUNICATION

S Situation	Assess what is currently happening in a short statement.	Patient presents as _____ Obtain information regarding Advanced Directive, living will, or health-care proxy in addition to pertinent health history.
B Background	Summarize important past assessment data for your patient here. Place lab results and medications on the concept map.	Age: Gender: Allergies: Fall Risk: Isolation:
A Assessment	Use the assessment data to complete your concept map.	**Nursing Diagnosis:** Place the Nursing Diagnoses in prioritized order on the concept map and add any needed for your specific patient. **Plan:** Place any further Nursing Interventions Classifications (NIC) needed on the map.

Implement Your Plan of Care

R Recommendation	Evaluate your nursing care and make recommendations related to the achievement of your desired outcomes. Were they met, or do new goals need to be established?	**EVALUATE YOUR CARE**	
		Diag / **Nursing Outcomes Classification (NOC)**	**Outcome met**
		1 Patient maintains VS within normal limits and urine output at least 30 mL/hr.	☐ Yes ☐ No
		2 Patient maintains adequate circulating fluid volume with palpable peripheral pulses of good quality, VS within normal limits.	☐ Yes ☐ No
		3 Patient maintains adequate oxygen exchange, ABGs within patient's normal range.	☐ Yes ☐ No
		4 Patient experiences no negative effects on physiologic clotting mechanisms or development of DIC.	☐ Yes ☐ No
		5	☐ Yes ☐ No

Nursing Diagnosis 1

Ineffective tissue perfusion related to hypovolemia and lactic acidosis evidenced by tachycardia, hypotension, hypoxemia, decreased urine output.

NIC:
1) Obtain culture and sensitivity of blood, urine, sputum, wounds, tips of catheters; **2)** Administer antimicrobials as prescribed; **3)** Assess for widened pulse pressure, decreasing BP, rate and character of pulse, changes in hemodynamic monitoring; **4)** Administer IV fluids (crystalloids/colloids) as ordered; **5)** Administer antimicrobials to treat infection and decrease release of inflammatory mediators; **6)** Administer vasopressors and positive inotropic agents to maintain adequate perfusion pressure and cardiac output.

Nursing Diagnosis 2

Risk for deficient fluid volume related to regulatory failure from systemic infection.

NIC:
1) Monitor hourly I&O; **2)** Review 24-hour I&O for deficit/excess and report findings; **3)** Administer IV therapy with isotonic crystalloid solutions to maintain circulatory volume; **4)** Monitor Hgb/Hct, BUN, creatinine levels; **5)** Administer packed RBCs for decreased Hct.

Nursing Diagnosis 3

Risk for impaired gas exchange related to altered oxygen-carrying capacity of blood.

NIC:
1) Administration oxygen and prepare for endotracheal intubation as needed; **2)** Monitor pulse oximetry readings, ABGs, skin color, changes in LOC; **3)** Implement measures to maintain adequate pulmonary tissue perfusion such as repositioning, low Fowler's, encouraging coughing and deep breathing, incentive spirometry, fluid resuscitation.

Nursing Diagnosis 4

Risk for disseminated intravascular coagulation (DIC) related to activation of clotting mechanisms of inflammatory mediators and acidosis.

NIC:
1) Assess and report signs of bleeding from IV sites, urinary catheters; **2)** Assess for black tarry stools; guaiac test as needed; **3)** Implement safety precautions to prevent further bleeding (injections, invasive procedures/lines); **4)** Administer antimicrobials, fresh frozen plasma, platelets as prescribed.

Condition:
Septic Shock
Age:

Link & Explain
• Nursing Interventions Classification (NIC)
• Laboratory and Diagnostic Procedures
• Medications

Nursing Diagnosis 5

NIC:

Medications

a. Antimicrobials

b. Vasopressors, positive inotropic agents, blood products, steroids

c. Recombinant activated protein

d.

Laboratory & Diagnostic Procedures

a. ABGs, blood cultures

b. Fibrin degradation products (FDP), D-dimer, fibrinogen-level platelet count

c. Prolonged activated partial thromboplastin time (APTT), prothrombin time (PT), and thrombin time (TT)

d. Liver function studies, BUN, creatinine, CBC, blood chemistry

CONDITION: Spinal Cord Trauma

PHYSIOLOGY: Spinal cord injury is an insult to the spinal cord from hyperflexion or hyperextension, compression, rotation, or a penetrating injury. Neurological involvement is dependent on the level of injury, degree of spinal shock, and degree of recovery. The injury is classified as:

1. Complete, which is total loss of sensation and voluntary motor function.
2. Incomplete, which is a mixed loss of sensation and voluntary motor function.

HANDOFF COMMUNICATION

S	Situation	Assess what is currently happening in a short statement.	Patient presents as _____
B	Background	Summarize important past assessment data for your patient here. Place lab results and medications on the concept map.	**Age:** **Gender:** **Allergies:** **Fall Risk:** **Isolation:**
A	Assessment	Use the assessment data to complete your concept map.	**Nursing Diagnosis:** Place the Nursing Diagnoses in prioritized order on the concept map and add any needed for your specific patient. **Plan:** Place any further Nursing Interventions Classifications (NIC) needed on the map.

Implement Your Plan of Care

		EVALUATE YOUR CARE		
	Evaluate your nursing care and make recommendations related to the achievement of your desired outcomes. Were they met, or do new goals need to be established?	**Diag**	**Nursing Outcomes Classification (NOC)**	**Outcome met**
R Recommendation		1	Patient maintains adequate ventilation, demonstrates appropriate behaviors to support respiratory effort.	☐ Yes ☐ No
		2	Patient maintains proper alignment of spine without further spinal cord damage.	☐ Yes ☐ No
		3	Patient maintains position of function evidenced by absence of contractures and footdrop.	☐ Yes ☐ No
		4	Patient identifies behaviors to compensate for deficits.	☐ Yes ☐ No
		5	Patient expresses feelings and progresses through stages of grief, focusing on one day at a time.	☐ Yes ☐ No

Nursing Diagnosis 1

Risk for ineffective breathing pattern related to impairment at or above C5 with complete or mixed loss of intercostal muscle function.

NIC:
1) Note the patient's spontaneous effort, use of accessory muscles, and quality of respirations; **2)** Auscultate breath sounds, noting areas of absent or decreased sounds and development of adventitious sounds; **3)** Assess strength and effectiveness of cough; **4)** Monitor diaphragmatic movement if phrenic pacemaker is implanted; **5)** Maintain airway patency, keep head midline; **6)** Suction as necessary. Monitor heart rate and pulse oximetry during suctioning; **7)** Assist with "quad cough" once patient is stable.

Nursing Diagnosis 2

Risk for additional spinal cord trauma related to instability of spinal column.

NIC:
1) Maintain bedrest and immobilization device; **2)** Monitor external stabilization devices (Gardner-Wells tongs) used for decompression of spinal fractures and stabilization of vertebral column; **3)** Elevate head of bed as indicated with traction. Ensure pulleys are aligned, weights hang freely. Check for correct weights as ordered; **4)** Use foam wedges, blanket rolls, pillows for positioning.

Nursing Diagnosis 3

Impaired physical mobility related to neuromuscular impairment evidenced by inability to perform purposeful movement, paralysis.

NIC:
1) Monitor motor function continuously; **2)** Perform or assist with ROM; **3)** Maintain ankles at 90 degrees with footboard; **4)** Assess for edema of ankles and feet, and raise lower extremities as indicated; **5)** Assess BP before and after activity until stable. Change positions slowly; **6)** Position periodically when sitting in chair; **7)** Prepare for weight-bearing activities such as the use of a tilt table; **8)** Inspect all skin surfaces for reddened areas by use of a mirror if necessary.

Nursing Diagnosis 4

Disturbed sensory perception related to destruction of sensory tracts with altered sensory reception, transmission, and integration evidenced by change in usual response to stimuli.

NIC:
1) Assess and document sensory function and deficit by means of touch, pinprick, heat, cold; **2)** Protect from bodily harm, such as falls, burns, and positioning; **3)** Assist the patient to recognize and compensate for alterations in sensation; **4)** Provide prism glasses to patient when prone on turning frame; **5)** Provide diversional activities such as television, music, pictures, visitors. Use a clock and calendar for orientation; **6)** Note changes or altered thought process, disorientation, and bizarre thinking.

Condition:
Spinal Cord Trauma
Age:

Link & Explain
• Nursing Interventions Classification (NIC)
• Laboratory and Diagnostic Procedures
• Medications

Nursing Diagnosis 5

Grieving related to perceived or actual loss of physiopsychosocial well-being evidenced by expressions of distress, denial, guilt, fear, sadness, altered affect.

NIC:
Identify signs of grieving such as shock, denial, anger, and depression. *Shock:* (1) Provide simple and accurate information to the patient without false reassurance. (2) Encourage expressions of sadness, grief, guilt, and fear. *Denial:* (1) Assist patient to verbalize feelings and avoid judgment. (2) Focus on present needs such as skin care, exercise, ROM. *Anger:* (1) Accept expressions of anger and hopelessness. Set limits on acting out with abusive language, sexual aggressive behavior. (2) Encourage patient to take control when able, such as of food choices and diversional activities. *Depression:* Note loss of interest in living, sleep disturbance, suicidal thoughts. Offer support.

Medications

a. Steroid: methylprednisolone (Depo-Medrol) (reduces cord edema and improves neurological outcome)
b. Vasopressors: dobutamine (Dobutrex) in acute phase (increase systolic BP greater than 100 mm Hg)
c. Muscle relaxants and antispasticity agents: diazepam (Valium), baclofen (Lioresal), dantrolene (Dantrium) (limit and reduce pain after acute phase)
d. Alpha-2-adrenoreceptor agonist: tizanidine (Zanaflex) (reduces spasticity)

Laboratory & Diagnostic Procedures

a. ABG and pulse oximetry to monitor status of ventilation and oxygenation
b. Spinal x-rays locate level of injury, determine alignment and reduction after traction or surgery
c. CT produces cross-section images to reveal fractures and damage to spinal canal
d. MRI reveals spinal cord damage, hemorrhage, and edema

CONDITION: Stroke/Brain Attack

PHYSIOLOGY: Cerebrovascular accident is an injury or death of parts of the brain caused by an interruption of blood flow to an area. The affected area may cause a disability such as paralysis or speech impairment.

Ischemic stroke is impaired cerebral circulation caused by partial or complete occlusion of a blood vessel categorized into thrombotic or embolic. Thrombotic stroke is caused by formation of a thrombus (clot) from atherosclerotic plaques that have already narrowed blood vessels. Embolic stroke occurs when an embolus (dislodged clot) occludes the cerebral artery of the brain. It originates from cardiac problems such as atrial fibrillation or valve disease.

Hemorrhagic stroke is bleeding into the brain from a ruptured aneurysm, arteriovenous malformation (AVM), infection, and arterial dissection. Hypertension leads to changes in the arterial wall that increase the risk of rupture. They are categorized as intracerebral or subarachnoid bleeds depending on the location.

HANDOFF COMMUNICATION

S Situation	Assess what is currently happening in a short statement.	Patient presents as _____ VS LOC	
B Background	Summarize important past assessment data for your patient here. Place lab results and medications on the concept map.	**Age:** **Allergies:** **Isolation:**	**Gender:** **Fall Risk:**
A Assessment	Use the assessment data to complete your concept map.	**Nursing Diagnosis:** Place the Nursing Diagnoses in prioritized order on the concept map and add any needed for your specific patient. **Plan:** Place any further Nursing Interventions Classifications (NIC) needed on the map.	

Implement Your Plan of Care

		EVALUATE YOUR CARE	
	R Recommendation — Evaluate your nursing care and make recommendations related to the achievement of your desired outcomes. Were they met, or do new goals need to be established?	**Diag**	**Nursing Outcomes Classification (NOC)**	**Outcome met**
		1	Patient maintains usual or improved LOC, cognition, sensory and motor function.	☐ Yes ☐ No
		2	Patient maintains optimal position of function evidenced by absence of contractures and footdrop.	☐ Yes ☐ No
		3	Patient demonstrates feeding methods appropriate for patient, maintains desired body weight.	☐ Yes ☐ No
		4	Patient indicates understanding of the communication problem, establishes a method of communication to express needs, and uses resources appropriately.	☐ Yes ☐ No
		5	Patient acknowledges presence of impairment.	☐ Yes ☐ No

Nursing Diagnosis 1

Ineffective cerebral tissue perfusion related to interruption of blood flow (occlusive disorder, hemorrhage) evidenced by altered LOC; changes in motor or sensory responses; deficits in language, intellectual, emotional status.

NIC:

1) Monitor neurological status and compare with baseline; **2)** Evaluate eye-opening (spontaneous, opens only to painful stimuli, keeps eyes closed). Document changes in vision such as blurred, alterations in visual field, or depth perception; **3)** Assess verbal response: note if alert, oriented to person, place, time, or is confused; uses inappropriate words and phrases that make little sense. If patient is alert, assess verbal and written communication; **4)** Assess motor response to simple commands, noting purposeful and non-purposeful movements. Document right and left sides separately; **5)** Evaluate pupils, noting size, shape, equality, and reaction to light; **6)** Monitor VS; BP, noting hypertension or hypotension; heart rate, noting regularity, rhythm and auscultate for murmurs; respirations, noting periods of apnea, Cheyne-Stokes respiration; **7)** Assess for nuchal rigidity, twitching; increased restlessness, seizures; **8)** Avoid activities that increase ICP or bleeding, such as straining at stool; **9)** Administer supplemental oxygen as needed.

Nursing Diagnosis 2

Impaired physical mobility related to neuromuscular involvement evidenced by inability to purposefully move within the environment.

NIC:

1) Provide flotation mattress. Position patient to avoid skin and tissue pressure damage. Turn at regular intervals; **2)** Assess functional ability and extent of impairment; **3)** Evaluate the need for positional aids such as pillow under axilla to abduct arm, hand rolls in palms of hands, trochanter roll to maintain leg in a neutral position, footboard to prevent footdrop; **4)** Begin active and passive ROM to all extremities; **5)** Monitor bowel elimination; **6)** Monitor urine output and inspect for color and odor of urine.

Nursing Diagnosis 3

Risk for impaired swallowing related to neuromuscular impairment.

NIC:

1) Have suction equipment available at bedside; **2)** Promote effective swallowing by using the following methods: place patient upright during and for 45 minutes after feedings, place foods of appropriate consistency in unaffected side of mouth, feed slowly over 30–45 minutes, provide a minimum of 30 minutes of rest before meals, offer liquids after patient is finished solid foods, provide oral care; **3)** Maintain accurate I&O and calorie count; **4)** Weigh patient periodically; **5)** Encourage participation in exercise and activity programs.

Nursing Diagnosis 4

Impaired verbal and/or written communication related to impaired cerebral circulation evidenced by impaired articulation, inability to comprehend written or spoken language.

NIC:

1) Assess type and degree of dysfunction, such as receptive aphasia, expressive aphasia; **2)** Differentiate aphasia from dysarthria; **3)** Ask patient to follow simple commands; **4)** Point to objects and have patient name them; **5)** Ask patient to write name; **6)** Ask patient to read a short sentence; **7)** Provide a special call bell if necessary; **8)** Provide alternative methods of communication, such as writing, felt board, pictures, gestures.

Condition:
Stroke/Brain Attack
Age:

Link & Explain
• Nursing Interventions Classification (NIC)
• Laboratory and Diagnostic Procedures
• Medications

Nursing Diagnosis 5

Unilateral neglect related to neuromuscular impairment evidenced by failure to move eyes, head, limbs despite stimulus in the space.

NIC:

1) Approach patient from unaffected side; **2)** Have patient touch affected side and bring across midline of body during care activities; **3)** Assist patient to position affected extremity with use of a mirror; **4)** Instruct caregiver to monitor skin regularly; **5)** Instruct caregiver to monitor alignment of limbs; **6)** Discuss environmental safety concerns and assist in developing a plan to correct risk factors.

Medications
a. Intravenous thrombolytics: tissue plasminogen activator (tPA), alteplase (Activase), recombinant prourokinase (Prourokinase) (minimize infarcted area with early treatment of ischemic stroke)
b. Anticoagulants: warfarin sodium (Coumadin), enoxaparin (Lovenox) (prevent further clotting)
c. Antiplatelet agents: aspirin (ASA) (used following ischemic stroke)
d. Antihypertensives (cautious management during stroke for patients with chronic hypertension)

Laboratory & Diagnostic Procedures
a. Prothrombin time (PT), partial thromboplastin time (PTT), international normalized ratio (INR) baseline information for anticoagulant therapy
b. CT scan indicates the size and location of the lesion
c. MRI determines the extent of brain injury
d. Angiography identifies the cerebrovascular occlusion, atherosclerotic plaque, and malformation of vessels

References and Resources

GENERAL

Deglin, J. H., Vallerand, A. H., & Sanoski, C. A. (2011). *Davis's drug guide for nurses* (12th ed.). Philadelphia: FA Davis.

DeSevo, M. (2009). *Maternal and newborn success: A course review applying critical thinking to test taking.* Philadelphia: FA Davis.

Doenges, M. E., Moorhouse, M. F., & Murr, A. C. (2011). *Nursing care plans: Guidelines for individualizing client care across the life span* (8th ed.). Philadelphia: FA Davis.

Dudek, S. G. (2010). *Nutrition essentials for nursing practice* (6th ed.). Philadelphia: Wolters Kluwer Health/Lippincott, Williams & Wilkins.

Jarvis, C. (2012). *Physical examination & health assessment* (6th ed.). St. Louis: Saunders/Elsevier.

Lehne, R. A. (2010). *Pharmacology for nursing care* (7th ed.). St. Louis: Saunders/Elsevier.

Pagana, K. D., & Pagana, T. J. (2011). *Mosby's diagnostic and laboratory test reference* (10th ed.). St. Louis: Saunders/Elsevier.

Schuster-McHugh, P. (2008). *Concept mapping: A critical-thinking approach to care planning* (2nd ed.). Philadelphia: FA Davis.

Smith, S. F., Duell, D. J., & Martin, B. C. (2011). *Clinical nursing skills* (8th ed.). Upper Saddle River, NJ: Prentice Hall.

Sommers, M. S. (2011). *Diseases and disorders: A nursing therapeutics manual* (4th ed.). Philadelphia: FA Davis.

Spratto, G. R., & Woods, A. L. (2010). *Delmar nurse's drug handbook.* Clifton Park, NY: Delmar Cengage.

Taber's Cyclopedic Medical Dictionary. (2009). (21st ed.). Philadelphia: FA Davis.

Van Leeuwen, A. M., Poelhuis-Leth, D., & Bladh, M. L. (2011). *Davis's comprehensive handbook of laboratory diagnostic tests with nursing implications* (4th ed.). Philadelphia: FA Davis.

Wilkinson, J. M. (2012). *Nursing process and critical thinking* (5th ed.). Upper Saddle River, NJ: Pearson Education.

MATERNAL AND NEWBORN

London, M. L., Ladewig, P. A., Ball, J. W., Bindler, R. C., & Cowen, K. J. (2011). *Maternal & child nursing care* (3rd ed.). Upper Saddle River, NJ: Pearson Education.

Ward, S., & Hinsley, S. (2009). *Maternal-child nursing care: Optimizing outcomes for mothers, children, and families.* Philadelphia: FA Davis.

Wittmann-Price, R. A. & Cornelius, F. (2011). *Maternal-child nursing test success: An unfolding case study review.* New York: Springer.

PEDIATRIC

Bindler, R. M., & Howry, L. B. (2006). *Pediatric drug guide with nursing implications.* Upper Saddle River, NJ: Prentice Hall.

Hockenberry, M. J., & Wilson, D. (2010). *Wong's nursing care of infants and children* (9th ed.). St. Louis: Mosby/Elsevier.

Hockenberry, M. J., & Wilson, D. (2009). *Wong's essentials of pediatric nursing* (8th ed.). St. Louis: Saunders/Elsevier.

Hogan, M. A., Brancato, V., Falkenstein, K., & White, J. E. (2007). *Child health nursing reviews and rationales.* (2nd ed.). Upper Saddle River, NJ: Prentice Hall.

MEDICAL-SURGICAL

DeLaune, S. C., & Ladner, P. K. (2011). *Fundamentals of nursing: Standards and practice* (4th ed.). Clifton Park, NY: Delmar Cengage.

DeLaune, S. C., & Ladner, P. K. (2011). *Skills checklist to accompany fundamentals of nursing: Standards and practice* (4th ed.). Clifton Park, NY: Delmar Cengage.

Ignatavicius, D. D., & Workman, M. L. (2010). *Medical-surgical nursing, patient-centered collaborative care* (6th ed.). St. Louis: Saunders/Elsevier.

Lewis, S. L., Ruff-Dirksen, S., McLean-Heitkemper, M., Bucher, L., & Camera, I. M. (2011). *Medical-surgical nursing, assessment and management of clinical problems* (8th ed.). St. Louis: Mosby/Elsevier.

Smeltzer, S. C., Bare, B. G., Hinkle, J. L., & Cheever, K. H. (2010). *Brunner and Suddarth's textbook of medical-surgical nursing* (12th ed.). Philadelphia: Wolters Kluwer Health/ Lippincott, Williams & Wilkins.

MENTAL HEALTH

Curtis, C. M., Fegley, A. B., & Tuzo, C. N. (2009). *Psychiatric mental health nursing success.* Philadelphia: FA Davis.

Varcarolis, E. M., Carson, V. B., & Shoemaker, N. C. (2010). *Foundations psychiatric mental health nursing a clinical approach.* St. Louis: Saunders/Elsevier.

COMMUNITY

Doenges, M. E., Moorhouse, M. F., & Geissler-Murr, A. C. (2004). *Nurse's pocket guide: Diagnoses, interventions, and rationales* (9th ed.). Philadelphia: FA Davis.

Heyman, D. (ed.). (2004). *Control of communicable diseases manual* (18th ed.). Washington, DC: American Public Health Association.

Maurer, F. A., & Smith, C. (2009). *Community/public health nursing practice: Health for families and populations* (4th ed). St. Louis: Saunders/Elsevier.

Stanhope, M., & Lancaster, J. (2008). *Public health nursing: Population-centered health care in the community* (7th ed.). St. Louis: Saunders/Elsevier.

LEADERSHIP

AHRQ (Agency for Healthcare Research and Quality). (2011). www.ahrq.gov/qual/patientsafetyix.htm.

AHRQ. (2008). AHRQ Innovations Exchange. www.innovations. ahrq.gov/content.aspx?id=2067.

ANA (American Nurses Association). (2005). *Principles for delegation*. Silver Spring, MD: ANA.

ANA. (2012). Safe staffing saves lives. www.safestaffingsaveslives.org.

ANA & NCSBN (National Council of State Boards of Nursing). (n.d.). Joint statement on delegation. https://www. ncsbn.org/Joint_statement.pdf.

Cohen, M. R. (2007). *Medication errors* (2nd ed.). Washington, DC: American Pharmacists Association.

Grossman, S. C., & Valiga, T. M. (2009). *The new leadership challenge: Creating the future of nursing* (3rd ed.). Philadelphia: F. A. Davis

ISMP (Institute of Safe Medication Practices). (2010). www. ismp.org.

Merriam-Webster Online Dictionary (2010). www.merriam-webster.com.

Motacki, K., & Burke, K. (2011). *Nursing delegation and management of patient care*. St. Louis: Saunders/Elsevier.

NCCMERP (National Coordinating Council for Medication Error Reporting and Prevention). (2010). www.nccmerp. org/aboutMedErrors.html.

NPSF (National Patient Safety Foundation). (2011). www. npsf.org/rc/mp/.

O'Daniel, M., & Rosenstein, A. H. (2008). Professional communication and team collaboration. In *Patient safety and quality: An evidence-based handbook for nurses* (ed. R. G. Hughs). Rockville, MD: Agency for Healthcare Research and Quality, ch. 33. www.ncbi.nlm.nih.gov/books/NBK2637/#top.

Pennsylvania Patient Safety Authority. (2010). Transfusion Process Map. http://patientsafetyauthority.org/EducationalTools/Patient SafetyTools/blood/Documents/process.pdf.

Pratt, S. D., Mann, S., Salisbury, M., Greenberg, P., Marcus, R., Stabile, B., McNamee, P., Nielsen, P., & Sachs B. P. (2007). Impact of CRM–based team training on obstetric outcomes and clinicians' patient safety attitudes. *Joint Commission Journal on Quality and Patient Safety*, *33*(12), 720–725. www.ncbi.nlm.nih.gov/books/NBK2637.

QSEN (Quality & Safety Education for Nurses). (2010). www.qsen.org/definition.php?id=5.

Rosenstein, A. H., & O'Daniel, M. (2005). Disruptive behavior and clinical outcomes: Perceptions of nurses and physicians. *American Journal of Nursing*, *105*(1), 54–64.

Rosenstein, A. H., & O'Daniel, M. (2008). A survey of the impact of disruptive behaviors and communication defects on patient safety. *Joint Commission Journal of Quality and Patient Safety*, *34*(8), 464–471.

U.S. Department of Veteran's Affairs. (n.d.). Safety huddle. www.visn8.va.gov/PatientSafetyCenter/safePtHandling/safet yhuddle_021110.pdf.

Whitehead, D. K., Weiss, S. A., & Tappen, R. M. (2010). *Essentials of nursing leadership and management* (5th ed.). Philadelphia: F. A. Davis

Wittmann-Price, R. A., & Reap Thompson, B. (eds.). (2010). *NCLEX-RN® EXCEL: Test success through unfolding case study review*. New York: Springer.

Wright, D. (2010). HHS REPORT: Infection prevention professionals, hospital representatives recommend steps to simplify and streamline federal HAI tracking system. *Joint Commission Perspectives*, *30*(2), 9–10. www.jointcommission. org/assets/1/18/S7-JCP-02-10.pdf.

Yoser-Wise, P.S. (2011). *Leading and managing in nursing*. St. Louis: Mosby/Elsevier.

Appendixes

APPENDIX A **REPORT WORKSHEET**

Report Worksheet

Nurse: _____

Patient Information					
Identifier:	**Age:**	Gender: _____	**Race:**	**DOA:**	PCP:

CC:	
Dx:	

Morning Report	

Report	**Medical**	**Surgical**

Scheduled Testing	**Radiology**	**Labs**	**Special Tests/Procedures**

Therapy	**Physical Therapy**	**Occupational Therapy**	**Speech Therapy**

Nursing Interventions	

Treatments	

Nursing Orders		**FSBS**
		Frequency:

Summary of Care	**Care Provided**	**Patient Response**

Clinical Assessment Tool

General Description

ADL	Activity Level	Bath	Eating

Vital Signs

Time: | **Frequency:**

BP	/	Location: ☐RUE ☐LUE ☐RLE ☐LLE
Pulse	beats per minute Characteristics:	
Resp	breaths per minute	☐Regular ☐Irregular ☐Labored ☐Non-Labored
Temp	F	☐Oral ☐Axillary ☐Rectal
Pain	___ /10	
SpO_2	%	

Integument

Color		Moisture		Temp	
Turgor	☐Brisk ☐Tenting (___ sec)	Texture		Condition	
Decubitus	Location:		Description:		

Wound Assessment	Type	Size	Location	Description

Head, Eyes, Ears, Nose, & Throat (HEENT)

Head	☐Normocephalic ☐Other:		

Eyes	Vision Correction	Discharge	Extraocular Movement
	☐None ☐Other:	☐None ☐Other:	☐Normal ☐Other:
	Sclera	Pupils	
	☐White ☐Other:	☐PERRL ☐Other:	

Ears	Position	Temperature/Moisture	Drainage
	☐Symmetrical ☐Other:	☐Warm ☐Moist ☐Dry ☐Other:	☐None ☐Other:
	Masses	Lesions	Hearing
	☐None ☐Other:	☐None ☐Other:	☐Normal ☐HOH ☐Aids

Nose	Discharge	Lesions	Olfactory Nerve
	☐None ☐Other:	☐None ☐Other:	☐Intact ☐Not Intact

Throat	Moisture	Color	Tenderness
	☐Moist ☐Dry	☐Pink ☐White ☐Red (Inflamed)	☐Non-Tender ☐Tender

Continued

Respiratory

Breath Sounds	☐ Bilaterally clear to auscultation ☐ Other:
O₂ Source	☐ Room Air ☐ Oxygen via: _____ @ ___ L/hr
Incentive Spirometer	☐ No ☐ Yes Frequency & Level:

Cardiovascular

Capillary Refill

Location	Seconds

Apical Pulse

☐ Regular ☐ Irregular
☐ Strong ☐ Weak
☐ S1S2 with RRR
☐ S3 ☐ S4
☐ Murmur
☐ Other:

IV Therapy — Site #1

☐ Central Line ☐ PICC ☐ Peripheral Line
Size:_____ Location:_____
Condition:_____
☐ Drip: _____ mL/hr ☐ Intermittent
Solution: _____ Date:_____
Amount: _____

Edema

☐ None
Location: _____
☐ 1+ ☐ 2+ ☐ 3+ ☐ 4+

Radial Pulse

☐ Regular ☐ Irregular
☐ Strong ☐ Weak

IV Therapy — Site #2

☐ Central Line ☐ PICC ☐ Peripheral Line
Size:_____ Location:_____
Condition:_____
☐ Drip: _____ mL/hr ☐ Intermittent
Solution: _____ Date:_____
Amount: _____

Telemetry

☐ Yes ☐ No
Reason:

Pedal Pulse

☐ Regular ☐ Irregular
☐ Strong ☐ Weak

Gastrointestinal & Genitourinary

NG Tube

Location	☐ Left Nare ☐ Right Nare
Suction	☐ Continuous ☐ Intermittent Suction @:
Characteristics	

Bowel Sounds

☐ Active
☐ Absent
☐ Hyperactive
☐ Hypoactive

Locations Heard:
☐ RUQ ☐ LUQ
☐ RLQ ☐ LLQ

Abdomen

☐ Soft ☐ Firm ☐ Distended
☐ Rigid ☐ Tender ☐ Pregnant
☐ Other:

GI

Last BM	
Appearance	
Normal Pattern	
Laxative Use	
Continence	

GU

Normal Pattern	
Color	
Character	
Frequency	
Continence	

Intake & Output

Diet

Type of Diet	Appetite	Gag Reflex
		☐ Intact ☐ Other:

Intake

PO	IV	Other

Output

Urine	Stool	Drainage	Other

Musculoskeletal

Gait		Aids		Strength	Arm		Leg	
					Right	___ /5	Right	___ /5
					Left	___ /5	Left	___ /5

ROM	☐ RUE ☐ LUE ☐ RLE ☐ LLE	Limitations
		N/A

Neurovascular

Sleep	Hours of Sleep	
	Trouble Falling/Staying Asleep	
	Sleep Aids	
	# of Pillows	
	Sleep Apnea	

Loss of Sensation	

Mental Status

Status	Memory	Language & Affect
☐ Alert ☐ Other: Oriented to: ☐ Person ☐ Place ☐ Time	☐ Recent Memory: ☐ Remote Memory:	Language: ☐ Appropriate ☐ Not Appropriate Affect: ☐ Congruent ☐ Non-Congruent

Treatments

Treatment	Time	Method	Rationale for Treatment	Evaluation

Developmental/Psychosocial Assessment

Developmental Stage	▼

Assessment	

APPENDIX C **PATIENT OVERVIEW**

Patient Overview

Student Name: **Date of Clinical:**

Patient Information

Identifier :

Room #:

Admission Date:

Age:

Gender:

Height:

Weight: lbs

Allergies: ☐ NKA

Marital Status:

Occupation:

Significant Past Medical History

Living Will: ☐ Yes ☐ No
Power of Attorney: ☐ Yes ☐ No
Resuscitate: ☐ Yes ☐ No

Surgical Procedures

Post-operative Days:

Name of Procedure

Description of Procedure

Summary of Present Illness

Summary of Present Illness

Chief Complaint

Medical Diagnosis & Definition

Pathophysiology

Expected Signs & Symptoms

How is this condition usually treated? How is this patient being treated?

APPENDIX D **LAB VALUES AND DIAGNOSTIC TESTS**

Lab Values

Test	Normal Value	Admission		Trends			Reason for Abnormal Value
ABG							
pH (Arterial)		☐	☐	☐	☐	☐	
Po$_2$ (Arterial)		☐	☐	☐	☐	☐	
Pco$_2$ (Arterial)		☐	☐	☐	☐	☐	
HCO$_3^-$		☐	☐	☐	☐	☐	
CBC							
WBC		☐	☐	☐	☐	☐	
RBC		☐	☐	☐	☐	☐	
Hemoglobin (Hgb)		☐	☐	☐	☐	☐	
Hematocrit (Hct)		☐	☐	☐	☐	☐	
Platelet Count		☐	☐	☐	☐	☐	
Coagulation							
PT		☐	☐	☐	☐	☐	
INR		☐	☐	☐	☐	☐	
PTT		☐	☐	☐	☐	☐	

Continued

Lab Values

	Test	Normal Value	Admission	Trends			Reason for Abnormal Value
Chemistry	Blood Glucose						
	Hemoglobin A1C						
	Sodium (Na)						
	Potassium (K)						
	Chloride (Cl)						
	Calcium (Ca)						
	BUN						
	Creatinine						
	Total Protein						
	Albumin						
	Total Cholesterol						
	LDL						

Lab Values

Test	Normal Value	Admission			Trends		Reason for Abnormal Value
HDL							
Triglycerides							
AST							
SGOT							
Bilirubin							
CK							
CK MB							
Troponin							
BNP							

Chemistry

Continued

Lab Values

Test	Normal Value	Admission	Trends			Reason for Abnormal Value
Color						
Character						
Specific Gravity						
Leukocytes						
Nitrite						
pH						
Protein						
Glucose						
Ketones						
Urobilinogen						

Diagnostic Tests

Name of Test	Date	Reason for Test	Interpretation of Results
Microbiology			
Radiology			
Ultrasound			
Cardiac Studies			

APPENDIX E **MEDICATIONS**

Medications

Brand Name							
Generic Name							
Classification							
Action							
Dose							
Route	▶	▶	▶	▶	▶	▶	▶
Frequency							
Reason this patient is taking							
Pharmacokinetics O P D ½ M E	O P D ½ M E	O P D ½ M E	O P D ½ M E	O P D ½ M E	O P D ½ M E	O P D ½ M E	O P D ½ M E
Contraindications							
Major Adverse Effects							
Nursing Considerations							
Patient Teaching							

APPENDIX F **NURSES' NOTES**

Nurses' Notes	
Time	

APPENDIX G NANDA-NURSING DIAGNOSES 2012 – 2014

DOMAIN 1: HEALTH PROMOTION

Class 1: Health Awareness

Deficient Diversional Activity

Definition: Decreased stimulation from (or interest or engagement in) recreational or leisure activities

Defining Characteristics: Reports feeling bored (e.g., wishes there was something to do, to read); Usual hobbies cannot be undertaken in the current setting

Related Factors: Environmental lack of diversional activity

Sedentary Lifestyle

Definition: Reports a habit of life that is characterized by a low physical activity level

Defining Characteristics: Chooses a daily routine lacking physical exercise; Demonstrates physical deconditioning; Reports preference for activities low in physical activity

Related Factors: Deficient knowledge of the health benefits of physical exercise; Lack of interest; Lack of motivation; Lack of resources (e.g., time, money, companionship, facilities); Lack of training for accomplishment of physical exercise

Class 2: Health Management

Deficient Community Health

Definition: Presence of one or more health problems or factors that deter wellness or increase the risk of health problems experienced by an aggregate

Defining Characteristics: Incidence of risks relating to hospitalization experienced by aggregates or populations; Incidence of risks relating to physiological states experienced by aggregates or populations; Incidence of risks relating to psychological states experienced by aggregates or populations; Incidence of health problems experienced by aggregates or populations; No program available to enhance wellness for an aggregate or population; No program available to prevent one or more health problems for an aggregate or population; No program available to reduce one or more health problems for an aggregate or population; No program available to eliminate one or more health problems for an aggregate or population

Related Factors: Lack of access to public healthcare providers; Lack of community experts; Limited resources; Program has inadequate budget; Program has inadequate community support; Program has inadequate consumer satisfaction; Program has inadequate evaluation plan; Program has inadequate outcome data; Program partly addresses health problem

Risk-Prone Health Behavior

Definition: Impaired ability to modify lifestyle/behaviors in a manner that improves health status

Defining Characteristics: Demonstrates nonacceptance of health status change; Failure to achieve optimal sense of control; Failure to take action that prevents health problems; Minimizes health status change

Related Factors: Excessive alcohol; Inadequate comprehension; Inadequate social support; Low self-efficacy; Low socioeconomic status; Multiple stressors; Negative attitude toward healthcare; Smoking

Ineffective Health Maintenance

Definition: Inability to identify, manage, and/or seek out help to maintain health

Defining Characteristics: Demonstrated lack of adaptive behaviors to environmental changes; Demonstrated lack of knowledge about basic health practices; History of lack of health-seeking behavior; Inability to take responsibility for meeting basic health practices; Impairment of personal support systems; Lack of expressed interest in improving health behaviors

Related Factors: Cognitive impairment; Complicated grieving; Deficient communication skills; Diminished fine motor skills; Diminished gross motor skills; Inability to make appropriate judgments; Ineffective family coping; Ineffective individual coping; Insufficient resources (e.g., equipment, finances); Lack of fine motor skills; Lack of gross motor skills; Perceptual impairment; Spiritual distress; Unachieved developmental tasks

Readiness for Enhanced Immunization Status

Definition A pattern of conforming to local, national, and/or international standards of immunization to prevent infectious disease(s) that is sufficient to protect a person, family, or community and can be strengthened

Defining Characteristics: Expresses desire to enhance behavior to prevent infectious disease; Expresses desire to enhance identification of possible problems associated with immunizations; Expresses desire to enhance identification of providers of immunizations; Expresses desire to enhance immunization status; Expresses desire to enhance knowledge of immunization standards; Expresses desire to enhance record-keeping of immunizations

*Note: This diagnosis will be removed from the next edition, as the diagnostic concept is contained within the diagnosis of **Readiness for Enhanced Self-Health Management.***

Ineffective Protection

Definition: Decrease in the ability to guard self from internal or external threats such as illness or injury

Defining Characteristics: Altered clotting; Anorexia; Chilling; Cough; Deficient immunity; Disorientation; Dyspnea; Fatigue; Immobility; Impaired healing; Insomnia; Itching; Maladaptive stress response; Neurosensory alteration; Perspiring; Pressure ulcers; Restlessness; Weakness

Related Factors: Abnormal blood profiles (e.g., leukopenia, thrombocytopenia, anemia, coagulation); Cancer; Extremes of age; Immune disorders; Inadequate nutrition; Pharmaceutical agents (e.g., antineoplastic, corticosteroid, immune, anticoagulant, thrombolytic); Substance abuse; Treatment-related side effects (e.g., surgery, radiation)

Ineffective Self-Health Management

Definition: Pattern of regulating and integrating into daily living a therapeutic regimen for the treatment of illness and its sequelae that is unsatisfactory for meeting specific health goals

Defining Characteristics: Failure to include treatment regimens in daily living; Failure to take action to reduce risk factors; Ineffective choices in daily living for meeting health goals; Reports desire to manage the illness; Reports difficulty with prescribed regimens

Related Factors: Complexity of healthcare system; Complexity of therapeutic regimen; Decisional conflicts; Deficient knowledge; Economic difficulties; Excessive demands made (e.g., individual, family); Family conflict; Family patterns of healthcare; Inadequate number of cues to action; Perceived barriers; Perceived benefits; Perceived seriousness; Perceived susceptibility; Powerlessness; Regimen; Social support deficit

Readiness for Enhanced Self-Health Management

Definition: A pattern of regulating and integrating into daily living a therapeutic regimen for the treatment of illness and its sequelae that is sufficient for meeting health-related goals and can be strengthened

Defining Characteristics: Choices of daily living are appropriate for meeting goals (e.g., treatment, prevention); Describes reduction of risk factors; Expresses desire to manage the illness (e.g., treatment, prevention of sequelae); Expresses little difficulty with prescribed regimens; No unexpected acceleration of illness symptoms

Ineffective Family Therapeutic Regimen Management

Definition: A pattern of regulating and integrating into family processes a program for the treatment of illness and its sequelae that is unsatisfactory for meeting specific health goals

Defining Characteristics: Acceleration of illness symptoms of a family member; Failure to take action to reduce risk factors; Inappropriate family activities for meeting health goals; Lack of attention to illness; Reports desire to manage the illness; Reports difficulty with prescribed regimen

Related Factors: Complexity of healthcare system; Complexity of therapeutic regimen; Decisional conflicts; Economic difficulties; Excessive demands; Family conflict

DOMAIN 2: NUTRITION

Class 1: Ingestion

Insufficient Breast Milk

Definition: Low production of maternal breast milk

Defining Characteristics: *Infant:* Constipation; Does not seem satisfied after sucking time; Frequent crying; Long breastfeeding time; Refuses to suck; Voids small amounts of concentrated urine (less than four to six times a day); Wants to suck very frequently; Weight gain is lower than 500 g in a month (comparing two measures)
Mother: Milk production does not progress; No milk appears when mother's nipple is pressed; Volume of expressed breast milk is less than prescribed volume

Related Factors: *Infant:* Ineffective latching on; Ineffective sucking; Insufficient opportunity to suckle; Rejection of breast; Short sucking time
Mother: Alcohol intake; Fluid volume depletion (e.g., dehydration, hemorrhage); Malnutrition; Medication side effects (e.g., contraceptives, diuretics); Pregnancy; Tobacco smoking

Ineffective Infant Feeding Pattern

Definition: Impaired ability of an infant to suck or coordinate the suck/swallow response resulting in inadequate oral nutrition for metabolic needs

Defining Characteristics: Inability to coordinate sucking, swallowing, and breathing; Inability to initiate an effective suck; Inability to sustain an effective suck

Related Factors: Anatomical abnormality; Neurological delay; Neurological impairment; Oral hypersensitivity; Prematurity; Prolonged nil by mouth (NPO) status

Imbalanced Nutrition: Less Than Body Requirements

Definition: Intake of nutrients insufficient to meet metabolic needs

Defining Characteristics: Abdominal cramping; Abdominal pain; Aversion to eating; Body weight 20% or more below ideal weight range; Capillary fragility; Diarrhea; Excessive hair loss; Hyperactive bowel sounds; Lack of food; Lack of information; Lack of interest in food; Loss of weight with adequate food intake; Misconceptions; Misinformation; Pale mucous membranes; Perceived inability to ingest food; Poor muscle tone; Reports altered taste sensation; Reports food intake less than recommended daily allowance (RDA); Satiety immediately after ingesting food; Sore buccal cavity; Steatorrhea; Weakness of muscles required for mastication; Weakness of muscles required for swallowing

Related Factors: Biological factors; Inability to absorb nutrients; Inability to digest food; Inability to ingest food; Insufficient finances; Psychological factors

Imbalanced Nutrition: More Than Body Requirements

Definition: Intake of nutrients that exceeds metabolic needs

Defining Characteristics: Concentrating food intake at the end of the day; Dysfunctional eating pattern (e.g., pairing food with other activities); Eating in response to external cues (e.g., time of day, social situation); Eating in response to internal cues other than hunger (e.g., anxiety); Sedentary lifestyle; Triceps skin fold >15mm in men; Triceps skin fold >25mm in women; Weight 20% over ideal for height and frame

Related Factors: Excessive intake in relation to metabolic need; Excessive intake in relation to physical activity (caloric expenditure);

Readiness for Enhanced Nutrition

Definition: A pattern of nutrient intake that is sufficient for meeting metabolic needs and can be strengthened

Defining Characteristics: Attitude toward drinking is congruent with health goals; Attitude toward eating is congruent with health goals; Consumes adequate fluid; Consumes adequate food; Eats regularly; Expresses knowledge of healthy fluid choices; Expresses knowledge of healthy food choices; Expresses willingness to enhance nutrition; Follows an appropriate standard for intake (e.g., the food pyramid or American Diabetic Association guidelines); Safe preparation of fluids; Safe preparation of food; Safe storage of fluids; Safe storage of food

Risk for Imbalanced Nutrition: More Than Body Requirements

Definition: At risk for an intake of nutrients that exceeds metabolic needs

Risk Factors: Concentrating food intake at the end of the day; Dysfunctional eating patterns; Eating in response to external cues (e.g., time of day, social situation); Eating in response to internal cues other than hunger (e.g., anxiety); Higher baseline weight at beginning of each pregnancy; Observed use of food as a comfort measure; Observed use of food as a reward; Pairing food with other activities; Parental obesity; Rapid transition across growth percentiles in children; Reports use of solid food as major food source before 5 months of age; Sedentary lifestyle

Impaired Swallowing

Definition: Abnormal functioning of the swallowing mechanism associated with deficits in oral, pharyngeal, or esophageal structure or function

Defining Characteristics: *Esophageal Phase Impairment:* Abnormality in esophageal phase by swallow study; Acidic-smelling breath; Bruxism; Epigastric pain; Food refusal; Heartburn; Hematemesis; Hyperextension of head (e.g., arching during or after meals); Nighttime awakening; Nighttime coughing; Observed evidence of difficulty in swallowing (e.g., stasis of food in oral cavity, coughing/choking); Odynophagia; Regurgitation of gastric contents (wet burps); Repetitive swallowing; Reports "something stuck"; Unexplained irritability surrounding mealtimes; Volume limiting; Vomiting; Vomitus on pillow

Oral Phase Impairment: Abnormality in oral phase of swallow study; Choking before a swallow; Coughing before a swallow; Drooling; Food falls from mouth; Food pushed out of mouth; Gagging before a swallow; Inability to clear oral cavity; Incomplete lip closure; Lack of chewing; Lack of tongue action to form bolus; Long meals with little consumption; Nasal reflux; Piecemeal deglutition; Pooling in lateral sulci; Premature entry of bolus; Sialorrhea; Slow bolus formation; Weak suck resulting in inefficient nippling

Pharyngeal Phase Impairment: Abnormality in pharyngeal phase by swallow study; Altered head positions; Choking; Coughing; Delayed swallow; Food refusal; Gagging; Gurgly voice quality; Inadequate laryngeal elevation; Multiple swallows; Nasal reflux; Recurrent pulmonary infections; Unexplained fevers

Related Factors: *Congenital Deficits:* Behavioral feeding problems; Conditions with significant hypotonia; Congenital heart disease; Failure to thrive; History of tube feeding; Mechanical obstruction (e.g., edema, tracheostomy tube, tumor); Neuromuscular impairment (e.g., decreased or absent gag reflex, decreased strength or excursion of muscles involved in mastication, perceptual impairment, facial paralysis); Protein–energy malnutrition; Respiratory disorders; Self-injurious behavior; Upper airway anomalies

Neurological Problems: Achalasia; Acquired anatomic defects; Cerebral palsy; Cranial nerve involvement; Developmental delay; Esophageal defects; Gastroesophageal reflux disease; Laryngeal abnormalities; Laryngeal defects; Nasal defects; Nasopharyngeal cavity defects; Oropharynx abnormalities; Prematurity; Tracheal defects; Traumas; Traumatic head injury; Upper airway anomalies

Class 2: Digestion

None at this time

Class 3: Absorption

None at this time

Class 4: Metabolism

Risk for Unstable Blood Glucose Level

Definition: At risk for variation of blood glucose/sugar levels from the normal range that may compromise health

Risk Factors: Deficient knowledge of diabetes management (e.g., action plan); Developmental level; Dietary intake; Inadequate blood glucose monitoring; Lack of acceptance of diagnosis; Lack of adherence to diabetes management plan (e.g., adhering to action plan); Lack of diabetes management (e.g., action plan); Medication management; Mental health status; Physical activity level; Physical health status; Pregnancy; Rapid growth periods; Stress; Weight gain; Weight loss

Neonatal Jaundice

Definition: The yellow–orange tint of the neonate's skin and mucous membranes that occurs after 24 hours of life as a result of unconjugated bilirubin in the circulation

Defining Characteristics: Abnormal blood profile (e.g., hemolysis; total serum bilirubin >2mg/dL; total serum bilirubin in the high-risk range on age in hour-specific nomogram); Abnormal skin bruising; Yellow mucous membranes; Yellow–orange skin; Yellow sclera

Related Factors: Abnormal weight loss (>7–8% in breastfeeding newborn, 15% in term infant); Feeding pattern not well established; Infant experiences difficulty making the transition to extrauterine life; Neonate age 1–7 days; Stool (meconium) passage delayed

Risk for Neonatal Jaundice

Definition: At risk for the yellow–orange tint of the neonate's skin and mucous membranes that occurs after 24 hours of life as a result of unconjugated bilirubin in the circulation

Risk Factors: Abnormal weight loss (>7–8% in breastfeeding newborn, 15% in term infant); Feeding pattern not well established; Infant experiences difficulty making the transition to extrauterine life; Neonate aged 1–7 days; Prematurity; Stool (meconium) passage delayed

Risk for Impaired Liver Function

Definition: At risk for a decrease in liver function that may compromise health

Risk Factors: Hepatotoxic medications (e.g., acetaminophen, statins); HIV coinfection; Substance abuse (e.g., alcohol, cocaine); Viral infection (e.g., hepatitis A, hepatitis B, hepatitis C, Epstein–Barr);

Class 5: Hydration

Risk for Electrolyte Imbalance

Definition: At risk for change in serum electrolyte levels that may compromise health

Risk Factors: Deficient fluid volume; Diarrhea; Endocrine dysfunction; Excess fluid volume; Impaired regulatory mechanisms (e.g., diabetes insipidus, syndrome of inappropriate secretion of antidiuretic hormone); Renal dysfunction; Treatment-related side effects (e.g., medications, drains); Vomiting

Readiness for Enhanced Fluid Balance

Definition: A pattern of equilibrium between the fluid volume and chemical composition of body fluids that is sufficient for meeting physical needs and can be strengthened

Defining Characteristics: Expresses willingness to enhance fluid balance; Good tissue turgor; Intake adequate for daily needs; Moist mucous membranes; No evidence of edema; No excessive thirst; Risk for deficient fluid volume; Specific gravity within normal limits; Stable weight; Straw-colored urine; Urine output appropriate for intake

Deficient Fluid Volume

Definition: Decreased intravascular, interstitial, and/or intracellular fluid. This refers to dehydration, water loss alone without change in sodium

Defining Characteristics: Change in mental status; Decreased blood pressure; Decreased pulse pressure; Decreased pulse volume; Decreased skin turgor; Decreased tongue turgor; Decreased urine output; Decreased venous filling; Dry mucous membranes; Dry skin; Elevated hematocrit; Increased body temperature; Increased pulse rate; Increased urine concentration; Sudden weight loss (except in third spacing); Thirst; Weakness

Related Factors: Active fluid volume loss; Failure of regulatory mechanisms

Excess Fluid Volume

Definition: Increased isotonic fluid retention

Defining Characteristics: Adventitious breath sounds; Anasarca; Anxiety; Azotemia; Blood pressure changes; Change in mental status; Changes in respiratory pattern; Decreased hematocrit; Decreased hemoglobin; Dyspnea; Edema; Electrolyte imbalance; Increased central venous pressure; Intake exceeds output; Jugular vein distension; Oliguria; Orthopnea; Pleural effusion; Positive hepatojugular reflex; Pulmonary artery pressure changes; Pulmonary congestion; Restlessness; Specific gravity changes; S3 heart sound; Weight gain over short period of time

Related Factors: Compromised regulatory mechanism; Excess fluid intake; Excess sodium intake

Risk for Deficient Fluid Volume

Definition: At risk for experiencing decreased intravascular, interstitial, and/or intracellular fluid. This refers to a risk for dehydration, water loss alone without change in sodium

Risk Factors: Active fluid volume loss; Deficient knowledge; Deviations affecting absorption of fluids; Deviations affecting access of fluids; Deviations affecting intake of fluids; Excessive losses through normal routes (e.g., diarrhea); Extremes of age; Extremes of weight; Factors influencing fluid needs (e.g., hypermetabolic state); Failure of regulatory mechanisms; Loss of fluid through abnormal routes (e.g., indwelling tubes); Pharmaceutical agents (e.g., diuretics)

Risk for Imbalanced Fluid Volume

Definition: At risk for a decrease, increase, or rapid shift from one to the other of intravascular, interstitial, and/or intracellular fluid that may compromise health. This refers to body fluid loss, gain, or both

Risk Factors: Abdominal surgery; Ascites; Burns; Intestinal obstruction; Pancreatitis; Receiving apheresis; Sepsis; Traumatic injury (e.g., fractured hip)

DOMAIN 3: ELIMINATION AND EXCHANGE

Class 1: Urinary Function

Functional Urinary Incontinence

Definition: Inability of a usually continent person to reach the toilet in time to avoid unintentional loss of urine

Defining Characteristics: Able to completely empty bladder; Amount of time required to reach toilet exceeds length of time between sensing the urge to void and uncontrolled voiding; Loss of urine before reaching toilet; May be incontinent only in the early morning; Senses need to void

Related Factors: Altered environmental factors; Impaired cognition; Impaired vision; Neuromuscular limitations; Psychological factors; Weakened supporting pelvic structures

Overflow Urinary Incontinence

Definition: Involuntary loss of urine associated with overdistension of the bladder

Defining Characteristics: Bladder distension; High post-void residual volume; Observed involuntary leakage of small volumes of urine; Reports involuntary leakage of small volumes of urine

Related Factors: Bladder outlet obstruct; Detrusor external sphincter dyssynergia; Detrusor hypocontractility; Fecal impaction; Severe pelvic prolapse; Side effects of anticholinergic medications; Side effects of calcium channel blockers; Side effects of decongestant medications; Urethral obstruction

Reflex Urinary Incontinence

Definition: Involuntary loss of urine at somewhat predictable intervals when a specific bladder volume is reached

Defining Characteristics: Inability to voluntarily inhibit voiding; Inability to voluntarily initiate voiding; Incomplete emptying with lesion above pontine micturition center; Incomplete emptying with lesion above sacral micturition center; No sensation of bladder fullness; No sensation of urge to void; No sensation of voiding; Predictable pattern of voiding; Sensation of urgency without voluntary inhibition of bladder contraction; Sensations associated with full bladder (e.g., sweating, restlessness, abdominal discomfort)

Related Factors: Neurological impairment above level of pontine micturition center; Neurological impairment above level of sacral micturition center; Tissue damage (e.g., due to radiation cystitis, inflammatory bladder conditions, radical pelvic surgery)

Stress Urinary Incontinence

Definition: Sudden leakage of urine with activities that increase intra-abdominal pressure

Defining Characteristics: Observed involuntary leakage of small amounts of urine in the absence of detrusor contraction; Observed involuntary leakage of small amounts of urine in the absence of an overdistended bladder; Observed involuntary leakage of small amounts of urine on exertion; Observed involuntary leakage of small amounts of urine with coughing; Observed involuntary leakage of small amounts of urine with laughing; Observed involuntary leakage of small amounts of urine with sneezing; Reports involuntary leakage of small amounts of urine in the absence of detrusor contraction; Reports involuntary leakage of small amounts of urine in the absence of an overdistended bladder; Reports involuntary leakage of small amounts of urine on exertion; Reports involuntary leakage of small amounts of urine with coughing; Reports involuntary leakage of small amounts of urine with laughing; Reports involuntary leakage of small amounts of urine with sneezing

Related Factors: Degenerative changes in pelvic muscles; High intra-abdominal pressure; Intrinsic urethral sphincter deficiency; Weak pelvic muscles

Urge Urinary Incontinence

Definition: Involuntary passage of urine occurring soon after a strong sense of urgency to void

Defining Characteristics: Observed inability to reach toilet in time to avoid urine loss; Reports inability to reach toilet in time to avoid urine loss; Reports involuntary loss of urine with bladder contractions; Reports involuntary loss of urine with bladder spasms; Reports urinary urgency

Related Factors: Alcohol intake; Atrophic urethritis; Atrophic vaginitis; Bladder infection; Caffeine intake; Decreased bladder capacity; Detrusor hyperactivity with impaired bladder contractility; Diuretic use; Fecal impaction

Risk for Urge Urinary Incontinence

Definition: At risk for involuntary passage of urine occurring soon after a strong sensation of urgency to void

Risk Factors: Atrophic urethritis; Atrophic vaginitis; Effects of alcohol; Effects of caffeine; Effects of pharmaceutical agents; Detrusor hyperactivity with impaired bladder contractility; Fecal impaction; Impaired bladder contractility; Ineffective toileting habits; Involuntary sphincter relaxation; Small bladder capacity

Impaired Urinary Elimination

Definition: Dysfunction in urine elimination

Defining Characteristics: Dysuria; Frequency; Hesitancy; Incontinence; Nocturia; Retention; Urgency

Related Factors: Anatomic obstruction; Multiple causality; Sensory motor impairment; Urinary tract infection

Readiness for Enhanced Urinary Elimination

Definition: A pattern of urinary functions that is sufficient for meeting eliminatory needs and can be strengthened

Defining Characteristics: Amount of output is within normal limits; Expresses willingness to enhance urinary elimination; Fluid intake is adequate for daily needs; Positions self for emptying of bladder; Specific gravity is within normal limits; Urine is odorless; Urine is straw colored

Urinary Retention

Definition: Incomplete emptying of the bladder

Defining Characteristics: Absence of urine output; Bladder distension; Dribbling; Dysuria; Frequent voiding; Overflow incontinence; Residual urine; Sensation of bladder fullness; Small voiding

Related Factors: Blockage; High urethral pressure; Inhibition of reflex arc; Strong sphincter

Class 2: Gastrointestinal Function

Constipation

Definition: Decrease in normal frequency of defecation accompanied by difficult or incomplete passage of stool and/or passage of excessively hard, dry stool

Defining Characteristics: Abdominal pain; Abdominal tenderness with palpable muscle resistance; Abdominal tenderness without palpable muscle resistance; Anorexia; Atypical presentations in older adults (e.g., change in mental status, urinary incontinence, unexplained falls, elevated body temperature); Borborygmi; Bright red blood with stool; Change in bowel pattern; Decreased frequency; Decreased volume of stool; Distended abdomen; Feeling of rectal fullness; Feeling of rectal pressure; Generalized fatigue; Hard, formed stool; Headache; Hyperactive bowel sounds; Hypoactive bowel sounds; Increased abdominal pressure; Indigestion; Nausea; Oozing liquid stool; Pain with defecation; Palpable abdominal mass; Palpable rectal mass; Percussed abdominal dullness; Presence of soft, paste-like stool in rectum; Severe flatus; Straining with defecation; Unable to pass stool; Vomiting

Related Factors: *Functional:* Abdominal muscle weakness; Habitual ignoring of urge to defecate; Inadequate toileting (e.g., timeliness, positioning for defecation, privacy); Insufficient physical activity; Irregular defecation habits; Recent environmental changes
Psychological: Depression; Emotional stress; Mental confusion
Pharmacological: Aluminum-containing antacids; Anticholinergics; Anticonvulsants; Antidepressants; Antilipemic agents; Bismuth salts; Calcium carbonate; Calcium channel blockers; Diuretics; Iron salts; Laxative abuse; Nonsteroidal anti-inflammatory agents; Opiates; Phenothiazines; Sedatives; Sympathomimetics
Mechanical: Electrolyte imbalance; Hemorrhoids; Hirschsprung's disease; Neurological impairment; Obesity; Postsurgical obstruction; Pregnancy; Prostate enlargement; Rectal abscess; Rectal anal fissures; Rectal anal stricture; Rectal prolapse; Rectal ulcer; Rectocele; Tumors
Physiological: Change in eating patterns; Change in usual foods; Decreased motility of gastrointestinal tract; Dehydration; Inadequate dentition; Inadequate oral hygiene; Insufficient fiber intake; Insufficient fluid intake; Poor eating habits

Perceived Constipation

Definition: Self-diagnosis of constipation combined with abuse of laxatives, enemas, and/or suppositories to ensure a daily bowel movement

Defining Characteristics: Expectation of a daily bowel movement; Expectation of passage of stool at the same time every day; Overuse of enemas; Overuse of laxatives; Overuse of suppositories

Related Factors: Cultural health beliefs; Family health beliefs; Faulty appraisal; Impaired thought processes

Risk for Constipation

Definition: At risk for a decrease in normal frequency of defecation accompanied by difficult or incomplete passage of stool and/or passage of excessively hard, dry stool

Risk Factors: *Functional:* Abdominal muscle weakness; Habitual ignoring of urge to defecate; Inadequate toileting (e.g., timeliness, positioning for defecation, privacy); Insufficient physical activity; Irregular defecation habits; Recent environmental changes
Psychological: Depression; Emotional stress; Mental confusion
Physiological: Change in usual eating patterns; Change in usual foods; Decreased motility of gastrointestinal tract; Dehydration; Inadequate dentition; Inadequate oral hygiene; Insufficient fiber intake; Insufficient fluid intake; Poor eating habits
Pharmacological: Aluminum-containing antacids; Anticholinergics; Anticonvulsants; Antidepressants; Antilipemic agents; Bismuth salts; Calcium carbonate; Calcium channel blockers; Diuretics; Iron salts; Laxative abuse; Nonsteroidal anti-inflammatory agents; Opiates; Phenothiazines; Sedatives; Sympathomimetics
Mechanical: Electrolyte imbalance; Hemorrhoids; Hirschsprung's disease; Neurological impairment; Obesity; Postsurgical obstruction; Pregnancy; Prostate enlargement; Rectal abscess; Rectal anal fissures; Rectal anal stricture; Rectal prolapse; Rectal ulcer; Rectocele; Tumors

Diarrhea

Definition: Passage of loose, unformed stools

Defining Characteristics: Abdominal pain; At least three loose liquid stools per day; Cramping; Hyperactive bowel sounds; Urgency

Related Factors: *Psychological:* Anxiety; High stress levels
Situational: Adverse effects of pharmaceutical agents; Alcohol abuse; Contaminants; Laxative abuse; Radiation; Toxins; Travel; Tube feedings
Physiological: Infectious processes; Inflammation; Irritation; Malabsorption; Parasites

Dysfunctional Gastrointestinal Motility

Definition: Increased, decreased, ineffective, or lack of peristaltic activity within the gastrointestinal system

Defining Characteristics: Abdominal cramping; Abdominal distension; Abdominal pain; Absence of flatus; Accelerated gastric emptying; Bile-colored gastric residual; Change in bowel sounds (e.g., absent, hypoactive, hyperactive); Diarrhea; Difficulty passing stool; Dry stool; Hard stool; Increased gastric residual; Nausea; Regurgitation; Vomiting

Related Factors: Aging; Anxiety; Enteral feedings; Food intolerance (e.g., gluten, lactose); Immobility; Ingestion of contaminates (e.g., food, water); Malnutrition; Pharmaceutical agents (e.g., narcotics/opiates, laxatives, antibiotics, anesthesia); Prematurity; Sedentary lifestyle; Surgery

Risk For Dysfunctional Gastrointestinal Motility

Definition: At risk for increased, decreased, ineffective, or lack of peristaltic activity within the gastrointestinal system

Risk Factors: Abdominal surgery; Aging; Anxiety; Change in food; Change in water; Decreased gastrointestinal circulation; Diabetes mellitus; Food intolerance (e.g., gluten, lactose); Gastroesophageal reflux disease (GERD); Immobility; Infection (e.g., bacterial, parasitic, viral); Pharmaceutical agents (e.g., antibiotics, laxatives, narcotics/opiates, proton pump inhibitors); Prematurity; Sedentary lifestyle; Stress; Unsanitary food preparation

Bowel Incontinence

Definition: Change in normal bowel habits characterized by involuntary passage of stool

Defining Characteristics: Constant dribbling of soft stool; Fecal odor; Fecal staining of bedding; Fecal staining of clothing; Inability to delay defecation; Inability to recognize urge to defecate; Inattention to urge to defecate; Recognizes rectal fullness but reports inability to expel formed stool; Red perianal skin; Self-report of inability to recognize rectal fullness; Urgency

Related Factors: Abnormally high abdominal pressure; Abnormally high intestinal pressure; Chronic diarrhea; Colorectal lesions; Dietary habits; Environmental factors (e.g., inaccessible bathroom); General decline in muscle tone; Immobility; Impaction; Impaired cognition; Impaired reservoir capacity; Incomplete emptying of bowel; Laxative abuse; Loss of rectal sphincter control; Lower motor nerve damage; Medications; Rectal sphincter abnormality; Stress; Toileting self-care deficit; Upper motor nerve damage

Class 3: Integumentary Function

None at this time

Class 4: Respiratory Function

Impaired Gas Exchange

Definition: Excess or deficit in oxygenation and/or carbon dioxide elimination at the alveolar–capillary membrane

Defining Characteristics: Abnormal arterial blood gases; Abnormal arterial pH; Abnormal breathing (e.g., rate, rhythm, depth); Abnormal skin color (e.g., pale, dusky); Confusion; Cyanosis (in neonates only); Decreased carbon dioxide; Diaphoresis; Dyspnea; Headache upon awakening; Hypercapnia; Hypoxemia; Hypoxia; Irritability; Nasal flaring; Restlessness; Somnolence; Tachycardia; Visual disturbances

Related Factors: Alveolar–capillary membrane changes; Ventilation–perfusion imbalance

DOMAIN 4: ACTIVITY/REST

Class 1: Sleep/Rest

Insomnia

Definition: A disruption in amount and quality of sleep that impairs functioning

Defining Characteristics: Increased absenteeism (e.g., work/school); Observed changes in affect; Observed lack of energy; Reports changes in mood; Reports decreased health status; Reports decreased quality of life; Reports difficulty concentrating; Reports difficulty falling asleep; Reports difficulty staying asleep; Reports dissatisfaction with sleep (current); Reports increased accidents; Reports lack of energy; Reports nonrestorative sleep; Reports sleep disturbances that produce next-day consequences; Reports waking up too early

Related Factors: Activity pattern (e.g., timing, amount); Anxiety; Depression; Environmental factors (e.g., ambient noise, daylight/darkness exposure, ambient temperature/humidity, unfamiliar setting); Fear; Frequent daytime naps; Gender-related hormonal shifts; Grief; Impairment of normal sleep pattern (e.g., travel, shift work); Inadequate sleep hygiene (current); Intake of alcohol; Intake of stimulants; Interrupted sleep; Parental responsibilities; Pharmaceutical agents; Physical discomfort (e.g., pain, shortness of breath, cough, gastroesophageal reflux, nausea, incontinence/urgency); Stress (e.g., ruminative pre-sleep pattern)

Sleep Deprivation

Definition: Prolonged periods of time without sleep (sustained natural, periodic suspension of relative consciousness)

Defining Characteristics: Acute confusion; Agitation; Anxiety; Apathy; Combativeness; Daytime drowsiness; Decreased ability to function; Fatigue; Fleeting nystagmus; Hallucinations; Hand tremors; Heightened pain sensitivity; Inability to concentrate; Irritability; Lethargy; Listlessness; Malaise; Perceptual disorders (e.g., disturbed body sensation, delusions, feeling afloat); Restlessness; Slowed reaction; Transient paranoia;

Related Factors: Aging-related sleep stage shifts; Dementia; Familial sleep paralysis; Idiopathic central nervous system hypersomnolence; Inadequate daytime activity; Narcolepsy; Nightmares; Nonsleep-inducing parenting practices; Periodic limb movement (e.g., restless leg syndrome, nocturnal myoclonus); Prolonged discomfort (e.g., physical, psychological); Prolonged use of dietary antisoporifics; Prolonged use of pharmacological agents; Sleep apnea; Sleep-related enuresis; Sleep-related painful erections; Sleep terror; Sleep walking; Sundowner's syndrome Sustained circadian asynchrony; Sustained environmental stimulation; Sustained inadequate sleep hygiene; Sustained uncomfortable sleep environment

Readiness for Enhanced Sleep

Definition: A pattern of natural, periodic suspension of consciousness that provides adequate rest, sustains a desired lifestyle, and can be strengthened

Defining Characteristics: Amount of sleep is congruent with developmental needs; Expresses willingness to enhance sleep; Follows sleep routines that promote sleep habits; Occasional use of pharmaceutical agents to induce sleep; Reports being rested after sleep

Disturbed Sleep Pattern

Definition: Time-limited interruptions of sleep amount and quality due to external factors

Defining Characteristics: Change in normal sleep pattern; Decreased ability to function; Dissatisfaction with sleep; Reports being awakened; Reports no difficulty falling asleep; Reports not feeling well rested

Related Factors: Ambient humidity; Ambient temperature; Caregiving responsibilities; Change in daylight–darkness exposure; Interruptions (e.g., for therapeutics, monitoring, lab tests); Lack of sleep control; Lack of sleep privacy; Lighting; Noise; Noxious odors; Physical restraint; Sleep partner; Unfamiliar sleep furnishings

Class 2: Activity/Exercise

Risk for Disuse Syndrome

Definition: At risk for deterioration of body systems as the result of prescribed or unavoidable musculoskeletal inactivity

Risk Factors: Altered level of consciousness; Mechanical immobilization; Paralysis; Prescribed immobilization; Severe pain
Note: Complications from immobility can include pressure ulcer, constipation, stasis of pulmonary secretions, thrombosis, urinary tract infection and/or retention, decreased strength or endurance, orthostatic hypotension, decreased range of joint motion, disorientation, body-image disturbance, and powerlessness.

Impaired Bed Mobility

Definition: Limitation of independent movement from one bed position to another

Defining Characteristics: Impaired ability to move from long sitting to supine; Impaired ability to move from prone to supine; Impaired ability to move from sitting to supine; Impaired ability to move from supine to long sitting; Impaired ability to move from supine to prone; Impaired ability to move from supine to sitting; Impaired ability to reposition self in bed; Impaired ability to turn from side to side

Related Factors: Cognitive impairment; Deconditioning; Deficient knowledge; Environmental constraints (e.g., bed size, bed type, treatment equipment, restraints); Insufficient muscle strength; Musculoskeletal impairment; Neuromuscular impairment; Obesity; Pain; Sedating pharmaceutical agents
Note: Specify level of independence using a standardized functional scale.

Impaired Physical Mobility

Definition: Limitation in independent, purposeful physical movement of the body or of one or more extremities

Defining Characteristics: Decreased reaction time; Difficulty turning; Engages in substitutions for movement (e.g., increased attention to other's activity, controlling behavior, focus on pre-illness disability/activity); Exertional dyspnea; Gait changes; Jerky movements; Limited ability to perform fine motor skills; Limited ability to perform gross motor skills; Limited range of motion; Movement-induced tremor; Postural instability; Slowed movement; Uncoordinated movements

Related Factors: Activity intolerance; Altered cellular metabolism; Anxiety; Body mass index above 75th age-appropriate percentile; Cognitive impairment; Contractures; Cultural beliefs regarding age-appropriate activity; Deconditioning; Decreased endurance; Decreased muscle control; Decreased muscle mass; Decreased muscle strength; Deficient knowledge regarding value of physical activity; Depressive mood state; Developmental delay; Discomfort; Disuse; Joint stiffness; Lack of environmental supports (e.g., physical or social); Limited cardiovascular endurance; Loss of integrity of bone structures; Malnutrition; Musculoskeletal impairment; Neuromuscular impairment; Pain; Pharmaceutical agents; Prescribed movement restrictions; Reluctance to initiate movement; Sedentary lifestyle; Sensoriperceptual impairments
Note: Specify level of independence using a standardized functional scale.

Impaired Wheelchair Mobility

Definition: Limitation of independent operation of wheelchair within environment

Defining Characteristics: Impaired ability to operate manual wheelchair on a decline; Impaired ability to operate manual wheelchair on an incline; Impaired ability to operate manual wheelchair on curbs; Impaired ability to operate manual wheelchair on even surface; Impaired ability to operate manual wheelchair on uneven surface; Impaired ability to operate power wheelchair on a decline; Impaired ability to operate power wheelchair on an incline; Impaired ability to operate power wheelchair on curbs; Impaired ability to operate power wheelchair on even surface; Impaired ability to operate power wheelchair on uneven surface

Related Factors: Cognitive impairment; Deconditioning; Deficient knowledge; Depressed mood; Environmental constraints (e.g., stairs, inclines, uneven surfaces, unsafe obstacles, distances, lack of assistive devices or person, wheelchair type); Impaired vision; Insufficient muscle strength; Limited endurance; Musculoskeletal impairment (e.g., contractures); Neuromuscular impairment; Obesity; Pain
Note: Specify level of independence using a standardized functional scale.

Impaired Transfer Ability

Definition: Limitation of independent movement between two nearby surfaces

Defining Characteristics: Inability to transfer between uneven levels; Inability to transfer from bed to chair; Inability to transfer from bed to standing; Inability to transfer from car to chair; Inability to transfer from chair to bed; Inability to transfer from chair to car; Inability to transfer from chair to floor; Inability to transfer from chair to standing; Inability to transfer from floor to chair; Inability to transfer from floor to standing; Inability to transfer from standing to bed; Inability to transfer from standing to chair; Inability to transfer from standing to floor; Inability to transfer in or out of bath tub; Inability to transfer in or out of shower; Inability to transfer on or off a commode; Inability to transfer on or off a toilet

Related Factors: Cognitive impairment; Deconditioning; Deficient knowledge; Environmental constraints (e.g., bed height, inadequate space, wheelchair type, treatment equipment, restraints); Impaired balance; Impaired vision; Insufficient muscle strength; Musculoskeletal impairment (e.g., contractures); Neuromuscular impairment; Obesity; Pain
Note: Specify level of independence using a standardized functional scale.

Impaired Walking

Definition: Limitation of independent movement within the environment on foot

Defining Characteristics: Impaired ability to climb stairs; Impaired ability to navigate curbs; Impaired ability to walk on a decline; Impaired ability to walk on an incline; Impaired ability to walk on uneven surfaces; Impaired ability to walk required distances

Related Factors: Cognitive impairment; Deconditioning; Depressed mood; Environmental constraints (e.g., stairs, inclines, uneven surfaces, unsafe obstacles, distances, lack of assistive devices or person, restraints); Fear of falling; Impaired balance; Impaired vision; Insufficient muscle strength; Lack of knowledge; Limited endurance; Musculoskeletal impairment (e.g., contractures); Neuromuscular impairment; Obesity; Pain
Note: Specify level of independence using a standardized functional scale.

Class 3: Energy Balance

Disturbed Energy Field

Definition: Disruption of the flow of energy surrounding a person's being that results in disharmony of the body, mind, and/or spirit

Defining Characteristics: Perceptions of changes in patterns of energy flow, such as: Movement (wave, spike, tingling, dense, flowing); Sounds (tone, words); Temperature change (warmth, coolness); Visual changes (image, color); Disruption of the field (deficit, hole, spike, bulge, obstruction, congestion, diminished flow in energy field)

Related Factors: Slowing or blocking of energy flows secondary to:
Maturational Factors: Age-related developmental crisis; Age-related developmental difficulties
Pathophysiological Factors: Illness; Injury; Pregnancy
Situational Factors: Anxiety; Fear; Grieving; Pain
Treatment-Related Factors: Chemotherapy; Immobility; Labor and delivery; Perioperative experience

Fatigue

Definition: An overwhelming sustained sense of exhaustion and decreased capacity for physical and mental work at the usual level

Defining Characteristics: Compromised concentration; Compromised libido; Decreased performance; Disinterest in surroundings; Drowsy; Increase in physical complaints; Increase in rest requirements; Introspection; Lack of energy; Lethargic; Listless; Perceived need for additional energy to accomplish routine tasks; Reports an overwhelming lack of energy; Reports an unremitting lack of energy; Reports feeling tired; Reports guilt over not keeping up with responsibilities; Reports inability to maintain usual level of physical activity; Reports inability to maintain usual routines; Reports inability to restore energy even after sleep

Related Factors:
Psychological: Anxiety; Depression; Reports boring lifestyle; Stress
Physiological: Anemia; Disease states; Increased physical exertion; Malnutrition; Poor physical condition; Pregnancy; Sleep deprivation
Environmental: Humidity; Lights; Noise; Temperature
Situational: Negative life events; Occupation

Wandering

Definition: Meandering, aimless, or repetitive locomotion that exposes the individual to harm; frequently incongruent with boundaries, limits, or obstacles

Defining Characteristics: Continuous movement from place to place; Frequent movement from place to place; Fretful locomotion; Getting lost; Haphazard locomotion; Hyperactivity; Inability to locate significant landmarks in a familiar setting; Locomotion into unauthorized/private spaces; Locomotion resulting in unintended leaving of a premises; Locomotion that cannot be easily dissuaded; Long periods of locomotion without an apparent destination; Pacing; Periods of locomotion interspersed with periods of nonlocomotion (e.g., sitting, standing, sleeping); Persistent locomotion in search of something; Scanning behaviors; Searching behaviors; Shadowing a caregiver's locomotion; Trespassing

Related Factors: Cognitive impairment (e.g., memory and recall deficits, disorientation, poor visuoconstructive or visuospatial ability, language defects); Cortical atrophy; Emotional state (e.g., frustration, anxiety, boredom, depression, agitation); Overstimulating environment; Physiological state or need (e.g., hunger, thirst, pain, urination, constipation); Premorbid behavior (e.g., outgoing, sociable personality, premorbid dementia); Sedation; Separation from familiar environment; Time of day

Class 4: Cardiovascular/Pulmonary Responses

Activity Intolerance

Definition: Insufficient physiological or psychological energy to endure or complete required or desired daily activities

Defining Characteristics: Abnormal blood pressure response to activity; Abnormal heart rate response to activity; EKG changes reflecting arrhythmias; EKG changes reflecting ischemia; Exertional discomfort; Exertional dyspnea; Reports fatigue; Reports feeling weak

Related Factors: Bed rest; Generalized weakness; Imbalance between oxygen supply/demand; Immobility; Sedentary lifestyle

Risk for Activity Intolerance

Definition: At risk for experiencing insufficient physiological or psychological energy to endure or complete required or desired daily activities

Risk Factors: Circulatory problems; Deconditioned status; History of previous activity intolerance; Inexperience with an activity; Respiratory problems

Ineffective Breathing Pattern

Definition: Inspiration and/or expiration that does not provide adequate ventilation

Defining Characteristics: Alterations in depth of breathing; Altered chest excursion; Assumption of three-point position; Bradypnea; Decreased expiratory pressure; Decreased inspiratory pressure; Decreased minute ventilation; Decreased vital capacity; Dyspnea; Increased anterior–posterior diameter; Nasal flaring; Orthopnea; Prolonged expiration phase; Pursed-lip breathing; Tachypnea; Use of accessory muscles to breathe

Related Factors: Anxiety; Body position; Bony deformity; Chest wall deformity; Fatigue; Hyperventilation; Hypoventilation syndrome; Musculoskeletal impairment; Neurological damage; Neurological immaturity; Neuromuscular dysfunction; Obesity; Pain; Respiratory muscle fatigue; Spinal cord injury

Decreased Cardiac Output

Definition: Inadequate blood pumped by the heart to meet the metabolic demands of the body

Defining Characteristics:
Altered Heart Rate/Rhythm: Arrhythmias; Bradycardia; EKG changes; Palpitations; Tachycardia
Altered Preload: Decreased central venous pressure (CVP); Decreased pulmonary artery wedge pressure (PAWP); Edema; Fatigue; Increased CVP; Increased PAWP; Jugular vein distension; Murmurs; Weight gain
Altered Afterload: Clammy skin; Decreased peripheral pulses; Decreased pulmonary vascular resistance (PVR); Decreased systemic vascular resistance (SVR); Dyspnea; Increased PVR; Increased SVR; Oliguria; Prolonged capillary refill; Skin color changes; Variations in blood pressure readings
Altered Contractility: Cough; Crackles; Decreased cardiac index; Decreased ejection fraction; Decreased left ventricular stroke work index (LVSWI); Decreased stroke volume index (SVI); Orthopnea; Paroxysmal nocturnal dyspnea; S3 sounds; S4 sounds;
Behavioral/Emotional: Anxiety; Restlessness
Related Factors: Altered afterload; Altered contractility; Altered heart rate; Altered preload; Altered rhythm; Altered stroke volume

Risk for Ineffective Gastrointestinal Perfusion

Definition: At risk for decrease in gastrointestinal circulation that may compromise health

Risk Factors: Abdominal aortic aneurysm; Abdominal compartment syndrome; Abnormal partial thromboplastin time; Abnormal prothrombin time; Acute gastrointestinal hemorrhage; Age >60 years; Anemia; Coagulopathy (e.g., sickle cell anemia); Diabetes mellitus; Disseminated intravascular coagulation; Female gender; Gastroesophageal varices; Gastrointestinal disease (e.g., duodenal or gastric ulcer, ischemic colitis, ischemic pancreatitis); Hemodynamic instability; Liver dysfunction; Myocardial infarction; Poor left ventricular performance; Renal failure; Smoking; Stroke; Trauma; Treatment-related side effects (e.g., cardiopulmonary bypass, pharmaceutical agents, gastric surgery); Vascular disease (e.g., peripheral vascular disease, aortoiliac occlusive disease)

Note: This diagnosis formerly held the label Ineffective Tissue Perfusion (Specify type: Gastrointestinal).

Risk for Ineffective Renal Perfusion

Definition: At risk for a decrease in blood circulation to the kidney that may compromise health

Risk Factors: Abdominal compartment syndrome; Advanced age; Bilateral cortical necrosis; Burns; Cardiac surgery; Cardiopulmonary bypass; Diabetes mellitus; Exposure to nephrotoxins; Female gender; Glomerulonephritis; Hypertension; Hypovolemia; Hypoxemia; Hypoxia; Infection (e.g., sepsis, localized infection); Interstitial nephritis; Malignancy; Malignant hypertension; Metabolic acidosis; Multitrauma; Polynephritis; Renal artery stenosis; Renal disease (polycystic kidney); Smoking; Substance abuse; Systemic inflammatory response syndrome; Treatment-related side effects (e.g., pharmaceutical agents, surgery); Vascular embolism; Vasculitis

Note: This diagnosis formerly held the label Ineffective Tissue Perfusion (Specify type: Renal).

Impaired Spontaneous Ventilation

Definition: Decreased energy reserves resulting in an inability to maintain independent breathing that is adequate to support life

Defining Characteristics: Decreased cooperation; Decreased Po_2; Decreased Sao_2; Decreased tidal volume; Dyspnea; Increased heart rate; Increased metabolic rate; Increased Pco_2; Increased restlessness; Increased use of accessory muscles; Reports apprehension

Related Factors: Metabolic factors; Respiratory muscle fatigue

Ineffective Peripheral Tissue Perfusion

Definition: Decrease in blood circulation to the periphery that may compromise health

Defining Characteristics: Absent pulses; Altered motor function; Altered skin characteristics (color, elasticity, hair, moisture, nails, sensation, temperature); Ankle-brachial index < 0.90; Blood pressure changes in extremities; Capillary refill time > 3 seconds; Claudication; Color does not return to leg on lowering it; Delayed peripheral wound healing; Diminished pulses; Edema; Extremity pain; Femoral bruit; Shorter total distances achieved in the six-minute walk test; Shorter pain free distances achieved in the six-minute walk test; Paresthesia; Skin color pale on elevation

Related Factors: Deficient knowledge of aggravating factors (e.g., smoking, sedentary lifestyle, trauma, obesity, salt intake, immobility); Deficient knowledge of disease process (e.g., diabetes, hyperlipidemia); Diabetes mellitus; Hypertension; Sedentary lifestyle; Smoking

Note: This diagnosis formerly held the label Ineffective Tissue Perfusion (Specify type: Peripheral).

Risk for Decreased Cardiac Tissue Perfusion

Definition: At risk for a decrease in cardiac (coronary) circulation that may compromise health

Risk Factors: Birth control pills; Cardiac surgery; Cardiac tamponade; Coronary artery spasm; Deficient knowledge of modifiable risk factors (e.g., smoking, sedentary lifestyle, obesity); Diabetes mellitus; Elevated C-reactive protein; Family history of coronary artery disease; Hyperlipidemia; Hypertension; Hypovolemia; Hypoxemia; Hypoxia; Substance abuse

Note: This diagnosis formerly held the label Ineffective Tissue Perfusion (Specify type: Cardiopulmonary).

Risk for Ineffective Cerebral Tissue Perfusion

Definition: At risk for a decrease in cerebral tissue circulation that may compromise health

Risk Factors: Abnormal partial thromboplastin time; Abnormal prothrombin time; Akinetic left ventricular segment; Aortic atherosclerosis; Arterial dissection; Atrial fibrillation; Atrial myxoma; Brain tumor; Carotid stenosis; Cerebral aneurysm; Coagulopathy (e.g., sickle cell anemia); Dilated cardiomyopathy; Disseminated intravascular coagulation; Embolism; Head trauma; Hypercholesterolemia; Hypertension; Infective endocarditis; Mechanical prosthetic valve; Mitral stenosis; Neoplasm of the brain; Recent myocardial infarction; Sick sinus syndrome; Substance abuse; Thrombolytic therapy; Treatment-related side effects (cardiopulmonary bypass, pharmaceutical agents)

Note: This diagnosis formerly held the label Ineffective Tissue Perfusion (Specify type: Cerebral).

Risk for Ineffective Peripheral Tissue Perfusion

Definition: At risk for a decrease in blood circulation to the periphery that may compromise health

Risk Factors: Age >60 years; Deficient knowledge of aggravating factors (e.g., smoking, sedentary lifestyle, trauma, obesity, salt intake, immobility); Deficient knowledge of disease process (e.g., diabetes, hyperlipidemia); Diabetes mellitus; Endovascular procedures; Hypertension; Sedentary lifestyle; Smoking

Note: This diagnosis formerly held the label Ineffective Tissue Perfusion (Specify type: Peripheral).

Dysfunctional Ventilatory Weaning Response

Definition: Inability to adjust to lowered levels of mechanical ventilator support that interrupts and prolongs the weaning process

Defining Characteristics:

Mild: Breathing discomfort; Fatigue; Increased concentration on breathing; Queries about possible machine malfunction; Reports feelings of increased need for oxygen; Restlessness; Slight increase of respiratory rate from baseline; Warmth

Moderate: Baseline increase in respiratory rate (<5 breaths/min); Color changes; Decreased air entry on auscultation; Diaphoresis; Hypervigilance to activities; Inability to cooperate; Inability to respond to coaching; Minimal respiratory accessory muscle use; Pale; Reports apprehension; Slight cyanosis; Slight increase from baseline blood pressure (<20 mmHg); Slight increase from baseline heart rate (<20 beats/min); Wide-eyed look

Severe: Adventitious breath sounds; Agitation; Asynchronized breathing with the ventilator; Audible airway secretions; Cyanosis; Decreased level of consciousness; Deterioration in arterial blood gases from current baseline; Full respiratory accessory muscle use; Gasping breaths; Increase from baseline blood pressure (≥20 mmHg); Increase from baseline heart rate (≥20 breaths/min); Paradoxical abdominal breathing; Profuse diaphoresis; Respiratory rate increases significantly from baseline; Shallow breaths

Related Factors:

Physiological: Inadequate nutrition; Ineffective airway clearance; Sleep pattern disturbance; Uncontrolled pain

Psychological: Anxiety; Decreased motivation; Decreased self-esteem; Deficient knowledge of the weaning process; Fear; Hopelessness; Insufficient trust in healthcare providers; Perceived inefficacy about ability to wean; Powerlessness

Situational: Adverse environment (e.g., noisy, active environment, negative events in the room, low nurse:patient ratio, unfamiliar nursing staff); History of multiple unsuccessful weaning attempts; History of ventilator dependence >4 days; Inadequate social support; Inappropriate pacing of diminished ventilator support; Uncontrolled episodic energy demands

Class 5: Self-Care

Impaired Home Maintenance

Definition: Inability to independently maintain a safe growth-promoting immediate environment

Defining Characteristics:

Objective: Disorderly surroundings; Inappropriate household temperature; Insufficient clothes; Insufficient linen; Lack of clothes; Lack of linen; Lack of necessary equipment; Offensive odors; Overtaxed family members; Presence of vermin; Repeated unhygienic disorders; Repeated unhygienic infections; Unavailable cooking equipment; Unclean surroundings

Subjective: Household members report difficulty in maintaining their home in a comfortable fashion; Household members report financial crises; Household members report outstanding debts; Household members request assistance with home maintenance

Related Factors: Deficient knowledge; Disease; Illness; Impaired functioning; Inadequate support systems; Injury; Insufficient family organization; Insufficient family planning; Insufficient finances; Lack of role modeling; Unfamiliarity with neighborhood resources

Readiness for Enhanced Self-Care

Definition: A pattern of performing activities for oneself that helps to meet health-related goals and can be strengthened

Defining Characteristics: Expresses desire to enhance independence in maintaining health; Expresses desire to enhance independence in maintaining life; Expresses desire to enhance independence in maintaining personal development; Expresses desire to enhance independence in maintaining well-being; Expresses desire to enhance knowledge of strategies for self-care; Expresses desire to enhance responsibility for self-care; Expresses desire to enhance self-care

Bathing Self-Care Deficit

Definition: Impaired ability to perform or complete bathing activities for self

Defining Characteristics: Inability to access bathroom; Inability to dry body; Inability to get bath supplies; Inability to obtain water source; Inability to regulate bath water; Inability to wash body

Related Factors: Cognitive impairment; Decreased motivation; Environmental barriers; Inability to perceive body part; Inability to perceive spatial relationship; Musculoskeletal impairment; Neuromuscular impairment; Pain; Perceptual impairment; Severe anxiety; Weakness

Note: Specify level of independence using a standardized functional scale.

*Note: This diagnosis formerly held the label **Bathing/Hygiene Self-care Deficit.***

Dressing Self-Care Deficit

Definition: Impaired ability to perform or complete dressing activities for self

Defining Characteristics: Impaired ability to fasten clothing; Impaired ability to obtain clothing; Impaired ability to put on necessary items of clothing; Impaired ability to put on shoes; Impaired ability to put on socks; Impaired ability to take off necessary items of clothing; Impaired ability to take off shoes; Impaired ability to take off socks; Inability to choose clothing; Inability to maintain appearance at a satisfactory level; Inability to pick up clothing; Inability to put clothing on lower body; Inability to put clothing on upper body; Inability to put on shoes; Inability to put on socks; Inability to remove clothes; Inability to remove shoes; Inability to remove socks; Inability to use assistive devices; Inability to use zippers

Related Factors: Cognitive impairment; Decreased motivation; Discomfort; Environmental barriers; Fatigue; Musculoskeletal impairment; Neuromuscular impairment; Pain; Perceptual impairment; Severe anxiety; Weakness

Note: Specify level of independence using a standardized functional scale.

*Note: This diagnosis formerly held the label **Dressing/Grooming Self-care Deficit.***

Feeding Self-Care Deficit

Definition: Impaired ability to perform or complete self-feeding activities

Defining Characteristics: Inability to bring food from a receptacle to the mouth; Inability to chew food; Inability to complete a meal; Inability to get food onto utensil; Inability to handle utensils; Inability to ingest food in a socially acceptable manner; Inability to ingest food safely; Inability to ingest sufficient food; Inability to manipulate food in the mouth; Inability to open containers; Inability to pick up cup or glass; Inability to prepare food for ingestion; Inability to swallow food; Inability to use assistive device

Related Factors: Cognitive impairment; Decreased motivation; Discomfort; Environmental barriers; Fatigue; Musculoskeletal impairment; Neuromuscular impairment; Pain; Perceptual impairment; Severe anxiety; Weakness

Note: Specify level of independence using a standardized functional scale.

Toileting Self-Care Deficit

Definition: Impaired ability to perform or complete toileting activities for self

Defining Characteristics: Inability to carry out proper toilet hygiene; Inability to flush toilet or commode; Inability to get to toilet or commode; Inability to manipulate clothing for toileting; Inability to rise from toilet or commode; Inability to sit on toilet or commode

Related Factors: Cognitive impairment; Decreased motivation; Environmental barriers; Fatigue; Impaired mobility status; Impaired transfer ability; Musculoskeletal impairment; Neuromuscular impairment; Pain; Perceptual impairment; Severe anxiety; Weakness

Note: Specify level of independence using a standardized functional scale.

Self-Neglect

Definition: A constellation of culturally framed behaviors involving one or more self-care activities in which there is a failure to maintain a socially accepted standard of health and well-being (Gibbons, Lauder & Ludwick, 2006)

Defining Characteristics: Inadequate environmental hygiene; Inadequate personal hygiene; Nonadherence to health activities

Related Factors: Capgras syndrome; Cognitive impairment (e.g., dementia); Depression; Executive processing ability; Fear of institutionalization; Frontal lobe dysfunction; Functional impairment; Learning disability; Lifestyle choice; Maintaining control; Major life stressor; Malingering; Obsessive–compulsive disorder; Paranoid personality disorders; Schizotypal personality disorders; Substance abuse

DOMAIN 5: PERCEPTION/COGNITION

Class 1: Attention

Unilateral Neglect

Definition: Impairment in sensory and motor response, mental representation, and spatial attention of the body, and the corresponding environment, characterized by inattention to one side and overattention to the opposite side. Left-side neglect is more severe and persistent than right-side neglect

Defining Characteristics: Appears unaware of positioning of neglected limb; Difficulty remembering details of internally represented familiar scenes that are on the neglected side; Displacement of sounds to the non-neglected side; Distortion of drawing on the half of the page on the neglected side; Failure to cancel lines on the half of the page on the neglected side; Failure to dress neglected side; Failure to eat food from portion of the plate on the neglected side; Failure to groom neglected side; Failure to move eyes in the neglected hemispace despite being aware of a stimulus in that space; Failure to move head in the neglected hemispace despite being aware of a stimulus in that space; Failure to move limbs in the neglected hemispace despite being aware of a stimulus in that space; Failure to move trunk in the neglected hemispace despite being aware of a stimulus in that space; Failure to notice people approaching from the neglected side; Lack of safety precautions with regard to the neglected side; Marked deviation* of the eyes to the non-neglected side to stimuli and activities on that side; Marked deviation* of the head to the non-neglected side to stimuli and activities on that side; Marked deviation* of the trunk to the non-neglected side to stimuli and activities on that side; Omission of drawing on the half of the page on the neglected side; Perseveration of visual motor tasks on the non-neglected side; Substitution of letters to form alternative words that are similar to the original in length when reading; Transfer of pain sensation to the non-neglected side; Use of only vertical half of page when writing

Related Factors: Brain injury from cerebrovascular problems; Brain injury from neurological illness; Brain injury from trauma; Brain injury from tumor; Hemianopsia; Left hemiplegia from cerebrovascular accident (CVA) of the right hemisphere;

As if drawn magnetically to stimuli and activities on that side.

Class 2: Orientation

Impaired Environmental Interpretation Syndrome

Definition: Consistent lack of orientation to person, place, time, or circumstances over more than 3–6 months necessitating a protective environment

Defining Characteristics: Chronic confusional states; Consistent disorientation; Inability to concentrate; Inability to follow simple directions; Inability to reason; Loss of occupation; Loss of social functioning; Slow in responding to questions

Related Factors: Dementia; Depression; Huntington's disease

Note: This diagnosis will retire from the NANDA-I Taxonomy in the 2015–2017 edition unless additional work is completed to bring it into compliance with the definition of syndrome diagnoses (requires two or more nursing diagnoses as defining characteristics/risk Factors).

Class 3: Sensation/Perception

None at this time

Class 4: Cognition

Acute Confusion

Definition: Abrupt onset of reversible disturbances of consciousness, attention, cognition, and perception that develop over a short period of time

Defining Characteristics: Fluctuation in cognition; Fluctuation in level of consciousness; Fluctuation in psychomotor activity; Hallucinations; Increased agitation; Increased restlessness; Lack of motivation to follow through with goal-directed behavior; Lack of motivation to follow through with purposeful behavior; Lack of motivation to initiate goal-directed behavior; Lack of motivation to initiate purposeful behavior; Misperceptions

Related Factors: Delirium; Dementia; Fluctuation in sleep–wake cycle; Over 60 years of age; Substance abuse

Chronic Confusion

Definition: Irreversible, longstanding, and/or progressive deterioration of intellect and personality characterized by decreased ability to interpret environmental stimuli and decreased capacity for intellectual thought processes, and manifested by disturbances of memory, orientation, and behavior

Defining Characteristics: Altered interpretation; Altered personality; Altered response to stimuli; Clinical evidence of organic impairment; Impaired long-term memory; Impaired short-term memory; Impaired socialization; Longstanding cognitive impairment; No change in level of consciousness; Progressive cognitive impairment

Related Factors: Alzheimer's disease; Cerebral vascular attack; Head injury; Korsakoff's psychosis; Multi-infarct dementia

Risk for Acute Confusion

Definition: At risk for reversible disturbances of consciousness, attention, cognition, and perception that develop over a short period of time

Risk Factors: Decreased mobility; Decreased restraints; Dementia; Fluctuation in sleep–wake cycle; History of stroke; Impaired cognition; Infection; Male gender; Metabolic abnormalities (Azotemia, Decreased hemoglobin, Dehydration, Electrolyte imbalances, Increased blood urea nitrogen (BUN)/creatinine, Malnutrition); Over 60 years of age; Pain; Pharmaceutical agents (Anesthesia, Anticholinergics, Diphenhydramine, Multiple medications, Opioids, Psychoactive drugs); Sensory deprivation; Substance abuse; Urinary retention

Ineffective Impulse Control

Definition: A pattern of performing rapid, unplanned reactions to internal or external stimuli without regard for the negative consequences of these reactions to the impulsive individual or to others

Defining Characteristics: Acting without thinking; Asking personal questions of others despite their discomfort; Inability to save money or regulate finances; Irritability; Pathological gambling; Sensation seeking; Sexual promiscuity; Sharing personal details inappropriately; Temper outbursts; Too familiar with strangers; Violence

Related Factors: Anger; Chronic low self-esteem; Co-dependency; Compunction; Delusion; Denial; Disorder of cognition; Disorder of development; Disorder of mood; Disorder of personality; Disturbed body image; Economically disadvantaged; Environment that might cause frustration; Environment that might cause irritation; Fatigue; Hopelessness; Ineffective coping; Insomnia; Organic brain disorders; Smoker; Social isolation; Stress vulnerability; Substance abuse; Suicidal feeling; Unpleasant physical symptoms

Deficient Knowledge

Definition: Absence or deficiency of cognitive information related to a specific topic

Defining Characteristics: Exaggerated behaviors; Inaccurate follow-through of instruction; Inaccurate performance of test; Inappropriate behaviors (e.g., hysterical, hostile, agitated, apathetic); Reports the problem

Related Factors: Cognitive limitation; Information misinterpretation; Lack of exposure; Lack of interest in learning; Lack of recall; Unfamiliarity with information resources

Readiness for Enhanced Knowledge

Definition: A pattern of cognitive information related to a specific topic, or its acquisition, that is sufficient for meeting health-related goals and can be strengthened

Defining Characteristics: Behaviors congruent with expressed knowledge; Describes previous experiences pertaining to the topic; Explains knowledge of the topic; Expresses an interest in learning

Impaired Memory

Definition: Inability to remember or recall bits of information or behavioral skills

Defining Characteristics: Forgets to perform a behavior at a scheduled time; Inability to learn new information; Inability to learn new skills; Inability to perform a previously learned skill; Inability to recall events; Inability to recall factual information; Inability to recall if a behavior was performed; Inability to retain new information; Inability to retain new skills; Reports experience of forgetting

Related Factors: Anemia; Decreased cardiac output; Electrolyte imbalance; Excessive environmental disturbances; Fluid imbalance; Hypoxia; Neurological disturbances

Class 5: Communication

Readiness for Enhanced Communication

Definition: A pattern of exchanging information and ideas with others that is sufficient for meeting one's needs and life's goals, and can be strengthened

Defining Characteristics: Able to speak a language; Able to write a language; Expresses feelings; Expresses satisfaction with ability to share ideas with others; Expresses satisfaction with ability to share information with others; Expresses thoughts; Expresses willingness to enhance communication; Forms phrases; Forms sentences; Forms words; Interprets nonverbal cues appropriately; Uses nonverbal cues appropriately

Impaired Verbal Communication

Definition: Decreased, delayed, or absent ability to receive, process, transmit, and/or use a system of symbols

Defining Characteristics: Absence of eye contact; Cannot speak; Difficulty expressing thoughts verbally (e.g., aphasia, dysphasia, apraxia, dyslexia); Difficulty forming sentences; Difficulty forming words (e.g., aphonia, dyslalia, dysarthria); Difficulty in comprehending usual communication pattern; Difficulty in maintaining usual communication pattern; Difficulty in selective attending; Difficulty in use of body expressions; Difficulty in use of facial expressions; Disorientation to person; Disorientation to space; Disorientation to time; Does not speak; Dyspnea; Inability to speak language of caregiver; Inability to use body expressions; Inability to use facial expressions; Inappropriate verbalization; Partial visual deficit; Slurring; Speaks with difficulty; Stuttering; Total visual deficit; Verbalizes with difficulty; Willful refusal to speak

Related Factors: Absence of significant others; Alteration in self-concept; Alteration of central nervous system; Altered perceptions; Anatomic defect (e.g., cleft palate, alteration of the neuromuscular visual system, auditory system, phonatory apparatus); Brain tumor; Chronic low self-esteem; Cultural differences; Decreased circulation to brain; Differences related to developmental age; Emotional conditions; Environmental barriers; Lack of information; Physical barrier (e.g., tracheostomy, intubation); Physiological conditions; Psychological barriers (e.g., psychosis, lack of stimuli); Situational low self-esteem; Stress; Treatment-related side effects (e.g., pharmaceutical agents); Weakened musculoskeletal system

DOMAIN 6: SELF-PERCEPTION

Class 1: Self-Concept

Hopelessness

Definition: Subjective state in which an individual sees limited or no alternatives or personal choices available and is unable to mobilize energy on own behalf

Defining Characteristics: Closing eyes; Decreased affect; Decreased appetite; Decreased response to stimuli; Decreased verbalization; Lack of initiative; Lack of involvement in care; Passivity; Shrugging in response to speaker; Sleep pattern disturbance; Turning away from speaker; Verbal cues (e.g., despondent content, "I can't," sighing)

Related Factors: Abandonment; Deteriorating physiological condition; Long-term stress; Lost belief in spiritual power; Lost belief in transcendent values; Prolonged activity restriction; Social isolation

Risk for Compromised Human Dignity

Definition: At risk for perceived loss of respect and honor

Risk Factors: Cultural incongruity; Disclosure of confidential information; Exposure of the body; Inadequate participation in decision-making; Loss of control of body functions; Perceived dehumanizing treatment; Perceived humiliation; Perceived intrusion by clinicians; Perceived invasion of privacy; Stigmatizing label; Use of undefined medical terms

Risk for Loneliness

Definition: At risk for experiencing discomfort associated with a desire or need for more contact with others

Risk Factors: Affectional deprivation; Cathectic deprivation; Physical isolation; Social isolation

Disturbed Personal Identity

Definition: Inability to maintain an integrated and complete perception of self

Defining Characteristics: Contradictory personal traits; Delusional description of self; Disturbed body image; Gender confusion; Ineffective coping; Ineffective relationships; Ineffective role performance; Reports feelings of emptiness; Reports feelings of strangeness; Reports fluctuating feelings about self; Unable to distinguish between inner and outer stimuli; Uncertainty about cultural values (e.g., beliefs, religion, moral questions); Uncertainty about goals; Uncertainty about ideological values (e.g., beliefs, religion, moral questions)

Related Factors: Chronic low self-esteem; Cult indoctrination; Cultural discontinuity; Discrimination; Dysfunctional family processes; Ingestion of toxic chemicals; Inhalation of toxic chemicals; Manic states; Multiple personality disorder; Organic brain syndromes; Perceived prejudice; Psychiatric disorders (e.g., psychoses, depression, dissociative disorder); Situational crises; Situational low self-esteem; Social role change; Stages of development; Stages of growth; Use of psychoactive pharmaceutical agents

Risk for Disturbed Personal Identity

Definition: Risk for the inability to maintain an integrated and complete perception of self

Risk Factors: Chronic low self-esteem; Cult indoctrination; Cultural discontinuity; Discrimination; Dysfunctional family processes; Ingestion of toxic chemicals; Inhalation of toxic chemicals; Manic states; Multiple personality disorder; Organic brain syndromes; Perceived prejudice; Psychiatric disorders (e.g., psychoses, depression, dissociative disorder); Situational crises; Situational low self-esteem; Social role change; Stages of development; Stages of growth; Use of psychoactive pharmaceutical agents

Readiness for Enhanced Self-Concept

Definition: A pattern of perceptions or ideas about the self that is sufficient for well-being and can be strengthened

Defining Characteristics: Accepts limitations; Accepts strengths; Actions are congruent with verbal expression; Expresses confidence in abilities; Expresses satisfaction with body image; Expresses satisfaction with personal identity; Expresses satisfaction with role performance; Expresses satisfaction with sense of worthiness; Expresses satisfaction with thoughts about self; Expresses willingness to enhance self-concept

Class 2: Self-Esteem

Chronic Low Self-Esteem

Definition: Longstanding negative self-evaluating/feelings about self or self-capabilities

Defining Characteristics: Dependent on others' opinions; Evaluation of self as unable to deal with events; Exaggerates negative feedback about self; Excessively seeks reassurance; Frequent lack of success in life events; Hesitant to try new situations; Hesitant to try new things; Indecisive behavior; Lack of eye contact; Nonassertive behavior; Overly conforming; Passive; Rejects positive feedback about self; Reports feelings of guilt; Reports feelings of shame

Related Factors: Ineffective adaptation to loss; Lack of affection; Lack of approval; Lack of membership in group; Perceived discrepancy between self and cultural norms; Perceived discrepancy between self and spiritual norms; Perceived lack of belonging; Perceived lack of respect from others; Psychiatric disorder; Repeated failures; Repeated negative reinforcement; Traumatic event; Traumatic situation

Situational Low Self-Esteem

Definition: Development of a negative perception of self-worth in response to a current situation

Defining Characteristics: Evaluation of self as unable to deal with events; Evaluation of self as unable to deal with situations; Indecisive behavior; Nonassertive behavior; Reports current situational challenge to self-worth; Reports helplessness; Reports uselessness; Self-negating verbalizations

Related Factors: Behavior inconsistent with values; Developmental changes; Disturbed body image; Failures; Functional impairment; Lack of recognition; Loss; Rejections; Social role changes

Risk for Chronic Low Self-Esteem

Definition: At risk for longstanding negative self-evaluating/feelings about self or self-capabilities

Risk Factors: Ineffective adaptation to loss; Lack of affection; Lack of membership in group; Perceived discrepancy between self and cultural norms; Perceived discrepancy between self and spiritual norms; Perceived lack of belonging; Perceived lack of respect from others; Psychiatric disorder; Repeated failures; Repeated negative reinforcement; Traumatic event; Traumatic situation

Risk for Situational Low Self-Esteem

Definition: At risk for developing a negative perception of self-worth in response to a current situation

Risk Factors: Behavior inconsistent with values; Decreased control over environment; Developmental changes; Disturbed body image; Failures; Functional impairment; History of abandonment; History of abuse; History of learned helplessness; History of neglect; Lack of recognition; Loss; Physical illness; Rejections; Social role changes; Unrealistic self-expectations

Class 3: Body Image

Disturbed Body Image

Definition: Confusion in mental picture of one's physical self

Defining Characteristics: Behaviors of acknowledgment of one's body; Behaviors of avoidance of one's body; Behaviors of monitoring one's body; Nonverbal response to actual change in body (e.g., appearance, structure, function); Nonverbal response to perceived change in body (e.g., appearance, structure, function); Reports feelings that reflect an altered view of one's body (e.g., appearance, structure, function); Reports perceptions that reflect an altered view of one's body in appearance

Objective: Actual change in function; Actual change in structure; Behaviors of acknowledging one's body; Behaviors of monitoring one's body; Change in ability to estimate spatial relationship of body to environment; Change in social involvement; Extension of body boundary to incorporate environmental objects; Intentional hiding of body part; Intentional overexposure of body part; Missing body part; Not looking at body part; Not touching body part; Trauma to nonfunctioning part; Unintentional hiding of body part; Unintentional overexposing of body part

Subjective: Depersonalization of loss by use of impersonal pronouns; Depersonalization of part by use of impersonal pronouns;

Emphasis on remaining strengths; Focus on past appearance; Focus on past function; Focus on past strength; Heightened achievement; Personalization of loss by name; Personalization of body part by name; Preoccupation with change; Preoccupation with loss; Refusal to verify actual change; Reports change in lifestyle; Reports fear of reaction by others; Reports negative feelings about body (e.g., feelings of helplessness, hopelessness, powerlessness)

Related Factors: Biophysical; Cognitive; Cultural; Developmental changes; Illness; Injury; Perceptual; Psychosocial; Spiritual; Surgery; Trauma; Treatment regimen

DOMAIN 7: ROLE RELATIONSHIPS

Class 1: Caregiving Roles

Ineffective Breastfeeding

Definition: Dissatisfaction or difficulty a mother, infant, or child experiences with the breastfeeding process

Defining Characteristics: Inadequate milk supply; Infant arching at the breast; Infant crying at the breast; Infant crying within the first hour after breastfeeding; Infant exhibiting fussiness within the first hour after breastfeeding; Infant inability to latch on to maternal breast correctly; Infant resisting latching on; Infant unresponsive to other comfort measures; Insufficient emptying of each breast per feeding; Insufficient opportunity for suckling at the breast; Lack of infant weight gain; No observable signs of oxytocin release; Perceived inadequate milk supply; Persistence of sore nipples beyond first week of breastfeeding; Sustained infant weight loss; Unsatisfactory breastfeeding process; Unsustained suckling at the breast

Related Factors: Deficient knowledge; Infant anomaly; Infant receiving supplemental feedings with artificial nipple; Interrupted breastfeeding; Maternal ambivalence; Maternal anxiety; Maternal breast anomaly; Nonsupportive family; Nonsupportive partner; Poor infant sucking reflex; Prematurity; Previous breast surgery; Previous history of breastfeeding failure

Interrupted Breastfeeding

Definition: Break in the continuity of the breastfeeding process as a result of inability or inadvisability to put baby to breast for feeding

Defining Characteristics: Deficient knowledge about expression of breast milk; Deficient knowledge about storage of breast milk; Infant receives no nourishment at the breast for some or all feedings; Maternal desire to provide breast milk for child's nutritional needs; Maternal desire to maintain breastfeeding for child's nutritional needs; Mother–child separation

Related Factors: Contraindications to breastfeeding (e.g., certain pharmaceutical agents); Infant illness; Infant prematurity; Maternal employment; Maternal illness; Need to abruptly wean infant

Readiness for Enhanced Breastfeeding

Definition: A pattern of proficiency and satisfaction of the mother–infant dyad that is sufficient to support the breastfeeding process and can be strengthened

Defining Characteristics: Adequate infant elimination patterns for age; Appropriate infant weight pattern for age; Eagerness of infant to nurse; Effective mother–infant communication patterns; Infant content after feeding; Mother able to position infant at breast to promote a successful latching-on response; Mother reports satisfaction with the breastfeeding process; Regular suckling at the breast; Regular swallowing at the breast;

Signs of oxytocin release are present; Sustained suckling at the breast; Sustained swallowing at the breast; Symptoms of oxytocin release are present
*Note: This diagnosis previously held the label, **Effective Breastfeeding**.*

Caregiver Role Strain

Definition: Difficulty in performing family/significant other caregiver role

Defining Characteristics:

Caregiving Activities: Apprehension about care receiver's care if caregiver unable to provide care; Apprehension about the future regarding caregiver's ability to provide care; Apprehension about the future regarding care receiver's health; Apprehension about possible institutionalization of care receiver; Difficulty completing required tasks; Difficulty performing required tasks; Dysfunctional change in caregiving activities; Preoccupation with care routine

Caregiver Health Status: **Physical:** Cardiovascular disease, Diabetes, Fatigue, Gastrointestinal upset, Headaches, Hypertension, Rash, Weight change; **Emotional:** Anger, Disturbed sleep pattern, Frustration, Impatience, Increased emotional lability, Increased nervousness, Ineffective coping, Lack of time to meet personal needs, Reports feeling depressed, Sleep deprivation, Somatization, Stress; **Socioeconomic:** Changes in leisure activities, Low work productivity, Refuses career advancement, Withdraws from social life

Caregiver–Care Receiver Relationship: Reports difficulty watching care receiver go through the illness; Reports grief regarding changed relationship with care receiver; Reports uncertainty regarding changed relationship with care receiver

Family Processes: Reports concerns about family members; Family conflict

Related Factors:

Care Receiver Health Status: Addiction; Co-dependency; Cognitive problems; Dependency; Illness chronicity; Illness severity; Increasing care needs; Instability of care receiver's health; Problem behaviors; Psychological problems; Substance abuse; Unpredictability of illness course

Caregiver Health Status: Co-dependency; Cognitive problems; Inability to fulfill one's own expectations; Inability to fulfill other's expectations; Marginal coping patterns; Physical problems; Psychological problems; Substance abuse; Unrealistic expectations of self

Caregiver–Care Receiver Relationship: History of poor relationship; Mental status of elder inhibiting conversation; Presence of abuse; Presence of violence; Unrealistic expectations of caregiver by care receiver

Caregiving Activities: 24-hour care responsibilities; Amount of activities; Complexity of activities; Discharge of family members to home with significant care needs; Ongoing changes in activities; Unpredictability of care situation; Years of caregiving

Family Processes: History of family dysfunction; History of marginal family coping

Resources: Caregiver is not developmentally ready for caregiver role; Deficient knowledge about community resources; Difficulty accessing community resources; Difficulty accessing formal assistance; Difficulty accessing formal support; Emotional strength; Inadequate community resources (e.g., respite services, recreational resources); Inadequate equipment for providing care; Inadequate informal assistance; Inadequate informal support; Inadequate physical environment for providing care (e.g., housing, temperature, safety); Inadequate transportation; Inexperience with caregiving; Insufficient finances; Insufficient time; Lack of caregiver privacy; Lack of support; Physical energy

Socioeconomic: Alienation from others; Competing role commitments; Insufficient recreation; Isolation from others

Risk for Caregiver Role Strain

Definition: At risk for caregiver vulnerability for felt difficulty in performing the family caregiver role

Risk Factors: Amount of caregiving tasks; Care receiver exhibits bizarre behavior; Care receiver exhibits deviant behavior; Caregiver health impairment; Caregiver is female; Caregiver is spouse; Caregiver isolation; Caregiver not developmentally ready for caregiver role; Caregiver's competing role commitments; Co-dependency; Cognitive problems in care receiver; Complexity of caregiving tasks; Congenital defect; Developmental delay of caregiver; Developmental delay of care receiver; Discharge of family member with significant home care needs; Duration of caregiving required; Family dysfunction before the caregiving situation; Family isolation; Illness severity of the care receiver; Inadequate physical environment for providing care (e.g., housing, transportation, community services, equipment); Inexperience with caregiving; Instability in the care receiver's health; Lack of recreation for caregiver; Lack of respite for caregiver; Marginal caregiver's coping patterns; Marginal family adaptation; Past history of poor relationship between caregiver and care receiver; Premature birth; Presence of abuse; Presence of situational stressors that normally affect families (e.g., significant loss, disaster or crisis, economic vulnerability, major life events); Presence of violence; Psychological problems in caregiver; Psychological problems in care receiver; Substance abuse; Unpredictable illness course

Impaired Parenting

Definition: Inability of the primary caretaker to create, maintain, or regain an environment that promotes the optimum growth and development of the child

Defining Characteristics:

Infant or Child: Behavioral disorders; Failure to thrive; Frequent accidents; Frequent illness; Incidence of abuse; Incidence of trauma (e.g., physical and psychological); Lack of attachment; Lack of separation anxiety; Poor academic performance; Poor cognitive development; Poor social competence; Runaway

Parental: Abandonment; Child abuse; Child neglect; Frequently punitive; Hostility to child; Inadequate attachment; Inadequate child health maintenance; Inappropriate caretaking skills; Inappropriate child care arrangements; Inappropriate stimulation (e.g., visual, tactile, auditory); Inconsistent behavior management; Inconsistent care; Inflexibility in meeting needs of child; Little cuddling; Maternal–child interaction deficit; Negative statements about child; Paternal–child interaction deficit; Rejection of child; Reports frustration; Reports inability to control child; Reports role inadequacy; Statements of inability to meet child's needs; Unsafe home environment

Related Factors:

Infant or Child: Altered perceptual abilities; Attention deficit hyperactivity disorder; Developmental delay; Difficult temperament; Handicapping condition; Illness; Multiple births; Not desired gender; Premature birth; Separation from parent; Temperamental conflicts with parental expectations

Knowledge: Deficient knowledge about child development; Deficient knowledge about child health maintenance; Deficient

knowledge about parenting skills; Inability to respond to infant cues; Lack of cognitive readiness for parenthood; Lack of education; Limited cognitive functioning; Poor communication skills; Preference for physical punishment; Unrealistic expectations

Physiological: Physical illness

Psychological: Closely spaced pregnancies; Depression; Difficult birthing process; Disability; Disturbed sleep pattern; High number of pregnancies; History of mental illness; History of substance abuse; Lack of prenatal care; Sleep deprivation; Young parental age

Social: Change in family unit; Chronic low self-esteem; Economically disadvantaged; Father of child not involved; Financial difficulties; History of being abused; History of being abusive; Inability to put child's needs before own; Inadequate child care arrangements; Job problems; Lack of family cohesiveness; Lack of parental role model; Lack of resources; Lack of social support networks; Lack of transportation; Lack of valuing of parenthood; Legal difficulties; Maladaptive coping strategies; Marital conflict; Mother of child not involved; Poor home environment; Poor parental role model; Poor problem-solving skills; Presence of stress (e.g., financial, legal, recent crisis, cultural move); Relocations; Role strain; Single parent; Situational low self-esteem; Social isolation; Unemployment; Unplanned pregnancy; Unwanted pregnancy

Readiness for Enhanced Parenting

Definition: A pattern of providing an environment for children or other dependent person(s) that is sufficient to nurture growth and development, and can be strengthened

Defining Characteristics: Children report satisfaction with home environment; Emotional support of children; Emotional support of other dependent person(s); Evidence of attachment; Exhibits realistic expectations of children; Exhibits realistic expectations of other dependent person(s); Expresses willingness to enhance parenting; Needs of children are met (e.g., physical and emotional); Needs of other dependent person(s) is/are met (e.g., physical and emotional); Other dependent person(s) express(es) satisfaction with home environment

Risk for Impaired Parenting

Definition: At risk for inability of the primary caretaker to create, maintain, or regain an environment that promotes the optimum growth and development of the child

Risk Factors:

Infant or Child: Altered perceptual abilities; Attention deficit hyperactivity disorder; Developmental delay; Difficult temperament; Handicapping condition; Illness; Multiple births; Not gender desired; Premature birth; Prolonged separation from parent; Temperamental conflicts with parental expectation

Knowledge: Deficient knowledge about child development; Deficient knowledge about child health maintenance; Deficient knowledge about parenting skills; Inability to respond to infant cues; Lack of cognitive readiness for parenthood; Low cognitive functioning; Low educational level; Poor communication skills; Preference for physical punishment; Unrealistic expectations of child

Physiological: Physical illness

Psychological: Closely spaced pregnancies; Depression; Difficult birthing process; Disability; High number of pregnancies; History of mental illness; History of substance abuse; Sleep deprivation; Sleep disruption; Young parental age

Social: Change in family unit; Chronic low self-esteem; Economically disadvantaged; Father of child not involved; Financial difficulties; History of being abused; History of being abusive; Inadequate child care arrangements; Job problems; Lack of access to resources; Lack of family cohesiveness; Lack of parental role model; Lack of prenatal care; Lack of resources; Lack of social support network; Lack of transportation; Lack of valuing of parenthood; Late prenatal care; Legal difficulties; Maladaptive coping strategies; Marital conflict; Mother of child not involved; Parent–child separation; Poor home environment; Poor parental role model; Poor problem-solving skills; Relocation; Role strain; Single parent; Situational low self-esteem; Social isolation; Stress; Unemployment; Unplanned pregnancy; Unwanted pregnancy

Class 2: Family Relationships

Risk for Impaired Attachment

Definition: At risk for disruption of the interactive process between parent/significant other and child that fosters the development of a protective and nurturing reciprocal relationship

Risk Factors: Anxiety associated with the parent role; Disorganized infant behavior; Ill child who is unable effectively to initiate parental contact; Inability of parent(s) to meet personal needs; Lack of privacy; Parental conflict resulting from disorganized infant behavior; Parent–child separation; Physical barriers; Premature infant; Substance abuse

Note: This diagnosis formerly held the label **Risk for Impaired Parent/Child Attachment***.*

Dysfunctional Family Processes

Definition: Psychosocial, spiritual, and physiological functions of the family unit are chronically disorganized, which leads to conflict, denial of problems, resistance to change, ineffective problem-solving, and a series of self-perpetuating crises

Defining Characteristics:

Behavioral: Agitation; Blaming; Broken promises; Chaos; Complicated grieving; Conflict avoidance; Contradictory communication; Controlling communication; Criticizing; Deficient knowledge about substance abuse; Denial of problems; Dependency; Difficulty having fun; Difficulty with intimate relationships; Difficulty with life cycle transitions; Diminished physical contact; Disturbances in academic performance in children; Disturbances in concentration; Enabling maintenance of substance use pattern (e.g., alcohol); Escalating conflict; Failure to accomplish developmental tasks; Family special occasions are substance-use centered; Harsh self-judgment; Immaturity; Impaired communication; Inability to accept a wide range of feelings; Inability to accept help; Inability to adapt to change; Inability to deal constructively with traumatic experiences; Inability to express a wide range of feelings; Inability to meet the emotional needs of its members; Inability to meet the security needs of its members; Inability to meet the spiritual needs of its members; Inability to receive help appropriately; Inadequate understanding of substance abuse; Inappropriate expression of anger; Ineffective problem-solving skills; Lack of reliability; Lying; Manipulation; Nicotine addiction; Orientation toward tension relief rather than achievement of goals; Paradoxical communication; Power struggles; Rationalization; Refusal to get help; Seeking affirmation; Seeking approval; Self-blaming; Social isolation; Stress-related physical illnesses; Substance abuse; Verbal abuse of children; Verbal abuse of parent; Verbal abuse of spouse

Feelings: Abandonment; Anger; Anxiety; Being different from other people; Being unloved; Chronic low self-esteem; Confuses love and pity; Confusion; Depression; Dissatisfaction; Distress; Embarrassment; Emotional control by others; Emotional isolation; Failure; Fear; Frustration; Guilt; Hopelessness; Hostility; Hurt; Insecurity; Lack of identity; Lingering resentment; Loneliness; Loss; Mistrust; Moodiness; Powerlessness; Rejection; Reports feeling misunderstood; Repressed emotions; Responsibility for substance abuser's behavior; Suppressed rage; Shame; Tension; Unhappiness; Vulnerability; Worthlessness

Roles and Relationships: Altered role function; Chronic family problems; Closed communication systems; Deterioration in family relationships; Disrupted family rituals; Disrupted family roles; Disturbed family dynamics; Economic problems; Family denial; Family does not demonstrate respect for autonomy of its members; Family does not demonstrate respect for individuality of its members; Inconsistent parenting; Ineffective spouse communication; Intimacy dysfunction; Lack of cohesiveness; Lack of skills necessary for relationships; Low perception of parental support; Marital problems; Neglected obligations; Pattern of rejection; Reduced ability of family members to relate to each other for mutual growth and maturation; Triangulating family relationships

Related Factors: Addictive personality; Biochemical influences; Family history of resistance to treatment; Family history of substance abuse; Genetic predisposition to substance abuse; Inadequate coping skills; Lack of problem-solving skills; Substance abuse

Note: This diagnosis formerly held the label **Dysfunctional Family Processes: Alcoholism***.*

Interrupted Family Processes

Definition: Change in family relationships and/or functioning

Defining Characteristics: Changes in assigned tasks; Changes in availability for affective responsiveness; Changes in availability for emotional support; Changes in communication patterns; Changes in effectiveness in completing assigned tasks; Changes in expressions of conflict with community resources; Changes in expressions of conflict within family; Changes in expressions of isolation from community resources; Changes in mutual support; Changes in participation in decision-making; Changes in participation in problem-solving; Changes in satisfaction with family; Changes in somatic complaints; Communication pattern changes; Intimacy changes; Pattern changes; Power alliance changes; Ritual changes; Stress-reduction behavior changes

Related Factors: Developmental crises; Developmental transition; Interaction with community; Modification in family finances; Modification in family social status; Power shift of family members; Shift in family roles; Shift in health status of a family member; Situation transition; Situational crises

Readiness for Enhanced Family Processes

Definition: A pattern of family functioning that is sufficient to support the well-being of family members and can be strengthened

Defining Characteristics: Activities support the growth of family members; Activities support the safety of family members; Balance exists between autonomy and cohesiveness; Boundaries of family members are maintained; Communication is adequate; Energy level of family supports activities of daily living; Expresses willingness to enhance family dynamics; Family adapts to change; Family functioning meets needs of family members; Family resilience is evident; Family roles are appropriate for developmental stages; Family roles are flexible for developmental stages; Family tasks are accomplished; Interdependent with community; Relationships are generally positive; Respect for family members is evident

Class 3: Role Performance

Ineffective Relationship

Definition: A pattern of mutual partnership that is insufficient to provide for each other's needs

Defining Characteristics: Does not identify partner as a key person; Does not meet developmental goals appropriate for family life-cycle stage; Inability to communicate in a satisfying manner between partners; No demonstration of mutual respect between partners; No demonstration of mutual support in daily activities between partners; No demonstration of understanding of partner's insufficient (physical, social, psychological) functioning; No demonstration of well-balanced autonomy between partners; No demonstration of well-balanced collaboration between partners; Reports dissatisfaction with complementary relation between partners; Reports dissatisfaction with fulfilling emotional needs between partners; Reports dissatisfaction with fulfilling physical needs between partners; Reports dissatisfaction with sharing of ideas between partners; Reports dissatisfaction with sharing of information between partners

Related Factors: Cognitive changes in one partner; Developmental crises; History of domestic violence; Incarceration of one partner; Poor communication skills; Stressful life events; Substance abuse; Unrealistic expectations

Readiness for Enhanced Relationship

Definition: A pattern of mutual partnership that is sufficient to provide for each other's needs and can be strengthened

Defining Characteristics: Demonstrates mutual respect between partners; Demonstrates mutual support in daily activities between partners; Demonstrates understanding of partner's insufficient (physical, social, psychological) function; Demonstrates well-balanced autonomy between partners; Demonstrates well-balanced collaboration between partners; Identifies each other as a key person; Meets developmental goals appropriate for family life-cycle stage; Reports desire to enhance communication between partners; Reports satisfaction with complementary relationship between partners; Reports satisfaction with fulfilling emotional needs by one's partner; Reports satisfaction with fulfilling physical needs by one's partner; Reports satisfaction with sharing of ideas between partners; Reports satisfaction with sharing of information between partners

Risk for Ineffective Relationship

Definition: Risk for a pattern of mutual partnership that is insufficient to provide for each other's needs

Risk Factors: Cognitive changes in one partner; Developmental crises; History of domestic violence; Incarceration of one partner; Poor communication skills; Stressful life events; Substance abuse; Unrealistic expectations

Parental Role Conflict

Definition: Parental experience of role confusion and conflict in response to crisis

Defining Characteristics: Anxiety; Demonstrates disruption in caretaking routines; Fear; Reluctant to participate in usual caretaking activities; Reports concern about changes in parental role; Reports concern about family (e.g., functioning, communication, health); Reports concern about perceived loss of control over decisions relating to child; Reports feelings of frustration; Reports feelings of guilt; Reports feeling of inadequacy to provide for child's needs (e.g., physical, emotional)

Related Factors: Change in marital status; Home care of a child with special needs; Interruptions of family life due to home care regimen (e.g., treatments, caregivers, lack of respite); Intimidation by invasive modalities (e.g., intubation); Intimidation by restrictive modalities (e.g., isolation); Parent–child separation due to chronic illness; Specialized care center

Ineffective Role Performance

Definition: Patterns of behavior and self-expression that do not match the environmental context, norms, and expectations

Defining Characteristics: Altered role perceptions; Anxiety; Change in capacity to resume role; Change in other's perception of role; Change in self-perception of role; Change in usual patterns of responsibility; Deficient knowledge; Depression; Discrimination; Domestic violence; Harassment; Inadequate adaptation to change; Inadequate confidence; Inadequate external support for role enactment; Inadequate motivation; Inadequate opportunities for role enactment; Inadequate self-management; Inadequate skills; Inappropriate developmental expectations; Ineffective coping; Ineffective role performance; Pessimism; Powerlessness; Role ambivalence; Role conflict; Role confusion; Role denial; Role dissatisfaction; Role overload; Role strain; System conflict; Uncertainty

Related Factors:

Knowledge: Inadequate role model; Inadequate role preparation (e.g., role transition, skill rehearsal, validation); Lack of education; Lack of role model; Unrealistic role expectations

Physiological: Body image alteration; Chronic low self-esteem; Cognitive deficits; Depression; Fatigue; Mental illness; Neurological defects; Pain; Physical illness; Situational low self-esteem; Substance abuse

Social: Conflict; Developmental level; Domestic violence; Economically disadvantaged; Inadequate role socialization; Inadequate support system; Inappropriate linkage with the healthcare system; Job schedule demands; Lack of resources; Lack of rewards; Stress; Young age

Impaired Social Interaction

Definition: Insufficient or excessive quantity or ineffective quality of social exchange

Defining Characteristics: Discomfort in social situations; Dysfunctional interaction with others; Family reports changes in interaction (e.g., style, pattern); Inability to communicate a satisfying sense of social engagement (e.g., belonging, caring, interest, shared history); Inability to receive a satisfying sense of social engagement (e.g., belonging, caring, interest, shared history); Use of unsuccessful social interaction behaviors;

Related Factors: Absence of significant others; Communication barriers; Deficit about ways to enhance mutuality (e.g., knowledge, skills); Disturbed thought processes; Environmental barriers; Limited physical mobility; Self-concept disturbance; Sociocultural dissonance; Therapeutic isolation

DOMAIN 8: SEXUALITY

Class 1: Sexual Identity

None at present time

Class 2: Sexual Function

Sexual Dysfunction

Definition: The state in which an individual experiences a change in sexual function during the sexual response phases of desire, excitation, and/or orgasm, which is viewed as unsatisfying, unrewarding, or inadequate

Defining Characteristics: Actual limitations imposed by disease; Actual limitations imposed by therapy; Alterations in achieving perceived sex role; Alterations in achieving sexual satisfaction; Change of interest in others; Change of interest in self; Inability to achieve desired satisfaction; Perceived alteration in sexual excitation; Perceived deficiency of sexual desire; Perceived limitations imposed by disease; Perceived limitations imposed by therapy; Seeking confirmation of desirability; Verbalization of problem

Related Factors: Absent role models; Altered body function (e.g., pregnancy, recent childbirth, drugs, surgery, anomalies, disease process, trauma, radiation); Altered body structure (e.g., pregnancy, recent childbirth, surgery, anomalies, disease process, trauma, radiation); Biopsychosocial alteration of sexuality; Deficient knowledge; Ineffectual role models; Lack of privacy; Lack of significant other; Misinformation; Physical abuse; Psychosocial abuse (e.g., harmful relationships); Values conflict; Vulnerability

Ineffective Sexuality Pattern

Definition: Expressions of concern regarding own sexuality

Defining Characteristics: Alteration in achieving perceived sex role; Alteration in relationship with significant other; Reports changes in sexual activities; Reports changes in sexual behaviors; Reports difficulties with sexual activities; Reports difficulties with sexual behaviors; Reports limitations in sexual activities; Reports limitations in sexual behaviors; Values conflict

Related Factors: Absent role model; Conflicts with sexual orientation; Conflicts with variant preferences; Deficient knowledge about alternative responses to health-related transitions, altered body function or structure, illness, or medical treatment; Fear of acquiring a sexually transmitted infection; Fear of pregnancy; Impaired relationship with a significant other; Ineffective role model; Lack of privacy; Lack of significant other; Skill deficit about alternative responses to health-related transitions, altered body function or structure, illness, or medical treatment

Class 3: Reproduction

Ineffective Childbearing Process

Definition: Pregnancy and childbirth process and care of the newborn* that does not match the environmental context, norms, and expectations

Defining Characteristics:

During Pregnancy: Does not access support systems appropriately; Does not report appropriate physical preparations; Does not report appropriate prenatal lifestyle (e.g., nutrition, elimination, sleep, bodily movement, exercise, personal hygiene); Does not report availability of support systems; Does not report managing unpleasant symptoms in pregnancy; Does not report realistic birth plan; Does not seek necessary knowledge (e.g., of labor and delivery, newborn care); Failure to prepare necessary newborn care items; Inconsistent prenatal health visits; Lack of prenatal visits; Lack of respect for unborn baby

During Labor and Delivery: Does not access support systems appropriately; Does not demonstrate attachment behavior to the newborn baby; Does not report availability of support systems;

Does not report lifestyle (e.g., diet, elimination, sleep, bodily movement, personal hygiene) that is appropriate for the stage of labor; Does not respond appropriately to onset of labor; Lacks proactivity during labor and delivery

After Birth:* Does not access support systems appropriately; Does not demonstrate appropriate baby feeding techniques; Does not demonstrate appropriate breast care; Does not demonstrate attachment behavior to the baby; Does not demonstrate basic baby care techniques; Does not provide safe environment for the baby; Does not report appropriate postpartum lifestyle (e.g., diet, elimination, sleep, bodily movement, exercise, personal hygiene); Does not report availability of support systems

Related Factors: Deficient knowledge (e.g., of labor and delivery, newborn care); Domestic violence; Inconsistent prenatal health visits; Lack of appropriate role models for parenthood; Lack of cognitive readiness for parenthood; Lack of maternal confidence; Lack of prenatal health visits; Lack of a realistic birth plan; Lack of sufficient support systems; Maternal powerlessness; Maternal psychological distress; Suboptimal maternal nutrition; Substance abuse; Unplanned pregnancy; Unsafe environment; Unwanted pregnancy

The original Japanese term for "childbearing" (shussan ikuji koudou), which encompasses both childbirth and rearing of the neonate. It is one of the main concepts of Japanese midwifery.

Readiness for Enhanced Childbearing Process*

Definition: A pattern of preparing for and maintaining a healthy pregnancy, childbirth process, and care of the newborn that is sufficient for ensuring well-being and can be strengthened

Defining Characteristics:

During Pregnancy: Attends regular prenatal health visits; Demonstrates respect for unborn baby; Prepares necessary newborn care items; Reports appropriate physical preparations; Reports appropriate prenatal lifestyle (e.g., nutrition, elimination, sleep, bodily movement, exercise, personal hygiene); Reports availability of support systems; Reports realistic birth plan; Reports managing unpleasant symptoms in pregnancy; Seeks necessary knowledge (e.g., of labor and delivery, newborn care)

During Labor and Delivery: Demonstrates attachment behavior to the newborn baby; Is proactive during labor and delivery; Reports lifestyle (e.g., diet, elimination, sleep, bodily movement, personal hygiene) that is appropriate for the stage of labor; Responds appropriately to onset of labor; Uses relaxation techniques appropriate for the stage of labor; Utilizes support systems appropriately

After Birth:* Demonstrates appropriate baby-feeding techniques; Demonstrates appropriate breast care; Demonstrates attachment behavior to the baby; Demonstrates basic baby care techniques; Provides safe environment for the baby; Reports appropriate postpartum lifestyle (e.g., diet, elimination, sleep, bodily movement, exercise, personal hygiene); Utilizes support system appropriately

The original Japanese term for "childbearing" (shussan ikuji koudou), which encompasses both childbirth and rearing of the neonate. It is one of the main concepts of Japanese midwifery.

Risk for Ineffective Childbearing Process

Definition: Risk for a pregnancy and childbirth process and care of the newborn* that does not match the environmental context, norms, and expectations

Risk Factors: Deficient knowledge (e.g., of labor and delivery, newborn care); Domestic violence; Inconsistent prenatal health visits; Lack of appropriate role models for parenthood; Lack of cognitive readiness for parenthood; Lack of maternal confidence; Lack of prenatal health visits; Lack of a realistic birth plan; Lack of sufficient support systems; Maternal powerlessness; Maternal psychological distress; Suboptimal maternal nutrition; Substance abuse; Unplanned pregnancy; Unwanted pregnancy

Risk for Disturbed Maternal–Fetal Dyad

Definition: At risk for disruption of the symbiotic maternal–fetal dyad as a result of comorbid or pregnancy-related conditions

Risk Factors: Complications of pregnancy (e.g., premature rupture of membranes, placenta previa or abruption, late prenatal care, multiple gestation); Compromised oxygen transport (e.g., anemia, cardiac disease, asthma, hypertension, seizures, premature labor, hemorrhage); Impaired glucose metabolism (e.g., diabetes, steroid use); Physical abuse; Substance abuse (e.g., tobacco, alcohol, drugs); Treatment-related side effects (e.g., pharmaceutical agents, surgery)

DOMAIN 9: COPING/STRESS TOLERANCE

Class 1: Post-Trauma Responses

Post-Trauma Syndrome

Definition: Sustained maladaptive response to a traumatic, overwhelming event

Defining Characteristics: Aggression; Alienation; Altered mood states; Anger; Anxiety; Avoidance; Compulsive behavior; Denial; Depression; Detachment; Difficulty concentrating; Enuresis (in children); Exaggerated startle response; Fear; Flashbacks; Gastric irritability; Grieving; Guilt; Headaches; Hopelessness; Horror; Hypervigilance; Intrusive dreams; Intrusive thoughts; Irritability; Neurosensory irritability; Nightmares; Palpitations; Panic attacks; Psychogenic amnesia; Rage; Reports feeling numb; Repression; Shame; Substance abuse

Related Factors: Being held prisoner of war; Criminal victimization; Disasters; Epidemics; Events outside the range of usual human experience; Physical abuse; Psychological abuse; Serious accidents (e.g., industrial, motor vehicle); Serious injury to loved ones; Serious injury to self; Serious threat to loved ones; Serious threat to self; Sudden destruction of one's community; Sudden destruction of one's home; Torture; Tragic occurrence involving multiple deaths; War; Witnessing mutilation; Witnessing violent death

Risk for Post-Trauma Syndrome

Definition: At risk for sustained maladaptive response to a traumatic, overwhelming event

Risk Factors: Diminished ego strength; Displacement from home; Duration of the event; Exaggerated sense of responsibility; Inadequate social support; Occupation (e.g., police, fire, rescue, corrections, emergency room staff, mental health worker); Perception of event; Survivor's role in the event; Unsupportive environment

Rape-Trauma Syndrome

Definition: Sustained maladaptive response to a forced, violent sexual penetration against the victim's will and consent

Defining Characteristics: Aggression; Agitation; Anger; Anxiety; Change in relationships; Chronic self-esteem; Confusion; Denial; Dependence; Depression; Disorganization; Dissociative disorders; Disturbed sleep pattern; Embarrassment; Fear; Guilt; Helplessness; Humiliation; Hyperalertness; Impaired decision-making; Mood

swings; Muscle spasms; Muscle tension; Nightmares; Paranoia; Phobias; Physical trauma; Powerlessness; Revenge; Self-blame; Sexual dysfunction; Shame; Shock; Substance abuse; Suicide attempts; Vulnerability

Related Factors: Rape

Relocation Stress Syndrome

Definition: Physiological and/or psychosocial disturbance following transfer from one environment to another

Defining Characteristics: Alienation; Aloneness; Anger; Anxiety (e.g., separation); Chronic low self-esteem; Concern over relocation; Dependency; Depression; Fear; Frustration; Increased illness; Increased physical symptoms; Increased verbalization of needs; Insecurity; Loneliness; Loss of identity; Loss of self-worth; Pessimism; Reports unwillingness to move; Situational low self-esteem; Sleep pattern disturbance; Withdrawal; Worry

Related Factors: Decreased health status; Impaired psychosocial health; Isolation; Lack of adequate support system; Lack of predeparture counseling; Language barrier; Losses; Move from one environment to another; Passive coping; Reports feelings of powerlessness; Unpredictability of experience

Risk for Relocation Stress Syndrome

Definition: At risk for physiological and/or psychosocial disturbance following transfer from one environment to another

Risk Factors: Decreased health status; Lack of adequate support system; Lack of predeparture counseling; Losses; Moderate-to-high degree of environmental change; Moderate mental competence; Move from one environment to another; Passive coping; Reports powerlessness; Unpredictability of experiences

Class 2: Coping Responses

Ineffective Activity Planning

Definition: Inability to prepare for a set of actions fixed in time and under certain conditions

Defining Characteristics: Failure pattern of behavior; History of procrastination; Lack of plan; Lack of resources; Lack of sequential organization; Reports excessive anxieties about a task to be undertaken; Reports fear toward a task to be undertaken; Reports worries about a task to be undertaken; Unmet goals for chosen activity

Related Factors: Compromised ability to process information; Defensive flight behavior when faced with proposed solution; Hedonism; Lack of family support; Lack of friend support; Unrealistic perception of events; Unrealistic perception of personal competence

Risk for Ineffective Activity Planning

Definition: At risk for an inability to prepare for a set of actions fixed in time and under certain conditions

Risk Factors: Compromised ability to process information; Defensive flight behavior when faced with proposed solution; Hedonism; History of procrastination; Ineffective support systems; Insufficient support systems; Unrealistic perception of events; Unrealistic perception of personal competence

Anxiety

Definition: Vague uneasy feeling of discomfort or dread accompanied by an autonomic response (the source often nonspecific or unknown to the individual); a feeling of apprehension caused by anticipation of danger. It is an alerting signal that warns of impending danger and enables the individual to take measures to deal with threat

Defining Characteristics:

Behavioral: Diminished productivity; Extraneous movement; Fidgeting; Glancing about; Insomnia; Poor eye contact; Reports concerns due to change in life events; Restlessness; Scanning; Vigilance

Affective: Anguish; Apprehensive; Distressed; Fear; Feelings of inadequacy; Focus on self; Increased wariness; Irritability; Jittery; Overexcited; Painful increased helplessness; Persistent increased helplessness; Rattled; Regretful; Uncertainty; Worried

Physiological: Facial tension; Hand tremors; Increased perspiration; Increased tension; Shakiness; Trembling; Voice quivering

Sympathetic: Anorexia; Cardiovascular excitation; Diarrhea; Dry mouth; Facial flushing; Heart pounding; Increased blood pressure; Increased pulse; Increased reflexes; Increased respiration; Pupil dilation; Respiratory difficulties; Superficial vasoconstriction; Twitching; Weakness

Parasympathetic: Abdominal pain; Decreased blood pressure; Decreased pulse; Diarrhea; Faintness; Fatigue; Nausea; Sleep disturbance; Tingling in extremities; Urinary frequency; Urinary hesitancy; Urinary urgency

Cognitive: Awareness of physiological symptoms; Blocking of thought; Confusion; Decreased perceptual field; Difficulty concentrating; Diminished ability to learn; Diminished ability to problem-solve; Fear of unspecified consequences; Forgetfulness; Impaired attention; Preoccupation; Rumination; Tendency to blame others

Related Factors: Change in: Economic status, Environment, Health status, Interaction patterns, Role function, Role status; Exposure to toxins; Familial association; Heredity; Interpersonal contagion; Interpersonal transmission; Maturational crises; Situational crises; Stress; Substance abuse; Threat of death; Threat to: Economic status, Environment, Health status, Interaction patterns, Role function, Role status, Self-concept; Unconscious conflict about essential goals of life; Unconscious conflict about essential values; Unmet needs

Defensive Coping

Definition: Repeated projection of falsely positive self-evaluation based on a self-protective pattern that defends against underlying perceived threats to positive self-regard

Defining Characteristics: Denial of obvious problems; Denial of obvious weaknesses; Difficulty establishing relationships; Difficulty in perception of reality testing; Difficulty maintaining relationships; Grandiosity; Hostile laughter; Hypersensitivity to criticism; Hypersensitivity to slight; Lack of follow-through in therapy; Lack of follow-through in treatment; Lack of participation in therapy; Lack of participation in treatment; Projection of blame; Projection of responsibility; Rationalization of failures; Reality distortion; Ridicule of others; Superior attitude toward others

Related Factors: Conflict between self-perception and value system; Deficient support system; Fear of failure; Fear of humiliation; Fear of repercussions; Lack of resilience; Low level of confidence in others; Low level of self-confidence; Uncertainty; Unrealistic expectations of self

Ineffective Coping

Definition: Inability to form a valid appraisal of the stressors, inadequate choices of practiced responses, and/or inability to use available resources

Defining Characteristics: Change in usual communication patterns; Decreased use of social support; Destructive behavior toward others; Destructive behavior toward self; Difficulty organizing information; Fatigue; High illness rate; Inability to attend to information; Inability to meet basic needs; Inability to meet role expectations; Inadequate problem-solving; Lack of goal-directed behavior; Lack of resolution of problem; Poor concentration; Reports inability to ask for help; Reports inability to cope; Risk-taking; Sleep pattern disturbance; Substance abuse; Use of forms of coping that impede adaptive behavior

Related Factors: Disturbance in pattern of appraisal of threat; Disturbance in pattern of tension release; Gender differences in coping strategies; High degree of threat; Inability to conserve adaptive energies; Inadequate level of confidence in ability to cope; Inadequate level of perception of control; Inadequate opportunity to prepare for stressor; Inadequate resources available; Inadequate social support created by characteristics of relationships; Maturational crisis; Situational crisis; Uncertainty

Readiness for Enhanced Coping

Definition: A pattern of cognitive and behavioral efforts to manage demands that is sufficient for well-being and can be strengthened

Defining Characteristics: Acknowledges power; Aware of possible environmental changes; Defines stressors as manageable; Seeks knowledge of new strategies; Seeks social support; Uses a broad range of emotion-oriented strategies; Uses a broad range of problem-oriented strategies; Uses spiritual resources

Ineffective Community Coping

Definition: Pattern of community activities for adaptation and problem-solving that is unsatisfactory for meeting the demands or needs of the community

Defining Characteristics: Community does not meet its own expectations; Deficits in community participation; Excessive community conflicts; High illness rates; Increased social problems (e.g., homicides, vandalism, arson, terrorism, robbery, infanticide, abuse, divorce, unemployment, poverty, militancy, mental illness); Reports of community powerlessness; Reports of community vulnerability; Stressors perceived as excessive

Related Factors: Deficits in community social support resources; Deficits in community social support services; Inadequate resources for problem-solving; Ineffective community systems (e.g., lack of emergency medical system, transportation system, disaster planning systems); Man-made disasters; Natural disasters; Nonexistent community systems

Readiness for Enhanced Community Coping

Definition: A pattern of community activities for adaptation and problem-solving that is sufficient for meeting the demands or needs of the community for the management of current and future problems/stressors and can be strengthened

Defining Characteristics: Active planning by community for predicted stressors; Active problem-solving by community when faced with issues; Agreement that community is responsible for stress management; Positive communication among community members; Positive communication between community/aggregates and larger community; Programs available for recreation; Programs available for relaxation; Resources sufficient for managing stressors

Compromised Family Coping

Definition: A usually supportive primary person (family member, significant other, or close friend) provides insufficient, ineffective, or compromised support, comfort, assistance, or encouragement that may be needed by the client to manage or master adaptive tasks related to his or her health challenge

Defining Characteristics:

Objective: Significant person attempts assistive behaviors with unsatisfactory results; Significant person attempts supportive behaviors with unsatisfactory results; Significant person displays protective behavior disproportionate to client's abilities; Significant person displays protective behavior disproportionate to client's need for autonomy; Significant person enters into limited personal communication with client; Significant person withdraws from client

Subjective: Client reports a complaint about significant person's response to health problem; Client reports a concern about significant person's response to health problem; Significant person reports an inadequate knowledge base, which interferes with effective supportive behaviors; Significant person reports an inadequate understanding, which interferes with effective supportive behaviors; Significant person reports preoccupation with personal reaction (e.g., fear, anticipatory grief, guilt, anxiety) to client's need

Related Factors: Coexisting situations affecting the significant person; Developmental crises that the significant person may be facing; Exhaustion of supportive capacity of significant people; Inadequate information available to a primary person; Inadequate understanding of information by a primary person; Incorrect information obtained by a primary person; Incorrect understanding of information by a primary person; Lack of reciprocal support; Little support provided by client, in turn, for primary person; Prolonged disease that exhausts supportive capacity of significant people; Situational crises that the significant person may be facing; Temporary family disorganization; Temporary family role changes; Temporary preoccupation by a significant person

Disabled Family Coping

Definition: Behavior of primary person (family member, significant other, or close friend) that disables his or her capacities and the client's capacities to effectively address tasks essential to either person's adaptation to the health challenge

Defining Characteristics: Abandonment; Aggression; Agitation; Carrying on usual routines without regard for client's needs; Client's development of dependence; Depression; Desertion; Disregarding client's needs; Distortion of reality regarding client's health problem; Family behaviors that are detrimental to well-being; Hostility; Impaired individualization; Impaired restructuring of a meaningful life for self; Intolerance; Neglectful care of client in regard to basic human needs; Neglectful care of client in regard to illness treatment; Neglectful relationships with other family members; Prolonged overconcern for client; Psychosomaticism; Rejection; Taking on illness signs of client

Related Factors: Arbitrary handling of family's resistance to treatment; Dissonant coping styles for dealing with adaptive tasks by the significant person and client; Dissonant coping styles among significant people; Highly ambivalent family relationships; Significant person with chronically unexpressed feelings (e.g., guilt, anxiety, hostility, despair)

Readiness for Enhanced Family Coping

Definition: A pattern of management of adaptive tasks by primary person (family member, significant other, or close friend) involved with the client's health challenge that is sufficient for health and growth, in regard to self and in relation to the client, and can be strengthened

Defining Characteristics: Chooses experiences that optimize wellness; Individual expresses interest in making contact with others who have experienced a similar situation; Significant person attempts to describe growth impact of crisis; Significant person moves in direction of enriching lifestyle; Significant person moves in direction of health promotion

Death Anxiety

Definition: Vague uneasy feeling of discomfort or dread generated by perceptions of a real or imagined threat to one's existence

Defining Characteristics: Reports concerns of overworking the caregiver; Reports deep sadness; Reports fear of developing terminal illness; Reports fear of loss of mental abilities when dying; Reports fear of pain related to dying; Reports fear of premature death; Reports fear of prolonged dying; Reports fear of suffering related to dying; Reports fear of the process of dying; Reports feeling powerless over dying; Reports negative thoughts related to death and dying; Reports worry about the impact of one's own death on significant others

Related Factors: Anticipating adverse consequences of general anesthesia; Anticipating impact of death on others; Anticipating pain; Anticipating suffering; Confronting the reality of terminal disease; Discussions on the topic of death; Experiencing dying process; Near-death experience; Nonacceptance of own mortality; Observations related to death; Perceived proximity of death; Uncertainty about an encounter with a higher power; Uncertainty about the existence of a higher power; Uncertainty about life after death; Uncertainty of prognosis

Ineffective Denial

Definition: Conscious or unconscious attempt to disavow the knowledge or meaning of an event to reduce anxiety and/or fear, leading to the detriment of health

Defining Characteristics: Delays seeking healthcare attention; Displaces fear of impact of the condition; Displaces source of symptoms to other organs; Displays inappropriate affect; Does not admit fear of death; Does not admit fear of invalidism; Does not perceive personal relevance of danger; Does not perceive personal relevance of symptoms; Makes dismissive comments when speaking of distressing events; Makes dismissive gestures when speaking of distressing events; Minimizes symptoms; Refuses healthcare attention; Unable to admit impact of disease on life pattern; Uses self-treatment

Related Factors: Anxiety; Fear of death; Fear of loss of autonomy; Fear of separation; Lack of competency in using effective coping mechanisms; Lack of control of life situation; Lack of emotional support from others; Overwhelming stress; Threat of inadequacy in dealing with strong emotions; Threat of unpleasant reality

Adult Failure to Thrive

Definition: Progressive functional deterioration of a physical and cognitive nature. The individual's ability to live with multisystem diseases, cope with ensuing problems, and manage his or her care is remarkably diminished

Defining Characteristics: Altered mood state; Anorexia; Apathy; Cognitive decline (Decreased perception, Demonstrated difficulty responding to environmental stimuli, Demonstrated difficulty with concentration, Demonstrated difficulty with decision-making, Demonstrated difficulty with judgment, Demonstrated difficulty with memory, Demonstrated difficulty with reasoning); Consumption of minimal to no food at most meals (e.g., consumes <75% of normal requirements); Decreased participation in activities of daily living; Decreased social skills; Frequent exacerbations of chronic health problems; Inadequate nutritional intake; Neglect of financial responsibilities; Neglect of home environment; Physical decline (e.g., fatigue, dehydration, incontinence of bowel and bladder); Reports desire for death; Reports loss of interest in pleasurable outlets; Self-care deficit; Social withdrawal; Unintentional weight loss (e.g., 5% in 1 month, 10% in 6 months)

Related Factors: Depression

Fear

Definition: Response to perceived threat that is consciously recognized as a danger

Defining Characteristics: Reports alarm; Reports apprehension; Reports being scared; Reports decreased self-assurance; Reports dread; Reports excitement; Reports increased tension; Reports jitteriness; Reports panic; Reports terror

Cognitive: Diminished learning ability; Diminished problem-solving ability; Diminished productivity; Identifies object of fear; Stimulus believed to be a threat

Behaviors: Attack behaviors; Avoidance behaviors; Impulsiveness; Increased alertness; Narrowed focus on the source of the fear

Physiological: Anorexia; Diarrhea; Dry mouth; Dyspnea; Fatigue; Increased perspiration; Increased pulse; Increased respiratory rate; Increased systolic blood pressure; Muscle tightness; Nausea; Pallor; Pupil dilation; Vomiting

Related Factors: Innate origin (e.g., sudden noise, height, pain, loss of physical support); Innate releasers (neurotransmitters); Language barrier; Learned response (e.g., conditioning, modeling from or identification with others); Phobic stimulus; Sensory impairment; Separation from support system in potentially stressful situation (e.g., hospitalization, hospital procedures); Unfamiliarity with environmental experience(s)

Grieving

Definition: A normal complex process that includes emotional, physical, spiritual, social, and intellectual responses and behaviors by which individuals, families, and communities incorporate an actual, anticipated, or perceived loss into their daily lives

Defining Characteristics: Alteration in activity level; Alterations in dream patterns; Alterations in immune function; Alterations in neuroendocrine function; Anger; Blame; Despair; Detachment; Disorganization; Disturbed sleep pattern; Experiencing relief; Maintaining the connection to the deceased; Making meaning of the loss; Pain; Panic behavior; Personal growth; Psychological distress; Suffering

Related Factors: Anticipatory loss of significant object (e.g., possession, job, status, home, parts and processes of body); Anticipatory loss of a significant other; Death of a significant other; Loss of significant object (e.g., possession, job, status, home, parts and processes of body)

Complicated Grieving

Definition: A disorder that occurs after the death of a significant other, in which the experience of distress accompanying bereavement fails to follow normative expectations and manifests in functional impairment

Defining Characteristics: Decreased functioning in life roles; Decreased sense of well-being; Depression; Experiencing somatic symptoms of the deceased; Fatigue; Grief avoidance; Longing for the deceased; Low levels of intimacy; Persistent emotional distress; Preoccupation with thoughts of the deceased; Reports anxiety; Reports distressful feelings about the deceased; Reports feeling dazed;

Reports feeling empty; Reports feeling in shock; Reports feeling stunned; Reports feelings of anger; Reports feelings of detachment from others; Reports feelings of disbelief; Reports feelings of mistrust; Reports lack of acceptance of the death; Reports persistent painful memories; Reports self-blame; Rumination; Searching for the deceased; Self-blame; Separation distress; Traumatic distress; Yearning

Related Factors: Death of a significant other; Emotional instability; Lack of social support

Risk for Complicated Grieving

Definition: At risk for a disorder that occurs after the death of a significant other, in which the experience of distress accompanying bereavement fails to follow normative expectations and manifests in functional impairment

Risk Factors: Death of a significant other; Emotional instability; Lack of social support

Readiness for Enhanced Power

Definition: A pattern of participating knowingly in change that is sufficient for well-being and can be strengthened

Defining Characteristics: Expresses readiness to enhance awareness of possible changes to be made; Expresses readiness to enhance freedom to perform actions for change; Expresses readiness to enhance identification of choices that can be made for change; Expresses readiness to enhance involvement in creating change; Expresses readiness to enhance knowledge for participation in change; Expresses readiness to enhance participation in choices for daily living; Expresses readiness to enhance participation in choices for health; Expresses readiness to enhance power

Note: Even though power (a response) and empowerment (an intervention approach) are different concepts, the literature related to both concepts supports the defining characteristics of this diagnosis.

Powerlessness

Definition: The lived experience of lack of control over a situation, including a perception that one's actions do not significantly affect an outcome

Defining Characteristics: Dependence on others; Depression over physical deterioration; Nonparticipation in care; Reports alienation; Reports doubt regarding role performance; Reports frustration over inability to perform previous activities; Reports lack of control; Reports shame

Related Factors: Illness-related regimen; Institutional environment; Unsatisfying interpersonal interactions

Risk for Powerlessness

Definition: At risk for the lived experience of lack of control over a situation, including a perception that one's actions do not significantly affect an outcome.

Risk Factors: Anxiety; Caregiving; Chronic low self-esteem; Deficient knowledge; Economically disadvantaged; Illness; Ineffective coping patterns; Lack of social support; Pain; Progressive debilitating disease; Situational low self-esteem; Social marginalization; Stigmatized condition; Stigmatized disease; Unpredictable course of illness

Impaired Individual Resilience

Definition: Decreased ability to sustain a pattern of positive responses to an adverse situation or crisis

Defining Characteristics: Decreased interest in academic activities; Decreased interest in vocational activities; Depression; Guilt; Isolation; Lower perceived health status; Low self-esteem; Renewed elevation of distress; Shame; Social isolation; Using maladaptive coping skills (i.e., drug use, violence, etc.)

Related Factors: Demographics that increase chance of maladjustment; Gender; Inconsistent parenting; Large family size; Low intelligence; Low maternal education; Minority status; Neighborhood violence; Parental mental illness; Poor impulse control; Poverty; Psychological disorders; Substance abuse; Violence; Vulnerability factors which encompass indices that exacerbate the negative effects of the risk condition

Readiness for Enhanced Resilience

Definition: A pattern of positive responses to an adverse situation or crisis that is sufficient for optimizing human potential and can be strengthened

Defining Characteristics: Access to resources; Demonstrates positive outlook; Effective use of conflict management strategies; Enhances personal coping skills; Expressed desire to enhance resilience; Identifies available resources; Identifies support systems; Increases positive relationships with others; Involvement in activities; Makes progress toward goals; Presence of a crisis; Reports enhanced sense of control; Reports self-esteem; Safe environment is maintained; Sets goals; Takes responsibilities for actions; Use of effective communication skills

Risk for Compromised Resilience

Definition: At risk for decreased ability to sustain a pattern of positive responses to an adverse situation or crisis

Risk Factors: Chronicity of existing crises; Multiple coexisting adverse situations; Presence of an additional new crisis (e.g., unplanned pregnancy, death of a spouse, loss of job, illness, loss of housing, death of family member)

Chronic Sorrow

Definition: Cyclical, recurring, and potentially progressive pattern of pervasive sadness experienced (by a parent, caregiver, individual with chronic illness or disability) in response to continual loss, throughout the trajectory of an illness or disability

Defining Characteristics: Reports feelings of sadness (e.g., periodic, recurrent); Reports feelings that interfere with ability to reach highest level of personal well-being; Reports feelings that interfere with ability to reach highest level of social well-being; Reports negative feelings (e.g., anger, being misunderstood, confusion, depression, disappointment, emptiness, fear, frustration, guilt, self-blame, helplessness, hopelessness, loneliness, low self-esteem, recurring loss, being overwhelmed)

Related Factors: Crises in management of the disability; Crises in management of the illness; Crises related to developmental stages; Death of a loved one; Experiences chronic disability (e.g., physical or mental); Experiences chronic illness (e.g., physical or mental); Missed opportunities; Missed milestones; Unending caregiving

Stress Overload

Definition: Excessive amounts and types of demands that require action

Defining Characteristics: Demonstrates increased feelings of anger; Demonstrates increased feelings of impatience; Reports a feeling of pressure; Reports a feeling of tension; Reports difficulty in functioning; Reports excessive situational stress (e.g., rates stress level as 7 or above on a 10-point scale); Reports increased feelings of anger; Reports increased feelings of impatience; Reports negative impact from stress (e.g., physical symptoms, psychological distress,

feeling of being sick or of going to get sick); Reports problems with decision-making

Related Factors: Inadequate resources (e.g., financial, social, education/knowledge level); Intense stressors (e.g., family violence, chronic illness, terminal illness); Multiple coexisting stressors (e.g., environmental threats/demands, physical threats/demands, social threats/demands); Repeated stressors (e.g., family violence, chronic illness, terminal illness)

Class 3: Neurobehavioral Stress

Autonomic Dysreflexia

Definition: Life-threatening, uninhibited sympathetic response of the nervous system to a noxious stimulus after a spinal cord injury at T7 or above

Defining Characteristics: Blurred vision; Bradycardia; Chest pain; Chilling; Conjunctival congestion; Diaphoresis (above the injury); Headache (a diffuse pain in different portions of the head and not confined to any nerve distribution area); Horner's syndrome; Metallic taste in mouth; Nasal congestion; Pallor (below the injury); Paresthesia; Paroxysmal hypertension; Pilomotor reflex; Red splotches on skin (above the injury); Tachycardia

Related Factors: Bladder distension; Bowel distension; Deficient caregiver knowledge; Deficient patient knowledge; Skin irritation

Risk for Autonomic Dysreflexia

Definition: At risk for life-threatening, uninhibited response of the sympathetic nervous system, postspinal shock, in an individual with spinal cord injury or lesion at T6 or above (has been demonstrated in patients with injuries at T7 and T8)

Risk Factors: An injury at T6 or above or a lesion at T6 or above AND at least one of the following noxious stimuli.

Cardiopulmonary Stimuli: Deep vein thrombosis; Pulmonary emboli

Gastrointestinal Stimuli: Bowel distension; Constipation; Difficult passage of feces; Digital stimulation; Enemas; Esophageal reflux; Fecal impaction; Gallstones; Gastric ulcers; Gastrointestinal system pathology; Hemorrhoids; Suppositories

Musculoskeletal–Integumentary Stimuli: Cutaneous stimulation (e.g., pressure ulcer, ingrown toenail, dressings, burns, rash); Fractures; Heterotopic bone; Pressure over bony prominences; Pressure over genitalia; Range-of-motion exercises; Spasm; Sunburns; Wounds

Neurological Stimuli: Irritating stimuli below level of injury; Painful stimuli below level of injury

Regulatory Stimuli: Extreme environmental temperatures; Temperature fluctuations

Reproductive Stimuli: Ejaculation; Labor and delivery; Menstruation; Ovarian cyst; Pregnancy; Sexual intercourse

Situational Stimuli: Constrictive clothing (e.g., straps, stockings, shoes); Narcotic/opiate withdrawal; Positioning; Reactions to pharmaceutical agents (e.g., decongestants, sympathomimetics, vasoconstrictors); Surgical procedure

Urological Stimuli: Bladder distension; Bladder spasm; Calculi; Catheterization; Cystitis; Detrusor sphincter dyssynergia; Epididymitis; Instrumentation; Surgery; Urethritis; Urinary tract infection

Disorganized Infant Behavior

Definition: Disintegrated physiological and neurobehavioral responses of infant to the environment

Defining Characteristics:

Attention–Interaction System: Abnormal response to sensory stimuli (e.g., difficult to soothe, unable to sustain alert status)

Motor System: Altered primitive reflexes; Changes to motor tone; Finger splaying; Fisting; Hands to face; Hyperextension of extremities; Jittery; Startles; Tremors; Twitches; Uncoordinated movement

Physiological: Arrhythmias; Bradycardia; Desaturation; Feeding intolerances; Skin color changes; Tachycardia; Time-out signals (e.g., gaze, grasp, hiccough, cough, sneeze, sigh, slack jaw, open mouth, tongue thrust)

Regulatory Problems: Inability to inhibit startle; Irritability

State–Organization System: Active–awake (fussy, worried gaze); Diffuse sleep; Irritable crying; Quiet–awake (staring, gaze aversion); State–oscillation

Related Factors:

Caregiver: Cue misreading; Deficient knowledge regarding behavioral cues; Environmental stimulation contribution

Environmental: Lack of containment within environment; Physical environment inappropriateness; Sensory deprivation; Sensory inappropriateness; Sensory overstimulation

Individual: Illness; Immature neurological system; Low postconceptual age; Prematurity

Postnatal: Feeding intolerance; Invasive procedures; Malnutrition; Motor problems; Oral problems; Pain

Prenatal: Congenital disorders; Genetic disorders; Teratogenic exposure

Readiness for Enhanced Organized Infant Behavior

Definition: A pattern of modulation of the physiological and behavioral systems of functioning (i.e., autonomic, motor, state–organization, self-regulatory, and attentional–interactional systems) in an infant that is sufficient for well-being and can be strengthened

Defining Characteristics: Definite sleep–wake states; Response to stimuli (e.g., visual, auditory); Stable physiological measures; Use of some self-regulatory behaviors

Risk for Disorganized Infant Behavior

Definition: At risk for alteration in integrating and modulation of the physiological and behavioral systems of functioning (i.e., autonomic, motor, state–organization, self-regulatory, and attentional–interactional systems)

Risk Factors: Environmental overstimulation; Invasive procedures; Lack of containment within environment; Motor problems; Oral problems; Pain; Painful procedures; Prematurity

Decreased Intracranial Adaptive Capacity

Definition: Intracranial fluid dynamic mechanisms that normally compensate for increases in intracranial volumes are compromised, resulting in repeated disproportionate increases in intracranial pressure (ICP) in response to a variety of noxious and non-noxious stimuli

Defining Characteristics: Baseline ICP ≥10 mmHg; Disproportionate increase in ICP following stimulus; Elevated P2 ICP waveform; Repeated increases of >10 mmHg for more than 5 minutes following any of a variety of external stimuli; Volume–pressure response test variation (volume:pressure ratio 2, pressure–volume index <10); Wide-amplitude ICP waveform

Related Factors: Brain injuries; Decreased cerebral perfusion ≤50–60 mmHg; Sustained increase in ICP of 10–15 mmHg; Systemic hypotension with intracranial hypertension

DOMAIN 10: LIFE PRINCIPLES

Class 1: Values

Readiness for Enhanced Hope

Definition: A pattern of expectations and desires for mobilizing energy on one's own behalf that is sufficient for well-being and can be strengthened

Defining Characteristics: Expresses desire to enhance ability to set achievable goals; Expresses desire to enhance belief in possibilities; Expresses desire to enhance congruency of expectations with desires; Expresses desire to enhance hope; Expresses desire to enhance interconnectedness with others; Expresses desire to enhance problem-solving to meet goals; Expresses desire to enhance sense of meaning to life; Expresses desire to enhance spirituality

Class 2: Beliefs

Readiness for Enhanced Spiritual Well-Being

Definition: A pattern of experiencing and integrating meaning and purpose in life through connectedness with self, others, art, music, literature, nature, and/or a power greater than oneself that is sufficient for well-being and can be strengthened

Defining Characteristics:

Connections to Self: Expresses desire for enhanced acceptance; Expresses desire for enhanced coping; Expresses desire for enhanced courage; Expresses desire for enhanced hope; Expresses desire for enhanced joy; Expresses desire for enhanced love; Expresses desire for enhanced meaning in life; Expresses desire for enhanced purpose in life; Expresses desire for enhanced satisfying philosophy of life; Expresses desire for enhanced self-forgiveness; Expresses desire for enhanced serenity (e.g., peace); Expresses desire for enhanced surrender; Meditation

Connections with Others: Provides service to others; Requests forgiveness of others; Requests interactions with significant others; Requests interactions with spiritual leaders

Connections with Art, Music, Literature, Nature: Displays creative energy (e.g., writing, poetry, singing); Listens to music; Reads spiritual literature; Spends time outdoors

Connections with Power Greater Than Self: Expresses awe; Expresses reverence; Participates in religious activities; Prays; Reports mystical experiences

Class 3: Value/Belief/Action Congruence

Readiness for Enhanced Decision-Making

Definition: A pattern of choosing a course of action that is sufficient for meeting short- and long-term health-related goals and can be strengthened

Defining Characteristics: Expresses desire to enhance congruency of decisions with goals; Expresses desire to enhance congruency of decisions with personal values; Expresses desire to enhance congruency of decisions with sociocultural goals; Expresses desire to enhance congruency of decisions with sociocultural values; Expresses desire to enhance decision-making; Expresses desire to enhance risk–benefit analysis of decisions; Expresses desire to enhance understanding of choices for decision-making; Expresses desire to enhance understanding of the meaning of choices; Expresses desire to enhance use of reliable evidence for decisions

Decisional Conflict

Definition: Uncertainty about course of action to be taken when choice among competing actions involves risk, loss, or challenge to values and beliefs

Defining Characteristics: Delayed decision-making; Physical signs of distress (e.g., increased heart rate, restlessness); Physical signs of tension; Questioning moral principles while attempting a decision; Questioning moral rules while attempting a decision; Questioning moral values while attempting a decision; Questioning personal beliefs while attempting a decision; Questioning personal values while attempting a decision; Self-focusing; Vacillation among alternative choices; Verbalizes feeling of distress while attempting a decision; Verbalizes uncertainty about choices; Verbalizes undesired consequences of alternative actions being considered

Related Factors: Divergent sources of information; Interference with decision-making; Lack of experience with decision-making; Lack of relevant information; Moral obligations require not performing action; Moral obligations require performing action; Moral principles support mutually inconsistent courses of action; Moral rules support mutually inconsistent courses of action; Moral values support mutually inconsistent courses of action; Multiple sources of information; Perceived threat to value system; Support system deficit; Unclear personal beliefs; Unclear personal values

Moral Distress

Definition: Response to the inability to carry out one's chosen ethical/moral decision/action

Defining Characteristics: Expresses anguish (e.g., powerlessness, guilt, frustration, anxiety, self-doubt, fear) over difficulty acting on one's moral choice

Related Factors: Conflict among decision-makers; Conflicting information guiding ethical decision-making; Conflicting information guiding moral decision-making; Cultural conflicts; End-of-life decisions; Loss of autonomy; Physical distance of decision-maker; Time constraints for decision-making; Treatment decisions

Noncompliance

Definition: Behavior of person and/or caregiver that fails to coincide with a health-promoting or therapeutic plan agreed on by the person (and/or family and/or community) and healthcare professional. In the presence of an agreed upon, health–promoting, or therapeutic plan, the person's or caregiver's behavior is fully or partially nonadherent and may lead to clinically ineffective or partially ineffective outcomes

Defining Characteristics: Behavior indicative of failure to adhere; Evidence of development of complications; Evidence of exacerbation of symptoms; Failure to keep appointments; Failure to progress; Objective tests provide evidence of failure to adhere (e.g., physiological measures, detection of physiological markers)

Related Factors:

Health System: Access to care; Communication skills of the provider; Convenience of care; Credibility of provider; Difficulty in client–provider relationship; Individual health coverage; Provider continuity; Provider regular follow-up; Provider reimbursement; Satisfaction with care; Teaching skills of the provider

Healthcare Plan: Complexity; Cost; Duration; Financial flexibility of plan; Intensity

Individual: Cultural influences; Deficient knowledge related to the regimen behavior; Developmental abilities; Health beliefs; Individual's value system; Motivational forces; Personal abilities; Significant others; Skill relevant to the regimen behavior; Spiritual values

Network: Involvement of members in health plan; Perceived beliefs of significant others; Social value regarding plan

Impaired Religiosity

Definition: Impaired ability to exercise reliance on beliefs and/or participate in rituals of a particular faith tradition

Defining Characteristics: Difficulty adhering to prescribed religious beliefs; Difficulty adhering to prescribed religious rituals (e.g., religious ceremonies, dietary regulations, clothing, prayer, worship/religious services, private religious behaviors/reading religious materials/media, holiday observances, meetings with religious leaders); Questions religious belief patterns; Questions religious customs; Reports a need to reconnect with previous belief patterns; Reports a need to reconnect with previous customs; Reports emotional distress because of separation from faith community

Related Factors:

Developmental and Situational: Aging; End-stage life crises; Life transitions

Physical: Illness; Pain

Psychological: Anxiety; Fear of death; Ineffective coping; Ineffective support; Lack of security; Personal crisis; Use of religion to manipulate

Sociocultural: Cultural barriers to practicing religion; Environmental barriers to practicing religion; Lack of social integration; Lack of sociocultural interaction

Spiritual: Spiritual crises; Suffering

Readiness for Enhanced Religiosity

Definition: A pattern of reliance on religious beliefs and/or participation in rituals of a particular faith tradition that is sufficient for well-being and can be strengthened

Defining Characteristics: Expresses desire to strengthen belief patterns that have provided religion in the past; Expresses desire to strengthen religious belief patterns that have provided comfort in the past; Expresses desire to strengthen religious customs that have provided comfort in the past; Questions belief patterns that are harmful; Questions customs that are harmful; Rejects belief patterns that are harmful; Rejects customs that are harmful; Requests assistance to expand religious options; Requests assistance to increase participation in prescribed religious beliefs (e.g., religious ceremonies, dietary regulations/rituals, clothing, prayer, worship/religious services, private religious behaviors, reading religious materials/media, holiday observances); Requests forgiveness; Requests meeting with religious leaders/facilitators; Requests reconciliation; Requests religious experiences; Requests religious materials

Risk for Impaired Religiosity

Definition: At risk for an impaired ability to exercise reliance on religious beliefs and/or participate in rituals of a particular faith tradition

Risk Factors:

Developmental: Life transitions

Environmental: Barriers to practicing religion; Lack of transportation

Physical: Hospitalization; Illness; Pain

Psychological: Depression; Ineffective caregiving; Ineffective coping; Ineffective support; Lack of security

Sociocultural: Cultural barrier to practicing religion; Lack of social interaction; Social isolation

Spiritual: Suffering

Spiritual Distress

Definition: Impaired ability to experience and integrate meaning and purpose in life through connectedness with self, others, art, music, literature, nature, and/or a power greater than oneself

Defining Characteristics:

Connections to Self: Anger; Expresses lack of acceptance; Expresses lack of courage; Expresses lack of hope; Expresses lack of love; Expresses lack of meaning in life; Expresses lack of purpose in life; Expresses lack of self-forgiveness; Expresses lack of serenity (e.g., peace); Guilt; Ineffective coping

Connections with Others: Expresses alienation; Refuses interactions with significant others; Refuses interactions with spiritual leaders; Verbalizes being separated from support system

Connections with Art, Music, Literature, and Nature: Disinterest in nature; Disinterest in reading spiritual literature; Inability to express previous state of creativity (e.g., singing/listening to music/ writing)

Connections with Power Greater than Self: Expresses anger toward power greater than self; Expresses feeling abandoned; Expresses hopelessness; Expresses suffering; Inability for introspection; Inability to experience the transcendent; Inability to participate in religious activities; Inability to pray; Requests to see a spiritual leader; Sudden changes in spiritual practices

Related Factors: Active dying; Anxiety; Chronic illness; Death; Life change; Loneliness; Pain; Self-alienation; Social alienation; Sociocultural deprivation

Risk for Spiritual Distress

Definition: At risk for an impaired ability to experience and integrate meaning and purpose in life through connectedness with self, others, art, music, literature, nature, and/or a power greater than oneself

Risk Factors:

Developmental: Life changes

Environmental: Environmental changes; Natural disasters

Physical: Chronic illness; Physical illness; Substance abuse

Psychosocial: Anxiety; Blocks to experiencing love; Change in religious rituals; Change in spiritual practices; Cultural conflict; Depression; Inability to forgive; Loss; Low self-esteem; Poor relationships; Racial conflict; Separated support systems; Stress

DOMAIN 11: SAFETY/PROTECTION

Class 1: Infection

Risk for Infection

Definition: At risk for being invaded by pathogenic organisms

Risk Factors: Chronic disease (Diabetes mellitus, Obesity); Deficient knowledge to avoid exposure to pathogens; Inadequate primary defenses (Altered peristalsis, Broken skin [e.g., intravenous catheter placement, invasive procedures], Change in pH of secretions, Decrease in ciliary action, Premature rupture of amniotic membranes, Prolonged rupture of amniotic membranes, Smoking, Stasis of body fluids, Traumatized tissue [e.g., trauma, tissue destruction]); Inadequate secondary defenses (Decreased hemoglobin; Immunosuppression [e.g., inadequate acquired immunity; pharmaceutical agents including immunosuppressants, steroids, monoclonal antibodies, immunomodulators], Leukopenia, Suppressed inflammatory response); Inadequate vaccination; Increased environmental exposure to pathogens (Outbreaks); Invasive procedures; Malnutrition

Class 2: Physical Injury

Ineffective Airway Clearance

Definition: Inability to clear secretions or obstructions from the respiratory tract to maintain a clear airway

Defining Characteristics: Absent cough; Adventitious breath sounds; Changes in respiratory rate; Changes in respiratory rhythm; Cyanosis; Difficulty vocalizing; Diminished breath sounds; Dyspnea; Excessive sputum; Ineffective cough; Orthopnea; Restlessness; Wide-eyed

Related Factors:

Environmental: Second-hand smoke; Smoke inhalation; Smoking

Obstructed Airway: Airway spasm; Excessive mucus; Exudate in the alveoli; Foreign body in airway; Presence of artificial airway; Retained secretions; Secretions in the bronchi

Physiological: Allergic airways; Asthma; Chronic obstructive pulmonary disease; Hyperplasia of the bronchial walls; Infection; Neuromuscular dysfunction

Risk for Aspiration

Definition: At risk for entry of gastrointestinal secretions, oropharyngeal secretions, solids, or fluids into the tracheobronchial passages

Risk Factors: Decreased gastrointestinal motility; Delayed gastric emptying; Depressed cough; Depressed gag reflex; Facial surgery; Facial trauma; Gastrointestinal tubes; Impaired swallowing; Incompetent lower esophageal sphincter; Increased gastric residual; Increased intragastric pressure; Neck surgery; Neck trauma; Oral surgery; Oral trauma; Presence of endotracheal tube; Presence of tracheostomy tube; Reduced level of consciousness; Situations hindering elevation of upper body; Treatment-related side effects (e.g., pharmaceutical agents); Tube feedings; Wired jaws

Risk for Bleeding

Definition: At risk for a decrease in blood volume that may compromise health

Risk Factors: Aneurysm; Circumcision; Deficient knowledge; Disseminated intravascular coagulopathy; History of falls; Gastrointestinal disorders (e.g., gastric ulcer disease, polyps, varices); Impaired liver function (e.g., cirrhosis, hepatitis); Inherent coagulopathies (e.g., thrombocytopenia); Postpartum complications (e.g., uterine atony, retained placenta); Pregnancy-related complications (e.g., placenta previa, molar pregnancy, placenta abruptio [placental abruption]); Trauma; Treatment-related side effects (e.g., surgery, medications, administration of platelet-deficient blood products, chemotherapy)

Impaired Dentition

Definition: Disruption in tooth development/eruption patterns or structural integrity of individual teeth

Defining Characteristics: Abraded teeth; Absent teeth; Asymmetrical facial expression; Crown caries; Erosion of enamel; Excessive calculus; Excessive plaque; Halitosis; Incomplete eruption for age (primary or permanent teeth); Loose teeth; Malocclusion; Missing teeth; Premature loss of primary teeth; Root caries; Tooth enamel discoloration; Tooth fracture(s); Tooth misalignment; Toothache; Worn-down teeth

Related Factors: Barriers to self-care; Bruxism; Chronic use of coffee; Chronic use of red wine; Chronic use of tea; Chronic use of tobacco; Chronic vomiting; Deficient knowledge regarding dental health; Dietary habits; Economically disadvantaged; Excessive intake of fluorides; Excessive use of abrasive cleaning agents; Genetic predisposition; Ineffective oral hygiene; Lack of access to professional care; Nutritional deficits; Selected prescription medications; Sensitivity to cold; Sensitivity to heat

Risk For Dry Eye

Definition: At risk for eye discomfort or damage to the cornea and conjunctiva due to reduced quantity or quality of tears to moisten the eye

Risk Factors: Aging; Autoimmune diseases (rheumatoid arthritis, diabetes mellitus, thyroid disease, gout, osteoporosis, etc.); Contact lenses; Environmental factors (air-conditioning, excessive wind, sunlight exposure, air pollution, low humidity); Female gender; History of allergy; Hormones; Lifestyle (e.g., smoking, caffeine use, prolonged reading); Mechanical ventilation therapy; Neurological lesions with sensory or motor reflex loss (lagophthalmos, lack of spontaneous blink reflex due to decreased consciousness and other medical conditions); Ocular surface damage; Place of living; Treatment-related side effects (e.g., pharmaceutical agents such as angiotensin-converting enzyme inhibitors, antihistamines, diuretics, steroids, antidepressants, tranquilizers, analgesics, sedatives, neuromuscular blockage agents; surgical operations); Vitamin A deficiency

Risk for Falls

Definition: At risk for increased susceptibility to falling that may cause physical harm

Risk Factors:

Adults: Age 65 or older; History of falls; Lives alone; Lower limb prosthesis; Use of assistive devices (e.g., walker, cane); Wheelchair use

Children: Age 2 or younger; Bed located near window; Lack of automobile restraints; Lack of gate on stairs; Lack of parental supervision; Lack of window guard; Male gender when <1 year of age; Unattended infant on elevated surface (e.g., bed, changing table)

Cognitive: Diminished mental status

Environment: Cluttered environment; Dimly lit room; Lacks antislip material in bath; Lacks antislip material in shower; Restraints; Throw rugs; Unfamiliar room; Weather conditions (e.g., wet floors, ice)

Medications: Alcohol use; Angiotensin-converting enzyme inhibitors; Antianxiety agents; Antihypertensive agents; Diuretics; Hypnotics; Narcotics/opiates; Tranquilizers; Tricyclic antidepressants

Physiological: Acute illness; Anemia; Arthritis; Decreased lower extremity strength; Diarrhea; Difficulty with gait; Faintness when extending neck; Faintness when turning neck; Foot problems; Hearing difficulties; Impaired balance; Impaired physical mobility; Incontinence; Neoplasms (i.e., fatigue/limited mobility); Neuropathy; Orthostatic hypotension; Postoperative conditions; Postprandial blood sugar changes; Proprioceptive deficits; Sleeplessness; Urinary urgency; Vascular disease; Visual difficulties

Risk for Injury

Definition: At risk for injury as a result of environmental conditions interacting with the individual's adaptive and defensive resources

Risk Factors:

External: Biological (e.g., immunization level of community, microorganism); Chemical (e.g., poisons, pollutants, drugs, pharmaceutical agents, alcohol, nicotine, preservatives, cosmetics, dyes); Human (e.g., nosocomial agents, staffing patterns, or cognitive, affective, psychomotor factors); Mode of transport; Nutritional (e.g., vitamins, food types); Physical (e.g., design, structure, and arrangement of community, building, and/or equipment)

Internal: Abnormal blood profile (e.g., leukocytosis/leukopenia, altered clotting factors, thrombocytopenia, sickle cell, thalassemia,

decreased hemoglobin); Biochemical dysfunction; Developmental age (physiological, psychosocial); Effector dysfunction; Immune/autoimmune dysfunction; Integrative dysfunction; Malnutrition; Physical (e.g., broken skin, altered mobility); Psychological (affective orientation); Sensory dysfunction; Tissue hypoxia

Impaired Oral Mucous Membrane

Definition: Disruption of the lips and/or soft tissue of the oral cavity

Defining Characteristics: Bleeding; Bluish masses (e.g., hemangiomas); Cheilitis; Coated tongue; Desquamation; Difficult speech; Difficulty eating; Difficulty swallowing; Diminished taste; Edema; Enlarged tonsils; Fissures; Geographic tongue; Gingival hyperplasia; Gingival pallor; Gingival recession; Halitosis; Hyperemia; Macroplasia; Mucosal denudation; Mucosal pallor; Nodules; Oral discomfort; Oral lesions; Oral pain; Oral ulcers; Papules; Pocketing deeper than 4 mm; Presence of pathogens; Purulent drainage; Purulent exudates; Red masses (e.g., hemangiomas); Reports bad taste in mouth; Smooth atrophic tongue; Spongy patches; Stomatitis; Vesicles; White, curd-like exudate; White patches; White plaques; Xerostomia

Related Factors: Barriers to oral self-care; Barriers to professional care; Chemical irritants (e.g., alcohol, tobacco, acidic foods, drugs, regular use of inhalers or other noxious agents); Cleft lip; Cleft palate; Decreased platelets; Decreased salivation; Deficient knowledge of appropriate oral hygiene; Dehydration; Depression; Diminished hormone levels (women); Ineffective oral hygiene; Infection; Immunocompromised; Immunosuppressed; Loss of supportive structures; Malnutrition; Mechanical factors (e.g., ill-fitting dentures, braces, tubes [endotracheal/nasogastric], surgery in oral cavity); Mouth breathing; Nil by mouth (NPO) for more than 24 hours; Stress; Treatment-related side effects (e.g., chemotherapy, pharmaceutical agents, radiation therapy); Trauma

Risk for Perioperative Positioning Injury

Definition: At risk for inadvertent anatomical and physical changes as a result of posture or equipment used during an invasive/surgical procedure

Risk Factors: Disorientation; Edema; Emaciation; Immobilization; Muscle weakness; Obesity; Sensory/perceptual disturbances due to anesthesia

Risk for Peripheral Neurovascular Dysfunction

Definition: At risk for disruption in the circulation, sensation, or motion of an extremity

Risk Factors: Burns; Fractures; Immobilization; Mechanical compression (e.g., tourniquet, cane, cast, brace, dressing, restraint); Orthopedic surgery; Trauma; Vascular obstruction

Risk for Shock

Definition: At risk for an inadequate blood flow to the body's tissues, which may lead to life-threatening cellular dysfunction

Risk Factors: Hypotension; Hypovolemia; Hypoxemia; Hypoxia; Infection; Sepsis; Systemic inflammatory response syndrome

Impaired Skin Integrity

Definition: Altered epidermis and/or dermis

Defining Characteristics: Destruction of skin layers; Disruption of skin surface; Invasion of body structures

Related Factors:

External: Chemical substance; Extremes of age; Humidity; Hyperthermia; Hypothermia; Mechanical factors (e.g., shearing forces, pressure, restraint); Moisture; Pharmaceutical agents; Physical immobilization; Radiation

Internal: Changes in fluid status; Changes in pigmentation; Changes in turgor; Developmental factors; Imbalanced nutritional state (e.g., obesity, emaciation); Immunological deficit; Impaired circulation; Impaired metabolic state; Impaired sensation; Skeletal prominence

Risk for Impaired Skin Integrity

Definition: At risk for alteration in epidermis and/or dermis

Risk Factors:

External: Chemical substance; Excretions; Extremes of age; Humidity; Hyperthermia; Hypothermia; Mechanical factors (e.g., shearing forces, pressure, restraint); Moisture; Physical immobilization; Radiation; Secretions

Internal: Changes in pigmentation; Changes in skin turgor; Developmental factors; Imbalanced nutritional state (e.g., obesity, emaciation); Immunological factors; Impaired circulation; Impaired metabolic state; Impaired sensation; Medications; Psychogenetic factors; Skeletal prominence

Note: Risk should be determined by use of a standardized risk assessment tool.

Risk for Sudden Infant Death Syndrome

Definition: At risk for sudden death of an infant under 1 year of age

Risk Factors:

Modifiable: Delayed prenatal care; Infant overheating; Infant overwrapping; Infant placed in prone position to sleep; Infant placed in side-lying position to sleep; Lack of prenatal care; Postnatal infant smoke exposure; Prenatal infant smoke exposure; Soft underlayment (loose articles in the sleep environment)

Potentially Modifiable: Low birth weight; Prematurity; Young maternal age

Nonmodifiable: Ethnicity (e.g., African–American or Native American); Infant age of 2–4 months; Male gender; Seasonality of sudden infant death syndrome deaths (e.g., winter and fall months)

Risk for Suffocation

Definition: At risk of accidental suffocation (inadequate air available for inhalation)

Risk Factors:

External: Children unattended in water; Discarding refrigerators without removing doors; Eating large mouthfuls of food; Hanging a pacifier around infant's neck; Household gas leaks; Inserting small objects into airway; Low-strung clothesline; Pillow in infant's crib; Playing with plastic bags; Propped bottle in infant's crib; Smoking in bed; Fuel-burning heaters not vented to outside; Vehicle warming in closed garage

Internal: Cognitive difficulties; Deficient knowledge regarding safe situations; Deficient knowledge regarding safety precautions; Disease process; Emotional difficulties; Injury process; Reduced motor abilities; Reduced olfactory sensation

Delayed Surgical Recovery

Definition: Extension of the number of postoperative days required to initiate and perform activities that maintain life, health, and well-being

Defining Characteristics: Difficulty in moving about; Evidence of interrupted healing of surgical area (e.g., red, indurated, draining, immobilized); Fatigue; Loss of appetite with nausea; Loss of appetite without nausea; Perception that more time is needed to recover; Postpones resumption of work/employment activities; Report of discomfort; Report of pain; Requires help to complete self-care

Related Factors: Extensive surgical procedure; Obesity; Pain; Postoperative surgical site infection; Preoperative expectations; Prolonged surgical procedure

Risk for Thermal Injury

Definition: At risk for damage to skin and mucous membranes due to extreme temperatures

Risk Factors: Cognitive impairment (e.g. dementia, psychoses); Developmental level (infants, aged); Exposure to extreme temperatures; Fatigue; Inadequate supervision; Inattentiveness; Intoxication (alcohol, drug); Lack of knowledge (patient, caregiver); Lack of protective clothing (e.g. flame-retardant sleepwear, gloves, ear covering); Neuromuscular impairment (e.g. stroke, amyotrophic lateral sclerosis, multiple sclerosis); Neuropathy; Smoking; Treatment-related side effects (e.g., pharmaceutical agents); Unsafe environment

Impaired Tissue Integrity

Definition: Damage to mucous membrane, corneal, integumentary, or subcutaneous tissues

Defining Characteristics: Damaged tissue (e.g., cornea, mucous membrane, integumentary, subcutaneous); Destroyed tissue

Related Factors: Altered circulation; Chemical irritants; Deficient fluid volume; Deficient knowledge; Excess fluid volume; Impaired physical mobility; Mechanical factors (e.g., pressure, shear, friction); Nutritional factors (e.g., deficit or excess); Radiation; Temperature extremes

Risk for Trauma

Definition: At risk of accidental tissue injury (e.g., wound, burn, fracture)

Risk Factors:

External: Accessibility of guns; Bathing in very hot water (e.g., unsupervised bathing of young children); Children playing with dangerous objects; Children riding in the front seat in car; Contact with corrosives; Contact with intense cold; Contact with rapidly moving machinery; Defective appliances; Delayed lighting of gas appliances; Driving a mechanically unsafe vehicle; Driving at excessive speeds; Driving while intoxicated; Driving without necessary visual aids; Entering unlighted rooms; Experimenting with chemicals; Exposure to dangerous machinery; Faulty electrical plugs; Flammable children's clothing; Flammable children's toys; Frayed wires; Grease waste collected on stoves; High beds; High-crime neighborhood; Inadequate stair rails; Inadequately stored combustibles (e.g., matches, oily rags); Inadequately stored corrosives (e.g., lye); Inappropriate call-for-aid mechanisms for bed-bound client; Knives stored uncovered; Lack of gate at top of stairs; Lack of protection from heat source; Lacks antislip material in bath; Lacks antislip material in shower; Large icicles hanging from roof; Misuse of necessary headgear; Misuse of seat restraints; Nonuse of seat restraints; Obstructed passageways; Overexposure to radiation; Overloaded electrical outlets; Overloaded fuse boxes; Physical proximity to vehicle pathways (e.g., driveways, lanes, railroad tracks); Playing with explosives; Pot handles facing toward front of stove; Potential igniting of gas leaks; Slippery floors (e.g., wet or highly waxed); Smoking in bed; Smoking near oxygen; Struggling with restraints; Throw rugs; Unanchored electric wires; Unsafe road; Unsafe walkways; Unsafe window protection in homes with young children; Use of cracked dishware; Use of unsteady chairs;

Use of unsteady ladders; Wearing flowing clothes around open flame

Internal: Balancing difficulties; Cognitive difficulties; Deficient knowledge regarding safe procedures; Deficient knowledge regarding safety precautions; Economically disadvantaged; Emotional difficulties; History of previous trauma; Poor vision; Reduced hand–eye coordination; Reduced muscle coordination; Reduced sensation; Weakness

Risk for Vascular Trauma

Definition: At risk for damage to a vein and its surrounding tissues related to the presence of a catheter and/or infused solutions

Risk Factors: Catheter type; Catheter width; Impaired ability to visualize the insertion site; Inadequate catheter fixation; Infusion rate; Insertion site; Length of insertion time; Nature of solution (e.g., concentration, chemical irritant, temperature, pH)

Class 3: Violence

Risk for Other-Directed Violence

Definition: At risk for behaviors in which an individual demonstrates that he or she can be physically, emotionally, and/or sexually harmful to others

Risk Factors: Availability of weapon(s); Body language (e.g., rigid posture, clenching of fists and jaw, hyperactivity, pacing, breathlessness, threatening stances); Cognitive impairment (e.g., learning disabilities, attention deficit disorder, decreased intellectual functioning); Cruelty to animals; Firesetting; History of childhood abuse; History of indirect violence (e.g., tearing off clothes, ripping objects off walls, writing on walls, urinating on floor, defecating on floor, stamping feet, temper tantrum, running in corridors, yelling, throwing objects, breaking a window, slamming doors, sexual advances); History of other-directed violence (e.g., hitting someone, kicking someone, spitting at someone, scratching someone, throwing objects at someone, biting someone, attempted rape, rape, sexual molestation, urinating/defecating on a person); History of substance abuse; History of threats of violence (e.g., verbal threats against property, verbal threats against person, social threats, cursing, threatening notes/letters, threatening gestures, sexual threats); History of violent antisocial behavior (e.g., stealing, insistent borrowing, insistent demands for privileges, insistent interruption of meetings, refusal to eat, refusal to take medication, ignoring instructions); History of witnessing family violence; Impulsivity; Motor vehicle offenses (e.g., frequent traffic violations, use of a motor vehicle to release anger); Neurological impairment (e.g., positive EEG, computed tomography, or magnetic resonance imaging scan, neurological findings, head trauma, seizure disorders); Pathological intoxication; Perinatal complications; Prenatal complications; Psychotic symptomatology (e.g., auditory, visual, command hallucinations; paranoid delusions; loose, rambling, or illogical thought processes); Suicidal behavior

Risk for Self-Directed Violence

Definition: At risk for behaviors in which an individual demonstrates that he or she can be physically, emotionally, and/or sexually harmful to self

Risk Factors: Age 15–19; Age 45 or older; Behavioral cues (e.g., writing forlorn love notes, directing angry messages at a significant other who has rejected the person, giving away personal items, taking out a large life insurance policy); Conflictual interpersonal relationships; Emotional problems (e.g., hopelessness, despair, increased anxiety, panic, anger, hostility); Employment problems

(e.g., unemployed, recent job loss/failure); Engagement in auto-erotic sexual acts; Family background (e.g., chaotic or conflictual, history of suicide); History of multiple suicide attempts; Lack of personal resources (e.g., poor achievement, poor insight, affect unavailable and poorly controlled); Lack of social resources (e.g., poor rapport, socially isolated, unresponsive family); Marital status (single, widowed, divorced); Mental health problems (e.g., severe depression, psychosis, severe personality disorder, alcoholism or drug abuse); Occupation (executive, administrator/owner of business, professional, semi-skilled worker); Physical health problems (e.g., hypochondriasis, chronic or terminal illness); Sexual orientation (bisexual [active], homosexual [inactive]); Suicidal ideation; Suicidal plan; Verbal cues (e.g., talking about death, "better off without me" asking questions about lethal dosages of drugs)

Self-Mutilation

Definition: Deliberate self-injurious behavior causing tissue damage with the intent of causing nonfatal injury to attain relief of tension

Defining Characteristics: Abrading; Biting; Constricting a body part; Cuts on body; Hitting; Ingestion of harmful substances; Inhalation of harmful substances; Insertion of object into body orifice; Picking at wounds; Scratches on body; Self-inflicted burns; Severing

Related Factors: Adolescence; Autistic individual; Battered child; Borderline personality disorder; Character disorder; Childhood illness; Childhood sexual abuse; Childhood surgery; Depersonalization; Developmentally delayed individual; Dissociation; Disturbed body image; Disturbed interpersonal relationships; Eating disorders; Emotional disorder; Family divorce; Family history of self-destructive behaviors; Family substance abuse; Feels threatened with loss of significant relationship; History of inability to plan solutions; History of inability to see long-term consequences; History of self-directed violence; Impulsivity; Inability to express tension verbally; Incarceration; Ineffective coping; Irresistible urge to cut self; Irresistible urge for self-directed violence; Isolation from peers; Labile behavior; Lack of family confidant; Living in nontraditional setting (e.g., foster, group, or institutional care); Low self-esteem; Mounting tension that is intolerable; Need for quick reduction of stress; Peers who self-mutilate; Perfectionism; Poor communication between parent and adolescent; Psychotic state (e.g., command hallucinations); Reports negative feelings (e.g., depression, rejection, self-hatred, separation anxiety, guilt, depersonalization); Sexual identity crisis; Substance abuse; Unstable body image; Unstable self-esteem; Use of manipulation to obtain nurturing relationship with others; Violence between parental figures

Risk for Self-Mutilation

Definition: At risk for deliberate self-injurious behavior causing tissue damage with the intent of causing nonfatal injury to attain relief of tension

Risk Factors: Adolescence; Autistic individuals; Battered child; Borderline personality disorders; Character disorders; Childhood illness; Childhood sexual abuse; Childhood surgery; Depersonalization; Developmentally delayed individuals; Dissociation; Disturbed body image; Disturbed interpersonal relationships; Eating disorders; Emotional disorder; Family divorce; Family history of self-destructive behaviors; Family substance abuse; Feels threatened with loss of significant relationship; History of inability to plan solutions; History of inability to see long-term consequences; History of self-directed violence; Impulsivity; Inability to express tension verbally; Inadequate coping; Incarceration; Irresistible urge for self-directed violence; Isolation from peers; Living in nontraditional setting (e.g., foster, group, or institutional care); Loss of control over problem-solving situations; Loss of significant relationship(s); Low self-esteem; Mounting tension that is intolerable; Need for quick reduction of stress; Peers who self-mutilate; Perfectionism; Psychotic state (e.g., command hallucinations); Reports negative feelings (e.g., depression, rejection, self-hatred, separation anxiety, guilt); Sexual identity crisis; Substance abuse; Unstable self-esteem; Use of manipulation to obtain nurturing relationship with others; Violence between parental figures

Risk for Suicide

Definition: At risk for self-inflicted, life-threatening injury

Risk Factors:

Behavioral: Buying a gun; Changing a will; Giving away possessions; History of prior suicide attempt; Impulsiveness; Making a will; Marked changes in attitude; Marked changes in behavior; Marked changes in school performance; Stockpiling medicines; Sudden euphoric recovery from major depression

Demographic: Age (e.g., elderly people, young adult males, adolescents); Divorced; Male gender; Race (e.g., white, Native American); Widowed

Physical: Chronic pain; Physical illness; Terminal illness

Psychological: Childhood abuse; Family history of suicide; Guilt; Homosexual youth; Psychiatric disorder; Psychiatric illness; Substance abuse

Situational: Adolescents living in nontraditional settings (e.g., juvenile detention center, prison, half-way house, group home); Economically disadvantaged; Institutionalization; Living alone; Loss of autonomy; Loss of independence; Presence of gun in home; Relocation; Retired

Social: Cluster suicides; Disciplinary problems; Disrupted family life; Grieving; Helplessness; Hopelessness; Legal problems; Loneliness; Loss of important relationship; Poor support systems; Social isolation

Verbal: States desire to die; Threats of killing oneself

Class 4: Environmental Hazards

Contamination

Definition: Exposure to environmental contaminants in doses sufficient to cause adverse health effects

Defining Characteristics: Defining characteristics are dependent on the causative agent. Agents cause a variety of individual organ responses as well as systemic responses.

Pesticides[1]: Dermatological effects of pesticide exposure; Gastrointestinal effects of pesticide exposure; Neurological effects of pesticide exposure; Pulmonary effects of pesticide exposure; Renal effects of pesticide exposure

Chemicals[2]: Dermatological effects of chemical exposure; Gastrointestinal effects of chemical exposure; Immunological effects of chemical exposure; Neurological effects of chemical exposure; Pulmonary effects of chemical exposure; Renal effects of chemical exposure

Biologics[3]: Dermatological effects of exposure to biologics; Gastrointestinal effects of exposure to biologics; Neurological effects of exposure to biologics; Pulmonary effects of exposure to biologics; Renal effects of exposure to biologics

Pollution[4]: Neurological effects of pollution exposure; Pulmonary effects of pollution exposure

Waste[5]: Dermatological effects of waste exposure; Gastrointestinal effects of waste exposure; Hepatic effects of waste exposure; Pulmonary effects of waste exposure

Radiation: External exposure through direct contact with radioactive material; Genetic effects of radiation exposure; Immunological effects of radiation exposure; Neurological effects of radiation exposure; Oncological effects of radiation exposure

Related Factors:

External: Chemical contamination of food; Chemical contamination of water; Economically disadvantaged (increases potential for multiple exposure, lack of access to healthcare, poor diet); Exposure through ingestion of radioactive material (e.g., food/water contamination); Exposure to bioterrorism; Exposure to disaster (natural or man-made); Exposure to radiation (occupation in radiology, employment in nuclear industries and electrical generating plants, living near nuclear industries and/or electrical generating plants); Flaking, peeling paint in presence of young children; Flaking, peeling plaster in presence of young children; Flooring surface (carpeted surfaces hold contaminant residue more than hard floor surfaces); Geographical area (living in area where high levels of contaminants exist); Household hygiene practices; Inadequate municipal services (trash removal, sewage treatment facilities); Inappropriate use of protective clothing; Lack of breakdown of contaminants once indoors (breakdown is inhibited without sun and rain exposure); Lack of protective clothing; Lacquer in poorly ventilated areas; Lacquer without effective protection; Paint in poorly ventilated areas; Paint without effective protection; Personal hygiene practices; Playing in outdoor areas where environmental contaminants are used; Presence of atmospheric pollutants; Unprotected contact with chemicals (e.g., arsenic); Unprotected contact with heavy metals (e.g., chromium, lead); Use of environmental contaminants in the home (e.g., pesticides, chemicals, environmental tobacco smoke)

Internal: Age (children <5 years, older adults); Concomitant exposures; Developmental characteristics of children; Female gender; Gestational age during exposure; Nutritional factors (e.g., obesity, vitamin and mineral deficiencies); Pre-existing disease states; Pregnancy; Previous exposures; Smoking

[1] *Major categories of pesticides: insecticides, herbicides, fungicides, antimicrobials, rodenticides; major pesticides: organophosphates, carbamates, organochlorines, pyrethrum, arsenic, glycophosphates, bipyridyls, chlorophenoxy compounds.*

[2] *Major chemical agents: petroleum-based agents, anticholinesterase type I agents act on proximal tracheobronchial portion of the respiratory tract; type II agents act on alveoli; type III agents produce systemic effects.*

[3] *Toxins from living organisms (bacteria, viruses, fungi).*

[4] *Major locations: air, water, soil; major agents: asbestos, radon, tobacco, heavy metal, lead, noise, exhaust fumes.*

[5] *Categories of waste: trash, raw sewage, industrial waste.*

Risk for Contamination

Definition: At risk for exposure to environmental contaminants in doses sufficient to cause adverse health effects

Risk Factors:

External: Chemical contamination of food; Chemical contamination of water; Economically disadvantaged (increases potential for multiple exposure, lack of access to healthcare, poor diet);

Exposure to bioterrorism; Exposure to disaster (natural or man-made); Exposure to radiation (occupation in radiography, employment in nuclear industries and electrical generating plants, living near nuclear industries and/or electrical generating plants); Flaking, peeling paint in presence of young children; Flaking, peeling plaster in presence of young children; Flooring surface (carpeted surfaces hold contaminant residue more than hard floor surfaces); Geographical area (living in area where high levels of contaminants exist); Household hygiene practices; Inadequate municipal services (e.g., trash removal, sewage treatment facilities); Inappropriate use of protective clothing; Lack of breakdown of contaminants once indoors (breakdown is inhibited without sun and rain exposure); Lack of protective clothing; Lacquer in poorly ventilated areas; Lacquer without effective protection; Paint, lacquer, etc. in poorly ventilated areas; Paint, lacquer, etc. without effective protection; Personal hygiene practices; Playing in outdoor areas where environmental contaminants are used; Presence of atmospheric pollutants; Unprotected contact with chemicals (e.g., arsenic); Unprotected contact with heavy metals (e.g., chromium, lead); Use of environmental contaminants in the home (e.g., pesticides, chemicals, environmental tobacco smoke

Internal: Age (children <5 years, older adults); Concomitant exposures; Developmental characteristics of children; Female gender; Gestational age during exposure; Nutritional factors (e.g., obesity, vitamin and mineral deficiencies); Pre-existing disease states; Pregnancy; Previous exposures; Smoking

Risk for Poisoning

Definition: At risk of accidental exposure to, or ingestion of, drugs or dangerous products in sufficient doses that may compromise health

Risk Factors:

External: Availability of illicit drugs potentially contaminated by poisonous additives; Dangerous products placed within reach of children; Dangerous products placed within reach of confused individuals; Large supplies of pharmaceutical agents in house; Pharmaceutical agents stored in unlocked cabinets accessible to children; Pharmaceutical agents stored in unlocked cabinets accessible to confused individuals

Internal: Cognitive difficulties; Deficient knowledge regarding pharmaceutical agents; Deficient knowledge regarding poisoning prevention; Emotional difficulties; Lack of proper precaution; Reduced vision; Reports occupational setting is without adequate safeguards

Class 5: Defensive Processes

Risk for Adverse Reaction to Iodinated Contrast Media

Definition: At risk for any noxious or unintended reaction associated with the use of iodinated contrast media that can occur within seven (7) days after contrast agent injection

Risk Factors: Anxiety; Concurrent use of medications (e.g., beta-blockers, interleukin-2, metformin, nephrotoxic medications); Dehydration; Extremes of age; Fragile veins (e.g., prior or actual chemotherapy treatment or radiation in the limb to be injected, multiple attempts to obtain intravenous access, indwelling intravenous lines in place for more than 24 hours, previous axillary lymph node dissection in the limb to be injected, distal intravenous access sites: hand, wrist, foot, ankle); Generalized debilitation; History of allergies; History of previous adverse effect from iodinated

contrast media; Physical and chemical properties of the contrast media (e.g., iodine concentration, viscosity, high osmolality, ion toxicity); Unconsciousness; Underlying disease (e.g., heart disease, pulmonary disease, blood dyscrasias, endocrine disease, renal disease, pheochromocytoma, autoimmune disease)

Latex Allergy Response

Definition: A hypersensitive reaction to natural latex rubber products

Defining Characteristics:

Life-Threatening Reactions Occurring in the First Hour After Exposure to Latex Protein: Bronchospasm; Cardiac arrest; Contact urticaria progressing to generalized symptoms; Dyspnea; Edema of the lips; Edema of the throat; Edema of the tongue; Edema of the uvula; Hypotension; Respiratory arrest; Syncope; Tightness in chest; Wheezing

Orofacial Characteristics: Edema of eyelids; Edema of the sclerae; Erythema of the eyes; Facial erythema; Facial itching; Itching of the eyes; Nasal congestion; Nasal erythema; Nasal itching; Oral itching; Rhinorrhea; Tearing of the eyes

Gastrointestinal Characteristics: Abdominal pain; Nausea

Generalized Characteristics: Flushing; Generalized discomfort; Generalized edema; Increasing complaint of total body warmth; Restlessness

Type IV Reactions Occurring 1 Hour or More After Exposure to Latex Protein: Discomfort reaction to additives such as thiurams and carbamates; Eczema; Irritation; Redness

Related Factors: Hypersensitivity to natural latex rubber protein

Risk for Allergy Response

Definition: Risk of an exaggerated immune response or reaction to substances

Risk Factors: Chemical products (e.g., bleach, cosmetics); Dander; Environmental substances (e.g., mold, dust, pollen); Foods (e.g., peanuts, shellfish, mushrooms); Insect stings; Pharmaceutical agents (e.g., penicillins); Repeated exposure to environmental substances

Risk for Latex Allergy Response

Definition: Risk of hypersensitivity to natural latex rubber products that may compromise health

Risk Factors: Allergies to avocados; Allergies to bananas; Allergies to chestnuts; Allergies to kiwis; Allergies to poinsettia plants; Allergies to tropical fruits; History of allergies; History of asthma; History of reactions to latex; Multiple surgical procedures, especially beginning in infancy; Professions with daily exposure to latex

Class 6: Thermoregulation

Risk for Imbalanced Body Temperature

Definition: At risk for failure to maintain body temperature within normal range

Risk Factors: Altered metabolic rate; Dehydration; Exposure to extremes of environmental temperature; Extremes of age; Extremes of weight; Illness affecting temperature regulation; Inactivity; Inappropriate clothing for environmental temperature; Pharmaceutical agents causing vasoconstriction; Pharmaceutical agents causing vasodilation; Sedation; Trauma affecting temperature regulation; Vigorous activity

Hyperthermia

Definition: Body temperature elevated above normal range

Defining Characteristics: Convulsions; Flushed skin; Increase in body temperature above normal range; Seizures; Skin warm to touch; Tachycardia; Tachypnea

Related Factors: Anesthesia; Decreased perspiration; Dehydration; Exposure to hot environment; Illness; Inappropriate clothing; Increased metabolic rate; Pharmaceutical agents; Trauma; Vigorous activity

Hypothermia

Definition: Body temperature below normal range

Defining Characteristics: Body temperature below normal range; Cool skin; Cyanotic nail beds; Hypertension; Pallor; Piloerection; Shivering; Slow capillary refill; Tachycardia

Related Factors: Aging; Consumption of alcohol; Damage to hypothalamus; Decreased ability to shiver; Decreased metabolic rate; Evaporation from skin in cool environment; Exposure to cool environment; Illness; Inactivity; Inadequate clothing; Malnutrition; Pharmaceutical agents; Trauma

Ineffective Thermoregulation

Definition: Temperature fluctuation between hypothermia and hyperthermia

Defining Characteristics: Cyanotic nail beds; Fluctuations in body temperature above and below the normal range; Flushed skin; Hypertension; Increase in body temperature above normal range; Increased respiratory rate; Mild shivering; Moderate pallor; Piloerection; Reduction in body temperature below normal range; Seizures; Skin cool to touch; Skin warm to touch; Slow capillary refill; Tachycardia

Related Factors: Extremes of age; Fluctuating environmental temperature; Illness; Trauma

DOMAIN 12: COMFORT

Class 1: Physical Comfort

Impaired Comfort*

Definition: Perceived lack of ease, relief, and transcendence in physical, psychospiritual, environmental, cultural, and social dimensions

Defining Characteristics: Anxiety; Crying; Disturbed sleep pattern; Fear; Inability to relax; Irritability; Moaning; Reports being cold; Reports being hot; Reports being uncomfortable; Reports distressing symptoms; Reports hunger; Reports itching; Reports lack of contentment in situation; Reports lack of ease in situation; Restlessness; Sighing

Related Factors: Illness-related symptoms; Insufficient resources (e.g., financial, social support); Lack of environmental control; Lack of privacy; Lack of situational control; Noxious environmental stimuli; Treatment-related side effects (e.g., medication, radiation)

This diagnosis belongs to all three classes of Domain 12: Comfort — Class 1: Physical Comfort; Class 2: Environmental Comfort; and Class 3: Social Comfort.

Readiness for Enhanced Comfort*

Definition: A pattern of ease, relief, and transcendence in physical, psychospiritual, environmental, and/or social dimensions that is sufficient for well-being and can be strengthened

Defining Characteristics: Expresses desire to enhance comfort; Expresses desire to enhance feeling of contentment; Expresses desire to enhance relaxation; Expresses desire to enhance resolution of complaints

This diagnosis belongs to all three classes of Domain 12: Comfort — Class 1: Physical Comfort; Class 2: Environmental Comfort; and Class 3: Social Comfort.

Nausea

Definition: A subjective phenomenon of an unpleasant feeling in the back of the throat and stomach that may or may not result in vomiting

Defining Characteristics: Aversion toward food; Gagging sensation; Increased salivation; Increased swallowing; Reports nausea; Reports sour taste in mouth

Related Factors:

Biophysical: Biochemical disorders (e.g., uremia, diabetic ketoacidosis); Esophageal disease; Gastric distension; Gastric irritation; Increased intracranial pressure; Intra-abdominal tumors; Labyrinthitis; Liver capsule stretch; Localized tumors (e.g., acoustic neuroma, primary or secondary brain tumors, bone metastases at base of skull); Ménière's disease; Meningitis; Motion sickness; Pain; Pancreatic disease; Pregnancy; Splenetic capsule stretch; Toxins (e.g., tumor-produced peptides, abnormal metabolites due to cancer)

Situational: Anxiety; Fear; Noxious odors; Noxious taste; Pain; Psychological factors; Unpleasant visual stimulation

Treatment: Gastric distension; Gastric irritation; Pharmaceutical agents

Acute Pain

Definition: Unpleasant sensory and emotional experience arising from actual or potential tissue damage or described in terms of such damage (International Association for the Study of Pain); sudden or slow onset of any intensity from mild to severe with an anticipated or predictable end and a duration of <6 months

Defining Characteristics: Changes in appetite; Changes in blood pressure; Changes in heart rate; Changes in respiratory rate; Coded report (e.g., use of pain scale); Diaphoresis; Distraction behavior (e.g., pacing, seeking out other people and/or activities, repetitive activities); Expressive behavior (e.g., restlessness, moaning, crying, vigilance, irritability, sighing); Facial mask (e.g., eyes lack luster, beaten look, fixed or scattered movement, grimace); Guarding behavior; Narrowed focus (e.g., altered time perception, impaired thought processes, reduced interaction with people and environment); Observed evidence of pain; Positioning to avoid pain; Protective gestures; Pupillary dilation; Reports pain; Self-focus; Sleep pattern disturbance

Related Factors: Injury agents (e.g., biological, chemical, physical, psychological)

Chronic Pain

Definition: Unpleasant sensory and emotional experience arising from actual or potential tissue damage or described in terms of such damage (International Association for the Study of Pain); sudden or slow onset of any intensity from mild to severe, constant or recurring without an anticipated or predictable end and with a duration of >6 months

Defining Characteristics: Altered ability to continue previous activities; Anorexia; Atrophy of involved muscle group; Changes in sleep pattern; Coded report (e.g., use of pain scale); Depression; Facial mask (e.g. eyes lack luster, beaten look, fixed or scattered movement, grimace); Fatigue; Fear of reinjury; Guarding behavior; Irritability; Observed protective behavior; Reduced interaction with people; Reports pain; Restlessness; Self-focusing; Sympathetic mediated responses (e.g., temperature, cold, changes of body position, hypersensitivity)

Related Factors: Chronic physical disability; Chronic psychosocial disability

Class 2: Environmental Comfort

Includes **Impaired Comfort** and **Readiness for Enhanced Comfort** *which were previously discussed.*

Class 3: Social Comfort

Also includes **Impaired Comfort** and **Readiness for Enhanced Comfort** *which were previously discussed.*

Social Isolation

Definition: Aloneness experienced by the individual and perceived as imposed by others and as a negative or threatening state

Defining Characteristics:

Objective: Absence of supportive significant other(s); Developmentally inappropriate behaviors; Dull affect; Evidence of handicap (e.g., physical, mental); Exists in a subculture; Illness; Meaningless actions; No eye contact; Preoccupation with own thoughts; Projects hostility; Repetitive actions; Sad affect; Seeks to be alone; Shows behavior unaccepted by dominant cultural group; Uncommunicative; Withdrawn

Subjective: Developmentally inappropriate interests; Experiences feelings of differences from others; Inability to meet expectations of others; Insecurity in public; Reports feelings of aloneness imposed by others; Reports feelings of rejection; Reports inadequate purpose in life; Reports values unacceptable to the dominant cultural group

Related Factors: Alterations in mental status; Alterations in physical appearance; Altered state of wellness; Factors contributing to the absence of satisfying personal relationships (e.g., delay in accomplishing developmental tasks); Immature interests; Inability to engage in satisfying personal relationships; Inadequate personal resources; Unaccepted social behavior; Unaccepted social values

DOMAIN 13: GROWTH/DEVELOPMENT

Class 1: Growth

Risk for Disproportionate Growth

Definition: At risk for growth above the 97th percentile or below the 3rd percentile for age, crossing two percentile channels

Risk Factors:

Caregiver: Abuse; Learning difficulties (mental handicap); Mental illness; Severe learning disability

Environmental: Deprivation; Economically disadvantaged; Lead poisoning; Natural disasters; Teratogen; Violence

Individual: Anorexia; Caregiver's maladaptive feeding behaviors; Chronic illness; Individual maladaptive feeding behaviors;

Infection; Insatiable appetite; Malnutrition; Prematurity; Substance abuse

Prenatal: Congenital disorders; Genetic disorders; Maternal infection; Maternal nutrition; Multiple gestation; Substance abuse; Teratogen exposure

Delayed Growth and Development*

Definition: Deviations from age-group norms

Defining Characteristics: Altered physical growth; Decreased response time; Delay in performing skills typical of age group; Difficulty in performing skills typical of age group; Flat affect; Inability to perform self-care activities appropriate for age; Inability to perform self-control activities appropriate for age; Listlessness

Related Factors: Effects of physical disability; Environmental deficiencies; Inadequate caretaking; Inconsistent responsiveness; Indifference; Multiple caretakers; Prescribed dependence; Separation from significant others; Stimulation deficiencies

*This diagnosis is also included in Class 2: Development.

Note: This diagnosis will retire from the NANDA-I Taxonomy in the 2015–2017 edition unless additional work is completed to separate the diagnostic foci of (1) growth, and (2) development into separate diagnostic concepts.

Class 2: Development

Also includes **Delayed Growth and Development** *which was previously discussed.*

Risk for Delayed Development

Definition: At risk for delay of 25% or more in one or more of the areas of social or self-regulatory behavior, or in cognitive, language, gross or fine motor skills

Risk Factors:

Prenatal: Economically disadvantaged; Endocrine disorders; Genetic disorders; Illiteracy; Inadequate nutrition; Inadequate prenatal care; Infections; Lack of prenatal care; Late prenatal care; Maternal age <15 years; Maternal age >35 years; Substance abuse; Unplanned pregnancy; Unwanted pregnancy

Individual: Adopted child; Behavior disorders; Brain damage (e.g., hemorrhage in postnatal period, shaken baby, abuse, accident); Chronic illness; Congenital disorders; Failure to thrive; Foster child; Frequent otitis media; Genetic disorders; Hearing impairment; Inadequate nutrition; Lead poisoning; Natural disasters; Positive drug screen(s); Prematurity; Seizures; Substance abuse; Technology dependent; Treatment-related side effects (e.g., chemotherapy, radiation therapy, pharmaceutical agents); Vision impairment

Environmental: Economically disadvantaged; Violence

Caregiver: Abuse; Learning disabilities; Mental illness; Severe learning disability

INDEX